Non-Neoplastic Diseases of the Central Nervous System

ATLAS OF NONTUMOR PATHOLOGY

AMERICAN REGISTRY OF PATHOLOGY 1976

ARMED FORCES INSTITUTE OF PATHOLOGY • 1949 •
founded as ARMY MEDICAL MUSEUM 1862

ARP PRESS™

Editorial & Production Manager: Mirlinda Q. Caton
Production Editor: Dian S. Thomas
Editorial Assistant: Melanie J. De Boer
Editorial Assistant: Magdalena C. Silva
Copyeditor: Audrey Kahn

ATLAS OF NONTUMOR PATHOLOGY

First Series
Fascicle 8

Non-Neoplastic Diseases of the Central Nervous System

David N. Louis, MD

Matthew P. Frosch, MD, PhD

Hernando Mena, MD

Elisabeth J. Rushing, MD

Alexander R. Judkins, MD

Published by the
American Registry of Pathology
Washington, DC
in collaboration with the
Armed Forces Institute of Pathology
Washington, DC

2009

ATLAS OF NONTUMOR PATHOLOGY

Available from the American Registry of Pathology
Armed Forces Institute of Pathology
Washington, DC 20306-6000
www.afip.org
ISBN: 1-933477-08-3
978-1-933477-08-4

INTRODUCTION TO SERIES

This is the eighth Fascicle of the Atlas of Nontumor Pathology, a complementary series to the Armed Forces Institute of Pathology (AFIP) Atlas of Tumor Pathology, first published in 1949.

For several years, various individuals in the pathology community have suggested the formation of a new series of monographs concentrating on this particular area. In 1998, an Editorial Board was appointed and outstanding authors were chosen shortly thereafter.

The purpose of the atlas is to provide surgical pathologists with ready expert reference material most helpful in their daily practice. The lesions described relate principally to medical non-neoplastic conditions. Many of these lesions represent complex entities and, when appropriate, we have included contributions from internists, radiologists, and surgeons. This has led to an increase in the size of the monographs, but the emphasis remains on diagnosis by the surgical pathologist.

Previously, the Fascicles have been available on CD-ROM format as well as in print. In order to provide the widest possible advantages of both modalities, we have formatted the print Fascicle on the World Wide Web. Use of the Internet allows cross-indexing within the Fascicles.

Our goal is to continue to provide expert information at the lowest possible cost. Therefore, marked reductions in pricing are available to residents and fellows as well as to pathology faculty and other staff members purchasing the Fascicles on a subscription basis.

We believe that the Atlas of Nontumor Pathology will serve as an outstanding reference for surgical pathologists as well as an important contribution to the literature of other medical specialties.

Donald West King, MD
William A. Gardner, MD
Leslie H. Sobin, MD
J. Thomas Stocker, MD
Bernard Wagner, MD

PREFACE

"The hesitating surgeon, knife in hand, uncertain whether to do a trifling operation or one terribly mutilating and severe, could always depend on the decision of his [the surgical pathologist's] master mind and experience, and a great number of men and women today owe their intact bodies or their lives to his quietly spoken opinion."

Surgical pathology has always been challenging, as shown by the above quote from 1921, written by two surgeons at the Massachusetts General Hospital, Drs. J.C. Warren and S.J. Mixter, in an obituary of Dr. William Fiske Whitney, the first surgical pathologist at the hospital. Dr. Whitney had practiced there from 1888 through 1916, and the quote illustrates that the characteristic challenges of surgical pathology were evident even then.

Of the various subspecialty areas in anatomic pathology, neuropathology tends to be one of the least familiar to general pathologists. Most surgical pathologists at institutions with neurosurgical practices gain quick familiarity with the common tumors of the central nervous system. Non-neoplastic diseases of the central nervous system, however, continue to remain a mystery to surgical pathologists, since non-neoplastic diseases of the nervous system represent a wide spectrum of relatively uncommon diseases that are not often biopsied. As a result, most surgical pathologists encounter non-neoplastic diseases of the nervous system only occasionally, making their diagnosis uniquely challenging.

Nearly all texts on surgical neuropathology rightly focus on neoplastic diseases, given their common occurrence. Indeed, most discussions of non-neoplastic diseases are found in textbooks geared toward general neuropathology, which are not often consulted by surgical pathologists. This text was created to fill that void: to provide a guide to the surgical pathology evaluation of non-neoplastic diseases of the central nervous system.

Given the large number of non-neoplastic diseases of the central nervous system, we have biased this Fascicle toward diseases that may be encountered in surgical pathology practice, and have not covered those entities only diagnosed by other means, such as autopsy. Moreover, we have tried to illustrate as many entities as possible with surgical material, and have used autopsy brains primarily to illustrate key macroscopic features of some diseases. We have not included non-neoplastic diseases of peripheral nerve or muscle; there are excellent books on biopsy diagnosis of nerve and muscle diseases, and such diseases are usually outside the bailiwick of general pathologists. Granted, decisions of inclusion and exclusion are difficult, but we feel that the current selection provides a broad and detailed guide to biopsy diagnosis of non-neoplastic diseases of the central nervous system, including uncommon conditions that may come to biopsy only rarely.

We hope that readers will find the book of use and comfort as they realize that the brain biopsy in front of them is not from a familiar neoplasm, but from one of the sometimes challenging and always fascinating non-neoplastic diseases of the central nervous system. Last, but certainly not least, we would strongly encourage the use of this book as well as comprehensive consultation with the neurosurgeon, neurologist, and neuroradiologist *prior to* biopsy in the setting of a suspected non-neoplastic disease of the central nervous system. As the old adage goes, "to be forewarned is to be forearmed."

David N. Louis, MD
Department of Pathology
Massachusetts General Hospital and Harvard Medical School

Matthew P. Frosch, MD, PhD
Department of Pathology
Massachusetts General Hospital and Harvard Medical School

Hernando Mena, MD
Office of the Chief Medical Examiner and
New York University School of Medicine

Elisabeth J. Rushing, MD
Division of Neuropathology and Ophthalmic Pathology
Armed Forces Institute of Pathology

Alexander R. Judkins, MD
Department of Pathology and Laboratory Medicine, Children's Hospital of
Philadelphia and University of Pennsylvania School of Medicine

Permission to use copyrighted illustrations has been granted by:

American Society of Neuroradiology
AJNR Am J Neuroradiol 1991;12:113-4. For figure 13-25.

Oxford University Press, Inc.
Principles and Practice of Neuropathology, 2003. For figure 5-22.

CONTENTS

1 MICROSCOPIC NEUROANATOMY

One of the greatest challenges in evaluating central nervous system (CNS) biopsies of non-neoplastic conditions is the extraordinary cytologic and architectural diversity of the CNS. Knowledge of this remarkable diversity is necessary for the proper evaluation of non-neoplastic biopsy specimens since recognition of pathologic features often entails comparison with a mental image of the normal structure of what has been biopsied.

Certain regions of the CNS are more amenable to biopsy than others because biopsy of some structures poses a high risk of neurologic morbidity and because neurosurgical access in some regions poses difficulties. Biopsies of neoplastic diseases must target the neoplastic mass, which is in many cases a single lesion. Even in the setting of probable neoplasm, however, some locations and clinicopathologic situations present problems that argue against biopsy, for example, in the case of a suspected diffuse pontine glioma or pineal germinoma. Non-neoplastic diseases less often feature a distinct single lesion, and thus sometimes allow more choice in terms of biopsy sites. In such situations, the neurosurgeon will select to biopsy a more readily accessible, less "eloquent" area, rather than biopsy a deep-seated nucleus or a region likely to lead to morbidity. As a result, some CNS regions are almost never biopsied. The following chapter reviews the cellular constituents of the CNS and its surroundings, as well as the architectural features of regions that are subject to biopsy.

REGIONAL NEUROANATOMY

The following section is oriented toward understanding the regional neuroanatomy of the CNS in the context of surgical neuropathology specimens. As such, the discussion is biased toward structures that are encountered by the pathologist when evaluating surgical specimens. Recognition of specific gray and white matter structures is important when interpreting neuropathologic findings, and can be of intraoperative help to neurosurgeons, particularly during stereotactically guided needle biopsies and microneurosurgical procedures.

By far the most common regions biopsied when non-neoplastic diseases are suspected are the meninges, cerebral cortex, and underlying white matter. In addition, the non-"eloquent" areas of the cerebrum are commonly removed for non-neoplastic processes, such as for epilepsy surgery or resections of infarcted or edematous brain. Although never resected, deep structures are sometimes biopsied, particularly if specific deep lesions suggest a greater likelihood of establishing a diagnosis. The following section discusses the architectural features of different regions that may be included in biopsy or resection material. For further information on neuroanatomy, the reader is referred to excellent reference texts (1,2).

Meninges

The meninges are the tripartite coverings of the CNS and are often included in biopsy material. The meninges may be the primary sites of certain infectious and inflammatory diseases, and are often biopsied to detect more global CNS conditions such as vasculitis. The meninges are composed of three layers: the dura mater, the arachnoid mater, and the pia mater.

The dura mater (pachymeninx) is the most external of the three membranes. In the cranial cavity, the dura is closely affixed to the overlying cranium, whereas in the vertebral cavity, the dura is free; as a result, there is only a potential epidural space in the head, but an actual spinal epidural space. The dura is a thick, densely collagenous, hypocellular structure composed of two layers (fig. 1-1). The two layers are histologically similar, but have collagen fibers running in different directions. Each layer features dense collagen, fibroblasts, and both arterial and venous blood vessels (fig. 1-2). In places where layers of the dura come together, large venous sinuses are

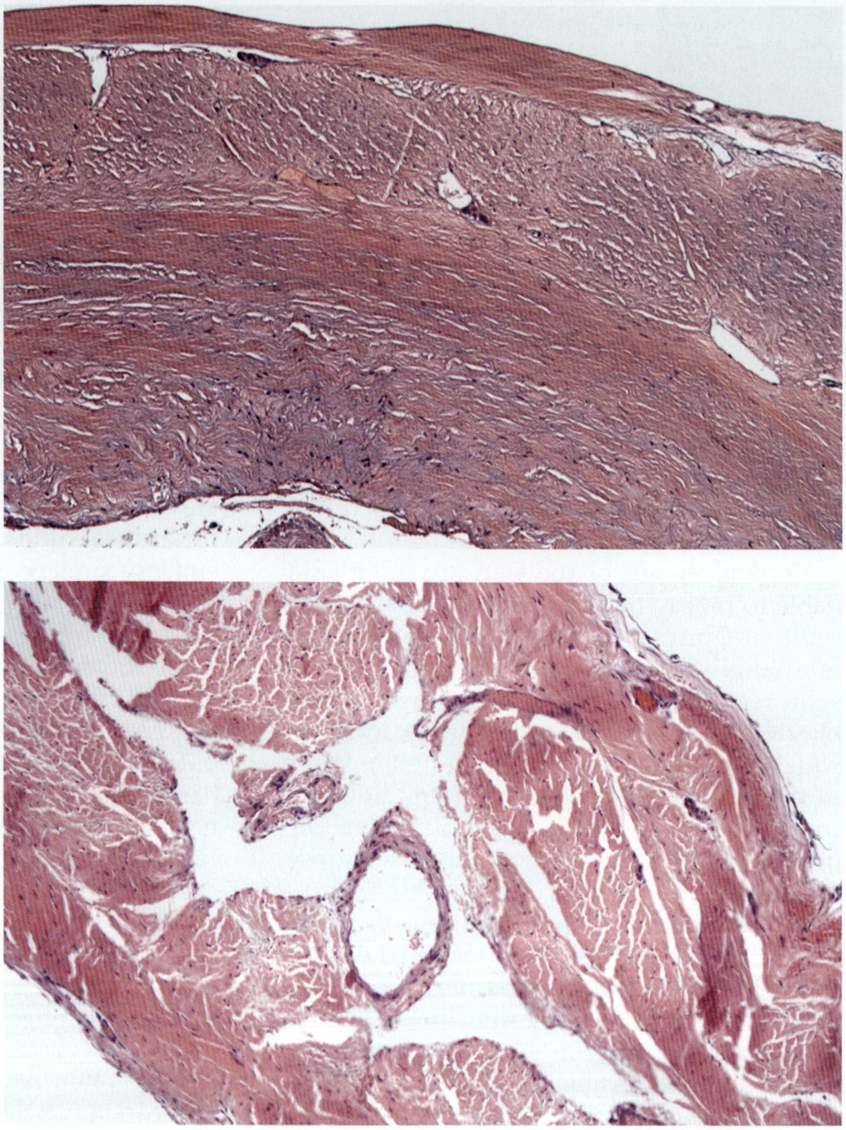

Figure 1-1

DURA MATER

Two layers and medium-sized blood vessels are seen.

present. These sinuses are lined by endothelial cells but are indented in places by arachnoid (pacchionian) granulations (see below).

The arachnoid mater (one of the leptomeninges) is not often biopsied by itself, but most biopsies of the cerebral cortex purposefully include the overlying arachnoid and the subarachnoid space (fig. 1-3). The arachnoid is a thin membrane, only a few cells thick, consisting of fibroblasts and arachnoidal cells (fig. 1-4). Arachnoidal cells vary from spindled to cuboidal. They resemble the cells commonly encountered by pathologists in meningiomas: cells that often have oval nuclei, open chromatin, and sometimes, intranuclear pseudoinclusions. Ultrastructurally, as in meningiomas, arachnoidal cells contain prominent intermediate filaments and desmosomes. In many places, they form small multicellular clusters (fig. 1-5); these clusters resemble little meningiomas, with prominent whorls and often with psammoma bodies. Along the large venous sinuses, the arachnoid aggregates further into granulations that protrude into the sinuses. These granulations feature arachnoidal cells, blood vessels, and a hyalinized, collagenous stroma (fig. 1-6). Scattered pigmented melanocytes are also present in the arachnoid and subarachnoid space (fig. 1-7), particularly along the base of the brain and in dark-skinned individuals.

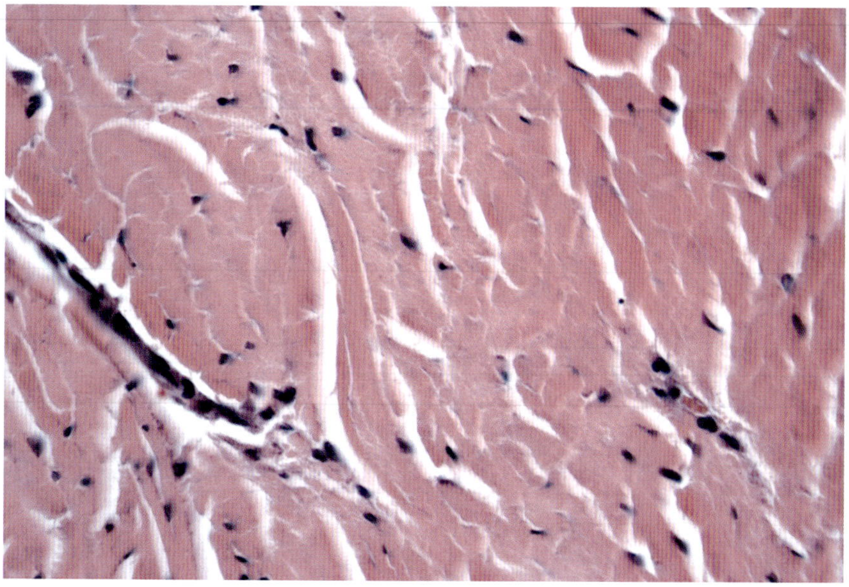

Figure 1-2

DURA MATER

Dense collagen bundles with scattered small blood vessels.

Figure 1-3

ARACHNOID MATER AND SUBARACHNOID SPACE

The subarachnoid space is found between the thin overlying arachnoid and the underlying pia mater at the surface of the cerebral cortex. The subarachnoid space contains medium-sized blood vessels and the cerebrospinal fluid.

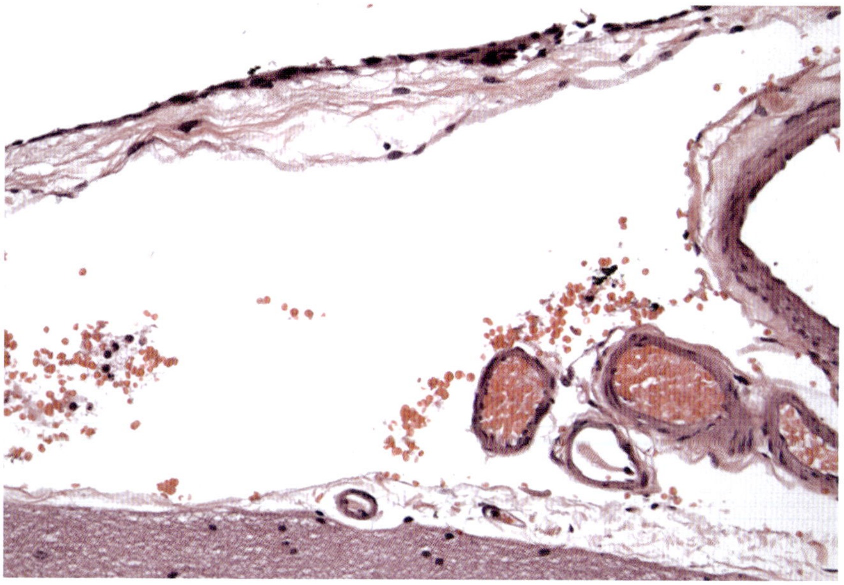

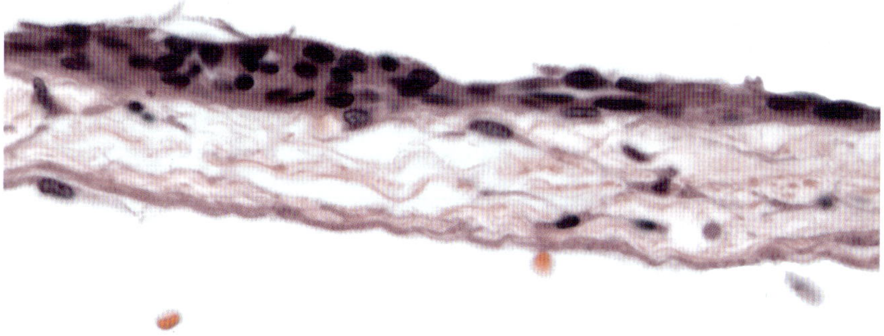

Figure 1-4

ARACHNOID MATER

The arachnoid is a thin membrane consisting of cuboidal to oval arachnoidal cells and fibroblasts.

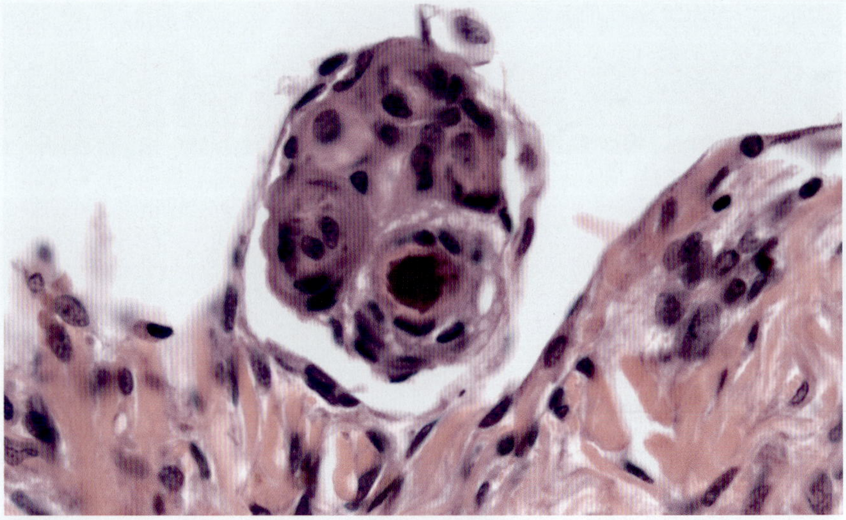

Figure 1-5

ARACHNOID MATER

Nests are formed by clusters of arachnoid cells, resembling small meningiomas, complete with whorls and psammoma bodies.

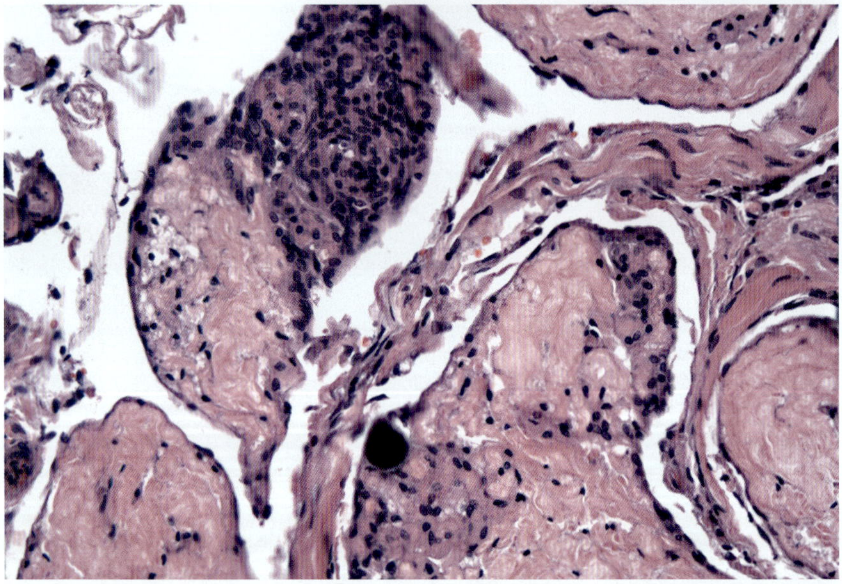

Figure 1-6

ARACHNOID GRANULATION

Fibrovascular cores with clusters of arachnoidal cells project into a dural sinus. A psammoma body is present.

The subarachnoid space is of major importance in surgical neuropathology, since it is targeted by many pathologic processes. The subarachnoid space primarily contains blood vessels and cerebrospinal fluid (CSF) (fig. 1-3). In older individuals, the subarachnoid space and overlying arachnoid may be fibrotic, particularly along the parasagittal convexities (fig. 1-8). The vessels are both arterial and venous. In surgical specimens that are compressed during removal, the subarachnoid vessels may be artifactually grouped closely together, mimicking vascular malformations. The surgical pathologist must be careful not to overcall a vascular malformation in such situations. In addition, occasional lymphocytes may be present in an otherwise unremarkable subarachnoid space.

The pia mater is not a separate membrane, but a layer of cells tightly affixed to the brain and spinal cord. Aside from maldevelopmental processes, there is little diagnostic pathology directly related to the pia mater.

Cerebral Cortex

Along with the meninges, the cerebral cortex is the single most frequently biopsied site for non-neoplastic diseases. In addition, along with the cerebellum, it is the only structure that is commonly removed as part of resection specimens, e.g., for epilepsy or stroke debulking. With

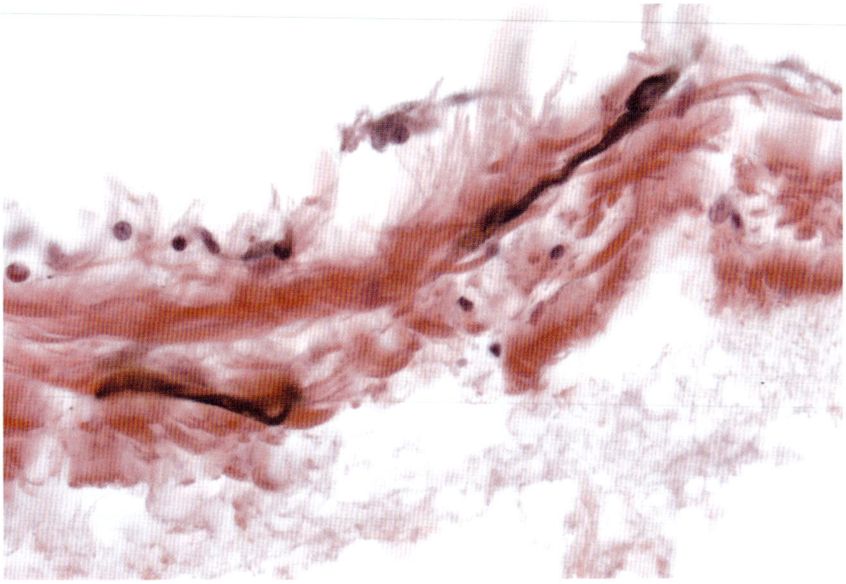

Figure 1-7

ARACHNOIDAL MELANOCYTES

Elongated, densely pigmented melanocytes are within the arachnoid membrane.

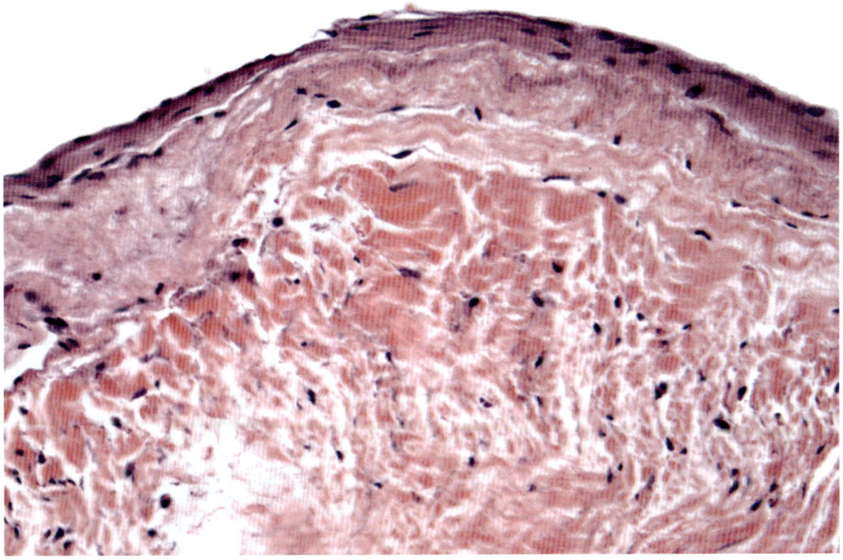

Figure 1-8

ARACHNOID MATER AND SUBARACHNOID SPACE

Fibrosis is common, particularly in the parasagittal regions of elderly patients.

the exception of the medial temporal lobe structures included in resection specimens (discussed below), nearly all sampled cortex is the six-layered neocortex. The neocortex varies from region to region, but has certain consistent features (figs. 1-9–1-13). Most strikingly, it is a laminated structure with large and medium-sized neurons "pointing" in the same direction: the apical dendrites, arising from the "tops" of the triangular (pyramidal) cells, are all oriented toward the cortical surface (fig. 1-11). This is readily apparent for the large pyramidal neurons, which are present in all cortical areas, but is not discernible for the smaller, more rounded granular neurons.

The six layers of neocortex are, beginning from the pial surface: 1) the cell-poor molecular layer; 2) the external granular cell layer; 3) the external pyramidal cell layer; 4) the internal granular cell layer; 5) the internal pyramidal cell layer; and 6) the polymorphous or transitional layer. Different regions of the brain have cortices that have different appearances, which are largely the result of variations in the prominence and cell types of the six different layers and the amount and pattern of myelin. Detailed

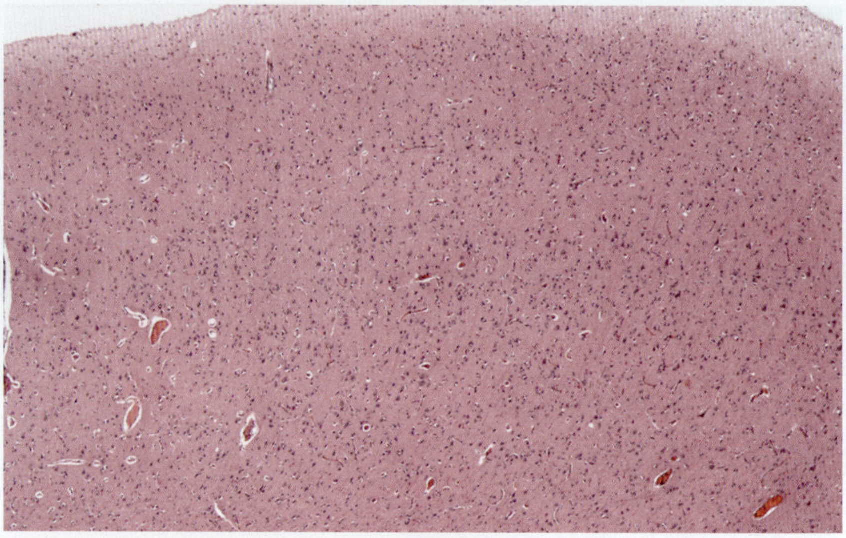

Figure 1-9

CEREBRAL CORTEX

Laminations and large neurons of frontal lobe cortex.

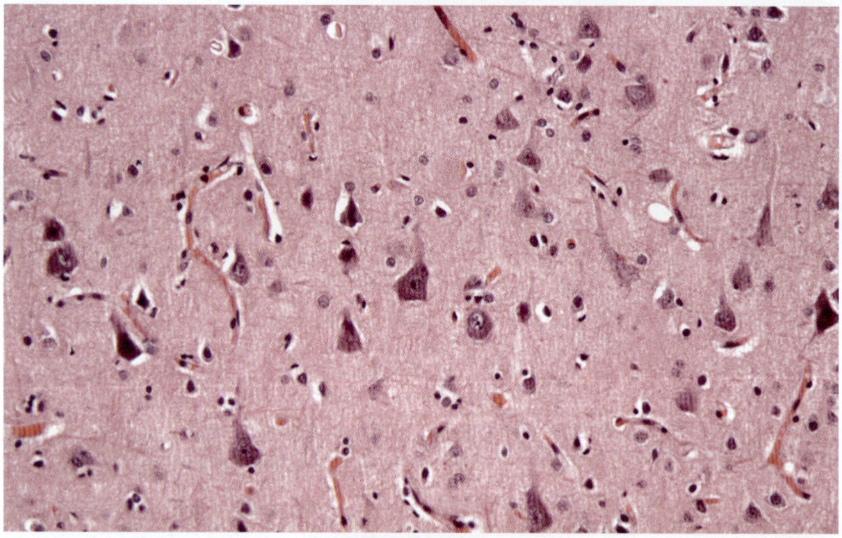

Figure 1-10

CEREBRAL CORTEX

Frontal cortex features large pyramidal neurons in layers 3 and 5.

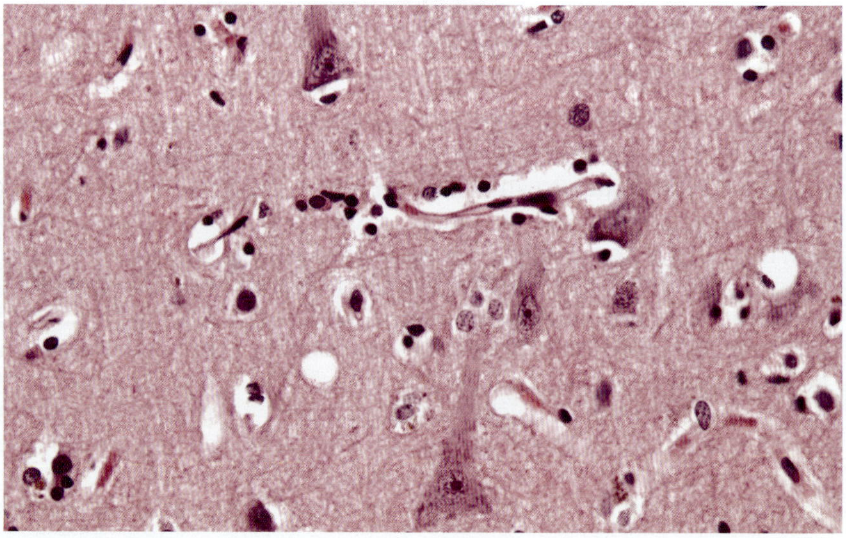

Figure 1-11

CEREBRAL CORTEX

Pyramidal neurons in frontal cortex point toward the pial surface.

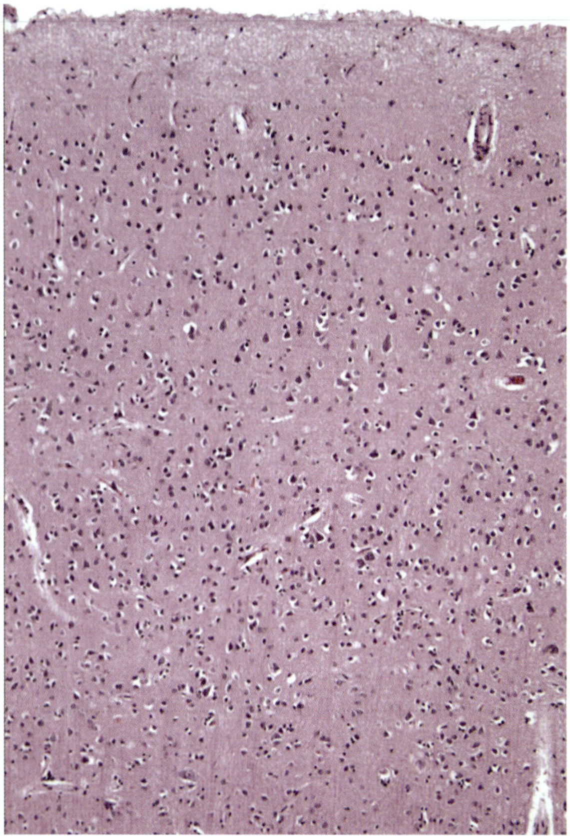

Figure 1-12

CEREBRAL CORTEX

Laminations and medium-sized neurons of occipital cortex.

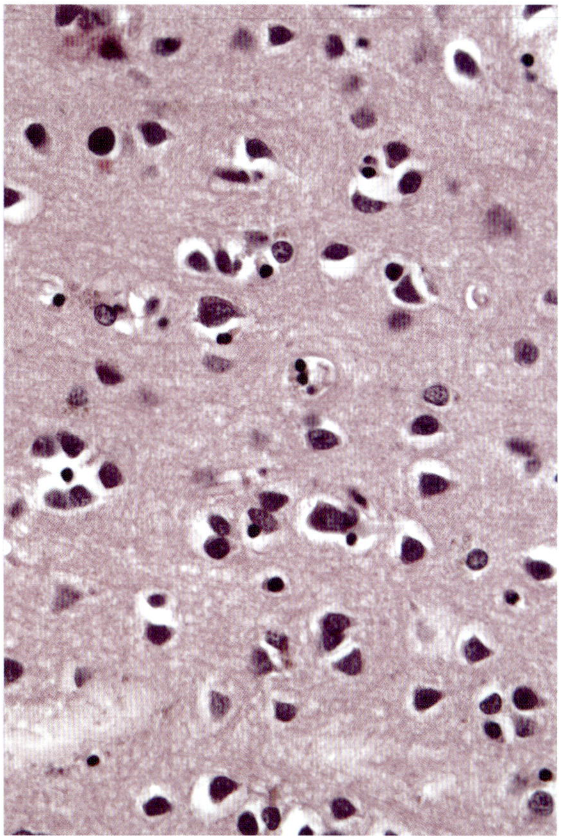

Figure 1-13

CEREBRAL CORTEX

Occipital lobe cortex features medium-sized and smaller neurons.

classifications of cortical cytoarchitecture and myeloarchitecture reflect these differences, the most famous of which is the Brodmann scheme (2). In general, however, cortices that subserve motor functions have prominent pyramidal cell layers. Most neurosurgical specimens that include the frontal lobe contain easily identifiable pyramidal cell layers (fig. 1-9). Although not often biopsied, the most striking example of such pyramidal cell prominence is the precentral motor cortex, with its extremely large Betz cells in the internal pyramidal layer (fig. 1-14). On the contrary, primary and secondary sensory cortices have smaller pyramidal cells and thicker granular cell layers. In general, samples of the parietal lobe have this more "sensory" appearance. Although not often biopsied, a striking example of this organization is found in the visual cortex of the occipital lobe (fig. 1-12).

The temporal lobe neocortex appears similar to other neocortical regions, with six layers and clearly discernible pyramidal cell layers. The only notable distinctions, which are primarily of significance in the differential diagnosis of infiltrating gliomas, are the presence of multiple perineuronal oligodendrocytes (which can mimic perineuronal satellitosis of glioma cells) and the presence of multiple neurons within the subcortical white matter. However, the non-neocortical medial temporal lobe structures, which are commonly encountered in surgical specimens for neoplastic and non-neoplastic conditions, have unique histologic features. The proper appreciation of the histologic architecture of these structures is dependent on the appropriate coronal orientation and cutting of these tissues on gross examination (see chapters 3 and 13), one of the few times in which

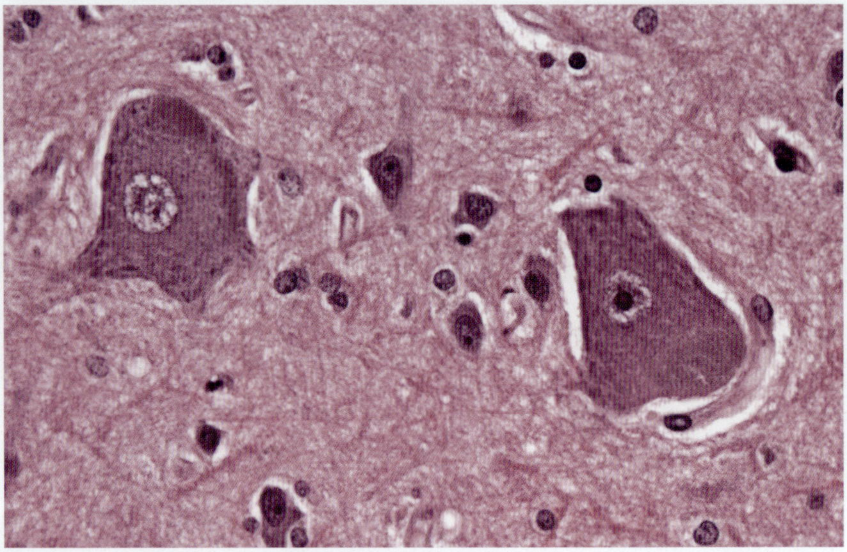

Figure 1-14

CEREBRAL CORTEX, BETZ CELLS

Betz cells are the largest neurons and are restricted to motor cortex.

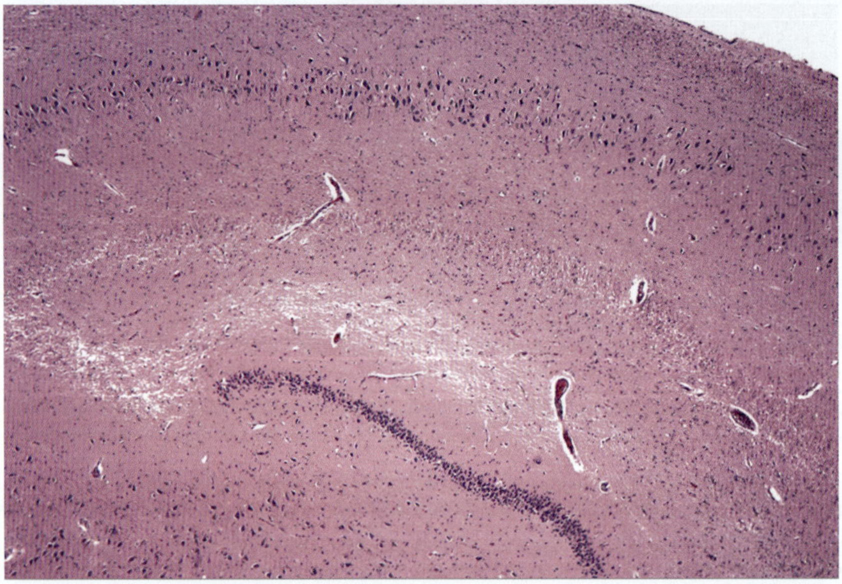

Figure 1-15

HIPPOCAMPUS

Pyramidal cells form a band (top) that circles the denser line of small cells comprising the dentate gyrus (middle, bottom) (also see figure 3-4).

macroscopic examination plays a crucial role in surgical neuropathology.

The hippocampus (fig. 1-15) is a multiply curved structure that has at least a superficial resemblance to a seahorse; hence the name. The medial temporal lobe structures of the hippocampus can be thought of as a skewed S-shaped combination of the entorhinal cortex/subiculum and cornu ammonis; the C-shaped dentate gyrus is located at the top of the skewed S (see chapter 3, fig. 3-4). On coronal sections, from lateral to medial, the temporal neocortex transitions to a cortical appearance in which clusters of large neurons ("clouds of Arnold") appear just below the pial surface. Proceeding into the cortical tissue immediately below the central part of the hippocampus, this primitive cortex becomes simpler, forming a three-layered area known as the subiculum. The subiculum, the "support" beneath the central hippocampus, consists of two relatively cell-free layers sandwiching large pyramidal neurons. The subiculum then transitions into the cornu ammonis (CA) of the hippocampus.

There are four distinct CA regions, CA1 to CA4, with CA1 directly adjacent to the subiculum; each contains prominent pyramidal cells (fig. 1-16). CA1 is known as the Sommer sector,

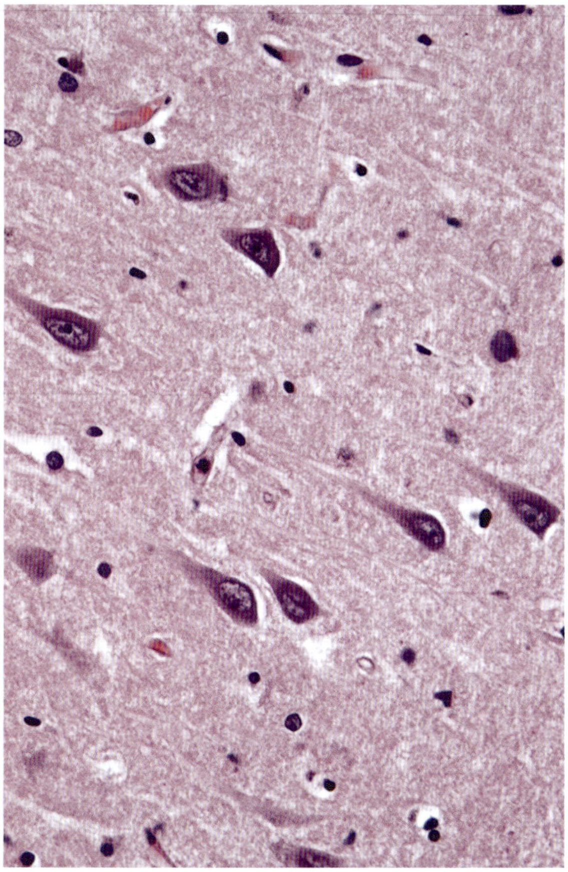

Figure 1-16

HIPPOCAMPUS

Pyramidal cells are directed inward, away from the ventricle and toward the dentate gyrus.

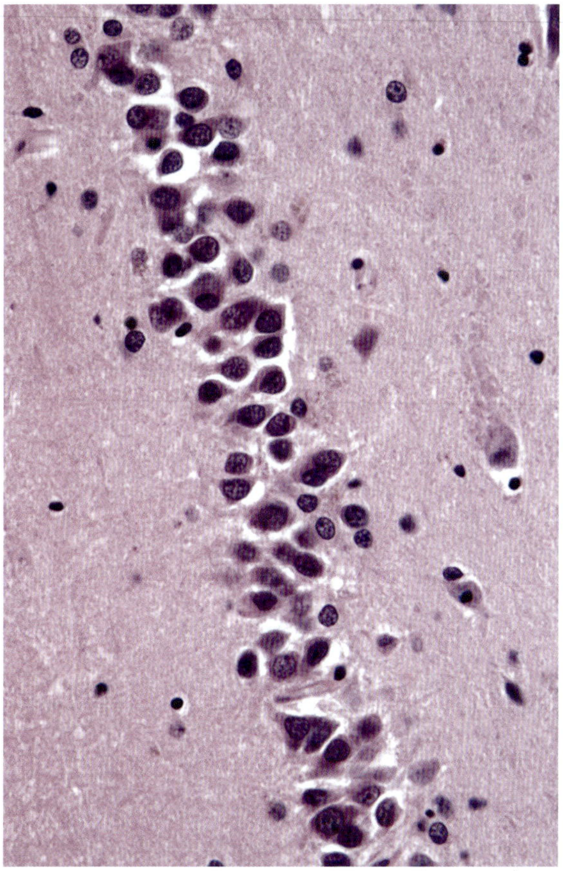

Figure 1-17

HIPPOCAMPUS

The dentate gyrus consists of small granular neurons in a few overlapping layers.

and is the region most sensitive to hypoxic damage and seizure-related changes (see chapter 13) as well as most affected in Alzheimer disease (see chapter 10). The central region of the hippocampus, following CA4, is the prominent dentate gyrus, consisting of a distinct line of small granular neurons (fig. 1-17).

The amygdala is located in the anterior temporal lobe, rostral to the hippocampus and temporal horn of the lateral ventricle. The structure is a combination of cortical and subcortical gray matter. Its histologic appearance is variable, but it is primarily composed of irregularly arranged globular, medium-sized neurons (fig. 1-18). White matter is sparse but in some areas is aggregated into small bundles that are reminiscent of the "pencils of Wilson" found in the striatum.

White Matter

The white matter is commonly sampled in neurosurgical procedures, in resection specimens, in cortical biopsies that include the underlying gyral white matter cores, and in deep needle biopsies. When stained with hematoxylin and eosin (H&E), white matter is characterized by numerous oligodendrocytes, often arranged in short lines of a few or more cells when sampled parallel to the direction of the axonal fibers (figs. 1-19, 1-20). Astrocytes are also present, but attention is drawn to the plentiful, dark oligodendrocyte nuclei. The background neuropil has a linear quality when the biopsy is parallel to the white matter tract, brought about by the parallel myelin sheaths and central, eosinophilic axons. When viewed

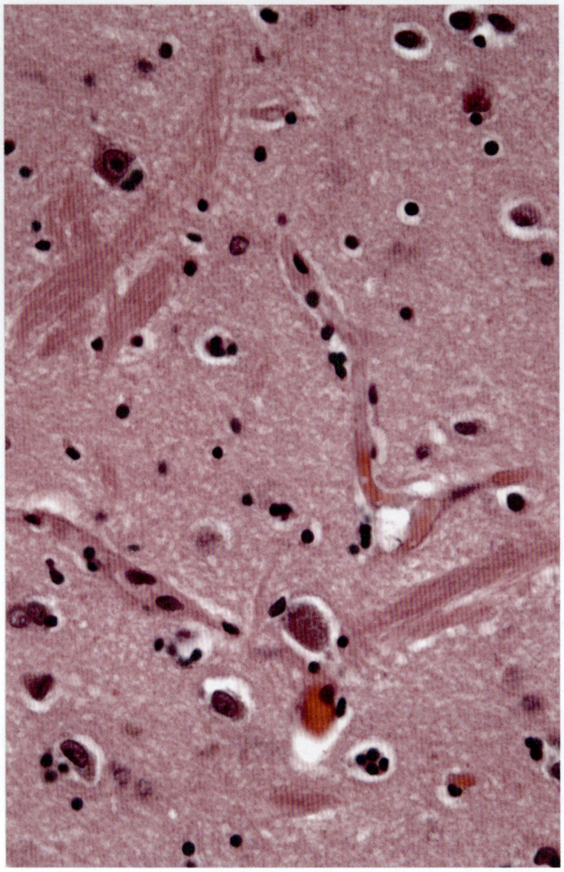

Figure 1-18

AMYGDALA

Medium-sized neurons are irregularly arranged, and bundles of white matter are often noted.

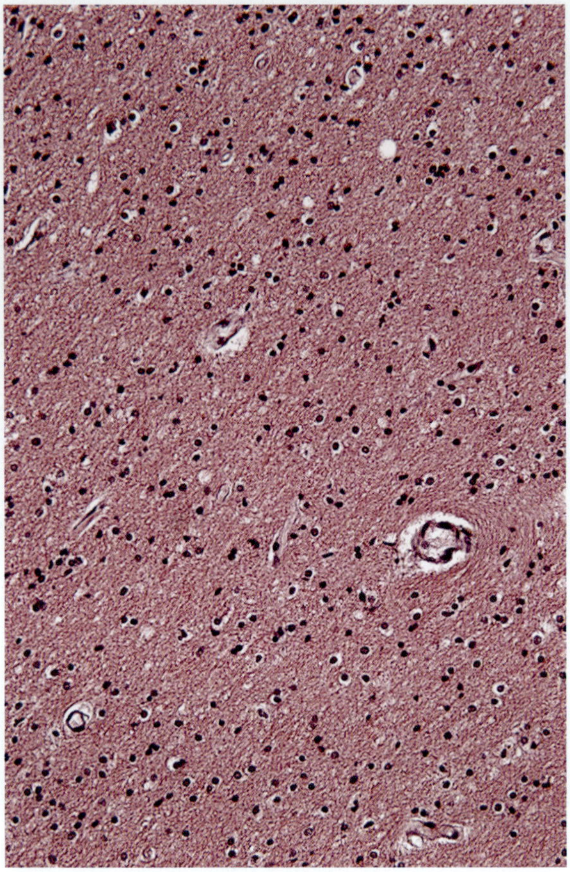

Figure 1-19

WHITE MATTER

Subcortical cerebral white matter contains numerous oligodendrocytes and small vessels.

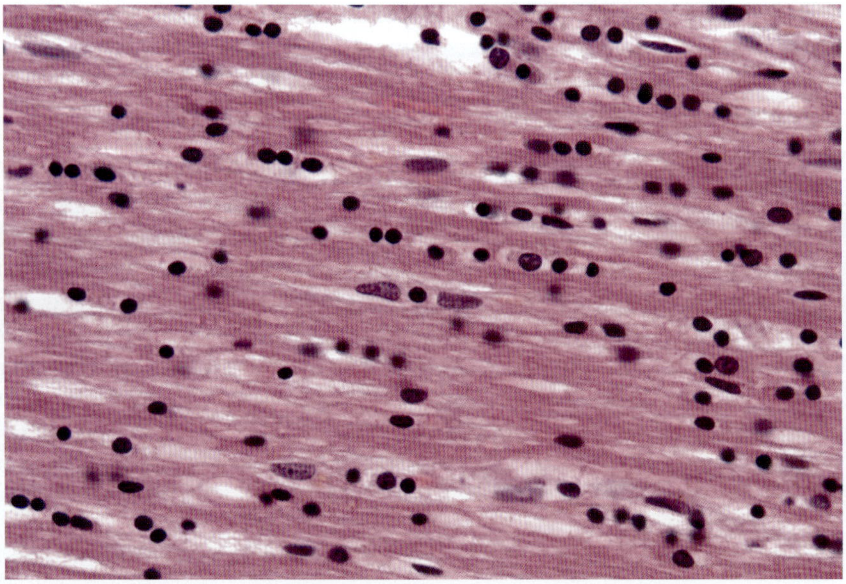

Figure 1-20

WHITE MATTER

Oligodendrocytes and astrocytes may be arrayed in lines in white matter bundles such as the anterior commissure.

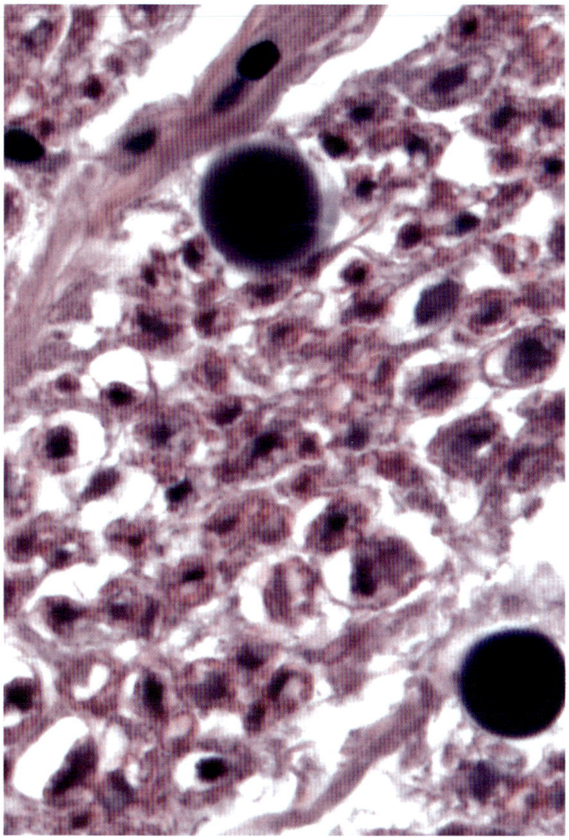

Figure 1-21

WHITE MATTER

In cross sections, as in this spinal cord, axons are recognized as dots within the retracted myelin sheaths. Corpora amylacea are present.

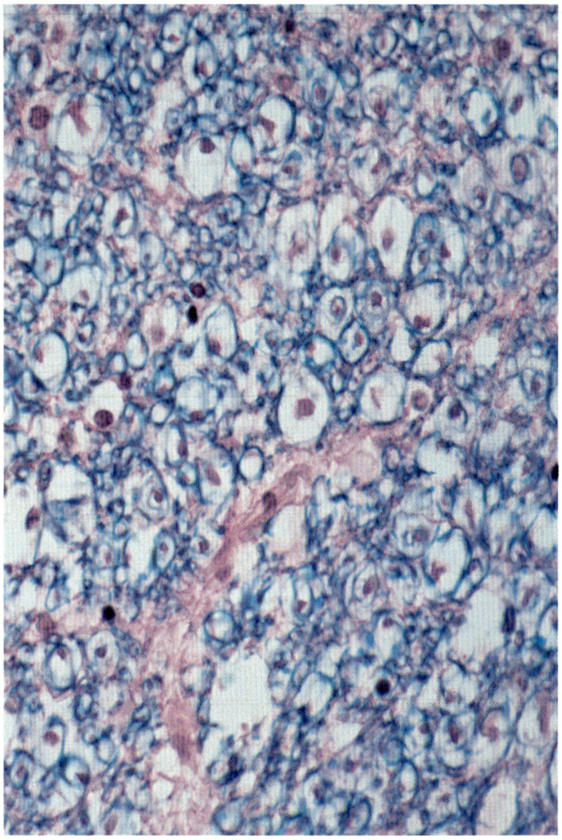

Figure 1-22

WHITE MATTER

Luxol fast blue stains myelin blue. Axons appear as central pink dots (Luxol fast blue-hematoxylin and eosin [H&E] stain).

perpendicular to the tract, there is a "vacuolar" quality that is occasioned by cross sectioning the myelin sheaths, which sometimes artifactually pull away from the central axons (fig. 1-21). Toluidine blue–stained, water-based frozen sections highlight the myelin debris as refractile purple-brown material. On paraffin sections, Luxol fast blue stains provide ready confirmation of myelin, and hence, of white matter tracts (fig. 1-22).

Some white matter areas have distinct features that suggest that region, and may therefore be of help in providing intraoperative guidance: the corpus callosum, internal capsule, and fornix (figs. 1-20, 1-23). Both the corpus callosum and the internal capsule are large and often-sampled white matter tracts that have similar histologic features. Perhaps because of their large size, longitudinal sections of these structures demonstrate longer rows of oligodendrocyte nuclei, with larger groups of myelinated fibers between the nuclear rows. Although only rarely sampled during surgical procedures, the fornix has a distinct organization when viewed in cross section. The white matter bundles are grouped into fascicles, in a manner reminiscent of the optic nerve (see below).

Deep Gray Matter

Although the various structures of the deep gray matter of the cerebral hemispheres differ markedly from one another in terms of their cytology and architecture (and obviously in their functions as well), they can be discussed together in the context of surgical neuropathology. Because of the unacceptable morbidity

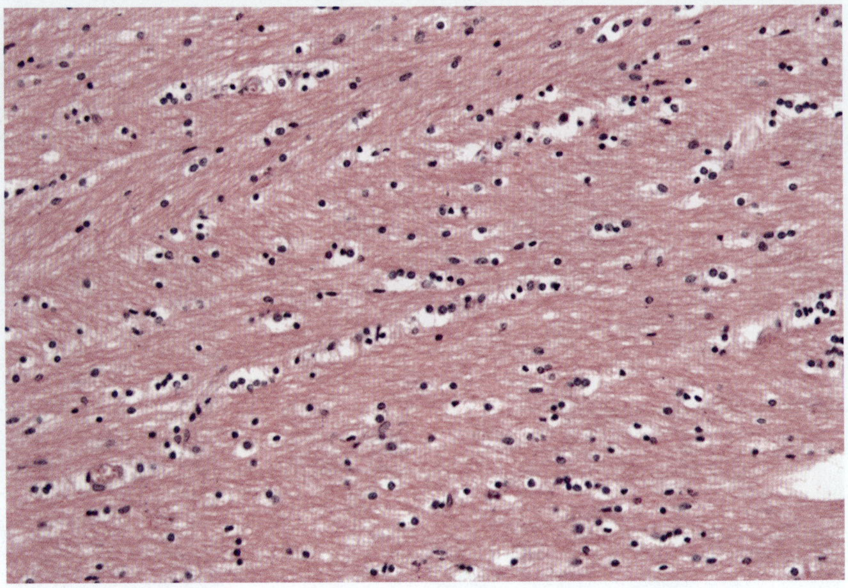

Figure 1-23

WHITE MATTER

The corpus callosum shows linear arrays of oligodendrocytes.

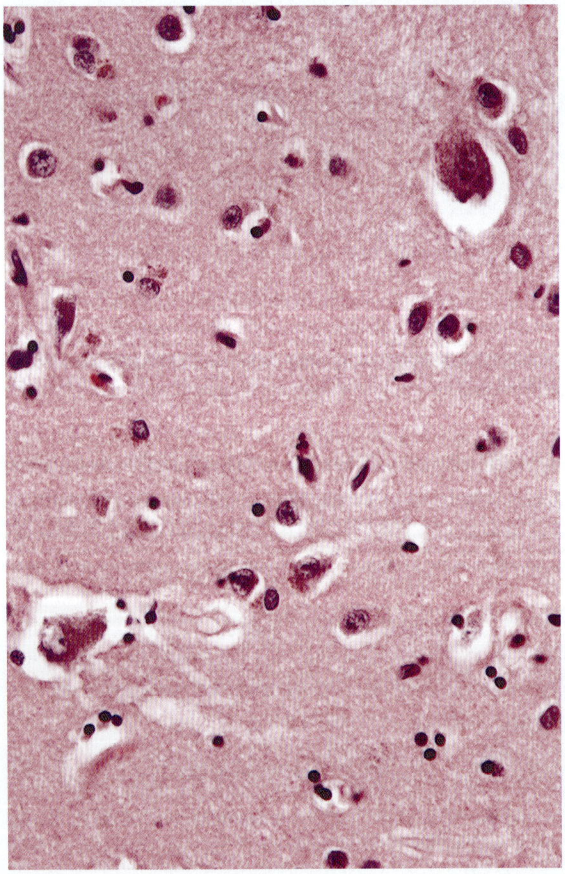

Figure 1-24

CAUDATE AND PUTAMEN

The striatum has many medium-sized neurons and scattered large neurons.

associated with any attempts to resect such structures, the deep gray matter nuclei are only visualized in small biopsy specimens. In fact, nearly all surgical specimens from deep gray matter are stereotactic needle biopsies. On the other hand, the more superficial gray matter regions that are not classic neocortex, such as the amygdala and hippocampus, are commonly included in temporal lobe resection specimens for either neoplastic or non-neoplastic conditions. These are discussed in the section on the cerebral cortex, above.

As a result of the small size of most deep gray matter biopsies, the architectural features of the three major deep gray matter regions—the basal ganglia, thalamus, and hypothalamus—are not often appreciated as they are depicted in standard neuroanatomy books. Nonetheless, cytologic features as well as some architectural features, such as the density of the neurons and the quality of the background neuropil, can hint at the origin of a deep gray matter specimen. Such information can be of substantial help to the neurosurgeon intraoperatively and to the interpretation of the final histologic sections. The three major regions are discussed below and illustrated in figures 1-24 to 1-28.

From the standpoint of surgical neuropathology, the basal ganglia consist of the caudate nucleus, putamen, and globus pallidus. Although standard neuroanatomy texts variably include a set of additional nuclei under the rubric of

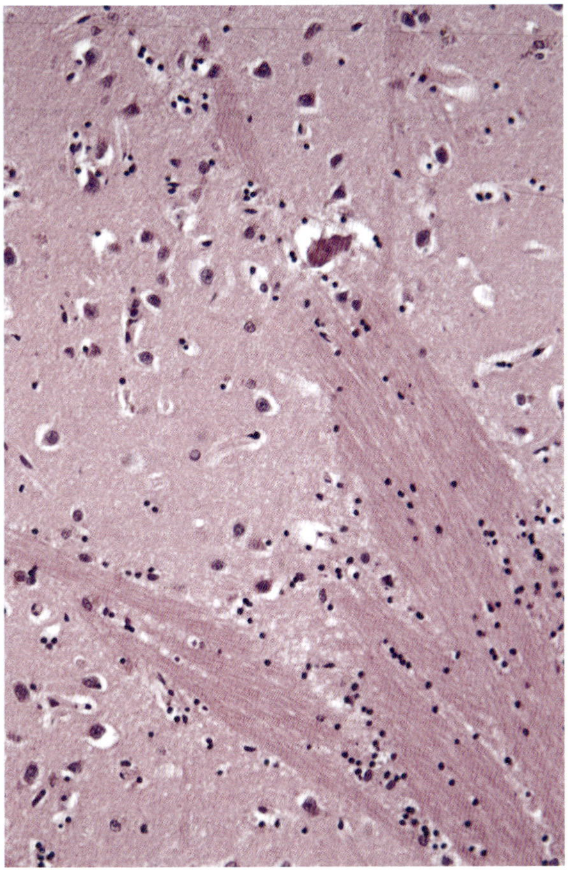

Figure 1-25

CAUDATE AND PUTAMEN

The striatum has conspicuous white matter bundles known as "pencils of Wilson" (lower right to middle).

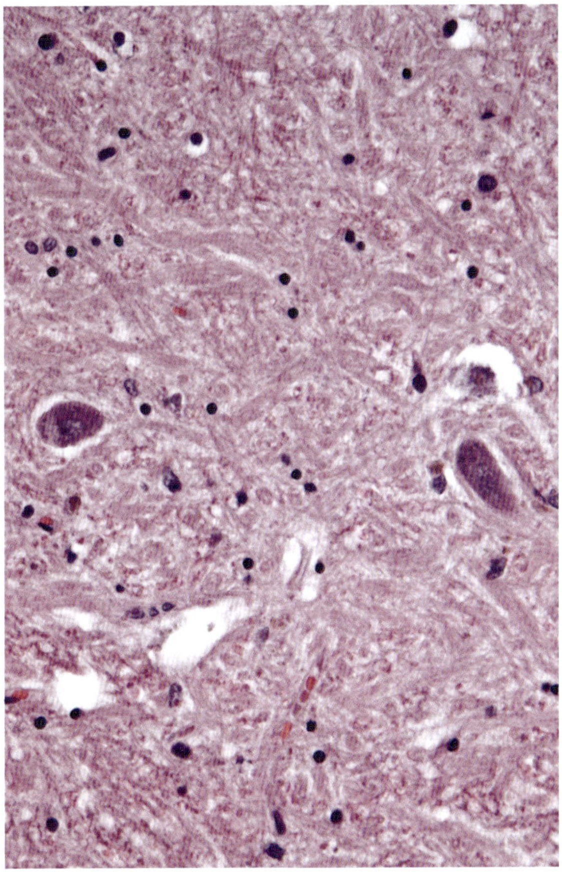

Figure 1-26

GLOBUS PALLIDUS

Scattered large neurons are in a background of numerous axons.

"basal ganglia," such as the subthalamic nucleus, these structures do not lend themselves to surgical biopsy. Histologically, the caudate and putamen are identical and the external and internal segments of the globus pallidus are very similar. For these reasons, there are two basic histologic patterns for surgical pathologists to recognize in the basal ganglia: that of the striatum (caudate nucleus and putamen) and that of the globus pallidus.

The caudate nucleus and putamen feature a combination of large and medium-sized neurons (fig. 1-24). These neurons are polygonal to rounded, are moderately densely packed (fig. 1-25), and are located in a neuropil that restricts myelin to fiber tracts known as "pencils of Wilson." These bundles are visible on H&E stains as small, short tracts of parallel fibers and arrays of oligodendrocytes; on Luxol fast blue stains, there is little visible myelin in the caudate and putamen except in these pencil fibers. This appearance contrasts markedly with the globus pallidus, which has a sparse collection of large, polygonal neurons in a neuropil that features numerous white matter fibers running in different directions (fig. 1-26). This abundance of myelinated fibers within a gray matter structure accounts for the relatively "pale" appearance of the globus pallidus on macroscopic examination; hence its name.

The thalamus and hypothalamus, in contrast to the caudate, putamen, and globus pallidus, are microscopically heterogeneous. Some regions of the thalamus, particularly the ventral (or laterally placed) tier of nuclei feature a background neuropil rich in myelinated fibers (fig. 1-27), whereas the remaining nuclear groups

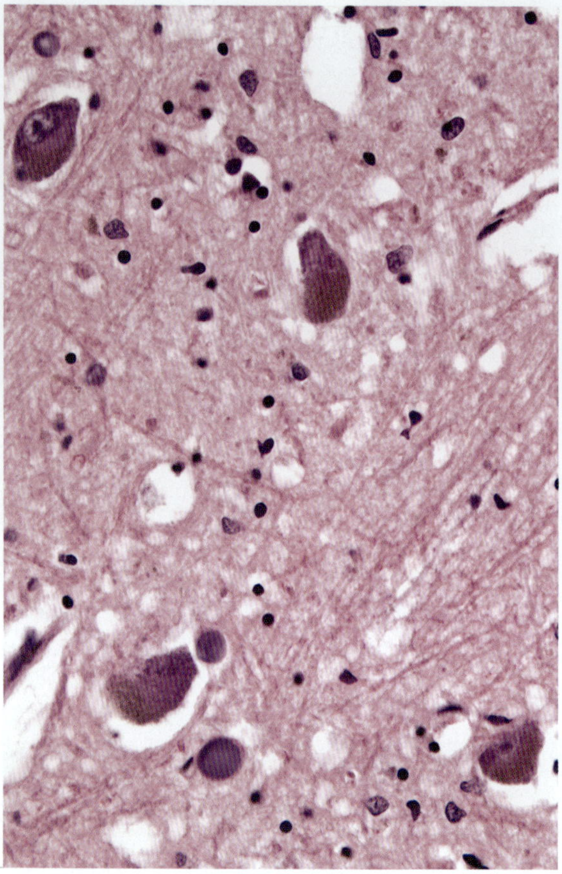

Figure 1-27

THALAMUS

Lateral thalamus features larger neurons with prominent axonal tracts.

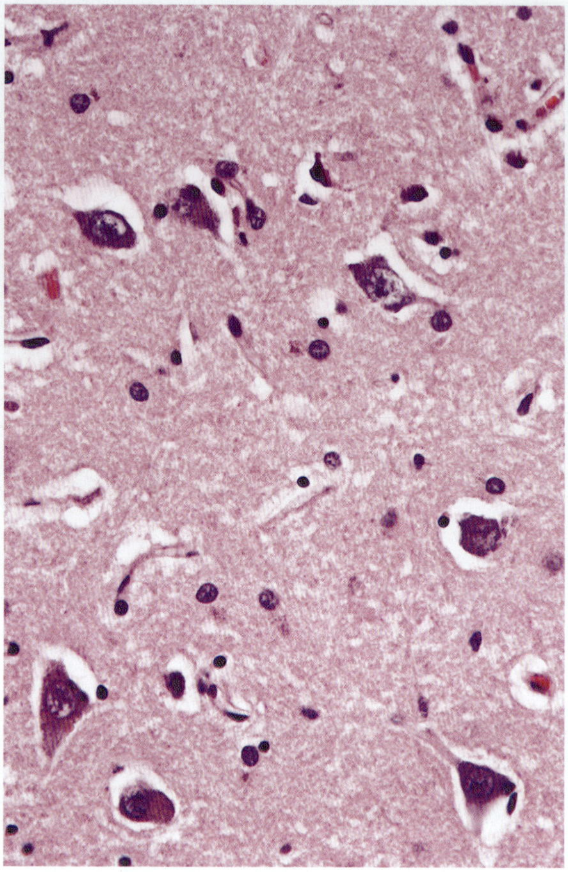

Figure 1-28

THALAMUS

Medial thalamus has irregularly arranged, medium-sized to large neurons.

tend to have more restricted white matter bundles and delicate neuropil (fig. 1-28). Most thalamic neurons are moderate in size, but they vary in shape and density from nucleus to nucleus. White matter lamina separate many of the thalamic nuclei from one another, but, with the exception of the mamillothalamic tract (tract of Vicq d'Azyr), are not prominent.

Similarly, the histologic appearance of the hypothalamus varies from region to region. Most hypothalamic neurons are moderate in size and range from polygonal to globular in shape. In some of the well-delineated hypothalamic nuclei, such as the supraoptic and paraventricular, the globular neurons are tightly packed together, but much of the more lateral hypothalamus features scattered neurons and moderate amounts of interspersed white matter.

Pineal Gland

A wide variety of non-neoplastic processes can involve the pineal region, and biopsies of the pineal gland are essentially always performed for tumor diagnosis or treatment. Occasionally, normal gland is sampled rather than tumor and so familiarity with the histology of the pineal gland is important for surgical pathologists. The pineal is composed of medium-sized neuronal cells as well as glia (fig. 1-29). The neuronal cells are polygonal, with short processes that can be highlighted with particular silver impregnations, such as the DeGirolami-Zvaigzne modification of the Achuccaro-Hortega method (3), as well as with immunohistochemistry for synaptophysin and retinal S-antigen. The important feature to appreciate is the lobularity of the normal pineal

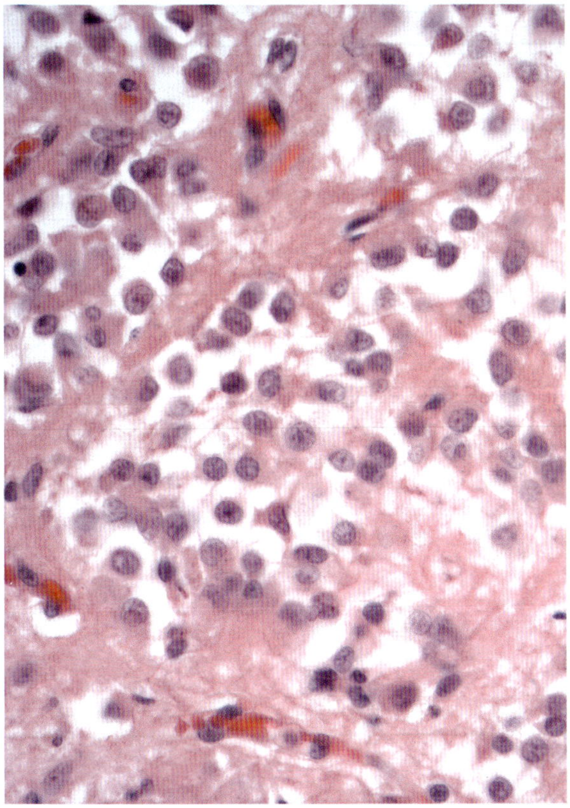

Figure 1-29

PINEAL GLAND

Rounded to carrot-shaped neuronal cells, some with visible processes.

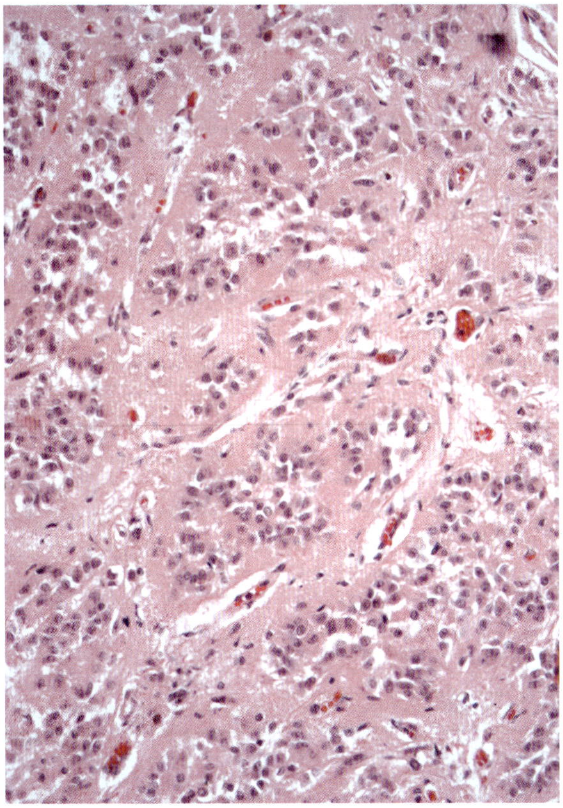

Figure 1-30

PINEAL GLAND

General clustering of cells by septa.

architecture, with cells packaged into large lobules by glial and vascular septa, and with large, irregular calcifications (fig. 1-30).

Brain Stem

The brain stem is seldom biopsied, for either suspected neoplasm or for non-neoplastic processes, because of the high risk of morbidity following biopsy. Occasional biopsies may target the middle cerebellar peduncle that joins the pons and deep cerebellar white matter. This white matter is indistinguishable from the deep hemispheric cerebral and cerebellar white matter. Rarely, exophytic lesions of the dorsal brain stem are biopsied via the fourth ventricle. In such situations, specimens may show the ependymal lining of the floor of the fourth ventricle, choroid plexus from the fourth ventricle itself, and occasional neurons from superficially located nuclei in the floor of the fourth ventricle. These are most often large neurons with typical neuronal cytologic features.

Cerebellum

The cerebellum is frequently included in posterior fossa biopsies, both as a target for biopsies and for access to deeper structures. It has a unique architecture that is easily recognized, but which can be mistaken for densely cellular pathologic processes in the setting of tiny biopsies and smear preparations.

The cerebellum is arranged in small folia: frond-like arrangements around a central white matter core (fig. 1-31). The cerebellar cortex has a trilaminar appearance, although at low power only the outer and inner layers are noticeable, given the thinness of the middle, Purkinje cell, layer. Beneath the pial surface is the outermost lamina, the paucicellular molecular layer (fig. 1-32). In addition to scattered glia, the molecular

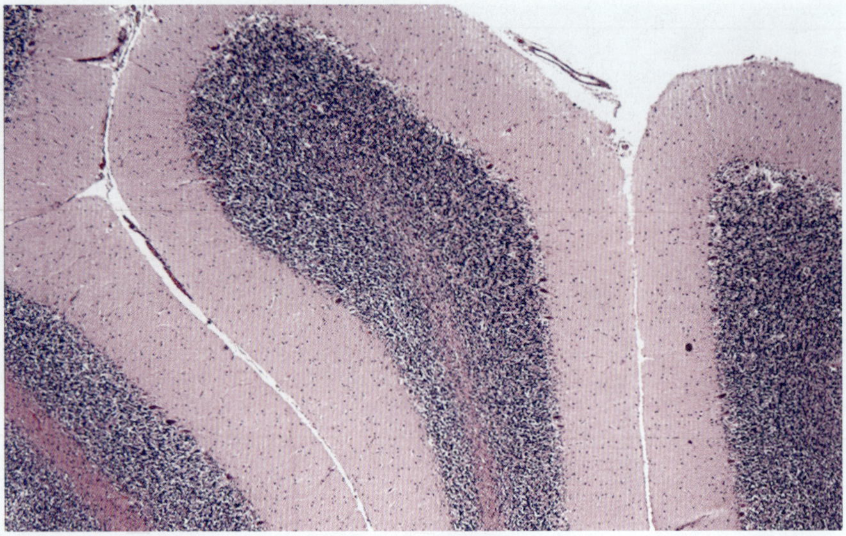

Figure 1-31

CEREBELLUM

Cerebellar cortex forms papillary folia.

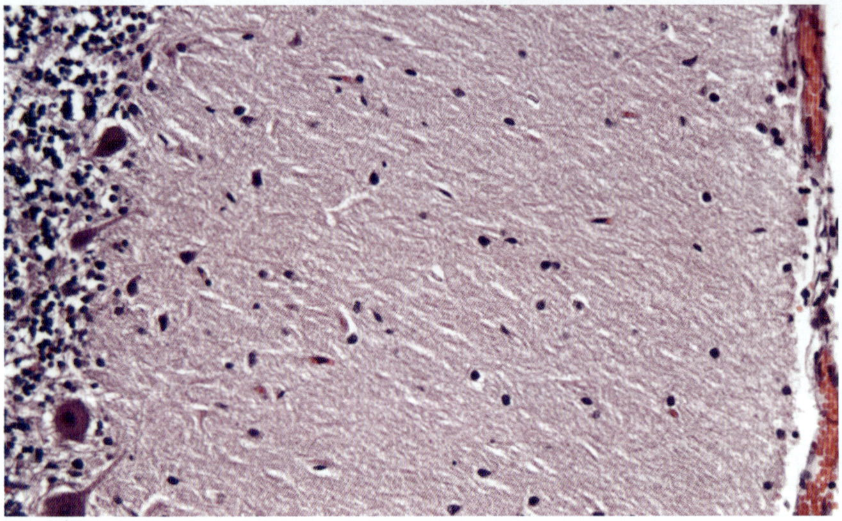

Figure 1-32

CEREBELLUM

The most superficial layer, the molecular layer, has few nuclei. Note the subarachnoid space on far right.

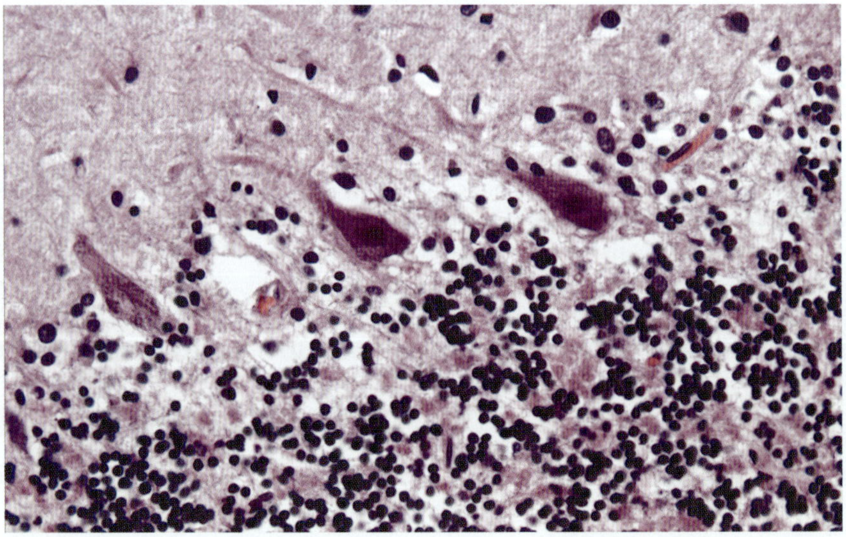

Figure 1-33

CEREBELLUM

Purkinje cells are large pyramidal and globoid cells between the molecular (top left) and granular (bottom right) layers.

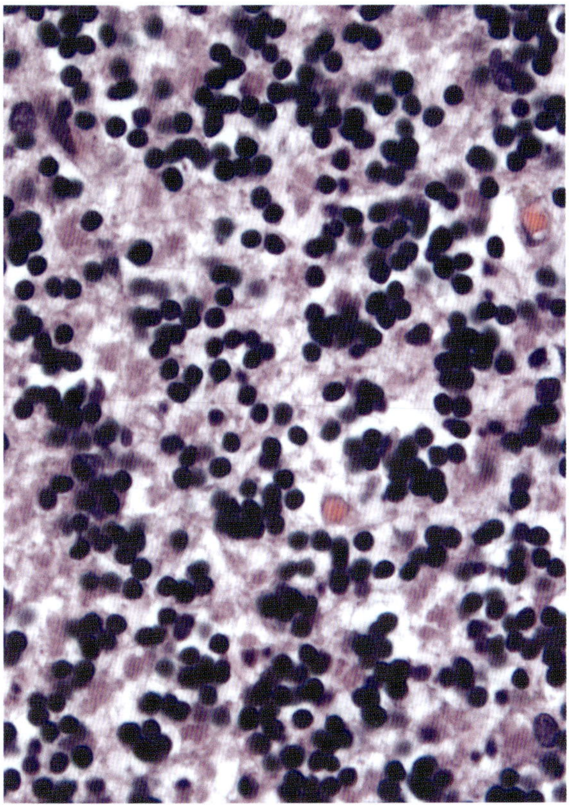

Figure 1-34

CEREBELLUM

The granular cell layer is composed of small neurons enmeshed in a delicate neuropil, with irregular rosettes.

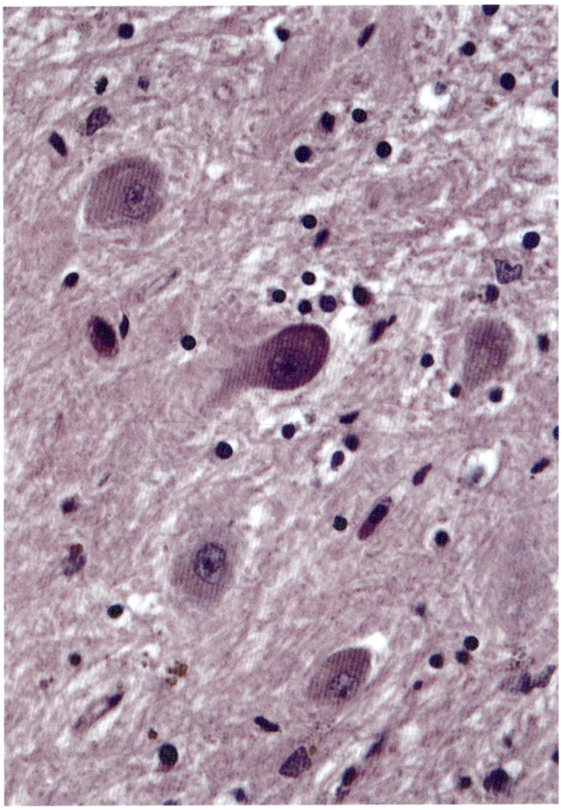

Figure 1-35

CEREBELLUM

The dentate gyrus of the cerebellum contains globoid neurons, often with lipofuscin.

layer includes two types of neurons, basket cells and outer stellate cells, as well as numerous axons (parallel fibers from the granular cells and dendrites of Purkinje cells). The thin Purkinje cell layer contains the large, pear-shaped Purkinje cells (fig. 1-33). Like other large neurons, these cells have round, euchromatic nuclei, each with a single, prominent nucleolus and amphophilic cytoplasm. Admixed with the Purkinje cells are the Bergmann glia, astrocytes that are usually inconspicuous but that respond by proliferating in the event of Purkinje cell loss. The innermost lamina is the granular cell layer, also known as the internal granular cell layer to distinguish it from the external granular cell layer (Obersteiner), which is a transient layer of small cells beneath the pial surface observed during fetal and infant life. The densely cellular granular cell layer features the small granular cells, with their hyperchromatic round nuclei and invisible cytoplasm (fig. 1-34). Granular neurons are arranged into small "glomeruli," in which the cells send processes into a central, nuclear-free region, nearly identical to the Homer-Wright rosettes seen in neuronal tumors. Golgi type II cells are also present in the granular layer, in the more superficial regions.

The cerebellar white matter is identical to white matter of the cerebral hemispheres. Deep cerebellar nuclei, specifically the dentate nucleus, are sometimes also included in biopsies. The dentate nucleus is comprised of large globular neurons (fig. 1-35), often with lipofuscin, arranged in a neuropil that forms an undulating layer. The finding of neurons in deep cerebellar biopsies, sometimes in an undulating linear arrangement (fig. 1-36), in the absence of features of cerebellar cortex, strongly suggests that the biopsy includes the cerebellar dentate nucleus.

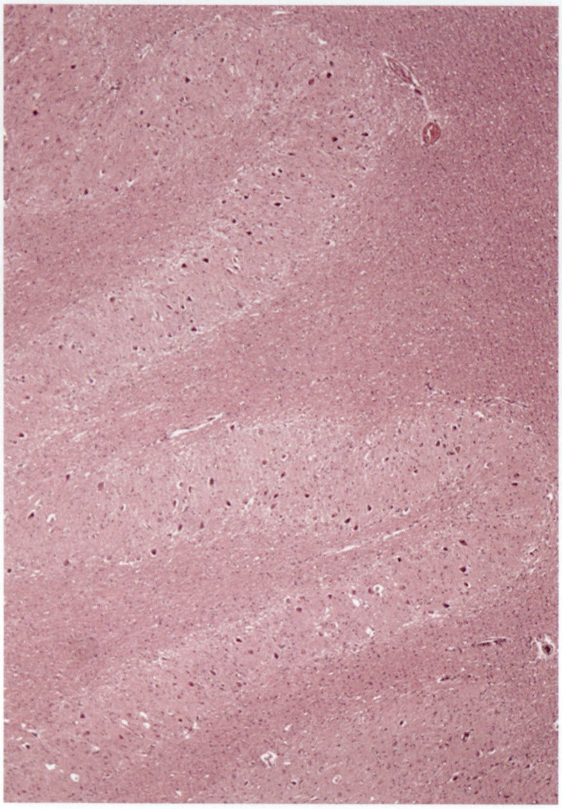

Figure 1-36

CEREBELLUM

The dentate gyrus of the cerebellum is an undulating structure.

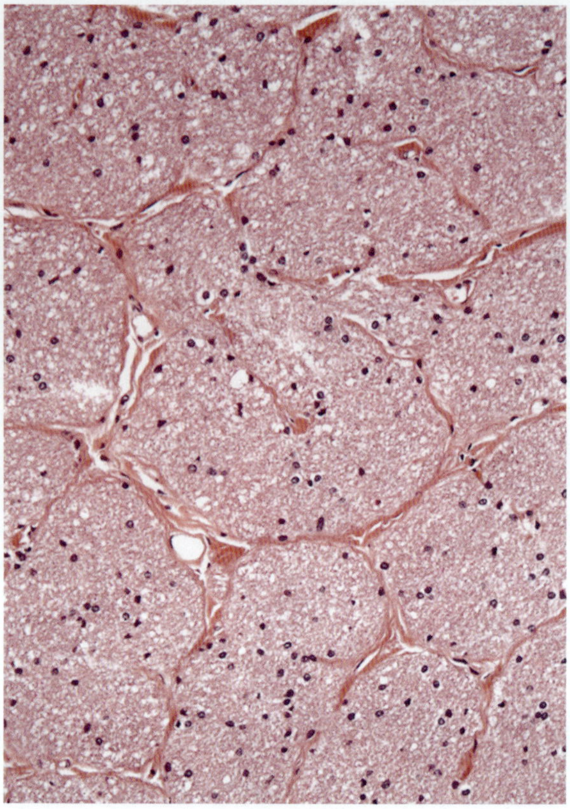

Figure 1-37

OPTIC NERVE

The fascicles of white matter are divided by fibrovascular septa.

The unique architecture of the cerebellum allows its ready identification, even in unusual situations. For example, necrotic cerebellar cortex has been recognized in the spinal subarachnoid space in the setting of brain death, sometimes as cellular debris in a spinal tap. More problematic, however, is mistaking the densely cellular granular layer for neoplastic cells or lymphocytes, particularly on smear preparations. Attention to the regularity of the nuclei and of the delicate neuropil usually allows distinction from small cell tumors of the cerebellum. The relative evenness of the smear and the neuropil helps in the distinction from lymphocytes, and immunohistochemistry for CD45 can solve any diagnostic questions.

Cranial Nerves

Cranial nerves are only rarely sampled in the setting of non-neoplastic diseases. Cranial nerves I and II, the olfactory and optic, are extensions of the CNS, with oligodendrocytes rather than Schwann cells (fig. 1-37). The remaining cranial nerves (III to XII) are peripheral nerves, with Schwann cells and peripheral nervous system (PNS) myelin (figs. 1-38, 1-39). For cranial nerves III to XII, the CNS-PNS junction (Obersteiner-Redlich zone) is sharp, and located, with the exception of cranial nerve VIII, just at the edge of the substance of the brain stem. For cranial nerve VIII, this junction is a few millimeters from the edge of the brain stem, closer to the internal acoustic meatus. Luxol fast blue–based stains can highlight this transition, since CNS and PNS myelin have different hues. The histology of the normal PNS and non-neoplastic diseases associated with it are discussed in detail elsewhere (4). The peripheral nerve intradural components are similar to those in the periphery, but are devoid of a perineurium or epineurium.

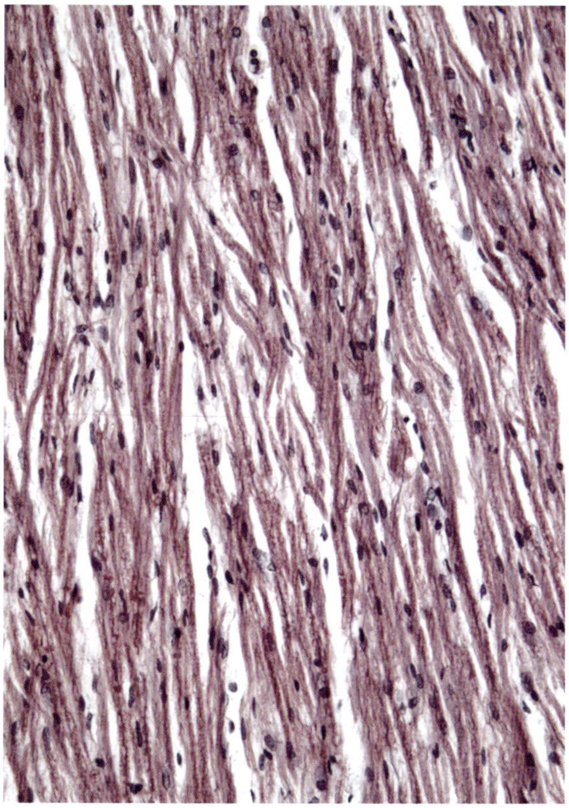

Figure 1-38

OCULOMOTOR NERVE

For cranial nerves III through XII, linear arrays of Schwann cells and axons are identical to those of peripheral nerves.

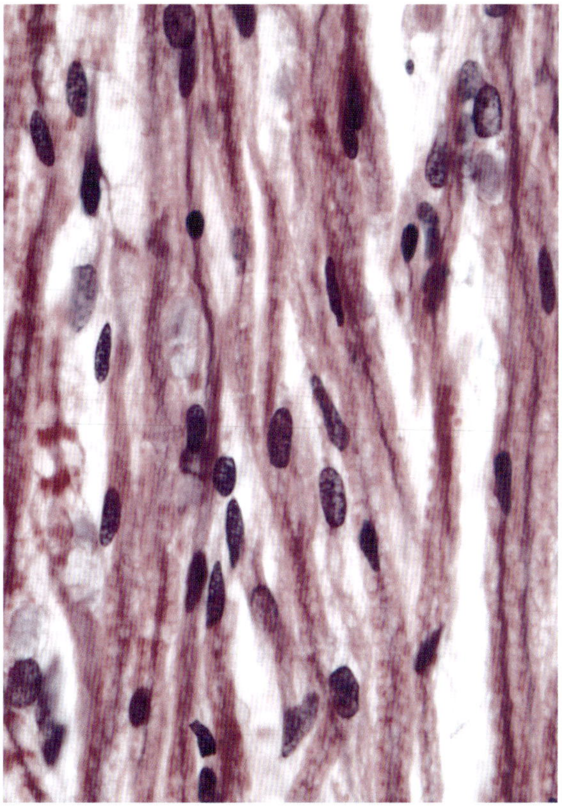

Figure 1-39

OCULOMOTOR NERVE

Schwann cells are present between axons, as in peripheral nerves.

The olfactory nerve is not, to our knowledge, ever found in surgical specimens, but the optic nerve is sampled, usually in the setting of tumor surgery. The optic nerve is ensheathed with meninges, including dura, arachnoid mater, and pia mater. The parenchyma of the optic nerve features parallel myelinated axons coursing along the length of the nerve, with intercalated astrocytes, oligodendrocytes, and capillaries. The ophthalmic artery runs down the approximate center of the nerve. The axons are packeted into partially separate groups by delicate fibrovascular septa (fig. 1-37). This packeting is unique among CNS white matter tracts.

Spinal Cord

Surgical specimens that include spinal cord tissue fall into two categories: minute biopsies for diagnostic purposes and resection specimens that include small amounts of adjacent spinal cord. The latter are most common in the setting of neoplastic disease, but occasional non-neoplastic lesions are resected if there is a high index of suspicion that the lesion is neoplastic. Importantly, in both situations, the amount of sampled spinal cord is exceedingly small.

Small cord biopsies sample the periphery of the cord and so are usually comprised entirely of white matter tracts (figs. 1-40, 1-41). More often than not, the tiny specimens suffer from some degree of crush artifact, complicating their interpretation. In such situations, artifactual hypercellularity should not be misdiagnosed as a primary neoplasm. In older patients, many corpora amylacea may be present.

Large cord biopsies, in the setting of presumed tumor, may include deeper structures, including gray matter. Unusually, large, Nissl substance–rich anterior horn cells are seen (fig. 1-42). More commonly, nondescript neurons are encountered (fig.

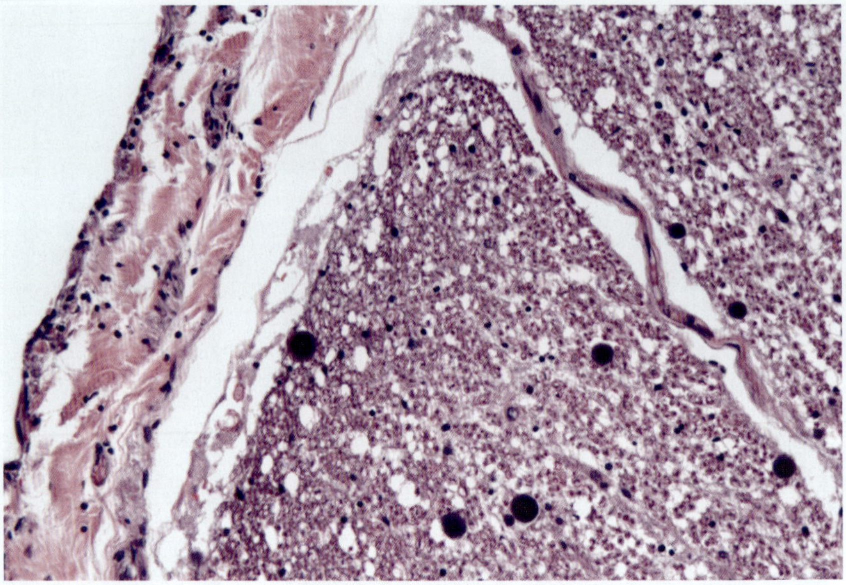

Figure 1-40

SPINAL CORD

The periphery of the dorsal columns is the region most commonly biopsied. The arachnoid (left) overlies white matter tracts with corpora amylacea.

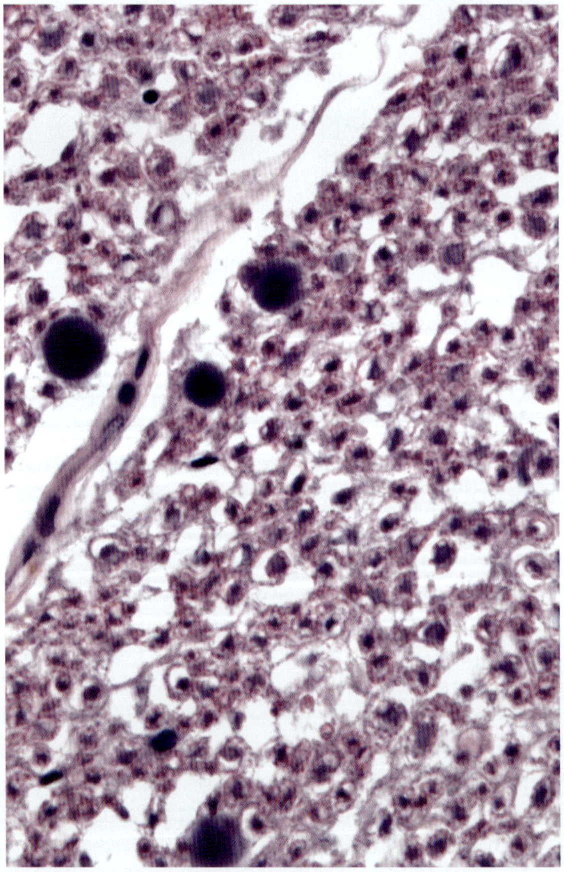

Figure 1-41

SPINAL CORD

Dorsal white matter tracts feature discernible axons and corpora amylacea.

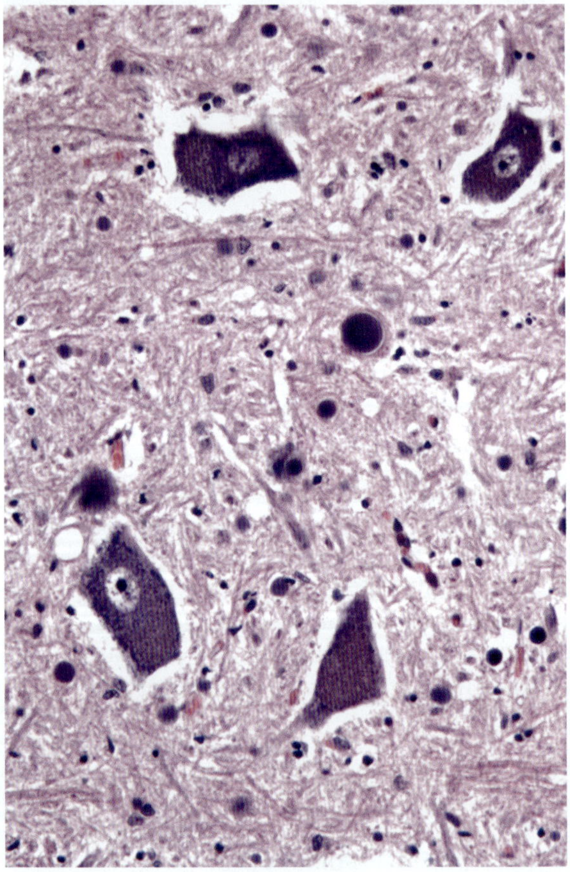

Figure 1-42

SPINAL CORD

Anterior horn cells have prominent Nissl substance, similar to other large motor neurons.

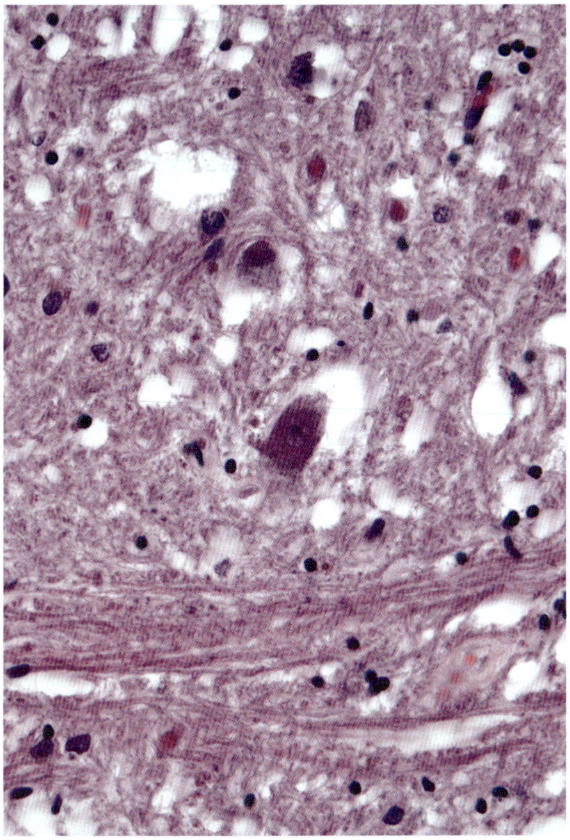

Figure 1-43

SPINAL CORD

Neurons in the dorsal horn are medium-sized with conspicuous background axons.

1-43), arranged in a neuropil that can be highlighted with synaptophysin staining.

CNS CELL TYPES

Neurons

Neurons are the most cytologically diverse cells in the entire human body. They range from huge cells with extremely long processes, such as the Betz cells of the motor cortex which extend axons as far as the lower spinal cord, to the small granular cells of the cerebellar cortex. So marked are the size differences that the nucleolus of a Betz cell is approximately the same size as the entire nucleus of a cerebellar granular cell.

Most neurons conform generally to one of three cytologic groups: large, usually triangular neurons with copious cytoplasm; medium-sized triangular to round neurons with some visible cytoplasm; and small, round neurons with little if any visible cytoplasm. The large neurons include those in the deeper layers of the cerebral cortex (including the Betz cells; figs. 1-11 and 1-14) and in many of the deep gray matter structures, brain stem nuclei, Purkinje cells of the cerebellar cortex (fig. 1-33) and cerebellar dentate nucleus (fig. 1-35), and spinal gray matter (fig. 1-42). They tend to have large, oval or rounded, euchromatic nuclei with a single, prominent nucleolus. Their cytoplasm is often amphophilic, with granular material, sometimes Nissl substance and sometimes lipofuscin (see below). Medium-sized neurons are widely distributed throughout the cerebral cortex (fig. 1-13) and particularly in deep gray matter structures (figs. 1-24, 1-26, 1-27). Their nuclei also feature prominent euchromatin, with single, small yet distinct nucleoli. Granular lipofuscin (see below) is sometimes noted in the cytoplasm. Small granular neurons are most often noted in the hippocampal dentate nucleus (fig. 1-34) and internal granular cell layer of the cerebellum (fig. 1-17). They have dense, hyperchromatic nuclei, without clear single nucleoli and little visible cytoplasm on standard stains.

Certain neurons have particular features that are relatively unique. The extremely large size of the deep-seated Betz cells has been commented on already. These cells, in addition to being large, have copious Nissl substance. These clumps of basophilic material, brought out with cresyl violet (Nissl) stains, represent rough endoplasmic reticulum, which is particularly pronounced in large motor neurons. Thus, motor neurons throughout the brain stem and spinal cord can be distinguished by their polygonal cell bodies harboring copious Nissl substance even on standard H&E-stained sections. The identification of such cells in a cortical biopsy taken from the pericentral region implies that the surgeon has biopsied the motor strip; their presence in a spinal cord biopsy means that the sample includes the anterior horn. Other neurons have a more globoid appearance, with rounded nuclei and eccentric rounded cytoplasm. These include neurons of the dorsal column of Clarke and the mesencephalic nucleus of the fifth cranial nerve, but these are seldom if ever present in biopsy specimens. Particular neuronal groups are deeply pigmented, at least

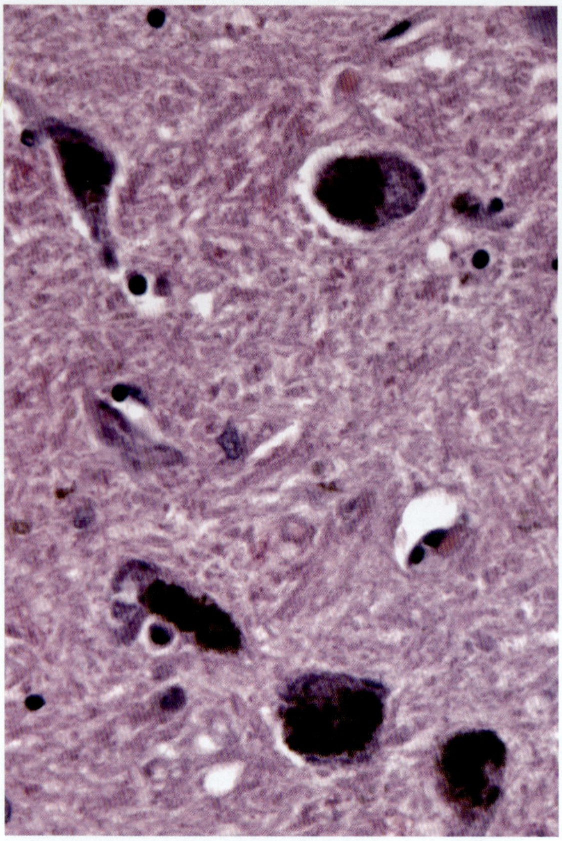

Figure 1-44

NEURONS, PIGMENT

Neuromelanin-containing neurons in the substantia nigra.

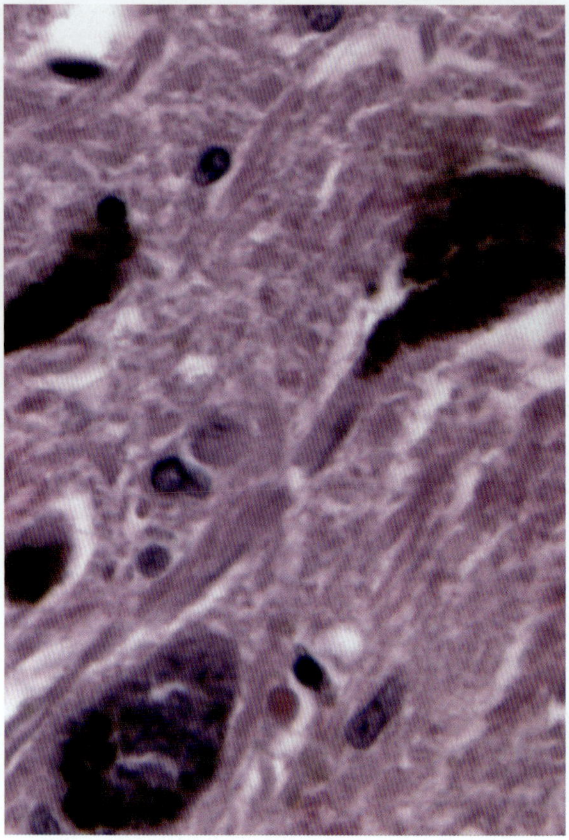

Figure 1-45

NEURONS, PIGMENT

Neuromelanin consists of evenly sized, dark brown granules.

in adults: those of the substantia nigra, locus ceruleus, and dorsal motor nucleus of the vagus, allowing their ready identification (figs. 1-44, 1-45). Again, however, these are rarely if ever included in surgical samples.

Lipofuscin accumulates in the cytoplasm of many neurons with age (fig. 1-46). Some neurons, such as those of the inferior olivary nucleus, acquire lipofuscin pigment early in life, whereas others only do so in adulthood. Neurons in the cerebral cortex, for example, progressively accumulate lipofuscin during adult life. On H&E stains, lipofuscin has a light brownish, refractile granularity and is often eccentrically located along the perikaryal edge. It is far lighter in color than either melanin or neuromelanin. In Luxol fast blue–stained tissues, it may acquire a bright blue appearance. Although not specific to neurons, since it accumulates in astrocytes as well, relatively extensive cytoplasmic lipofuscin can be a convenient "marker" for neurons in smear preparations, frozen sections, and paraffin sections.

Neurons are usually recognizable because of their unique cytologic appearance. Pathologic processes, however, may distort the tissue architecture and surgical artifact may compress cells. As a result, there may be a need for special stains and immunohistochemistry to highlight neuronal cell bodies and processes. Because of its ability to highlight Nissl substance, which is so prominent in neurons, a cresyl violet stain may highlight neurons, enabling their identification as well as the evaluation of their architecture in structures such as the cerebral cortex. For example, in epilepsy resection specimens (see chapter 13), it is often necessary to determine whether the cerebral cortex is normally formed or dysplastic. Nissl staining is a convenient means for doing this.

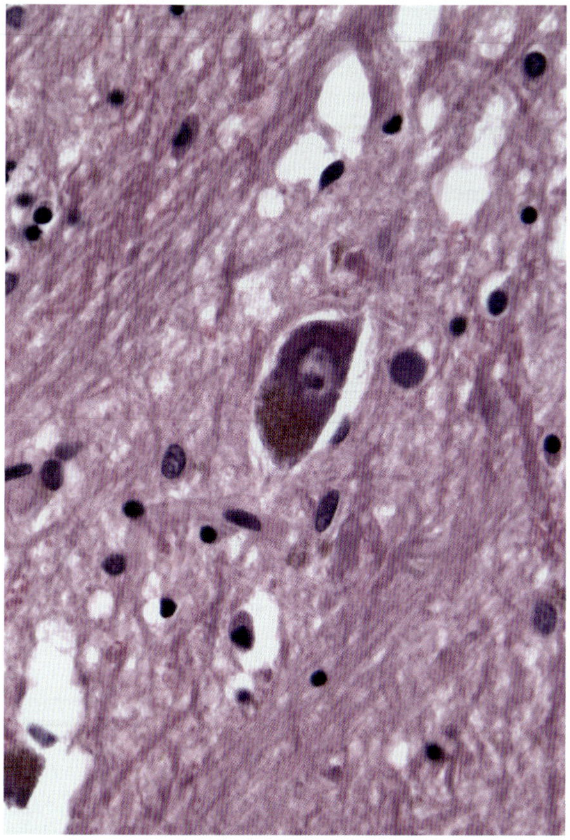

Figure 1-46

NEURONS, LIPOFUSCIN

Aging pigment is commonly noted as granular, amphophilic cytoplasmic material, as in this neuron from the lateral thalamus.

Immunohistochemistry also plays a major role in the identification and evaluation of neurons. The three proteins most commonly studied using immunohistochemical means are NeuN, synaptophysin, and neurofilament. NeuN is a nuclear marker of mature neurons. Most normal neurons stain strongly for NeuN. As such, assays for NeuN provide a convenient means for identifying questionable cells as neurons and for evaluating neuronal organization in epilepsy specimens. Synaptophysin labels synaptic vesicles, and is therefore present in a diffuse granular pattern within the gray matter. In general, it is not found in great amounts in neuronal cell bodies, but rather highlights the background neuropil. In neuronal neoplasms, however, synaptophysin may stain the neoplastic neuronal cell bodies. In biopsies of non-neoplastic processes, synaptophysin immunohistochemistry is a convenient method to confirm the presence of neuropil. Neurofilament immunohistochemistry is typically performed with a "cocktail" of antibodies to the low-, medium- and high-molecular weight neurofilaments, the intermediate filaments specific to neurons. Intermediate neurofilaments are almost exclusively found in neuronal cell processes rather than cell bodies, and their antibodies are therefore used to stain axons. In certain conditions, such as demyelinating diseases, the visualization of axons is crucial to establishing a correct diagnosis.

On ultrastructural examination, neurons display a wide variety of appearances (5). Common to the different cells, however, is the presence of processes with microtubules and synaptic vesicles. In the neuropil of the gray matter, these processes constitute almost the entirety of the tissue. In the white matter, the axons feature numerous microtubules and neurofilaments, surrounded by dense myelin sheaths (see below).

Astrocytes

Astrocytes subserve a number of different functions in the brain. From a surgical pathology point of view, their most salient function is their nearly universal reaction to injury, making them a prominent feature of nearly all neuropathologic processes (chapter 2). Despite the fact that they vastly outnumber neurons in the CNS and that they participate so extensively in reacting to brain injury, astrocytes are fairly inconspicuous on standard stains. Astrocytes are located throughout both gray and white matter, but are generally passed over as the eye focuses on the impressive neurons and the small, dark oligodendrocytes. They extend foot processes to the pial surface (the glia limitans) as well as to blood vessels. They have oval nuclei with euchromatin and no visible cytoplasm (fig. 1-47); indeed, the presence of discernible eosinophilic cytoplasm strongly suggests that the astrocyte is reactive. In some sites, in which "reaction" to cellular stresses may be an ongoing process during life, such as the pial surface or subependymal region, astrocytic foot processes may be visible as slightly coarse fibrils. In addition, in certain places such as the subependymal

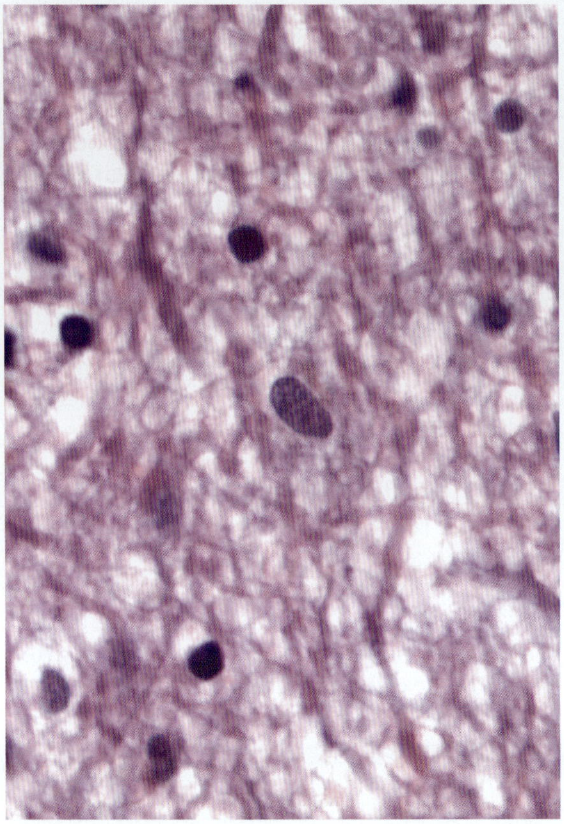

Figure 1-47

ASTROCYTES AND OLIGODENDROCYTES

An astrocyte (center) has oval, euchromatic nucleus and lacks visible cytoplasm. Oligodendrocytes also lack discernible cytoplasm but have rounded, hyperchromatic nuclei.

regions, a chronic astrocytic reaction results in the accumulation of corpora amylacea in the astrocytic processes. These concentric, rounded collections of polysaccharide-containing material, appear basophilic on H&E stains (figs. 1-21, 1-41) and strongly positive on periodic acid–Schiff (PAS) stains. The often striking and diagnostically important reactive features of astrocytes are discussed in the next chapter.

Normal astrocytes are not easily labeled immunohistochemically, since glial fibrillary acidic protein (GFAP) is not present in detectable quantities except in subpial and some perivascular astrocytes. Reactive astrocytes, on the other hand, are robustly labeled with antibodies to GFAP, S-100 protein, or vimentin (see chapter 2). Ultrastructurally, the most characteristic feature of astrocytes is their cytoplasmic processes with GFAP-positive intermediate filaments.

Oligodendrocytes and Myelin

Oligodendrocytes send out complex processes to axons to provide myelin sheaths. As such, they are copious in the white matter but are present in gray matter as well. In large white matter tracts, such as the corpus callosum and internal capsule, oligodendrocytes are aligned in rows alongside the myelinated fibers. In gray matter, particularly in temporal lobe neocortex, they satellite around neurons and are in the intervening neuropil. Their nuclei are dark and round, and regular in appearance, and they lack visible cytoplasm on H&E-stained sections (fig. 1-47).

Myelin is the visible evidence of oligodendrocyte processes in the CNS. The visualization of myelin is often of great importance in the evaluation of brain biopsies, particularly if the differential diagnosis includes demyelinating diseases. On frozen sections stained with water-based methods, such as toluidine blue, myelin can be seen as granular, purple-brown, slightly refractile material. But myelin is most readily demonstrated using specific myelin stains. Of these, the most commonly used is the Luxol fast blue, either in combination with H&E (LHE) or with cresyl violet (Kluver-Barrera stain). With Luxol fast blue, myelin has a bright blue appearance; with LHE at high power, myelin consists of tubes surrounding eosinophilic axons (fig. 1-48). Peripheral myelin, with its slightly different lipoprotein constituents, has a more purplish color on LHE stains, allowing easy visualization of the CNS-PNS border (Obersteiner-Redlich zone).

Ultrastructurally, oligodendrocytes are most notable for their cytoplasmic processes that contain microtubules and for the myelin sheaths. The compact, concentrically oriented myelin represents the flattened and rolled cell membranes and attenuated cytoplasm of oligodendrocytes. Some immunohistochemical stains label oligodendrocytes, such as CNPase, but these do not work well on fixed, embedded tissues and have not to date found a role in surgical neuropathology.

Ependyma

Ependymal cells are glial in origin, despite their epithelial appearance. They line the ventricles of the brain and, as such, are frequently present in periventricular biopsies. Indeed,

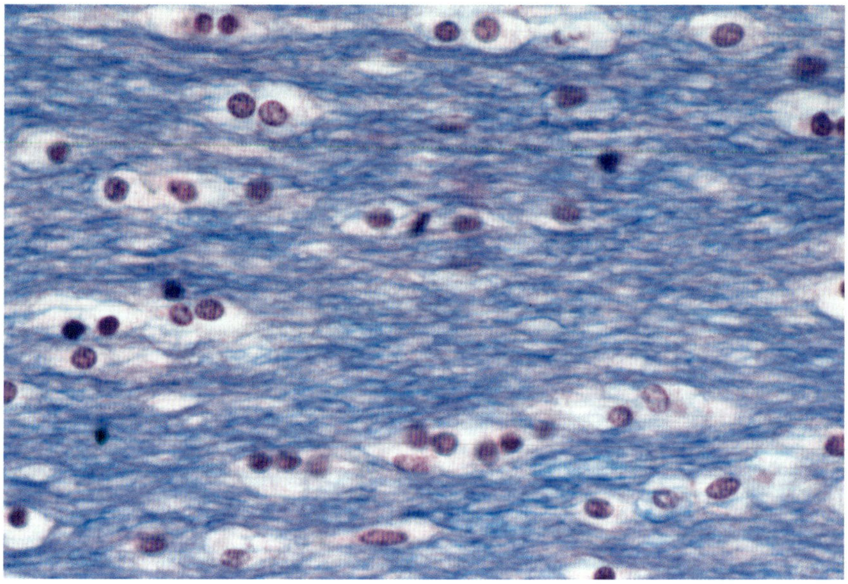

Figure 1-48

OLIGODENDROCYTES AND MYELIN

Myelin is highlighted with the Luxol fast blue stain.

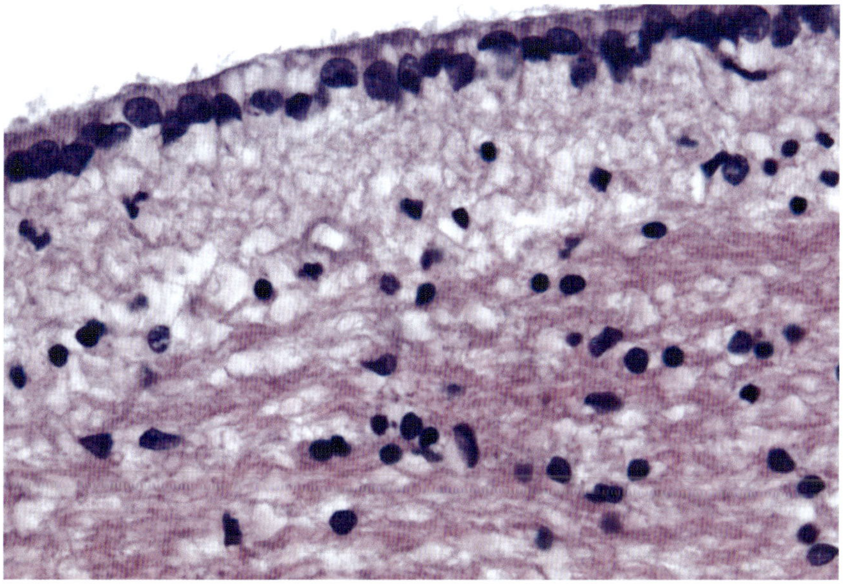

Figure 1-49

EPENDYMA

Ependymal cells are cuboidal, sometimes with visible cilia.

the presence of ependymal cells can alert the pathologist to the site of origin of a specimen, which is useful information to relay to the neurosurgeon intraoperatively. Ependymal cells are usually cuboidal, with round to elongated nuclei having coarse chromatin (fig. 1-49). In children, the cells are more columnar and often ciliated (fig. 1-50). On ultrastructural analysis, ependymal cells feature microvilli and cilia as well as complex intercellular junctions.

Ependymal cells may also be arranged in subventricular clusters, so-called subependymal nests (fig. 1-51). These are particularly common in the inferior reaches of the frontal horns of the lateral ventricles, as residua of the embryonal olfactory ventricle. In the spinal cord, as the central canal collapses during adult life, the ependymal cells form similar clusters (fig. 1-52). Again, the presence of these cells can be a useful indicator of location in biopsy material. In older adults and in patients who have had prior ventricular inflammation (typically from remote meningitis), the ependymal lining may be discontinuous and associated with a subependymal astrocytic proliferation. In some of these cases, there may be glial bands

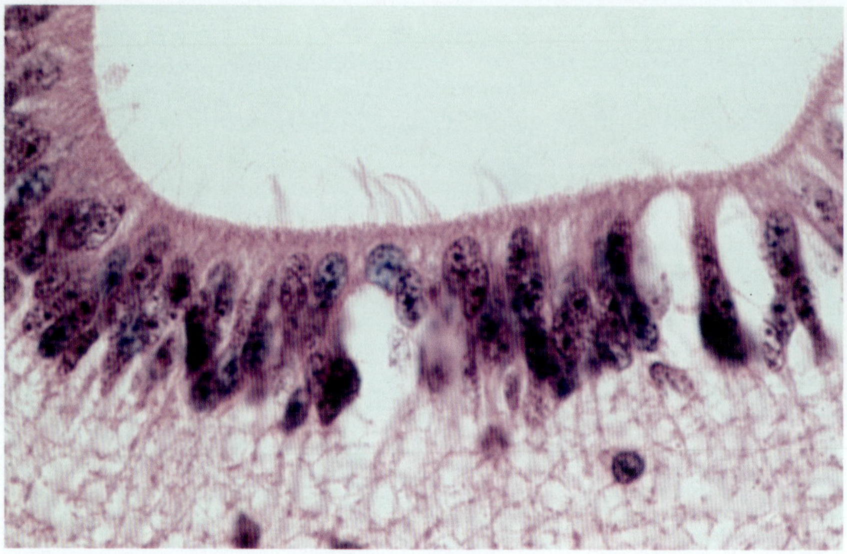

Figure 1-50

EPENDYMA

In children, ependymal cells are more columnar, often with cilia.

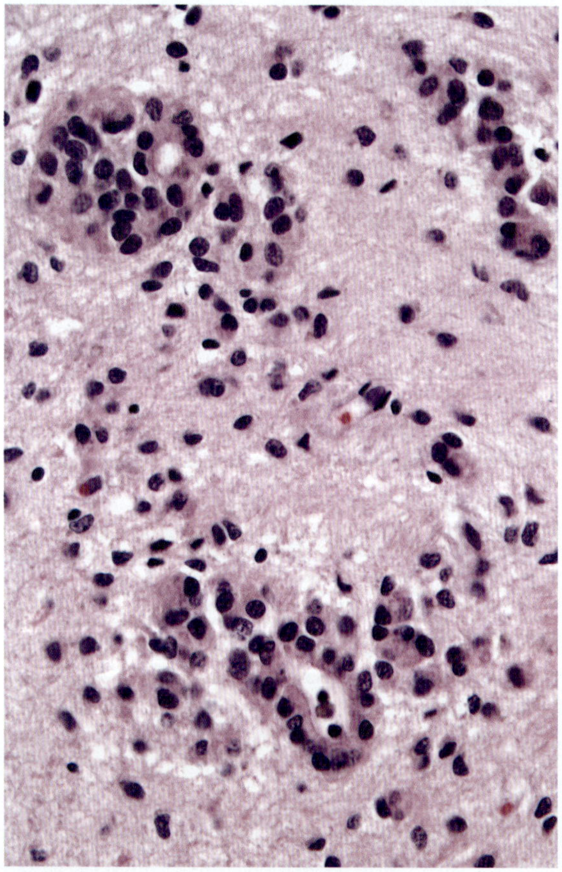

Figure 1-51

EPENDYMA

Ependymal nests are often found in the subependymal regions, particularly near the lateral ventricles. Small rosettes are sometimes formed.

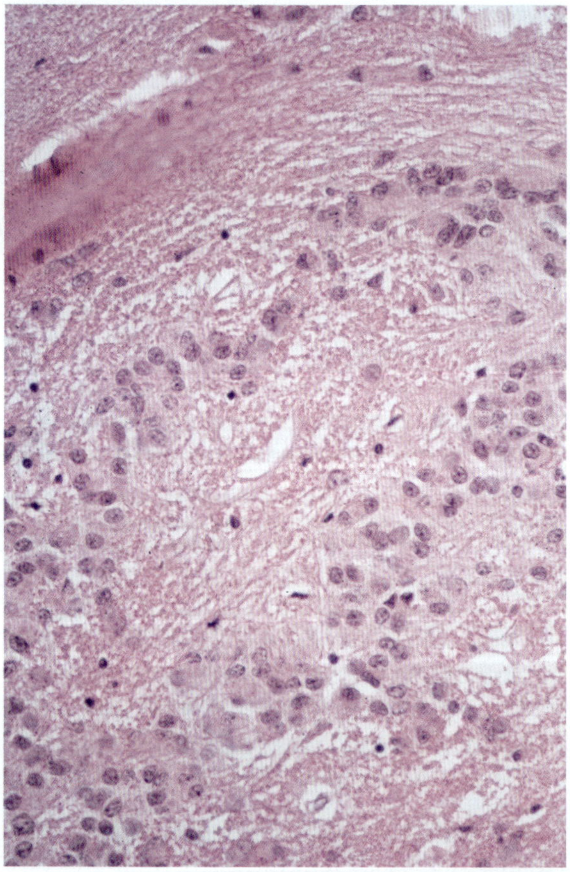

Figure 1-52

EPENDYMA

In the adult spinal cord, the central canal is usually collapsed, leaving clusters of ependymal cells.

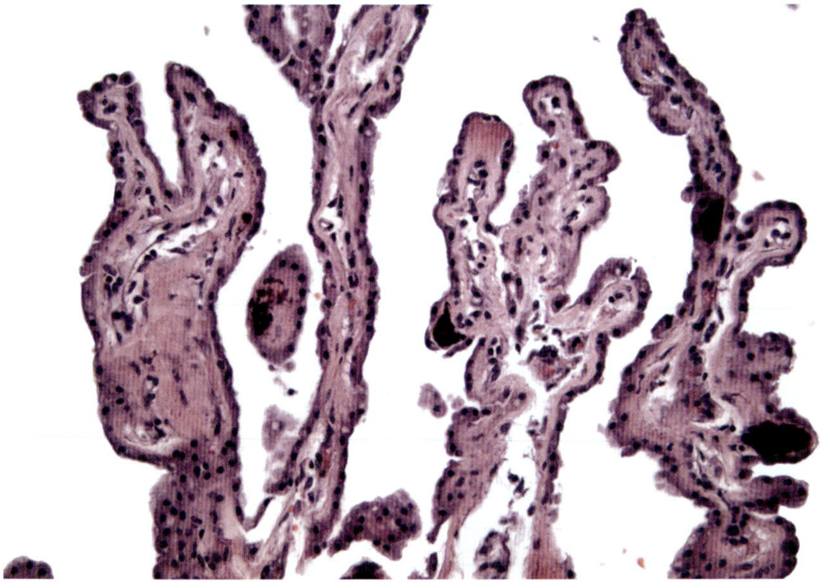

Figure 1-53

CHOROID PLEXUS

Papillary fronds with mineralizations.

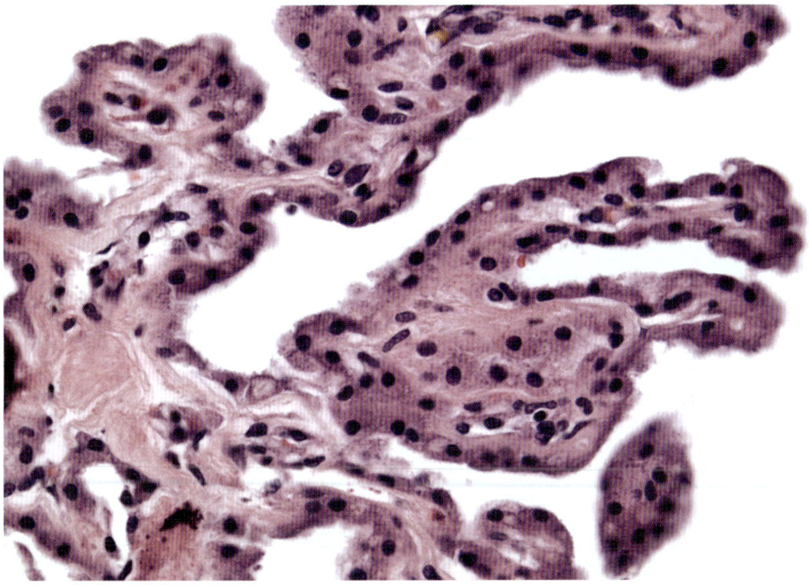

Figure 1-54

CHOROID PLEXUS

Nonoverlapping cuboidal epithelial cells line the papillae.

crossing from one side of the ventricle to the other, which are known as synechia. In most situations, such changes are unrelated to other pathologic processes.

Choroid Plexus

The choroid plexus is the most epithelially differentiated of the glia-derived structures. It is composed of cuboidal cells with round nuclei on fibrovascular stalks (fig. 1-53). The cells often have a rounded apical side, producing a somewhat "hobnail" appearance, and they do not overlap one another (fig. 1-54). Their arrangement on fibrovascular cores forms the typical papillary structure of the choroid plexus. The core of the papillae may contain meningothelial cells as well as irregular calcifications. In older patients, evidence of prior hemorrhage with xanthogranuloma formation is common (see chapter 8).

The choroid plexus is found in most of the lateral ventricles (with the exception of the frontal horns), in the roof of the third ventricle, and in the fourth ventricle where it extends into the foramina, and out the foramina of Luschka into the cerebellopontine angle ("flower basket of Bochdalek"). The presence of choroid plexus can therefore offer localization information that may be of help for both the pathologist in interpreting the findings and for the surgeon intraoperatively.

Normal choroid plexus is commonly encountered and easily recognized in surgical material. With aging and after therapies such as radiation and surgery, the choroid plexus can be hyalinized and calcified, with attenuation and loss of the lining cells. In extreme instances, the tissue just consists of cauterized-appearing fibrovascular stalks with occasional calcifications. The pathologist needs to be aware of this variation in appearance for the correct identification of location and the correct interpretation of the histologic findings from ventricular specimens.

Microglia

Microglia are the resident macrophages of the brain. Like astrocytes, they become prominent in many pathologic processes (see chapter 2). In the normal brain stained with H&E or LHE, microglia are not easily defined. Some have argued that the microglia that become conspicuous during tissue reactions are not endogenous to the brain, but represent recruitment of bone marrow cells at the time of injury.

Vasculature

At the light microscopic level, the vasculature of the CNS is similar to the systemic vasculature. CNS vessels encountered in surgical pathology specimens range from the large arteries at the base of the brain to small arterioles coursing through the subarachnoid space and CNS parenchyma. Included are the venous sinuses of the dura mater, veins and venules in many locations, and the extensive capillaries of the CNS itself. Subarachnoid vessels are commonly included in surgical specimens. When artifactually crushed and cauterized, these vessels cluster together and raise the possibility of a vascular malformation.

The small CNS capillaries are ubiquitous in surgical material, but are fairly inconspicuous on standard H&E-stained sections. In most settings, the capillaries collapse in surgical biopsies; particular prominence of capillary lumens should prompt close examination of vessel walls and for intraluminal material. At an ultrastructural level, CNS capillaries are different from systemic capillaries since they include fenestrated endothelial cells.

REFERENCES

1. Haines DE. Neuroanatomy: an atlas of structures, sections, and systems, 5th ed. Philadephia: Lippincott Williams & Wilkins; 2000.
2. Parent A. Carpenter's human neuroanatomy, 9th ed. Baltimore: Williams & Wilkins; 1996.
3. De Girolami U, Zvaigzne O. Modification of the Achucarro-Hortega pineal stain for paraffin-embedded formalin-fixed tissue. Stain Technol 1973;48:48-50.
4. Scheithauer BW, Woodruff JM, Erlandson RA. Tumors of the peripheral nervous system. AFIP Atlas of Tumor Pathology, 3rd Series, Fascicle 24. Washington, DC: American Registry of Pathology; 1999.
5. Peters A, Palay SL, Webster HD. Fine structure of the nervous system: neurons and their supporting cells, 3rd ed. New York: Oxford University Press; 1991.

2 MICROSCOPIC NEUROPATHOLOGY

The cells of the brain and spinal cord, like those of other organs, react in a stereotypical manner to a broad range of insults. The reactive changes in the cells of the central nervous system (CNS), however, often differ from those in other organs, and the range of changes may be daunting. For example, neurons often respond to pathologic processes by forming cellular inclusions, but the morphologic and molecular nature of the inclusions varies between neuropathologic entities.

This chapter reviews the general neuropathologic changes that the pathologist may encounter when evaluating biopsies from the CNS and adjacent meninges. By far the most common cell to demonstrate pathologic changes is the astrocyte, and many surgical neuropathology specimens feature reactive astrocytes. Unfortunately, although a few reactive astrocytic changes are relatively specific, most are nonspecific. Neurons also show pathologic changes and, in contrast to astrocytes, some of these may be diagnostic of particular conditions. The other elements of the CNS, such as the meninges and the vasculature, have more limited features that overlap with pathologic processes seen in the rest of the body. Inflammatory changes may be primary or secondary to many pathologic conditions in the CNS, and may feature the unique microglial cell. It is important to consider certain general processes, such as edema, which have severe consequences given the "closed" environment created by the blood-brain barrier and the limited intracranial space.

The pathologist must be familiar with the broad range of cellular changes seen in brain biopsies. It is useful to provide an overview of such histopathologic features. These cytologic and microenvironmental processes are discussed in this chapter, as well as in subsequent chapters that address specific conditions.

GLIA

The macroglia, notably the astrocytes, are the most common cells to display reactive changes in surgical biopsy specimens. Indeed, the vast majority of biopsies—whether for tumor, infection, or metabolic condition—have reactive astrocytes if one looks diligently. In common parlance, the terms *gliosis* and *astrocytosis*, defined below, are used interchangeably, with gliosis being the less specific, but more commonly used, phrase.

Astrocytosis

Astrocytosis is defined either as an increase in the number of astrocytes or as a conversion of astrocytes from a "resting" to a "reactive" state. In many cases, the number of astrocytes is within normal limits, but they appear cytologically reactive (see below). In other situations, the number of astrocytes is increased, but never to the degree of hypercellularity that mimics malignant tumors. It is uncommon to note mitotic activity in reactive astrocytes, with the exception of the Creutzfeldt cells that accompany acute demyelinating conditions.

In general, astrocytes respond to injury in a local manner; that is, reactive astrocytes are found within or surrounding a pathologic process. This is helpful in surgical biopsies, particularly during intraoperative consultations. A series of biopsies that progresses from showing unremarkable brain to gliotic brain strongly suggests that the surgeon is getting closer to the site of interest. The exception to this rule is metabolic disease, in which astrocytosis is typically diffuse.

Acute Astrocytosis. Within a day of injury, astrocytes begin to display features of acute reaction. Such changes are marked within a week of injury, and typically persist, depending on the exact nature of the process, for at least a few months before converting to a more chronic appearance. Given that most brain biopsies are performed at least 1 day and often many days after a neurologic process has begun, most biopsies demonstrate acute reactive astrocytes.

Normal astrocytes (see chapter 1) do not have discernible cytoplasm on standard histologic

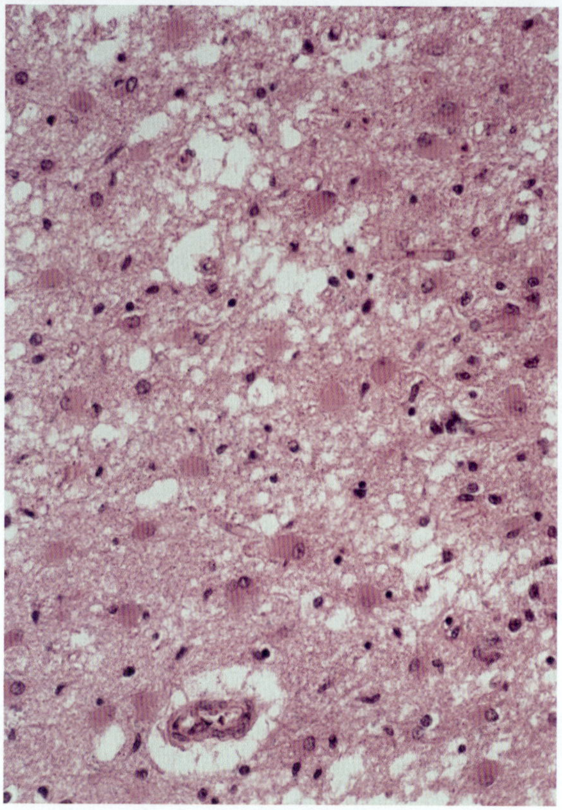

Figure 2-1

REACTIVE ASTROCYTES

Hematoxylin and eosin (H&E) stains reactive astrocytes, which are evenly distributed cells with star-like eosinophilic processes.

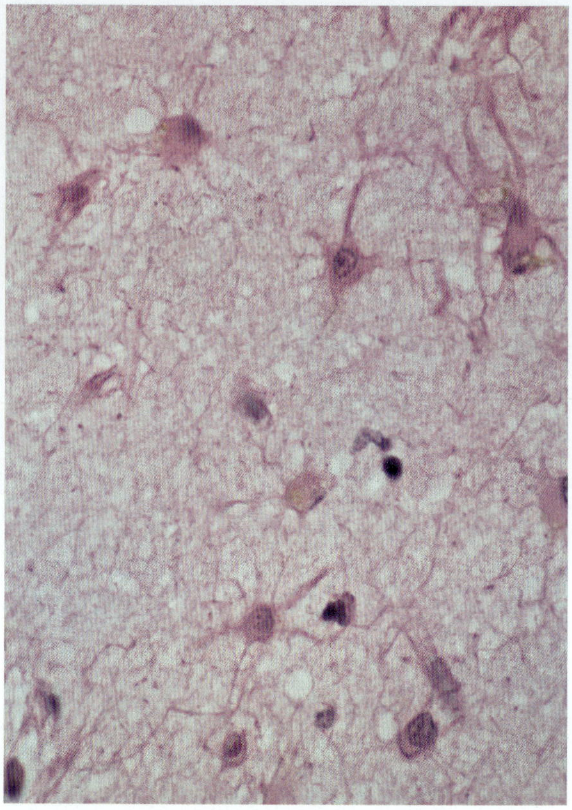

Figure 2-2

REACTIVE ASTROCYTES

The nuclei tend to be rounded, with even nuclear contours, euchromatin, and single prominent nucleoli. The cytoplasm is prominent and has eosinophilic processes.

stains, and have oval nuclei with euchromatic nuclei and inconspicuous nucleoli. Acute reactive changes in astrocytes include prominent expansion of the cytoplasm and cytoplasmic processes that appear eosinophilic with hematoxylin and eosin (H&E) stains and that are strikingly highlighted immunohistochemically with glial fibrillary acidic protein (GFAP) (figs. 2-1–2-9). Immunohistochemistry for vimentin or S-100 protein produces a similar striking picture. With their long processes, astrocytes have a remarkable appearance that exaggerates the normal "star-like" shape of the cells; hence the term astrocyte (figs. 2-1–2-9). In fact, simple visibility of eosinophilic cytoplasm and processes with standard H&E stains can be interpreted as representing astrocytosis in biopsy specimens. The nuclei of reactive astrocytes are larger and rounder that those of normal astrocytes, and often feature single prominent nucleoli (figs. 2-2, 2-3, 2-6, 2-7).

In acute astrocytosis, there is often a relatively even distribution of reactive cells, with the long processes of one cell seeming to respect the territory of the next reactive cell (figs. 2-1–2-7). The cell processes may extend down to a small blood vessel or to the pial surface, but in most cases such attachments are not easily appreciated.

A number of histologic features help to distinguish reactive from neoplastic astrocytic processes. The even distribution of reactive astrocytes can often be appreciated on low-power microscopic evaluation. The open, round nuclei of reactive astrocytes do not resemble the hyperchromatic, irregular nuclei of neoplastic astrocytes. Although some neoplastic astrocytes, such as in gemistocytic astrocytomas, may have

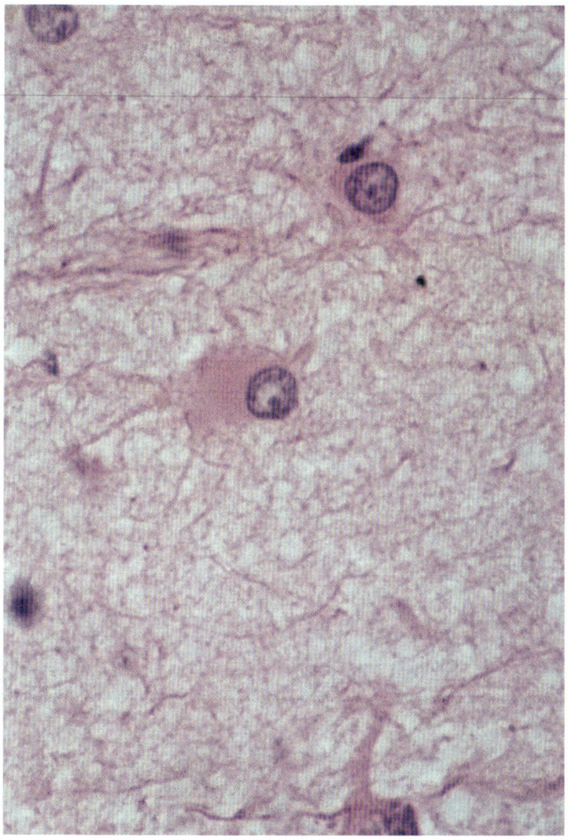

Figure 2-3

REACTIVE ASTROCYTES

Rounded nuclei, single prominent nucleoli, and eosinophilic processes are seen.

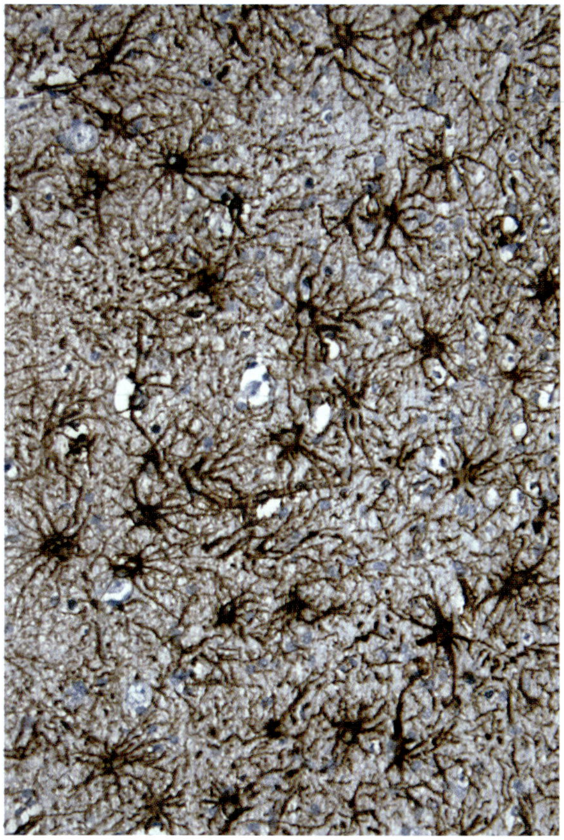

Figure 2-4

REACTIVE ASTROCYTES

Glial fibrillary acidic protein (GFAP) immunohistochemistry highlights the even distribution of reactive astrocytes, as well as their long, stellate processes.

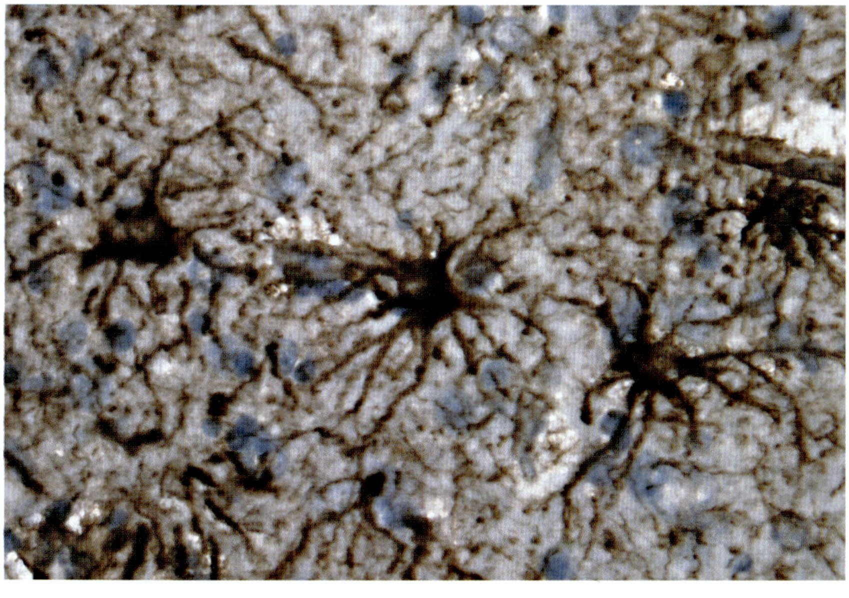

Figure 2-5

REACTIVE ASTROCYTES

High-power microscopy reveals elongated, stellate processes (GFAP immunohistochemistry).

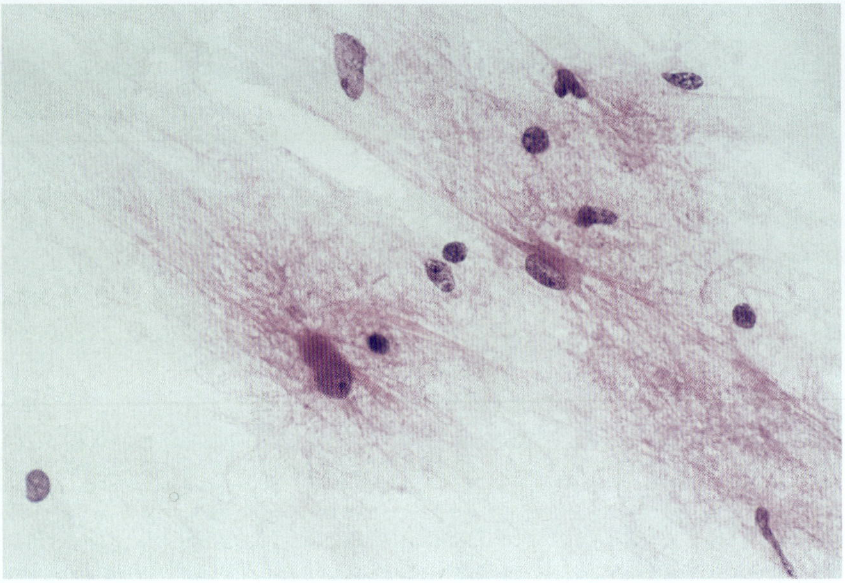

Figure 2-6

REACTIVE ASTROCYTES

The cytologic features of reactive astrocytes are clearly demonstrated on a smear preparation. A single reactive astrocyte appears to "hold together" a patch of neuropil.

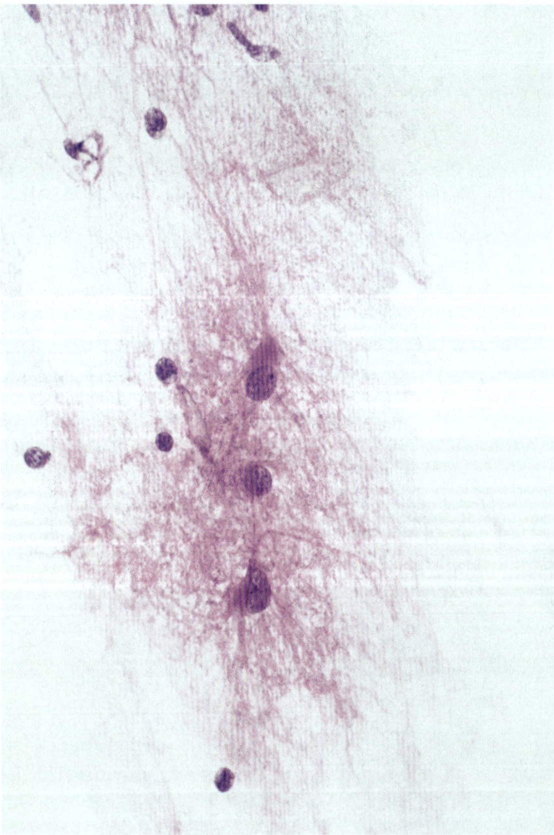

Figure 2-7

REACTIVE ASTROCYTES

Rounded nuclei, single nucleoli, and elongated processes are easily noted on smear preparation.

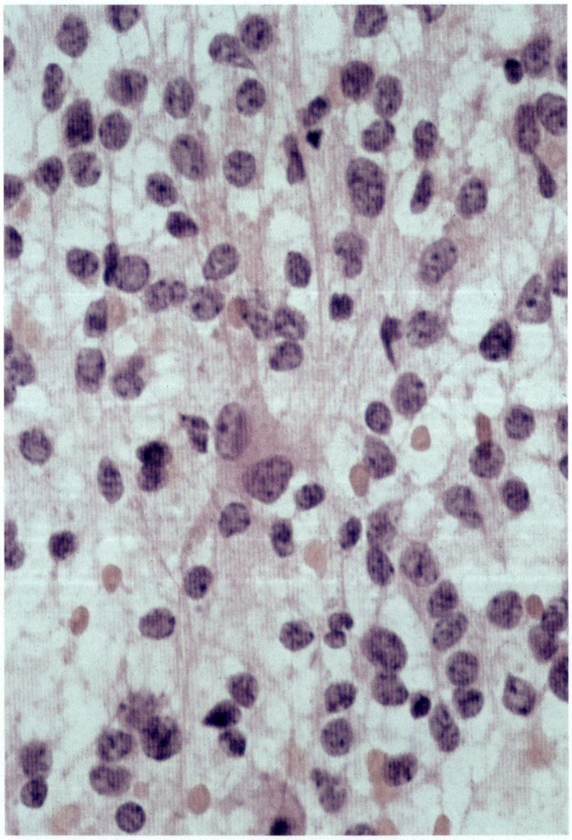

Figure 2-8

REACTIVE ASTROCYTES

On smear preparations of neoplasms such as this oligodendroglioma, reactive astrocytes stand out with their eosinophilic cytoplasm and elongated processes (center).

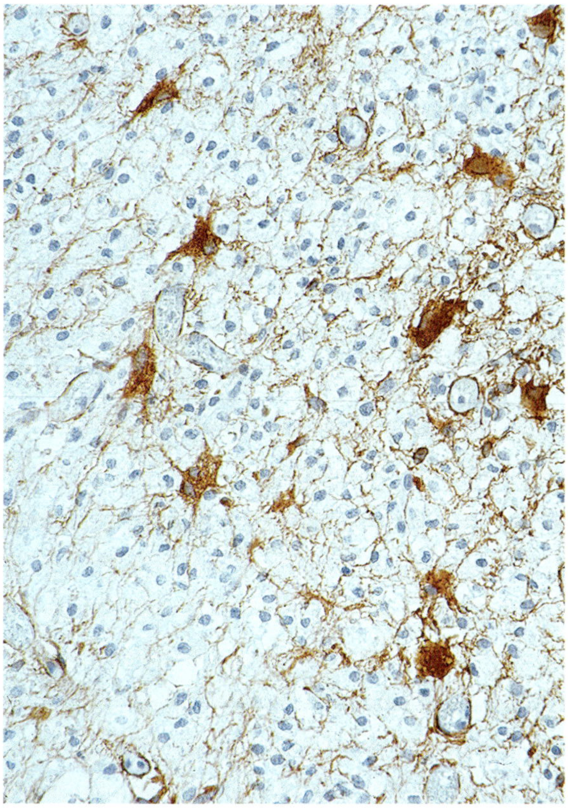

Figure 2-9

REACTIVE ASTROCYTES

Reactive astrocytes in the background of this oligodendroglioma are highlighted by GFAP.

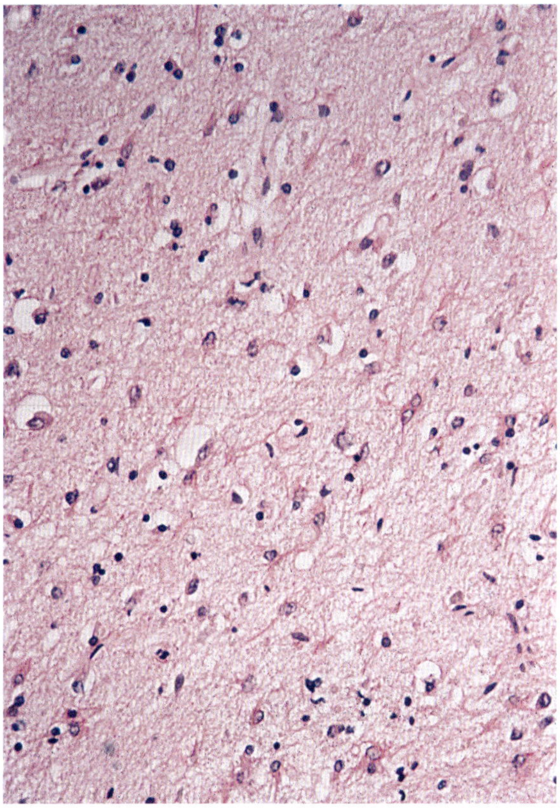

Figure 2-10

REACTIVE ASTROCYTES

Chronic reactive astrocytosis features elongated processes without copious eosinophilic cytoplasm.

copious eosinophilic cytoplasm, these neoplastic cells almost never feature long cytoplasmic processes. Thus, careful attention to the cytologic features, both nuclear and cytoplasmic, is usually sufficient to differentiate reactive and neoplastic astrocytes.

Chronic Astrocytosis. As the lesion ages, the astrocytic reaction changes accordingly. It is difficult to assign an exact time line to such changes but, in general, they occur after a few months. Nonetheless, infarcts sampled at autopsy years or even decades after their formation may have some reactive astrocytes that appear acute in nature. Furthermore, there may be differences in the timing of the transition from acute to chronic gliosis, depending on the nature of the process and the location of the lesion within the CNS.

In most chronic situations, reactive astrocytes eventually lose their copious eosinophilic cytoplasm and begin to emphasize their cellular processes (fig. 2-10). As a result, the gliotic neuropil becomes coarser, as it is filled with long, stout astrocytic processes filled with GFAP. GFAP immunohistochemistry no longer emphasizes the prominent perikarya of these cells, but instead highlights the coarse background. In addition, astrocytic nuclei typically become more elongated in chronic settings.

Longstanding astrocytosis may be accompanied by particular characteristic histologic changes. The presence of these features offers strong evidence that the lesion has been in existence for a long time, often on the order of years. These characteristic features all involve cytoplasmic alterations in the astrocytic processes. The three hallmark changes are Rosenthal fibers, eosinophilic granular bodies, and corpora amylacea.

Rosenthal fibers are brightly eosinophilic, rounded or sausage-shaped structures that are

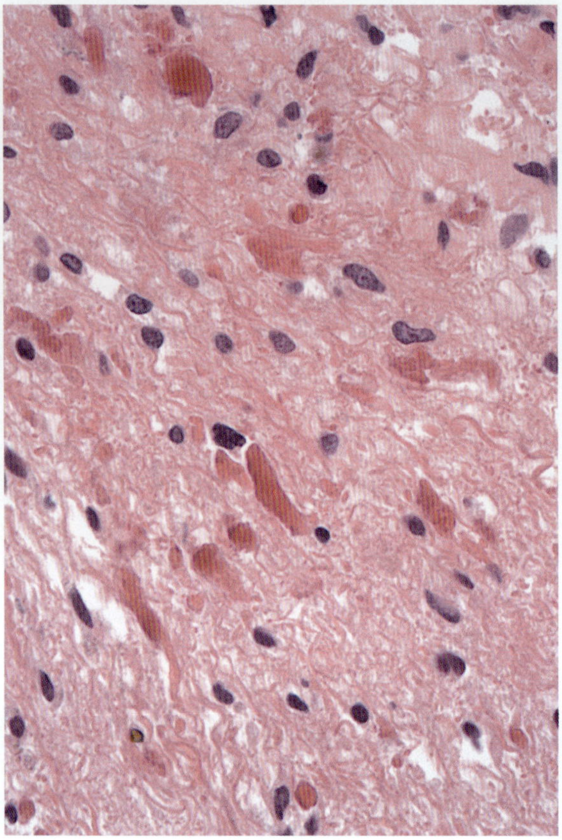

Figure 2-11

REACTIVE ASTROCYTOSIS

Rosenthal fibers are eosinophilic, rounded to elongated structures that are irregularly distributed in areas of chronic gliosis.

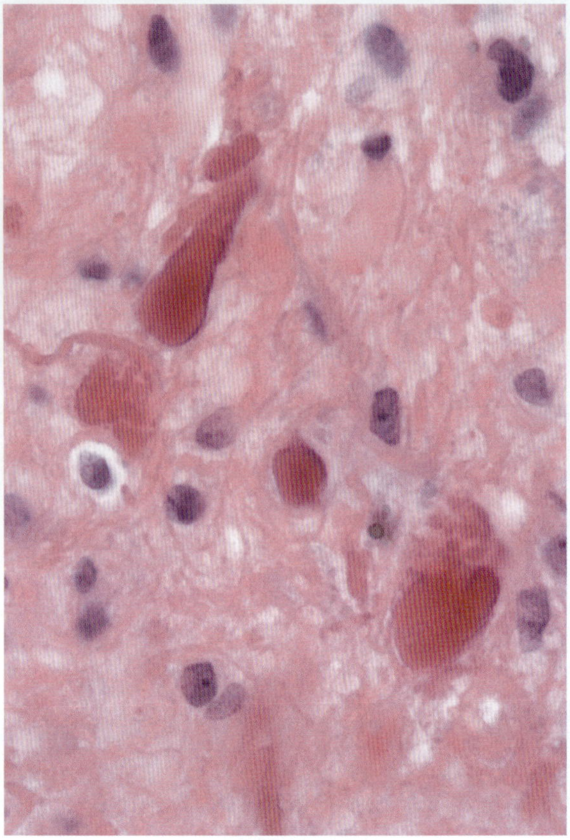

Figure 2-12

REACTIVE ASTROCYTOSIS

High-power microscopy shows the irregular shape and refractile appearance of Rosenthal fibers.

usually no more than a few microns in diameter but that may extend for many microns in length (figs. 2-11, 2-12). Although not apparently related to astrocytes at the light microscopic level, electron microscopy demonstrates their presence in astrocytic processes. Ultrastructurally, they are composed of densely osmiophilic material in which intermediate filaments of GFAP surround the osmiophilic core. Typically, the core does not stain for GFAP although the surrounding filaments do. The core reacts with antibodies to alpha-B-crystallin and ubiquitin.

Rosenthal fibers are most common in long-standing reactive conditions that involve deep-seated structures near the midline, for instance, surrounding the third and fourth ventricles and in the spinal cord. They are often present in the gliotic reaction to slow-growing midline masses, such as craniopharyngiomas, hemangioblastomas, and syringomyelic cavities. Indeed, in these settings, Rosenthal fiber deposition may be massive, exceeding by far the number of Rosenthal fibers found in low-grade glial tumors. This discrepancy in number is useful in differentiating a pilocytic astrocytoma and a glial reaction to another tumor. In addition, Rosenthal fibers can be found in a wide variety of reactive processes as well as in Alexander disease and other rare conditions (see chapters 12 and 13).

Eosinophilic granular bodies (EGBs), also known simply as *granular bodies,* or eponymically as *granular bodies of Zülch*, are anuclear collections of small particles that are also found in chronic gliosis (fig. 2-13). EGBs range from the size of a macrophage to almost 100 µm in diameter; individual granules vary in size, but are typically just a few microns in width. The

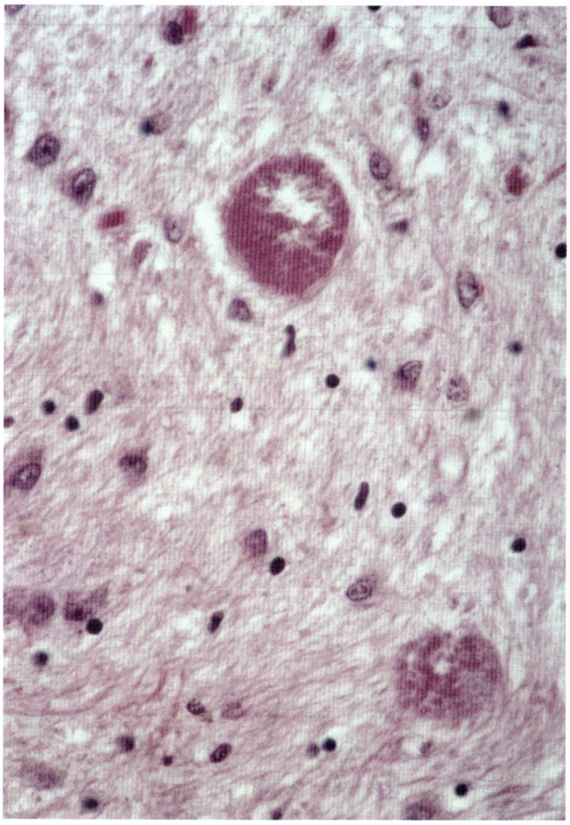

Figure 2-13

REACTIVE ASTROCYTOSIS

Eosinophilic granular bodies accompany chronic gliosis as globular aggregates of light pink to dark red granular material.

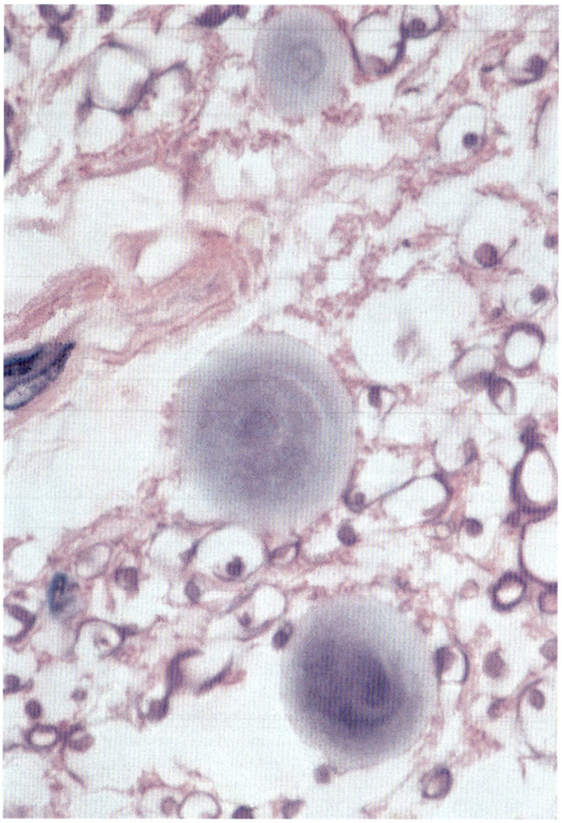

Figure 2-14

REACTIVE ASTROCYTOSIS

Corpora amylacea are basophilic, concentric structures found in regions of chronic gliosis, including in the normal subpial region.

granules are always eosinophilic, but range from pale to bright with the H&E stain. EGBs are usually not strongly positive for GFAP, but are immunopositive for nonspecific markers such as alpha-1-antichymotrypsin. Like Rosenthal material, EGBs are not obviously related to astrocytes on light microscopic examination, but appear to represent dilatations of astrocytic processes on electron microscopy. The granules correspond to stuffed lysosomal structures. Again, as with Rosenthal fibers, EGBs bespeak chronicity and may be found in reactive as well as low-grade neoplastic processes. EGBs, for example, are common in pilocytic astrocytomas and pleomorphic xanthoastrocytomas. Unlike Rosenthal fibers, however, their occurrence is not known to be more frequent in particular regions of the brain.

Corpora amylacea are refractile, basophilic, round, anuclear masses that stain strongly with periodic acid–Schiff (PAS) or other stains that recognize carbohydrates (figs. 2-14, 2-15). They are histologically identical to the polyglucosan bodies and Lafora bodies found in specific metabolic diseases (see chapter 12). Corpora amylacea are composed of complex carbohydrate moieties. As with Rosenthal fibers and EGBs, they are not obviously of astrocytic origin on standard light microscopy, but can be demonstrated to be expanding astrocytic processes on electron microscopy. Corpora amylacea are particularly common in reactive conditions that affect the pial surface of the brain and spinal cord as well as the periventricular regions. In most older individuals, perhaps as a result of a chronic reaction to molecules in the cerebrospinal fluid, there are collections of corpora amylacea in the subpial regions of the brain and spinal cord and surrounding the ventricles.

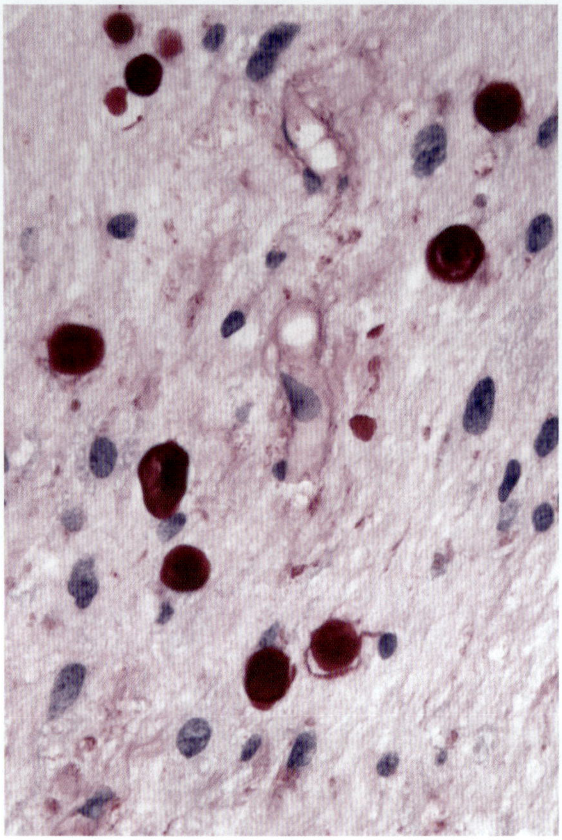

Figure 2-15

REACTIVE ASTROCYTOSIS

Corpora amylacea are strongly positive with the periodic acid–Schiff (PAS) stain.

A particular pattern of astrocytosis is found in the Purkinje cell layer of the cerebellum. In response to the loss of cerebellar neurons, particularly in association with the loss of Purkinje cells, there is a proliferation of Bergmann cells, the glia that are native to the Purkinje cell layer. This reaction is known as *Bergmann gliosis* (fig. 2-16).

Astrocytic Reaction in Specific Conditions. The astrocytic reaction to most conditions is stereotypical, but astrocytes in some diseases have specific histopathologic features. Although each feature is rare, each is highly suggestive of a particular disease or set of diseases. Since some of these conditions are occasionally biopsied, recognition of such astrocytic changes is of importance to the surgical pathologist.

Alzheimer type II astrocytes are found in many types of metabolic encephalopathy and are most prominent in longstanding *hepatic encephalopathy*, regardless of the cause of the hepatic failure. They are not related to Alzheimer disease, except in their being also named after Alois Alzheimer. Alzheimer type II cells are reactive astrocytes that are different than the standard reactive astrocytes discussed above. Alzheimer type II astrocytes have irregular, sometimes lobated, extremely euchromatic nuclei; the nucleus has a "washed out" appearance; and abundant glycogen is noted on electron microscopy (figs. 2-17, 2-18). In addition, these cells have no discernible cytoplasm

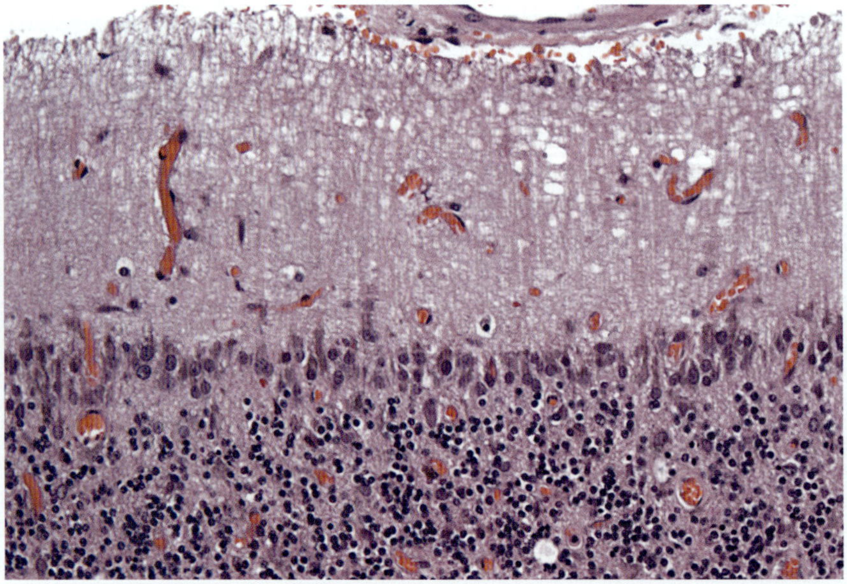

Figure 2-16

REACTIVE ASTROCYTES

Bergmann gliosis is characterized by a proliferation of astrocytes in the Purkinje cell layer, typically with loss of Purkinje cells. (Also see fig. 5-9.)

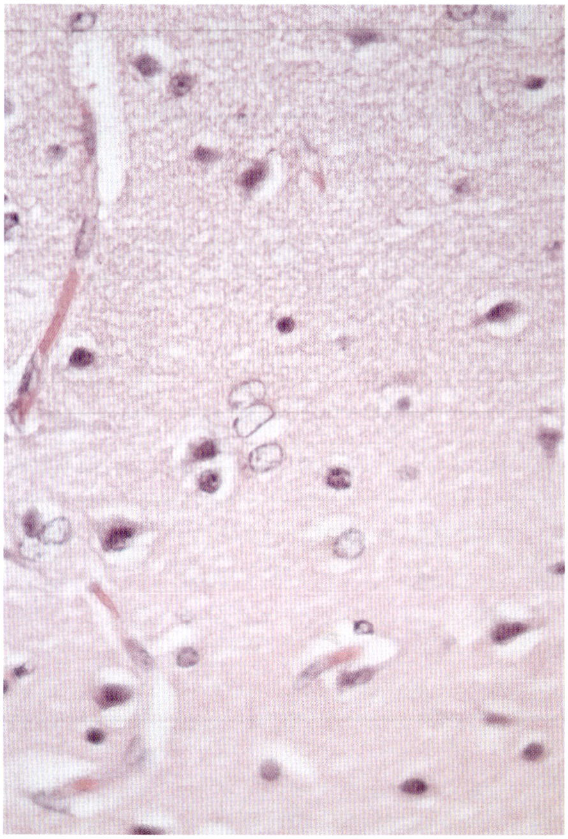

Figure 2-17

REACTIVE ASTROCYTES

Alzheimer type II astrocytes are characterized by watery nuclei having irregular contours and no discernible cytoplasm.

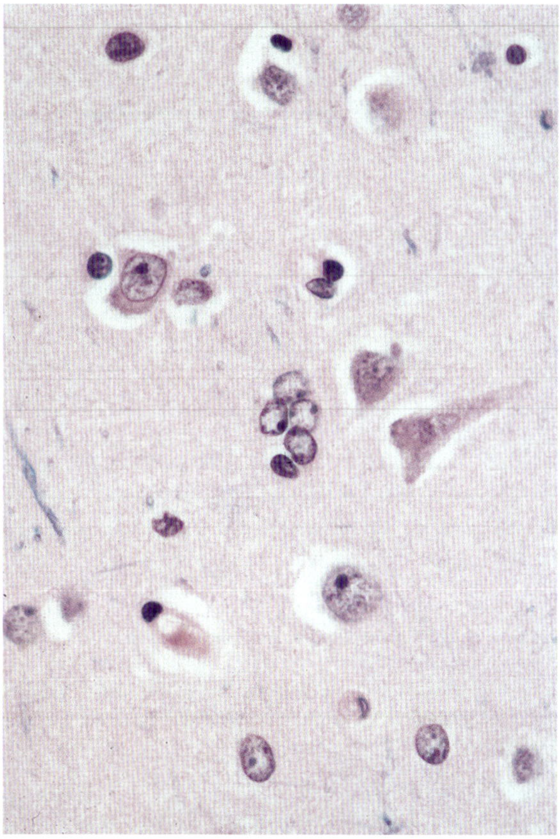

Figure 2-18

REACTIVE ASTROCYTES

Alzheimer type II astrocytes are often clustered in 2-, 3-, and 4-cell groups (Luxol fast blue-H&E stain).

and accordingly do not stain for GFAP or S-100 protein. Alzheimer type II cells are most numerous in the gray matter of the cerebral cortex and basal ganglia, and are often found as clusters of nuclei in pairs, triplets, or even quadruplets.

In *progressive multifocal leukoencephalopathy* (PML; see chapter 7), which is caused by infection of glia with the JC virus, astrocytes may become markedly enlarged, with bizarre and sometimes hyperchromatic nuclei and visible cytoplasm (fig. 2-19). So pleomorphic are the nuclei that they suggest malignant glioma. These cells are usually found in the brain parenchyma adjacent to demyelinated foci. The correct diagnosis can be surmised if such cells are found in the setting of a multifocal white matter disease in an immunocompromised patient. The diagnosis of PML is established with certainty if the characteristic enlarged, basophilic oligodendrocytes are also found and if the virus can be demonstrated with either immunohistochemistry or electron microscopy. Fortunately, the bizarre astrocytes often are found in the same regions as the pathognomonic oligodendrocytes.

Similar enlarged, cytologically bizarre cells may be found in the setting of prior *radiation therapy*. Within weeks of radiation, astrocytes enlarge, acquiring large, irregular nuclei and copious cytoplasm (see chapter 14), in a manner similar to radiation-exposed cells in other areas of the body. Given that radiation therapy is often used for malignant gliomas, the presence of these cells can create diagnostic confusion with recurrent glioma. Indeed, most neurosurgical specimens that have histologic features of

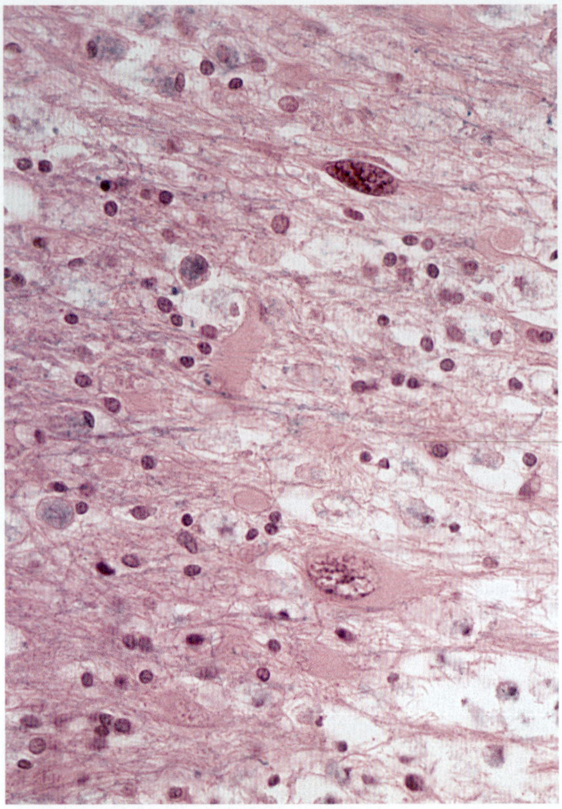

Figure 2-19

REACTIVE ASTROCYTES

In progressive multifocal leukoencephalopathy, large astrocytes may have a neoplastic appearance (Luxol fast blue-H&E stain).

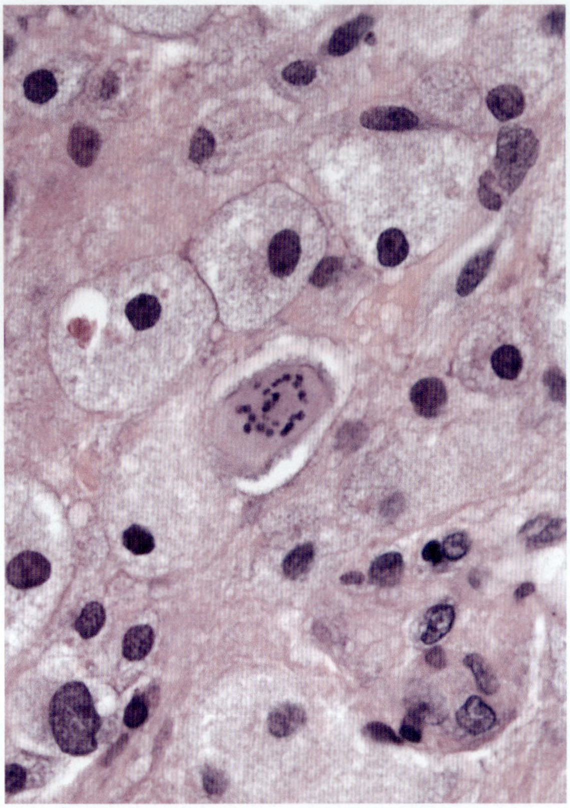

Figure 2-20

REACTIVE ASTROCYTES

In acute demyelinating conditions, astrocytes with "exploded" nuclei (Creutzfeldt cells) are characteristic. Note the numerous macrophages.

radiation are sampled to determine whether the clinical process is recurrent malignant glioma or radiation necrosis, and radiated reactive-appearing astrocytes may well coexist with malignant astrocytic cells. This differential diagnosis is discussed at greater length in chapter 14.

Creutzfeldt cells are curious-looking astrocytes that are almost pathognomonic of *acute demyelinating diseases*. They are cells with eosinophilic, astrocytic-appearing cytoplasm and an "exploded" nucleus that either resembles scattered chromosomes or multiple micronuclei (fig. 2-20). Such cells label immunohistochemically with GFAP, confirming their astrocytic nature, and sometimes with MIB-1, suggesting that they are, in fact, actively dividing cells. Creutzfeldt cells must not be misinterpreted as neoplastic; indeed, they can be one of the many histologic miscues that result in the incorrect diagnosis of glioma in the setting of acute demyelination (see chapter 9). It is unclear why these cells form in the setting of acute demyelinating conditions.

In *neurofibromatosis 2* (NF2), *astrocytic hamartomas* are often found in the cerebral cortex and other gray matter structures (see chapter 13). These hamartomas are irregular clusters of astrocytes that have enlarged, somewhat irregular, often euchromatic nuclei and visible cytoplasm with processes (figs. 2-21, 2-22).

In *tuberous sclerosis,* the cortical tubers are composed of diverse cells, including large neurons, astrocytes, and cells with intermediate features (fig. 2-23; see chapter 13). The astrocytes are often large, with extensive cytoplasm and irregular, usually euchromatic nuclei. Similarly atypical, large astrocytes are found in sporadic *focal cortical dysplasia* (see chapter 13). The lesions of tuberous sclerosis and focal cortical

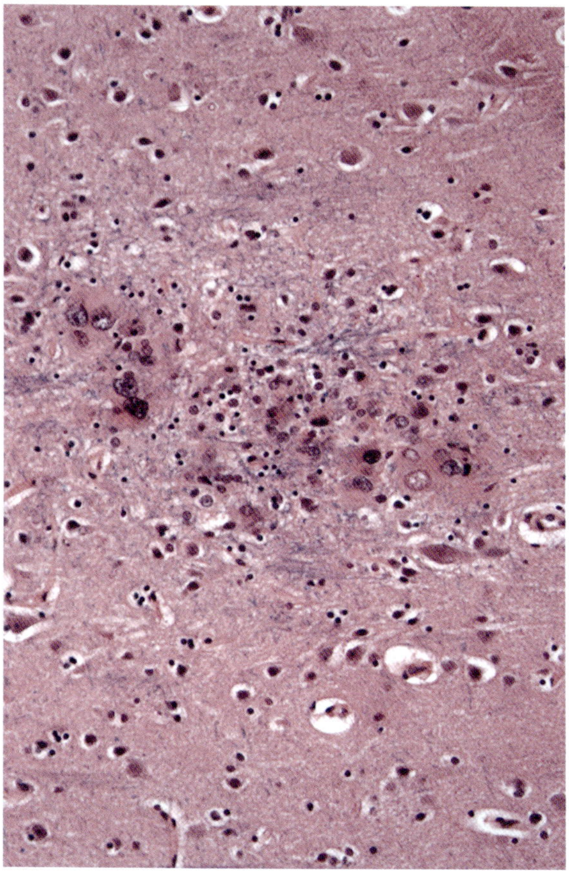

Figure 2-21

MALFORMATIVE GLIA

In neurofibromatosis 2, clusters of irregular glial cells are scattered in the cerebral cortex.

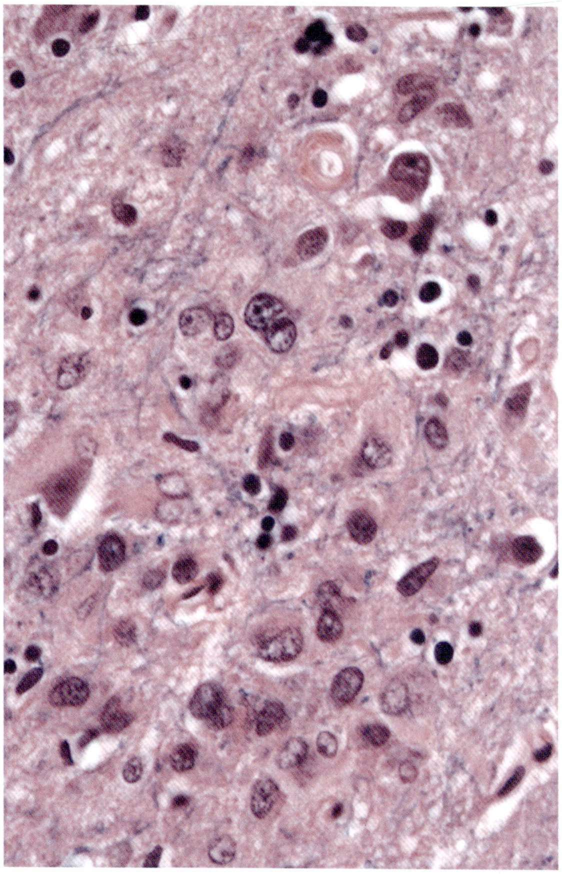

Figure 2-22

MALFORMATIVE GLIA

In neurofibromatosis 2, glial cells often have irregular, euchromatic nuclei and eosinophilic cytoplasm.

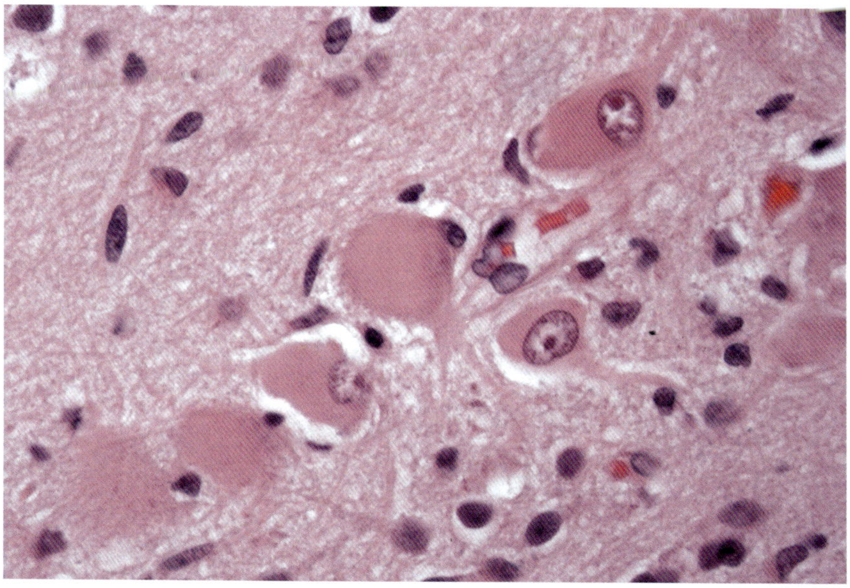

Figure 2-23

MALFORMATIVE GLIA

In tuberous sclerosis, large cells that have the cytologic features of both glia and neurons populate the cortex.

Table 2-1

DIAGNOSTICALLY USEFUL CELLULAR INCLUSIONS IN THE CENTRAL NERVOUS SYSTEM

Cell Type	Category	Inclusion	Disease	Neuroanatomic Predilection	Cellular Location	Hematoxylin & Eosin Appearance	Content	Chapter
Neuron	Neurodegenerative	NFT[a]	AD, aging	Cerebral cortex	C[b]	Flame or globose	Tau, ubiquitin	10
		Neuritic plaques	AD, aging	Cerebral cortex	C (dp)[c]	Eosinophilic, irregular	Tau	10
		Pick bodies	Pick disease	Temporal lobe	C	Eosinophilic	Tau, ubiquitin, neurofilament	10
		Lewy bodies	PD, DLBD	Pigmented neurons, cerebral cortex	C	Eosinophilic with halo	Ubiquitin, alpha-synuclein	10
		Hirano bodies	AD, aging, Pick disease	Hippocampus, CA1	C,E	Eosinophilic, elongated	Actin	10
		GVD	AD, aging, Pick disease	Hippocampus, CA1	C	Granule in vacuole	Tau	10
		Skeins	ALS	Upper and lower motor neurons	C	Eosinophilic	Ubiquitin	10
		Hyaline inclusions	ALS	Upper and lower motor neurons	C	Pale	Ubiquitin	10
		Ubiquitin inclusions	ALS with dementia	Cerebral cortex, hippocampus	C	Eosinophilic	Ubiquitin	10
		Bunina bodies	ALS	Spinal motor neurons	C	Eosinophilic	Cystatin-C	10
		"Intranuclear inclusions"	HD	Cerebral cortex > caudate	N	(requires immunohistochemistry)	Ubiquitin, huntingtin	10
		Eosinophilic thalamic inclusions	Myotonic dystrophy	Thalamus	C	Eosinophilic		
		Rod-like cytoplasmic inclusions	Myotonic dystrophy	Caudate	C	Eosinophilic		
	Viral	Cowdry type A	HSVE, CMVE, SSPE		N	Eosinophilic with halo	HSV, CV, measles	7
		Negri bodies	Rabies	Cerebellar Purkinje cells, brain stem	C	Eosinophilic, multiple	Rabies virus	7
		Other viral inclusions			N	Smudged nucleus	Viral particles	7
	Prion	Membrane-bound vacuole	Prion diseases, e.g., CJD	Cerebral cortex	C	Vacuoles		10
	Metabolic	Lafora bodies	Lafora body disease	Many regions	C	Basophilic	Polyglucosan	12
		Storage disorders	See chapter 12		C	Vacuoles	See chapter 12	12
	Normal	Marinesco body	Normal	Substantia nigra	N	Eosinophilic	Nuclear filaments	
		Eosinophilic thalamic inclusions	Normal	Thalamus	C	Eosinophilic		
		Rod-like cytoplasmic inclusions	Normal	Caudate	C	Eosinophilic		
		Hirano bodies	Normal aging	Hippocampus, CA1	C,E	Eosinophilic	Actin	10
		GVD	Normal aging	Hippocampus, CA1	C	Granule in vacuole	Tau	10

[a]NFT = neurofibrillary tangle; AD = Alzheimer disease; PD = Parkinson disease; DLBD = diffuse Lewy body disease; GVD = granulovacuolar degeneration; ALS = amyotrophic lateral sclerosis; HD = Huntington disease; HSVE = herpes simplex encephalitis; CMVE = cytomegalovirus encephalitis; SSPE = subacute sclerosing panencephalitis; CJD = Creutzfeldt-Jacob disease; PSP = progressive supranuclear palsy; CBD = cortical basal ganglionic degeneration; PML = progressive multifocal leukoencephalopathy; CMV = cytomegalovirus; H&E = hematoxylin and eosin.

[b]Cellular location: C = cytoplasmic; E = extracellular; N = nuclear.

[c]dp = distal process.

Table 2-1, continued

Cell Type	Category	Inclusion	Disease/ Neuroanatomic Predilection	Cellular Location	Hematoxylin & Eosin Appearance	Content	Chapter
Astrocyte	Reactive	Rosenthal fibers	Gliosis, glial tumors, Alexander disease/periventricular	C	Eosinophilic, pleomorphic	GFAP, alpha B-crystallin, ubiquitin	2
		Eosinophilic granular	Gliosis, glial tumors	C	Eosinophilic, granular	Alpha-antichymotrypsin	
		Corpora amylacea	Gliosis/periventricular, subpial	C	Basophilic, round	Polyglucosans	1,2
	Neurode-generative	Glial cytoplasmic	Multiple system atrophy/white matter	C	Eosinophlic	Tau	10
		Glial fibrillary tangles	PSP, Pick disease, CBD	C		Tau	10
		Astrocytic plaques	CBD	C[c]		Tau	10
		Tufted astrocytes	PSP, Pick disease	C		Tau	10
		Coils and threads	PSP, CBD			Tau	10
Oligoden-drocyte	Neurode-generative	Glial cytoplasmic	Multiple system atrophy	C, wm[c]	Eosinophilic	Tau	10
		Interfascicular threads	PSP, CBD	C, wm		Tau	10
	Viral	Inclusion	PML	N, wm	Basophilic	JC virus	7
Epend.[c] Cell	Viral	Cowdry type A	CMV	N	Eosinophilic with halo	CMV	
Endothe-lial Cell	Metabolic	Lysomal storage material	Fabry disease	C			12
	Viral		Zoster	N			

[c]dp = distal process; wm = white matter.
[d]Epend. = Ependymal.

dysplasia come to neurosurgical attention for seizure control, and are therefore frequently encountered in hospitals specializing in epilepsy surgery. The cortical lesions of NF2 are only rarely encountered, since removal of cortical tissues is not often necessary in the management of NF2-associated neoplasms.

In the rare metabolic condition, *Wilson disease*, characteristic astrocytes are found, predominantly in the degenerated lenticular nucleus. These large *Opalski cells* are characterized by large, irregular nuclei and copious cytoplasm. They stain immunohistochemically for GFAP and S-100 protein. These cells should not come to neurosurgical attention unless patients with Wilson disease are being biopsied for other reasons.

Other Glial Cells

Other glial cells participate in pathologic processes in characteristic ways. These are far more restricted than the common and general participation of astrocytes, but their typical features once again require familiarity by the pathologist.

Oligodendrocytes are less versatile than astrocytes in their responses to pathologic conditions. In the setting of ischemia and edema, oligodendrocytes may acquire discernible cytoplasm, often eccentrically placed and amphophilic in nature. Ischemic changes may also manifest as hyperchromatic, shrunken nuclei (see chapter 5). Oligodendrocytes are not known to proliferate in response to injury, but are increased in oligodendrocytes seen adjacent to vascular malformations and possibly surrounding demyelinating lesions. Oligodendrocytes may also accumulate material to form inclusions. This is most striking in multiple system atrophies in which small, sometimes flame-shaped, argyrophilic inclusions eccentrically expand oligodendrocyte cell bodies (Table 2-1; see chapter 10), and in progressive multifocal leukoencephalopathy in which virus-laden oligodendrocyte nuclei are enlarged, "glassy," and basophilic (Table 2-1, fig. 2-24; see chapter 7).

Ependymal cells have a limited set of responses to injury. When damaged, the ependymal surface becomes denuded, and subependymal astrocytes proliferate to form small protuberances, so-called *granular ependymitis*. In normal development and aging, ependymal cells surrounding the lateral ventricles, particularly near the inferior reaches of the frontal horns, may form

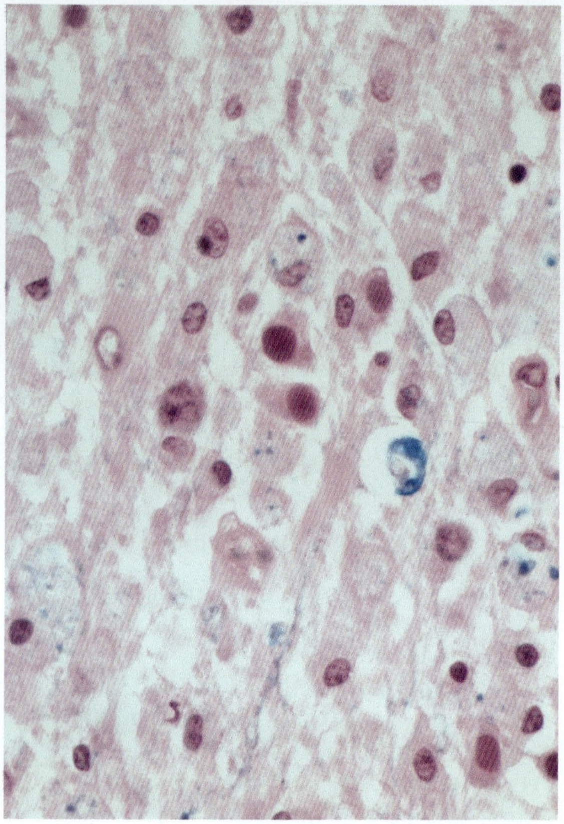

Figure 2-24

OLIGODENDROCYTE INCLUSIONS

In progressive multifocal leukoencephalopathy, oligodendrocytes are enlarged and basophilic, with "glassy" nuclei (Luxol fast blue-H&E stain).

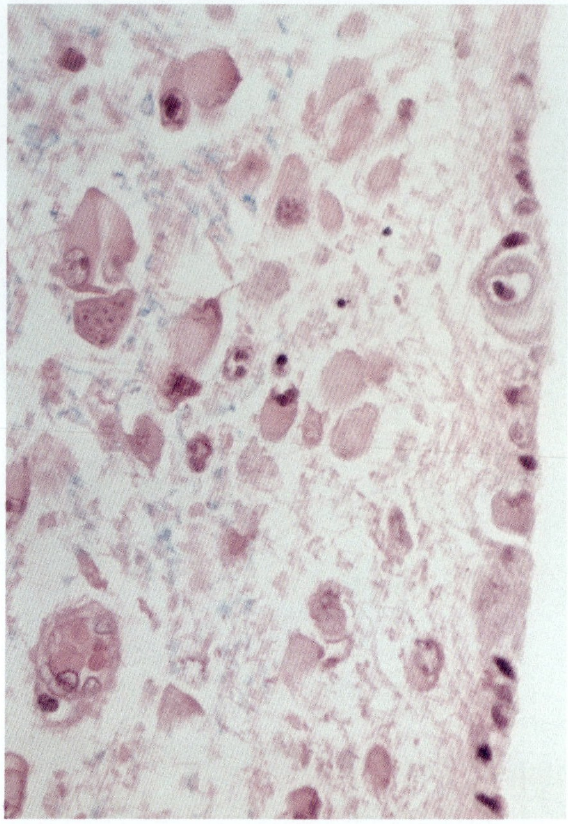

Figure 2-25

EPENDYMAL INCLUSIONS

Cytomegalovirus infection enlarges ependymal cells, as well as subependymal cells, with large Cowdry type A inclusions in the cells (Luxol fast blue-H&E stain).

buried ependymal nests that sometimes have small central cavities (see chapter 1). In adults, the central canal of the spinal cord is typically collapsed, with an irregular, disorganized nest of ependymal cells marking its location. Both types of ependymal nests can be present in surgical biopsy specimens. Ependymal cells may be a major site of cytomegalovirus infection; the cells are markedly enlarged and have prominent Cowdry type A intranuclear inclusions (fig. 2-25).

The *choroid plexus* reacts in limited ways. In response to chronic injury, for instance, radiation or irritation from adjacent neoplasms, the choroid plexus epithelium can become denuded and the vascular core can become hyalinized. Calcifications may be present as well. As a result, the traumatized choroid plexus may appear as a vaguely papillary structure composed of fibrous, vascular structures. Xanthomatous changes are also common, as is seen with normal aging, leading in extreme examples to frank xanthogranulomas (see chapter 14).

NEURONS

Neurons are highly sensitive to many types of injury, with the common endpoint being cell death. Neuronal dropout is a cardinal feature of many neuropathologic processes, and is often attended by reactive astrocytosis. Neuronal gigantism may be found in focal cortical dysplasia (fig. 2-26; see chapter 13). In the setting of chronic insult, shy of cell death, neurons have a broad range of intracellular responses, with many involving the formation of inclusions (figs. 2-27, 2-28). Certain neuronal responses to pathologic processes are virtually pathognomonic of a particular disease and are therefore of importance to the surgical pathologist (Table 2-1).

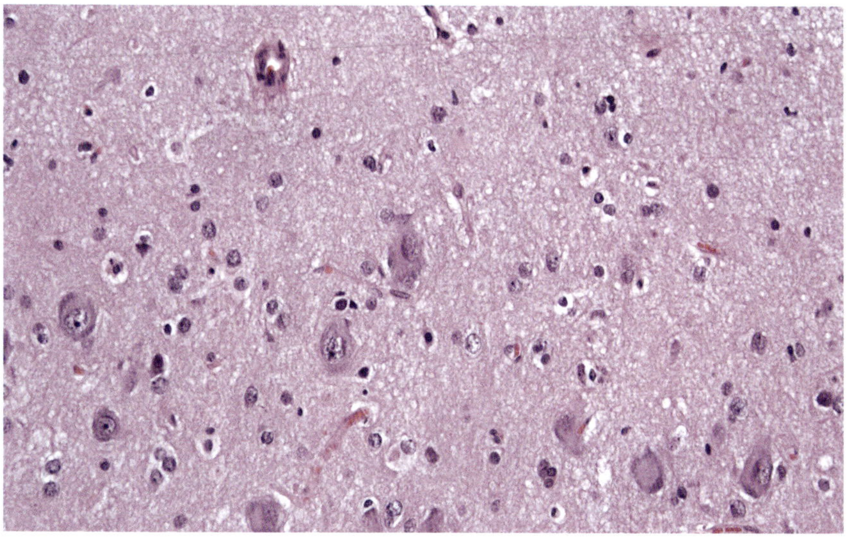

Figure 2-26

NEURONAL GIGANTISM

Giant, morphologically normal neurons are present high in layer 2 of the frontal cortex in a case of focal cortical dysplasia.

Hypoxia/Ischemia

The most common neuronal injury detected in neurosurgical biopsy specimens is hypoxic-ischemic change. Neurons respond to hypoxic-ischemic insults in a characteristic manner: nuclei become dark and angular, and the cytoplasm becomes eosinophilic (fig. 2-29). Such cells are variably referred to as having undergone "red neuron," or Spielmeyer, change. As discussed in chapter 5, hypoxic-ischemic damage includes a number of other histologic features that enable proper diagnosis. These other changes are important to consider, since neurons may acquire dark nuclei ("dark neurons") simply as a result of surgical manipulation (fig. 2-30); such artifactual changes, however, are not associated with reddened cytoplasm or with other histologic findings of hypoxic-ischemic damage.

Mineralization

Neurons may undergo mineralization or ferrugination, most commonly in the setting of hypoxic-ischemic change in infants. The residual neurons appear darkly basophilic and often fractured on H&E-stained sections (fig. 2-31).

Spongiform Change

Vacuolar change surrounding neurons, in which the neuropil "pulls away" from the neurons, is a common artifact, particularly after ischemic injury to the cerebral cortex. Vacuolar change in the neuropil as a result of extensive astrocytosis, so-called status spongiosus, is nonspecific. True *spongiform change*, however, is a specific alteration that raises the strong consideration of spongiform encephalopathies such as Creutzfeldt-Jakob disease (see chapter 10). True spongiform change is characterized by intraneuronal vacuoles; at the ultrastructural level, the cytoplasmic vacuoles are membrane bound and filled with clear material or slightly granular debris. On light microscopic examination, the vacuoles are rounded and vary in size substantially, most ranging from 3 to 20 µm in diameter. In contrast to artifactual vacuoles, not all true spongiform vacuoles extend through the thickness of the tissue section. Although many of the vacuoles are found in the surrounding neuropil, those immediately adjacent to neuronal cell bodies often indent the perikaryon, an uncommon feature in artifactual vacuoles.

Chromatolysis

In response to transection of its axon or to specific degenerative and metabolic insults (e.g., pellagra and corticobasal ganglionic degeneration), neurons undergo a process known as *chromatolysis*. The term derives from the loss of the "colored" Nissl substance (rough endoplasmic reticulum). Neurons show a rounding of the usually triangular cell body, accompanied by a washing out of the cytoplasm, with the Nissl substance becoming either inapparent or marginalized to the edge of the perikaryon (fig. 2-32). Chromatolysis is more often encountered in autopsy specimens than in biopsies.

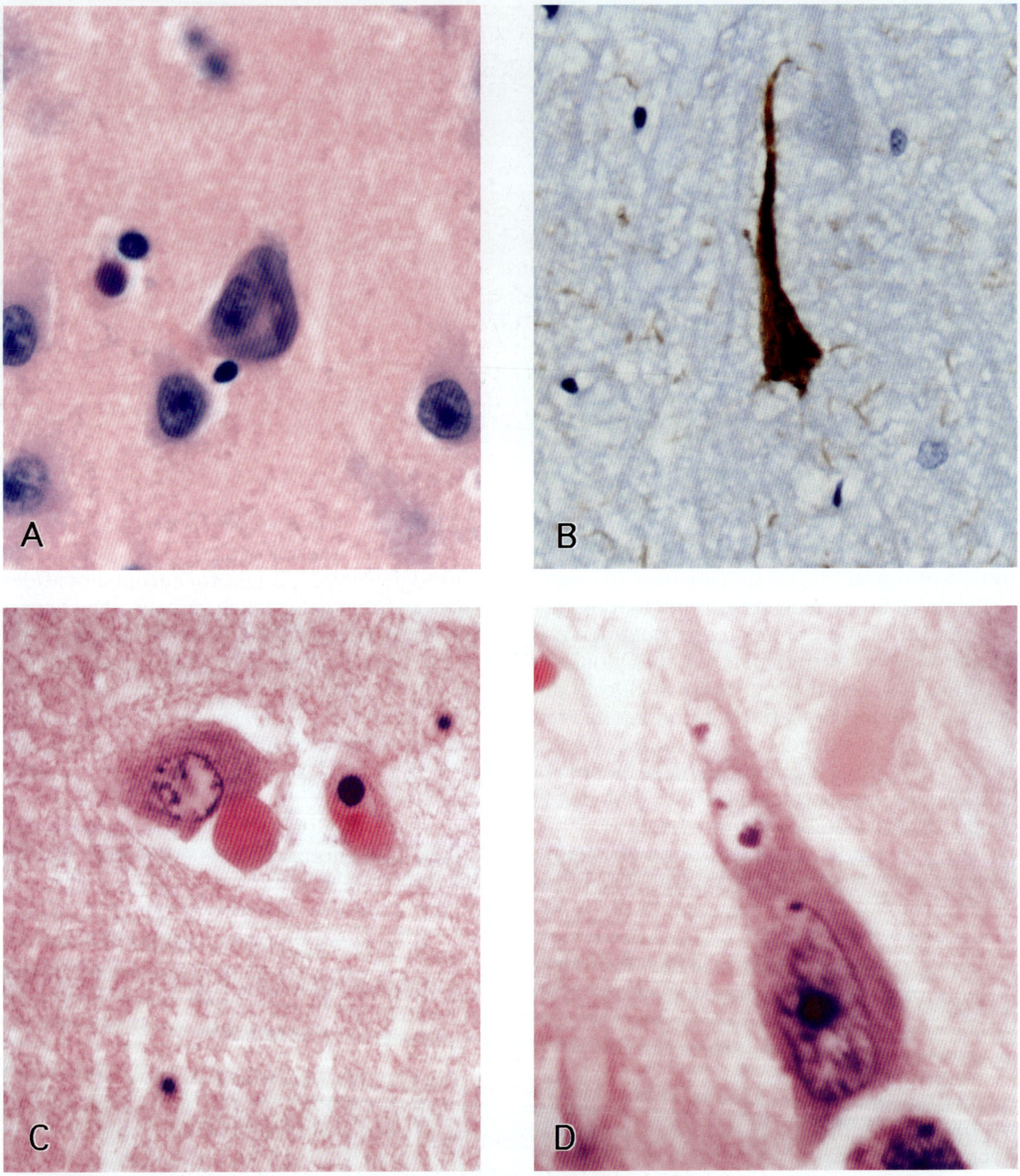

Figure 2-27

NEURONAL INCLUSIONS

Inclusions are common alterations in neurons, particularly in neurodegenerative diseases.

A: A neurofibrillary tangle, characteristic but not diagnostic of Alzheimer disease, is noted in this cortical neuron, but can be difficult to see with standard H&E stains.

B: Neurofibrillary tangles stain strongly for tau protein on immunohistochemistry.

C: Hirano bodies are brightly eosinophilic inclusions of different sizes and shapes that often appear "extracellular" on light microscopy; they are found in the hippocampus in Alzheimer disease and in aging.

D: Granulovacuolar degeneration is common in pyramidal hippocampal neurons in Alzheimer disease and aging.

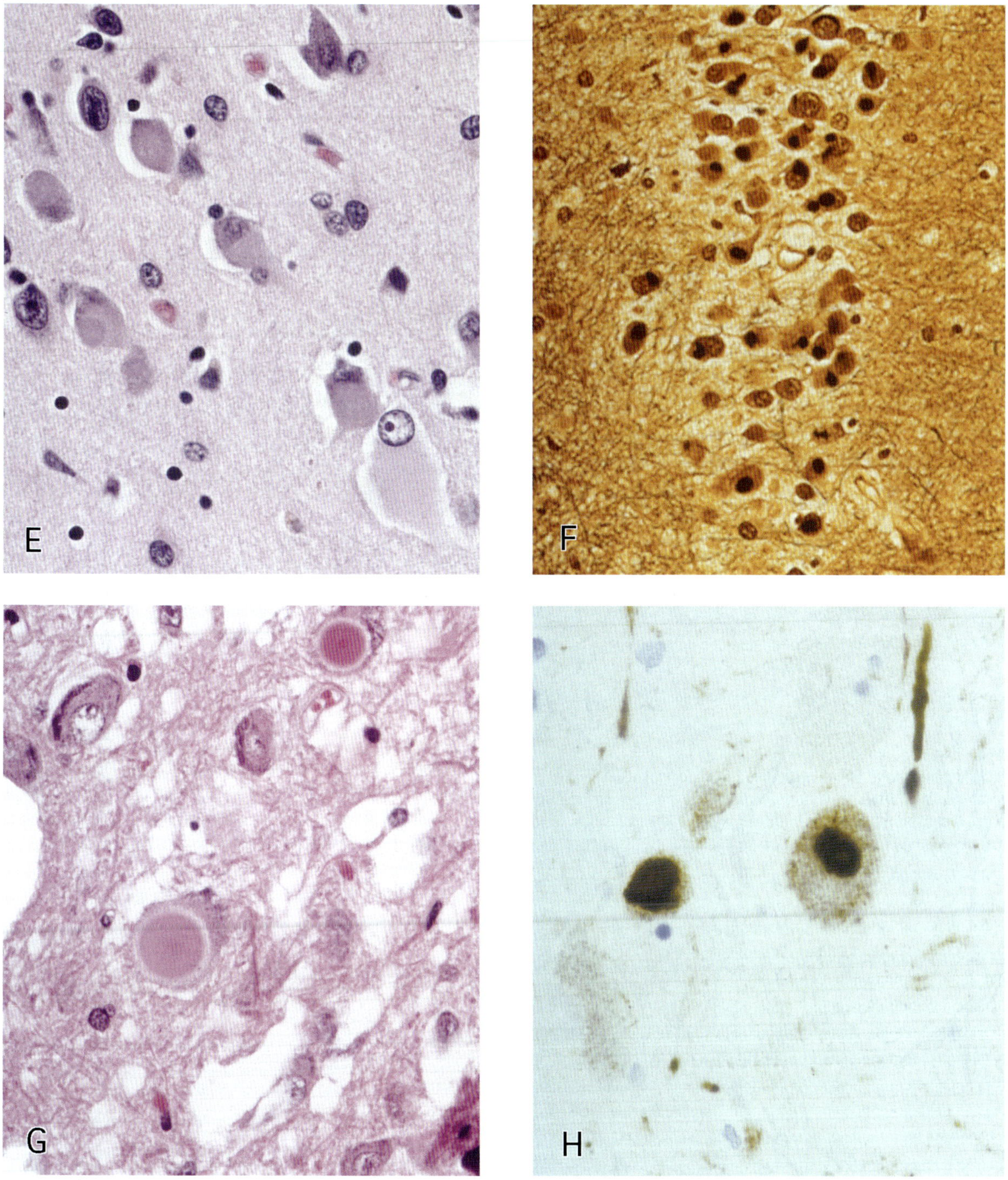

Figure 2-27 (continued)

E: Pick bodies (center and upper left) are rounded eosinophilic cytoplasmic inclusions that are often associated with achromasic neurons (lower right) in Pick disease.

F: Pick bodies are highlighted with Bielschowsky silver impregnations; note black inclusions in small neurons of the hippocampal dentate gyrus.

G: Cortical Lewy bodies either appear as classic Lewy bodies, with a round eosinophilic cytoplasmic inclusion surrounded by a clear halo, or as smaller, irregular cytoplasmic inclusions without halos.

H: Lewy bodies stain strongly on alpha-synuclein immunohistochemistry.

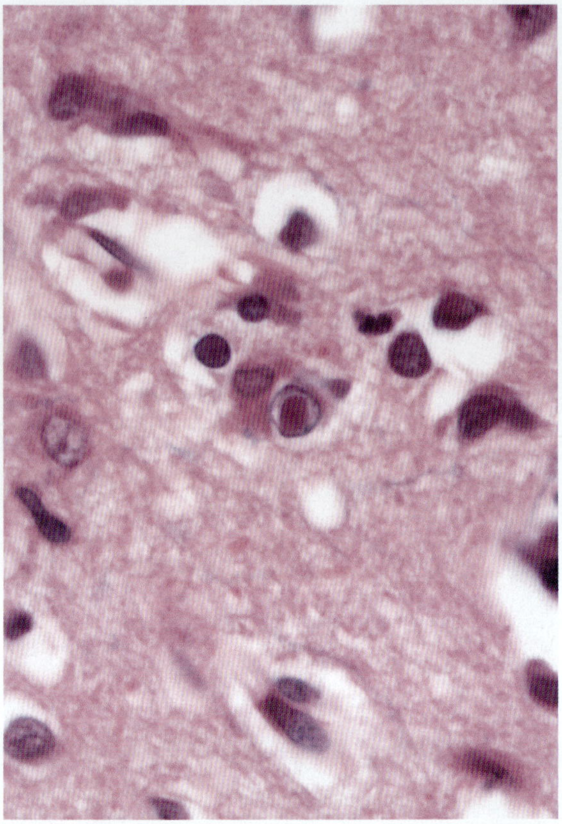

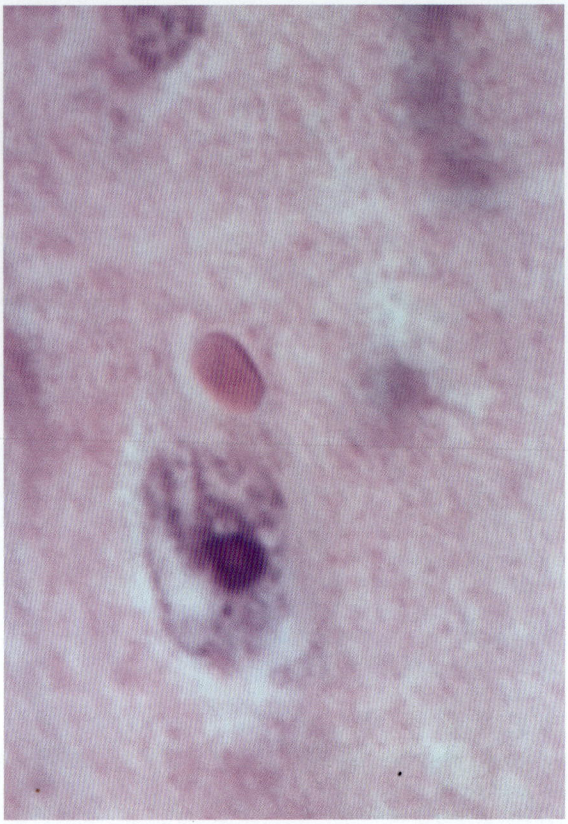

Figure 2-28

NEURONAL INCLUSIONS

Neuronal inclusions are common alterations in infectious diseases.

Left: A Cowdry type A inclusion in a case of subacute sclerosing panencephalitis is a large, round, eosinophilic nuclear inclusion with a perinuclear halo. Similar inclusions are found in herpes encephalitis and cytomegalovirus infection.

Right: A Negri body in a patient with rabies is an irregular, eosinophilic cytoplasmic inclusion.

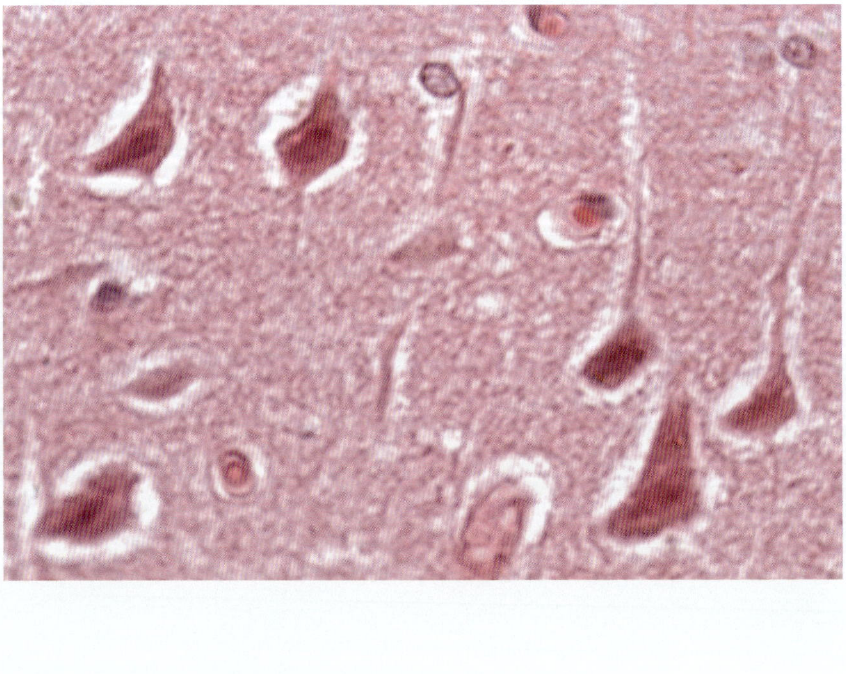

Figure 2-29

NEURONAL ISCHEMIA

Ischemic neurons, as in this example from the cerebral cortex, have an eosinophilic hue to their cytoplasm, with shrunken, darkened nuclei; this is usually referred to as "red neuron" change.

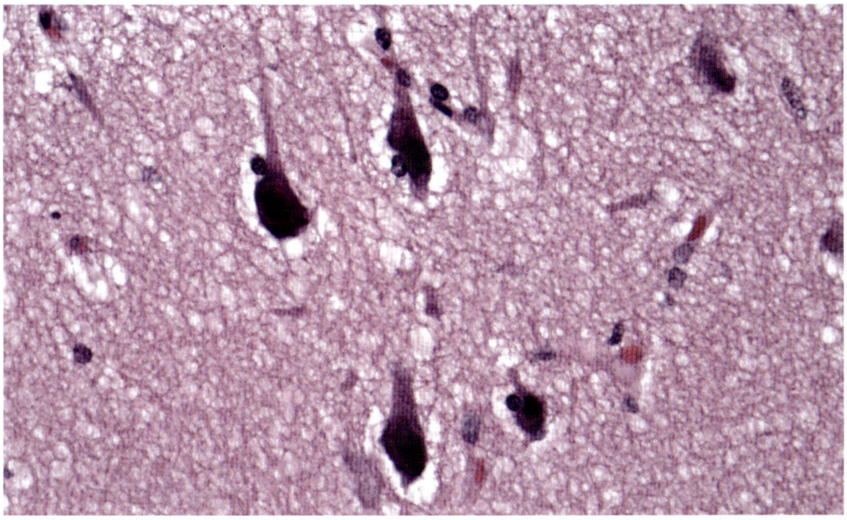

Figure 2-30

NEURONAL SURGICAL ARTIFACT

An artifact of surgical manipulation is a "dark neuron" change, in which nuclei are dark, but the cytoplasm appears normal and no other changes are found in the tissue to suggest ischemic damage.

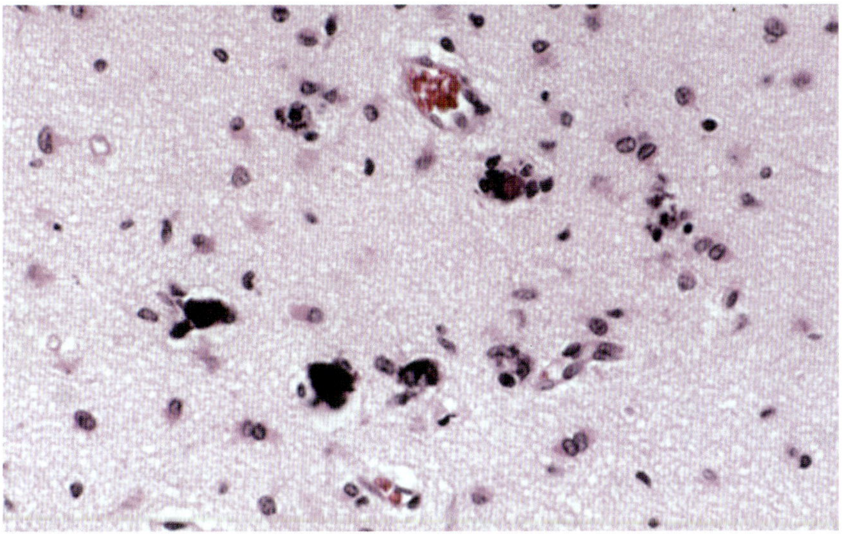

Figure 2-31

NEURONAL MINERALIZATION

After ischemic injury, neurons may become mineralized.

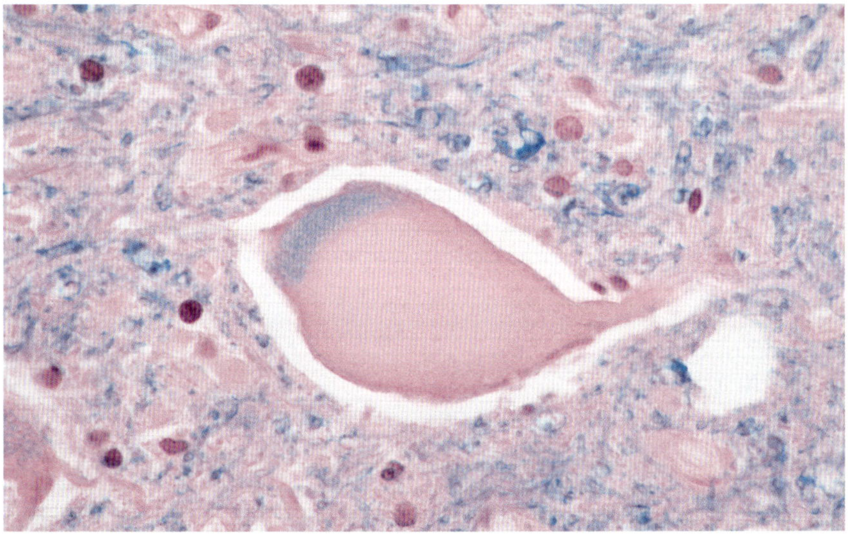

Figure 2-32

NEURONAL CHROMATOLYSIS

Chromatolysis represents a stereotypical response to axonal damage, with clearing of Nissl substance to the periphery of the perikaryon (Luxol fast blue-H&E stain).

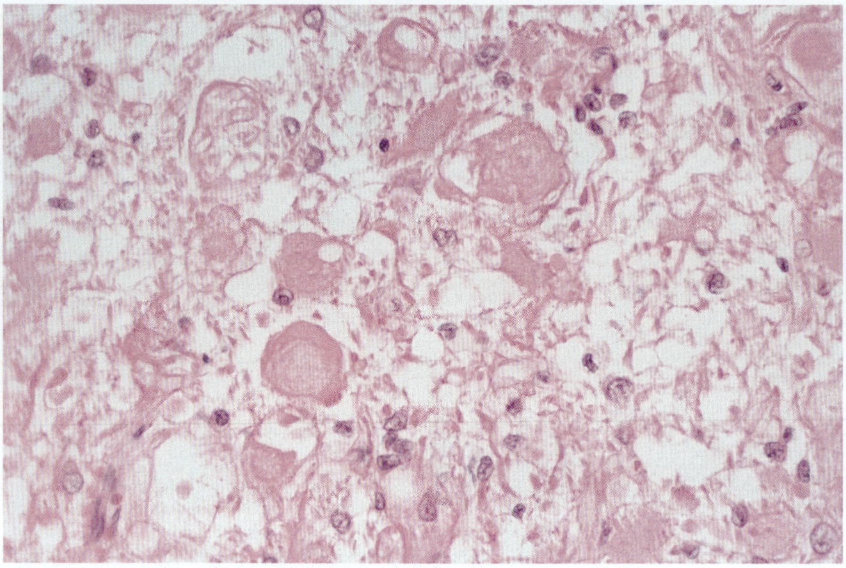

Figure 2-33

NEURONAL SPHEROIDS

Spheroidal expansion of axons occurs following axonal transection or other forms of axonal disruption.

Axonal Spheroids

Transection of an axon or a specific toxic, metabolic, or degenerative injury to an axon (e.g., chemotherapy/radiation therapy effect, vitamin E deficiency) can result in the dilatation of axons into globose spheroids (*axonal spheroids*). Such spheroids are eosinophilic on H&E-stained specimens and can be highlighted with silver impregnations and immunohistochemistry for neurofilaments (figs. 2-33–2-35). Electron microscopy demonstrates that most spheroids are disorganized collections of axonal contents, sometimes with lysosomal structures as well. In the cerebellum, spheroids forming in the major Purkinje cell efferents, typically detected within the internal granular cell layer, are known as "torpedoes."

Axonal spheroids generally form proximal to axonal transections within days of injury. In surgical neuropathology specimens, they are most commonly encountered at the edge of acute infarcts; the infarct destroys the axons, leading to spheroid formation in the viable adjacent neuropil.

Wallerian Degeneration

After neuronal death or axonal transection, axons degenerate distal to the injury in a process known as *Wallerian degeneration*. The axonal degeneration is attended by myelin breakdown, foamy macrophages that clear the cellular debris, and astrocytes that react to the process. Wallerian degeneration begins fairly soon after injury, but takes weeks to months to reach full effect. Wallerian degeneration is not often detected in surgical neuropathology specimens, but can be found in resection specimens, including tissue surrounding a chronic process. For example, resections of arteriovenous malformations or of longstanding cerebellar tumors that include some underlying white matter may reveal degenerating white matter that reflects Wallerian change.

Central Neuroma

Attempted regenerative growth of axons, with resulting traumatic neuroma formation, is common in the peripheral nervous system, but has not been clearly documented in the CNS. A curious, rare phenomenon is the presence of *central neuromas* in the central tegmental tract of the brain stem. These irregular tangles of axons, which resemble small traumatic neuromas, are found only in the central tegmental tract caudal to small destructive lesions such as infarcts. Because of their location in a structure that is not amenable to biopsy, central neuromas have not been noted in surgical pathology specimens.

Neuronophagia and Other Signs of Neuronal Loss

In some processes, neuronal death is attended by small macrophage groups surrounding and presumably ingesting neuronal cell remnants. This process is known as *neuronophagia*. In some

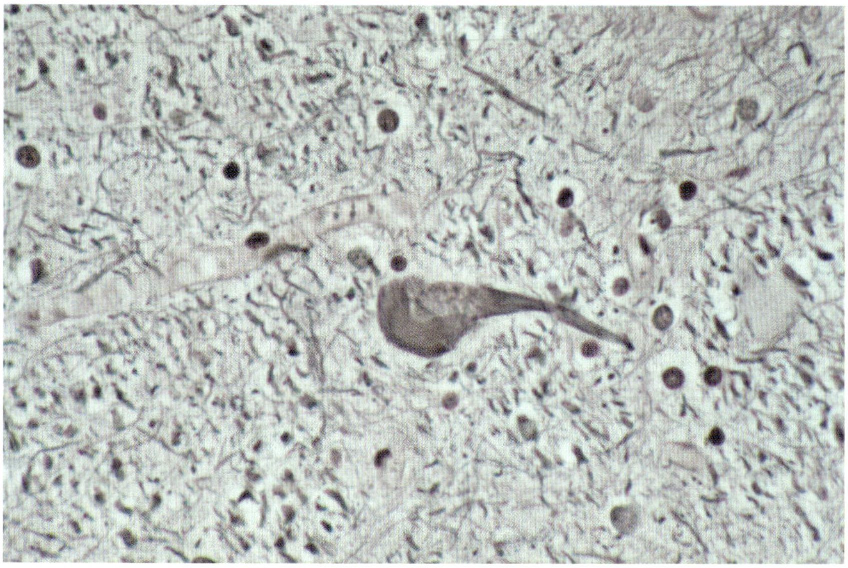

Figure 2-34

NEURONAL SPHEROID

Bodian silver impregnation highlights the relationship of the spheroidal dilation to the remaining axon.

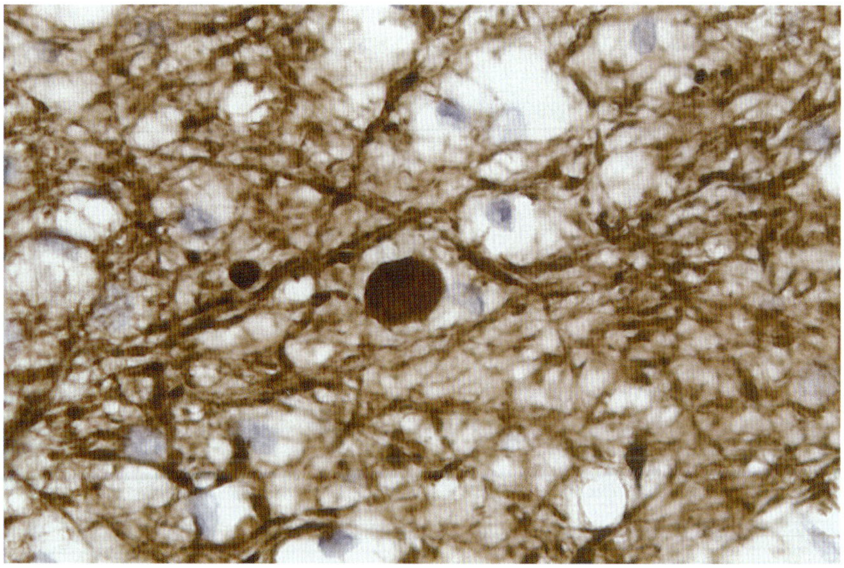

Figure 2-35

NEURONAL SPHEROID

Neurofilament immunohistochemistry most clearly demonstrates spheroids.

situations, only macrophages are present, providing a "tombstone" to mark what has most likely transpired. Neuronophagia and residual tombstone macrophages may be seen in infectious and inflammatory processes (e.g., poliomyelitis) and in degenerative conditions (e.g., residual pigmented macrophages in the setting of nigral degeneration). Neuronophagia is only rarely found in surgical specimens, most often in the setting of viral infection. A parallel situation is found in the dorsal root ganglia, in which neuronal loss is accompanied by exaggeration of the surrounding satellite cells, forming a so-called *nodule of Nageotte*.

Aging and Pigment

Many neurons acquire *lipofuscin* in their cytoplasm with aging. Lipofuscin is particularly common in sites that are only rarely or essentially never neurosurgically sampled, such as the cerebellar dentate nucleus and the inferior olivary nucleus, but accumulates to easily detectable levels in the cerebral cortex as well. As a result, lipofuscin is often noted in biopsies that include the cerebral cortex. H&E stains lipofuscin a greenish brown color (see chapter 1, fig. 1-46); this is often dark blue with a Luxol fast blue stain. On toluidine blue–stained frozen

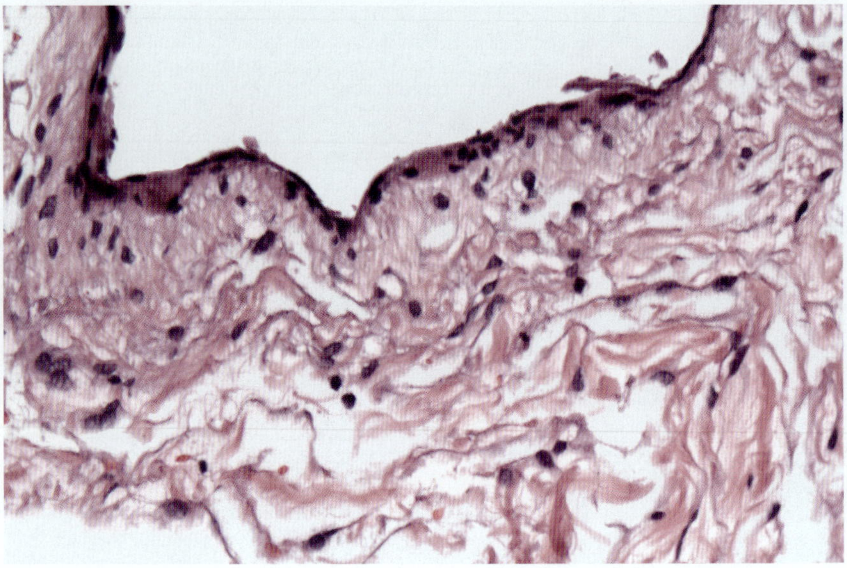

Figure 2-36

ARACHNOIDAL FIBROSIS

Arachnoidal fibrosis is a common accompaniment of aging. Fibrosis is also a reaction to local injury.

sections, its refractile nature can help identify neurons. Ultrastructurally, lipofuscin consists of membrane-bound material with a mixed dense osmiophilic and lipid appearance.

Neuromelanin is a derivative of catecholamine metabolism. It is found in certain pigmented nuclei, most notably the substantia nigra, locus ceruleus, and dorsal motor nucleus of the vagus nerve (see chapter 1, figs. 1-44, 1-45). Neuromelanin is usually not detectable microscopically until the latter half of the first decade of life. In elderly adults, neuromelanin can be found in macrophages if there is loss of the pigmented cells. Since these structures are rarely if ever biopsied, neuromelanin is not encountered in surgical specimens.

Inclusions and Storage Material

Inclusions and storage of particular materials are the most colorful and potentially the most specific of neuronal reactions. They occur in a wide variety of conditions, from infectious to toxic to degenerative. *Neuronal inclusions* occur in both the cytoplasm and the nucleus. Some are readily visible with standard H&E stains, others only with specific immunohistochemical stains, and some only with electron microscopy. None of the neuronal inclusions is commonly encountered in surgical material, but their presence is often of great diagnostic importance. These inclusions are illustrated in figures 2-27 and 2-28 and listed in Table 2-1; they are discussed in individual chapters.

MENINGES

The dura mater responds to injury in a manner that is similar to that of other densely collagenous structures in the rest of the body. Chronic processes affecting the dura may result in collagenous thickening, which can be noted on neuroimaging studies. Neoplastic and inflammatory/infectious diseases are the most common conditions that result in surgical sampling of the dura mater. In many institutions, samples of the cerebral cortex and leptomeninges for possible vasculitis or other inflammatory conditions often include dura mater. Of particular importance to surgical pathologists is involvement of the dura mater by metastatic breast cancer, hematopoietic conditions (including lymphoma), and a variety of granulomatous processes (including rheumatoid arthritis) that preferentially target the dura.

The arachnoid also typically responds to injury by collagen deposition (fig. 2-36). The normally thin arachnoid can thicken, and extensive collagen can expand the subarachnoid space. At autopsy, arachnoidal thickening can be found locally after relatively minor insults. Identical changes occur with normal aging, primarily over the cerebral convexities, near the midline. Caution must be exercised, therefore, when attributing arachnoidal fibrosis to particular pathologic causes in surgical material.

The arachnoid also responds to injury with proliferation of the arachnoidal cells. In some

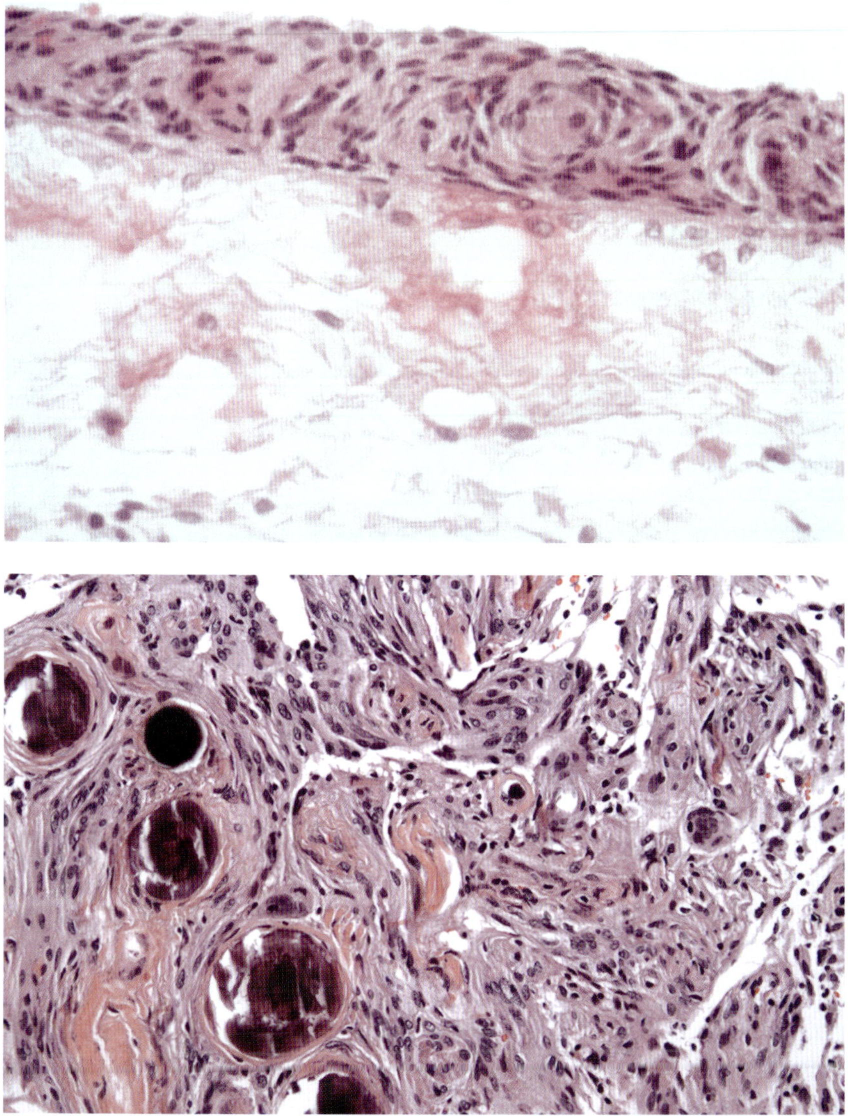

Figure 2-37

ARACHNOIDAL HYPERPLASIA

Top: Arachnoidal hyperplasia is the exuberant proliferation of arachnoidal cells in response to a local lesion, typically a neoplasm.

Bottom: Small biopsies may mimic meningiomas, and include psammoma bodies, as in this example found adjacent to a metastasis.

instances, this can lead to impressive *arachnoidal hyperplasia* (fig. 2-37). Such foci are histologically indistinguishable from small meningothelial meningiomas, and can lead to diagnostic confusion on biopsies. Arachnoidal hyperplasia may mislead the pathologist in two locations: surrounding the optic nerve and in the sellar region, in both situations because of underlying tumors. Superficial biopsies in these locations may result in an erroneous diagnosis of meningioma, rather than optic glioma or a sellar neoplasm. Careful correlation with neuroimaging findings helps to avoid possible misdiagnoses in these settings. Although not typically a diagnostic challenge, hyperplasia can be differentiated from normal arachnoid tissue using immunohistochemistry for the detection of progesterone receptor, since hyperplasias are often positive whereas normal arachnoid is not (1).

The arachnoid is frequently sampled in neurosurgical specimens, typically intact over the underlying cerebral cortex or, less commonly, spinal cord parenchyma. These samples provide an opportunity to examine the subarachnoid space, for instance, for neoplastic or inflammatory cells, as well as the prominent subarachnoid vasculature. In most situations in which the arachnoid is sampled incidentally in neurosurgical material, the arachnoid and subarachnoid space appear within normal limits.

The pia mater itself does not demonstrate any stereotypic responses to injury. Disruption of the pial-glial interface (glia limitans) occurs in malformative lesions that may be resected for seizure control (see chapter 13). In these situations, ectopic neuroglial tissue may be present in the subarachnoid space. Disruption of the glia limitans can also be found in neoplasms that erupt into the subarachnoid space and is particularly notable in pilocytic astrocytomas of the cerebellum.

BLOOD VESSELS

The cerebral vasculature is nearly always sampled as part of neurosurgical specimens. Despite differences that account for the blood-brain barrier, these vessels undergo pathologic changes similar to vessels in other areas of the body. Nonetheless, the cerebral vasculature can be the site of pathognomonic changes in a number of diverse conditions, such as vasculitis, cerebral amyloid angiopathy, and cerebral autosomal dominant arteriopathy with subcortical infarcts and leukoencephalopathy (CADASIL; see chapter 6), that may come to biopsy (see Table 2-1).

Because medium-sized vessels penetrate deep into the brain, into the Virchow-Robin spaces, which are extensions of the subarachnoid space, examination of pathologic processes must carefully evaluate whether inflammatory cells, for example, are within the wall of the blood vessel or in the subarachnoid space proper. Care must also be taken not to overinterpret the normal subarachnoid vasculature as a vascular malformation in surgical materials; the normal subarachnoid vessels often "contract" together after resection and this artifactual congerie of lumens can resemble a superficial arteriovenous malformation.

SCHWANN CELLS

Schwann cells are components of peripheral nerves, not of the CNS. Non-neoplastic conditions of the peripheral nervous system that may come to the attention of a surgical pathologist are discussed elsewhere (2). Nonetheless, it is important to recall that small peripheral nerves accompany larger blood vessels into the cerebral parenchyma. Schwann cells can therefore react to injury within the substance of the CNS, a process known as *schwannosis*.

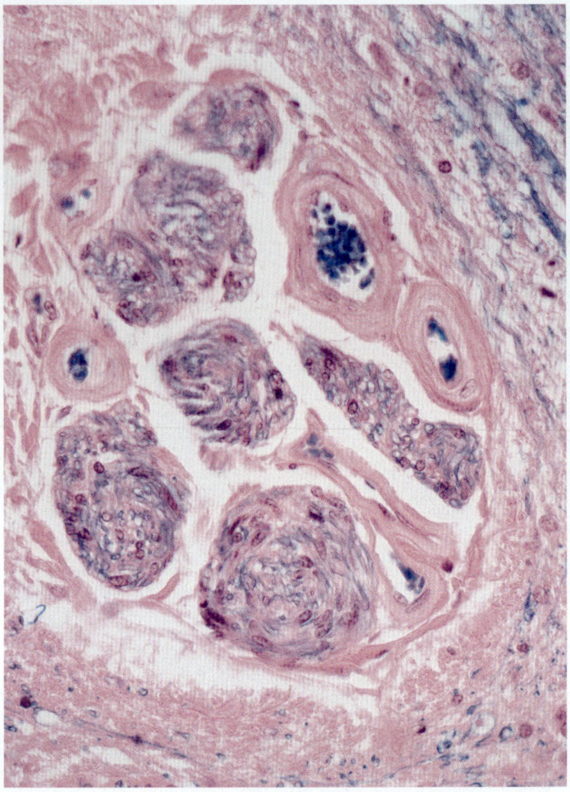

Figure 2-38

SCHWANNOSIS

Schwannosis is a proliferation of Schwann cells in the CNS, usually surrounding blood vessels in the spinal cord (Luxol fast blue-H&E stain).

Schwannosis is a common and nonspecific finding at autopsy (3) but is not often encountered in surgical specimens. It is more common in patients with neurofibromatosis 2 (4,5) and in the spinal cord after trauma (6). Typically located in the superficial parenchyma of the brain stem or spinal cord, sometimes near the dorsal root entry zones, schwannosis consists of small perivascular, irregularly whorled collections of Schwann cells (fig. 2-38). Like other Schwann cells, they stain strongly for S-100 protein.

INFLAMMATION

Inflammatory changes in the brain are largely similar to those in other organs, with a spectrum from acute to chronic infiltrates, and have the same connotations about disease processes. The most notable exception to this similarity is the microglial cell. *Microglia* are unique to

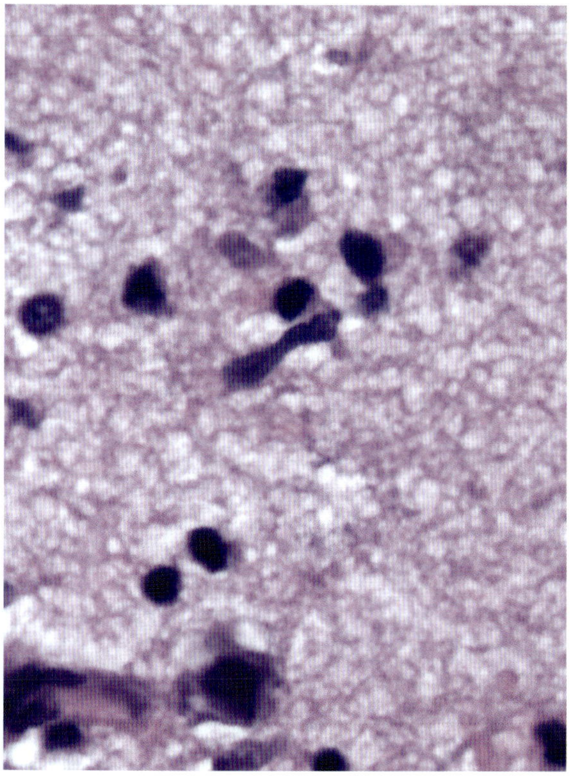

Figure 2-39

MICROGLIA

Microglia are elongated cells with thin, curved nuclei.

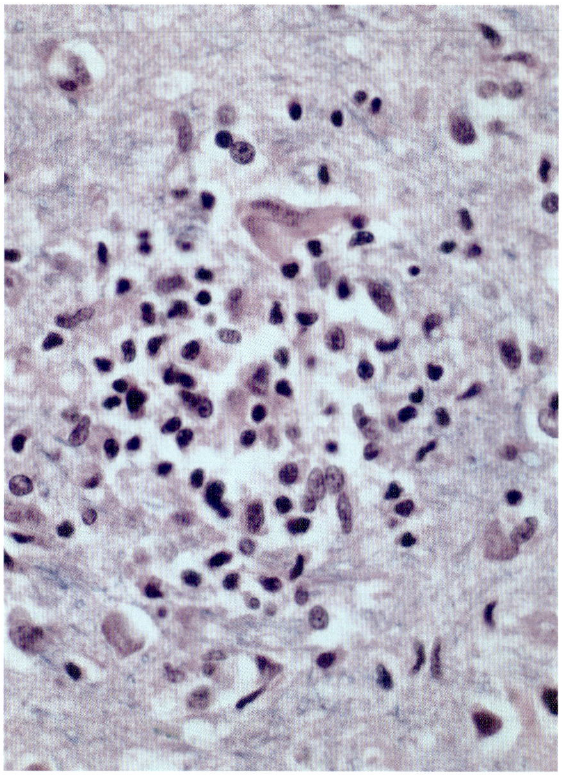

Figure 2-40

MICROGLIA

Microglia often cluster with other inflammatory cells into microglial nodules (Luxol fast blue-H&E stain).

the CNS. These delicate, elongated cells can be found in many pathologic processes but are particularly prominent in the setting of certain infectious conditions (see chapter 7), most notably viral encephalitis and syphilis, as well as in inflammatory diseases, such as paraneoplastic encephalitis and subacute sclerosing panencephalitis. In viral conditions, microglia may also form *microglial nodules*, vaguely nodular aggregates of microglia and lymphocytes that should raise the strong diagnostic consideration of a viral condition. (In rabies encephalitis, brain stem microglial nodules are referred to as *Babes nodules*.)

Microglia may be histologically similar to infiltrating neoplastic astrocytes, creating diagnostic difficulties. In general, microglia are thinner, more delicate, and more elongated than astrocytoma cells (fig. 2-39) and may be associated with microglial nodules (fig. 2-40), which are rare in gliomas. In some situations, immunohistochemistry is useful in distinguishing these cell types, with microglia staining for macrophage markers such as CD68 (fig. 2-41) and neoplastic astrocytes sometimes staining for GFAP.

Large numbers macrophages, particularly foamy macrophages or "gitter cells," are remarkably common in CNS processes (fig. 2-42). It is likely that such cells are derived from resident microglia. The presence of numerous macrophages in surgical neuropathology specimens should immediately alert the pathologist to the possibility of a reactive condition, such as acute demyelinating disease or a subacute cerebral infarct. These cells can be highlighted with special stains that highlight their cytoplasmic contents, such as Luxol fast blue for myelin. On frozen sections, oil red O staining identifies macrophages during intraoperative consultation. In addition, as with peripheral macrophages, these cells stain immunohistochemically for markers such as CD68 (fig. 2-43).

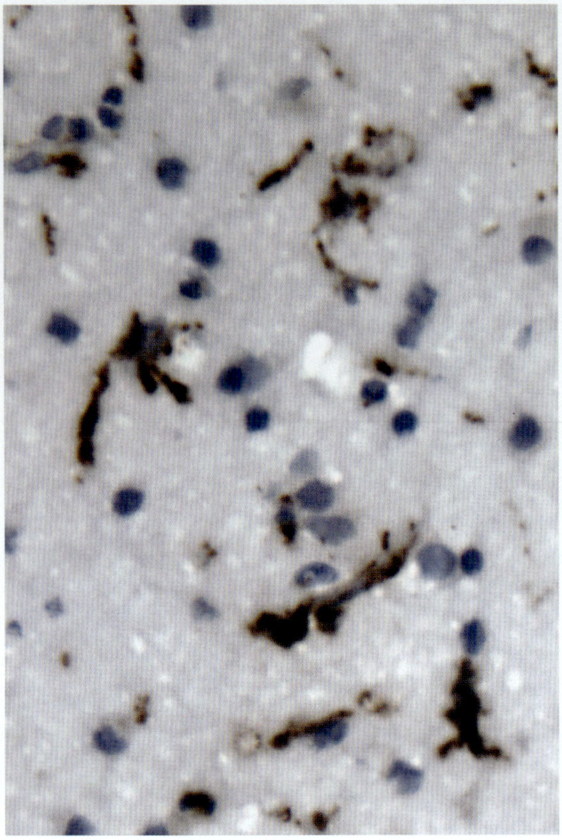

Figure 2-41

MICROGLIA

CD68 immunohistochemistry highlights microglia. Note the elongated cells with branching processes.

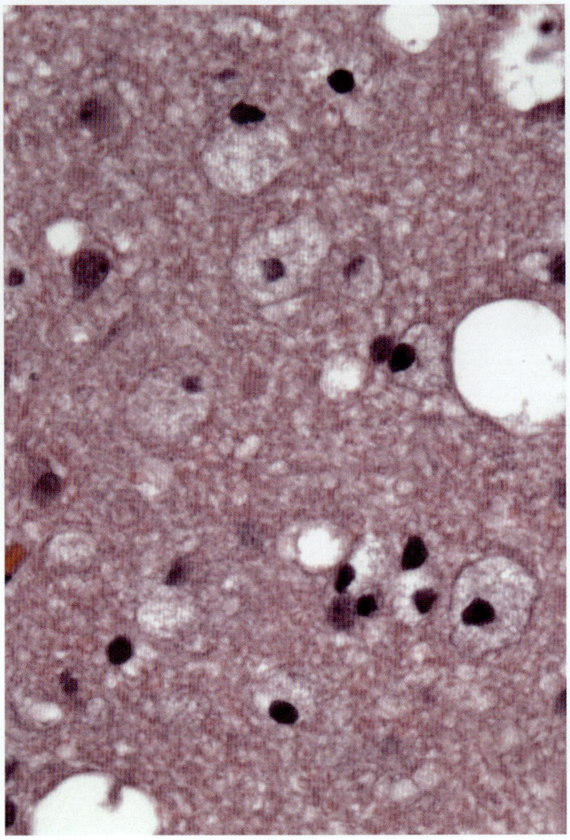

Figure 2-42

MACROPHAGES

Macrophages appear in the CNS as cells with clearly defined borders and granular cytoplasm.

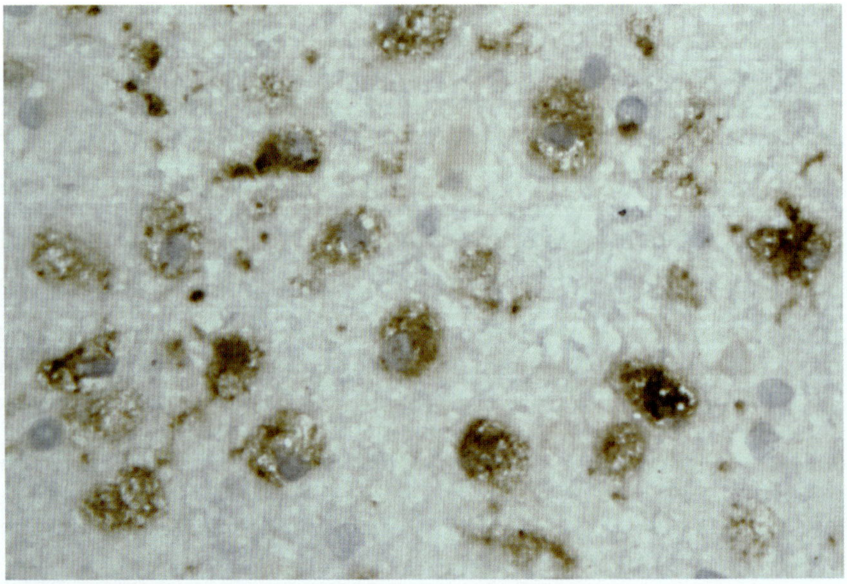

Figure 2-43

MACROPHAGES

CD68 immunohistochemistry highlights macrophages.

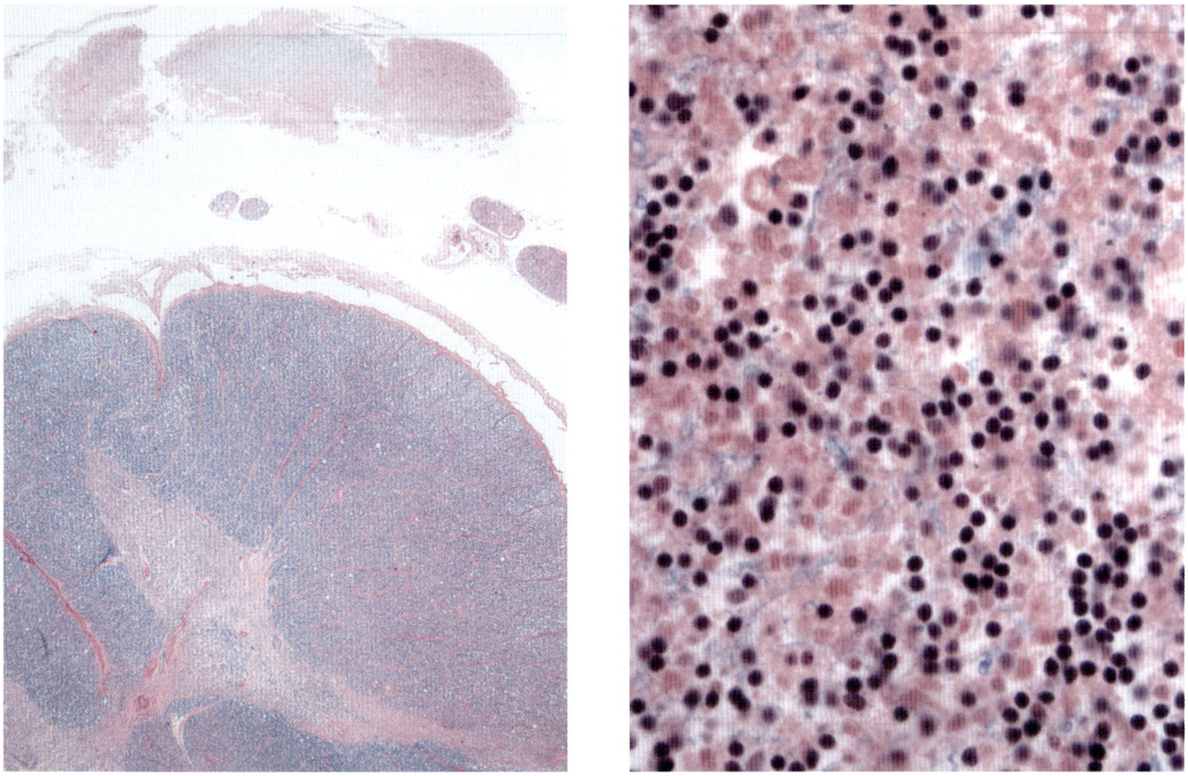

Figure 2-44

CEREBELLAR HERNIATION

Left: In tonsillar herniation, necrotic cerebellum can be found in the spinal subarachnoid space.
Right: Higher power shows a necrotic internal granular layer (Luxol fast blue-H&E stain).

CEREBRAL EDEMA

Cerebral edema is a common accompaniment to those processes coming to neurosurgical attention and, as a result, is often found in neurosurgical materials submitted for pathologic examination. In some situations in which acute trauma or cerebral infarction has necessitated partial lobectomy to prevent cerebral herniation, the histologic changes of edema may be the only findings.

In contrast to its catastrophic clinical effects and its striking appearance at autopsy, acute cerebral edema produces rather subtle microscopic changes. Ultrastructurally, different types of edema have different appearances, but the common feature is swelling of the myelin sheaths. At the light microscopic level, this appears as vacuolation of the gray and white matter, and is more prominent in the white matter. The vacuoles are small to large, seemingly extracellular, openings. Accordingly, there is pallor of the white matter with myelin stains such as Luxol fast blue. On frozen sections, acute cerebral edema often produces marked accentuation of the usual bubbles produced by freezing artifact. In acute edema that has been ongoing for many days, early reactive astrocytes may be noted.

In chronic situations, cerebral edema leads to marked astrocytosis as well as a diffuse, partial decrease in myelin. This is often accompanied by a gross yellowing of the white matter, which can be appreciated on macroscopic examination of white matter fragments by the pathologist.

The most ominous complication of edema is cerebral herniation and brain death. In rare situations in which patients are maintained on life support after brain death, fragments of necrotic cerebellar tissue may "drop" into the spinal subarachnoid space, and may be sampled during spinal tap (fig. 2-44). In such a situation, the pathologist may be asked to confirm the presence of necrotic cerebellar tissue.

REFERENCES

1. Perry A, Lusis EA, Gutmann DH. Meningothelial hyperplasia: a detailed clinicopathologic, immunohistochemical and genetic study of 11 cases. Brain Pathol 2005;15:109-115.
2. Scheithauer BW, Woodruff JM, Erlandson RA. Tumors of the peripheral nervous system. AFIP Atlas of Tumor Pathology, 3rd Series, Fascicle 24. Washington, DC: American Registry of Pathology; 1999.
3. Adelman LS, Aronson SM. Intramedullary nerve fiber and Schwann cell proliferation within the spinal cord (schwannosis). Neurology 1972;22:726-731.
4. Rubinstein LJ. The malformative central nervous system lesions in the central and peripheral forms of neurofibromatosis. A neuropathological study of 22 cases. Ann N Y Acad Sci 1986;486:14-29.
5. Louis DN, Ramesh V, Gusella JF. Neuropathology and molecular genetics of neurofibromatosis 2 and related tumors. Brain Pathol 1995;5:163-172.
6. Bruce JH, Norenberg MD, Kraydieh S, Puckett W, Marcillo A, Dietrich D. Schwannosis: role of gliosis and proteoglycan in human spinal cord injury. J Neurotrauma 2000;17:781-788.

3 TECHNICAL CONSIDERATIONS IN THE HANDLING OF SURGICAL SPECIMENS

BASIC APPROACHES

As in other areas of surgical pathology, proper processing of specimens is essential to derive necessary diagnostic information. For neurosurgical specimens, the small size of most biopsies and the reliance on stereotactic methods to target many lesions place a premium on proper handling. For some epilepsy surgeries, specimens must be correctly oriented or certain conditions will elude diagnosis. Potential problems from improper handling are, in fact, most distressing in the setting of non-neoplastic diseases of the nervous system since tumors are relatively easy to process in a simple, uniform manner and rarely require detailed orientation. The present chapter presents a suggested approach to the handling of neurosurgical specimens from non-neoplastic conditions. The reader is also referred to other references on this subject (1–3).

Specimen Triage

Optimal specimen triage always involves a discussion with the neurosurgeon and often other physicians caring for the patient, as well as knowledge of the neuroradiologic findings. This is particularly important in the setting of non-neoplastic diseases, since the surgical pathology approach to different differential diagnoses may in turn differ, for example, in the need for processing tissue for special infectious studies or electron microscopy. The neurosurgeon, usually more accustomed to obtaining specimens from neoplastic processes, may overlook the need for special processing. Furthermore, the neurologist or infectious disease specialist may have a long list of diagnostic considerations that has not been shared in detail with the neurosurgeon. Knowledge of all considered entities will ensure adequate processing to evaluate each. It is therefore prudent to undertake preoperative and intraoperative consultation with the neurosurgeon, neuroradiologist, and other physicians on all biopsies for suspected non-neoplastic processes.

For each specimen, based on such consultations, the questions that must be answered prior to processing are shown in Table 3-1. Careful answers to these questions will determine the proper approach to specimen triage, and prevent mistakes of omission that could necessitate additional biopsies in the future.

Frozen Section

While intraoperative consultations are essential in the setting of non-neoplastic diseases, frozen sections are not always necessary. Frozen sections are only necessary in the following situations.

Frozen sections are needed to confirm that abnormal tissue has been sampled, particularly for stereotactic biopsies. If the frozen section does not demonstrate abnormal tissue, the neurosurgeon must obtain further tissue. In some situations, whether because of bleeding complications or cardiovascular instability, the neurosurgeon may have already elected to take a single set of biopsies only; in this situation, if the only goal is to confirm abnormal tissue, there is no need to perform a frozen section.

Table 3-1

QUESTIONS THAT NEED TO BE ADDRESSED PRIOR TO PROCESSING SPECIMENS

1. What is the proper orientation of the specimen?
2. What portion of the specimen will be required for standard formalin fixation and paraffin embedding?
3. Should a frozen section be undertaken?
4. Should tissue be saved frozen?
5. Should tissue be fixed for electron microscopy?
6. Should tissue be fixed in fixatives other than standard formalin?
7. Should tissue be sent to the microbiology laboratory by the neurosurgeon?
8. Should tissue be saved in other ways, e.g., in culture medium, as frozen sections, or as smears?

Frozen sections are also needed to gain information that may alter how a sample is processed. For example, the differential diagnosis may involve a series of neoplastic and non-neoplastic conditions, some requiring special studies and others not.

Finally, frozen section provides rapid feedback to the treating physician about certain diseases, notably acute infectious diseases, that may require urgent therapy.

If the above issues are considered and there is no need for a frozen section, the pathologist should not perform one since freezing of tissue introduces extensive tissue artifacts that may preclude adequate assessment of the final fixed, embedded specimens. An example of this situation is in the setting of a demented patient being biopsied to evaluate the possibility of prion diseases. A frozen section in this case will undoubtedly create artifacts that complicate the adequate evaluation of the tissue for true spongiform change.

Once the decision to perform a frozen section is made, it is nonetheless essential not to freeze all material provided, that is, it is mandatory to save some tissues for proper fixation and other potential processing. For the portion chosen for freezing, standard approaches are used. Staining of formalin-fixed sections with hematoxylin and eosin (H&E) and of alcohol-fixed sections with toluidine blue is valuable. The toluidine blue–stained, alcohol-fixed sections are particularly useful for evaluating myelin and nuclear features. Oil red O stains demonstrate the presence of lipid-laden macrophages.

Smear Preparation

Smear preparations are extremely practical for evaluating cytologic details and sometimes for detecting infectious organisms. The decision to proceed with a smear preparation follows the same decision-making process discussed above for frozen sections. If a decision has been made to do a frozen section, then a smear should also be made.

The details of proper smear preparation are illustrated in figure 3-1, and are discussed in more detail elsewhere (1–3). Use of tissues less than 1 mm^3 is optimal, with intermediate pressure applied for the smear, and immediate fixation to prevent air drying artifacts. Fixation in alcohol followed by standard H&E staining ensures good cytologic detail. After fixation, smears can also be saved for further use.

Electron Microscopy

Electron microscopy is an essential technique for the evaluation of some non-neoplastic conditions of the central nervous system (CNS). As discussed throughout this Fascicle, a number of diseases, ranging from infectious to metabolic in nature, have characteristic ultrastructural changes that are diagnostically useful. Preservation of tissue in appropriate fixative is best accomplished during the intraoperative consultation. In some situations in which this is not possible—for example, a specimen already processed in formalin—tissue can be retrieved from other fixatives and from paraffin blocks and reprocessed for electron microscopy. While not optimal, such tissue can still yield key diagnostic information concerning minute structures such as viral particles.

Snap Freezing

Snap freezing of tissues is a prudent method for saving tissue that can subsequently be used for a wide range of studies, including molecular and metabolic evaluations. Snap freezing is best accomplished by immersing tissue in liquid nitrogen or in isopentane cooled in liquid nitrogen; in most instances, this is most readily done by freezing in Optimal Cutting Temperature (OCT) compound. The use of a rim of OCT around the tissue makes it easier for sections to be obtained in the future, prior to specialized studies which require histologic confirmation of the saved tissues. Indeed, in situations in which the process could be focal, it may be useful to perform a frozen section biopsy on the snap frozen tissue immediately after freezing to ensure that lesional tissue is being saved. After snap freezing, the tissue is optimally saved in liquid nitrogen. If such facilities are not available, the tissue should be saved at -80°C. Careful identification of the specimen is of the utmost importance; with some chronic non-neoplastic conditions, tissue may be requested many months or sometimes years after the initial biopsy for additional testing as new clinical features suggest other possibilities or as new diagnostic tests are developed.

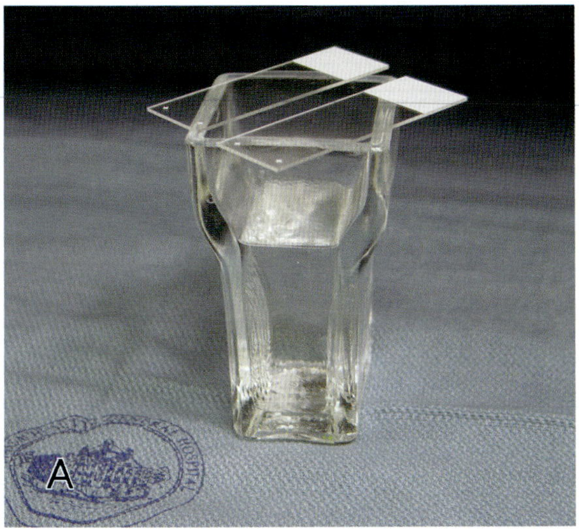

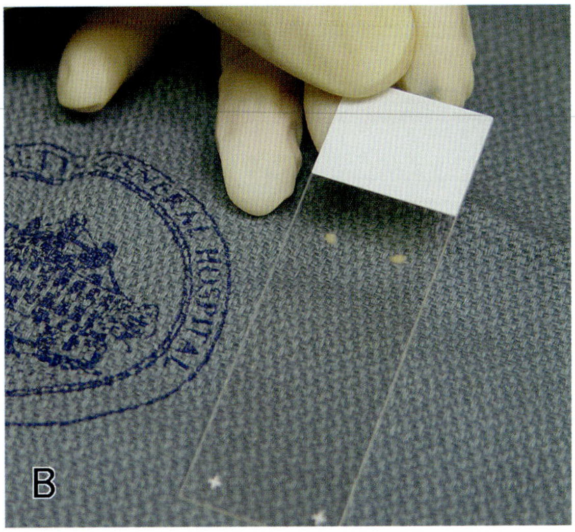

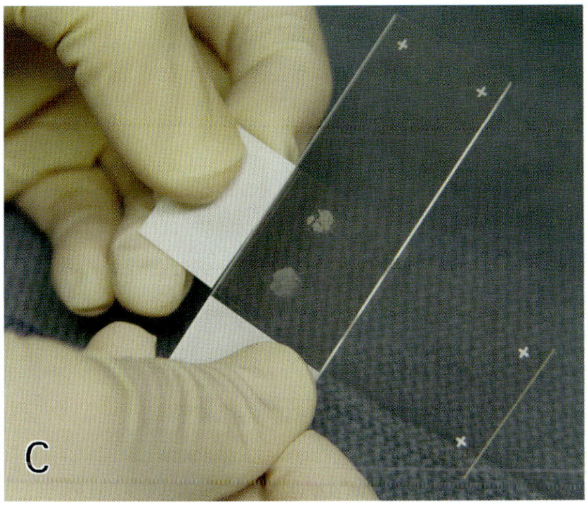

Figure 3-1

SMEAR PREPARATION

A: Step 1. Two slides are necessary, as well as fixative solution close at hand.

B: Step 2. Two fragments are placed near the label end of the slide; for stereotactic needle cores, the two fragments should sample each end of the core (see fig. 3-2).

C: Step 3. Using gentle but firm pressure, a second slide is placed on top in order to compress the tissue fragments against the bottom slide.

D: Step 4. With gentle but firm pressure, the top slide is dragged across the bottom slide, "smearing" the two tissue fragments along the length of the bottom slide.

E: Step 5. The lower slide, which has most of the smeared tissue, is placed immediately in fixative.

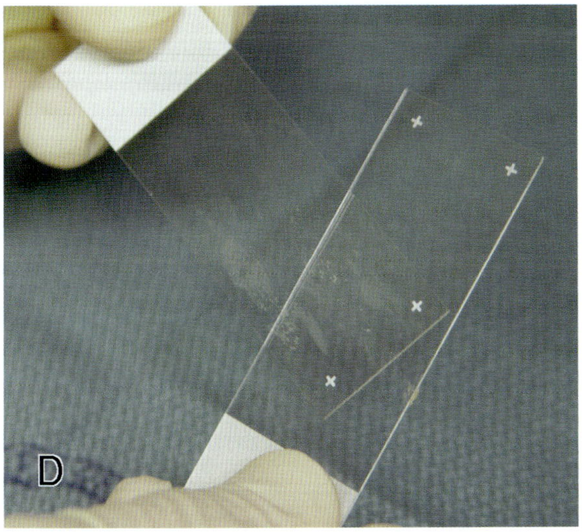

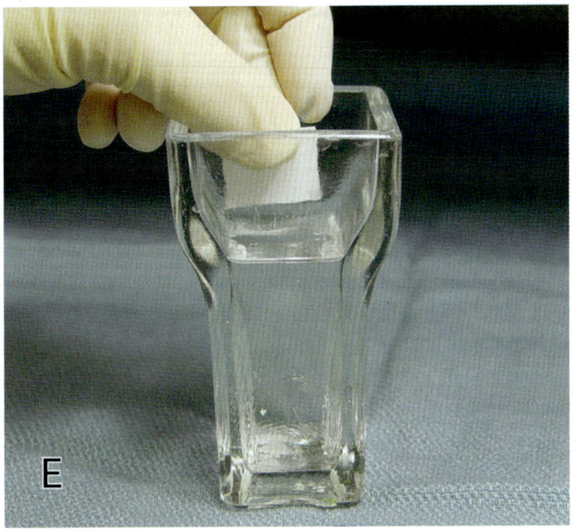

Table 3-2

STAINS

Cell Type	Assay	Stain	Target	Localization	Pathological Process
Neuron	Immunohistochemistry	NeuN	Nuclear Ag[a]	N	Cortical malformations
		Neurofilament	Intermediate filament	C, axons	Axon status
		Synaptophysin	Synaptic protein	C, neuropil	Neuropil identification
		Tau	Microtubule-associated protein	C	NFT, Pick bodies
		Ubiquitin	Proteolytic protein	C	Lewy body
		Alpha-synuclein	Presynaptic protein	C	Lewy body, glial cytoplasmic inclusions
	Silver impregnation	Bielschowsky	Multiple	C, processes	NFT, neuritic plaques
		Bodian	Multiple	C, axons	Axon status
	Special stain	Nissl	Rough endoplasmic reticulum	C, clumps	
Astrocyte	Immunohistochemistry	GFAP	Intermediate filament	C	Reactive astrocytes
		Ubiquitin	Proteolytic protein	C	Rosenthal fibers
		Alpha-B-crystallin	Lens protein	C	Rosenthal fibers
	Special stain	PTAH	Glial cell processes	C	Reactive astrocytes, Rosenthal fibers
Oligodendrocyte	Silver impregnation	Gallyas		C	Glial cytoplasmic inclusions
	Special stain	Luxol fast blue	Myelin	C, myelin sheaths	
Other	Special stain	Congo red	Amyloid	E	Neuritic plaque cores, angiopathy
		PAS	Multiple	E	CADASIL, basement membrane abnormalities
		Trichrome	Multiple	neuropil/collagen	Neuropil/collagen identification

[a]Ag = antigen; NFT = neurofibrillary tangle; GFAP = glial fibrillary acidic protein; PTAH = phosphotungstic acid hematoxylin; PAS = periodic acid–Schiff; N = nuclear; C = cytoplasmic; E = endothelial/vascular.

Fixation and Processing

In nearly all cases, standard buffered formalin is the preferred fixative for tissue that is not destined for special processing (freezing, glutaraldehyde-based fixation for electron microscopy, culturing). Formalin fixation allows excellent tissue preservation for standard light microscopic examination and is optimal for most special stains and for standard clinical immunohistochemical assays.

Staining

The role of special stains and immunohistochemistry in guiding the differential diagnosis of non-neoplastic disorders of the CNS parallels the role of these techniques in similar systemic diseases. Certain stains, silver impregnations, and immunohistochemical assays are also powerful methods for evaluating specific CNS elements. A list of the most useful stains, along with their applications, is given in Table 3-2.

SPECIMEN TYPES

Different types of neurosurgical specimens require different approaches to processing. The three major types of brain specimen obtained for non-neoplastic disorders are stereotactic biopsies, open biopsies, and resection/lobectomy specimens. Spinal cord specimens are always small open biopsies, as are meningeal samplings.

The most challenging specimens are stereotactic and open biopsies, since they are small specimens invariably taken for diagnostic purposes. They are, therefore, the most difficult specimens for the surgical pathologist, from the point of view of both gross processing and histologic assessment. Resection/lobectomy specimens are for therapy of lesions such as vascular malformations or seizure foci, and so are less challenging for the pathologist. The proper approach to processing neurosurgical specimens from the pituitary gland is discussed elsewhere (4).

Stereotactic Biopsies

Stereotactic biopsies are small core specimens that typically measure less than 1 cm in length and less than 2 mm in diameter. They are obtained through a burr hole in the skull based on radiologic guidance. Although the systems that enable targeting of brain lesions are accurate, it is important for the pathologist to understand that they are not perfect, that it is still possible for a stereotactic biopsy to "miss" a lesion. For this reason, the pathologist must have a good idea of the clinical and neuroradiologic differential diagnosis in order to determine whether the histologic findings appear representative of the possible entities considered.

For stereotactic biopsies, after detailed discussions with the neurosurgeon, neuroradiologist, and other physicians regarding the differential diagnosis and any urgency in obtaining a preliminary diagnosis, a decision must be made concerning performing a frozen section and retaining tissues in particular ways (see above). In many instances, a frozen section and special processing is indicated, necessitating that the tiny specimen be divided into multiple, even smaller pieces.

Most stereotactic biopsies can have the final millimeter of each end removed for a smear (fig. 3-2). If the neurosurgeon orients the core, indicating which end is deep, it is useful to smear each end independently, designating one as "deep" and the other as "superficial." Since these represent the ends of the specimen, the presence of abnormalities in the deeper part could indicate that the biopsy comes from the edge of the specimen and that additional, deeper passes might prove more diagnostic.

The remaining core can often be bisected longitudinally down the middle, with half for freezing and half for formalin fixation (fig. 3-2). This often requires great care on the part of the pathologist in order to place the tiny half core into a cassette in a protected manner and on the part of the technicians handling the tiny half cores for processing and embedding. A prudent approach is to label the cassette to indicate that the technician should automatically cut 10 unstained sections in addition to the standard H&E sections when first facing the paraffin block. Doing so ensures that cutting the initial H&E section does not waste the small amount of tissue and that the first cutting already provides unstained sections for future special stains and immunohistochemistry.

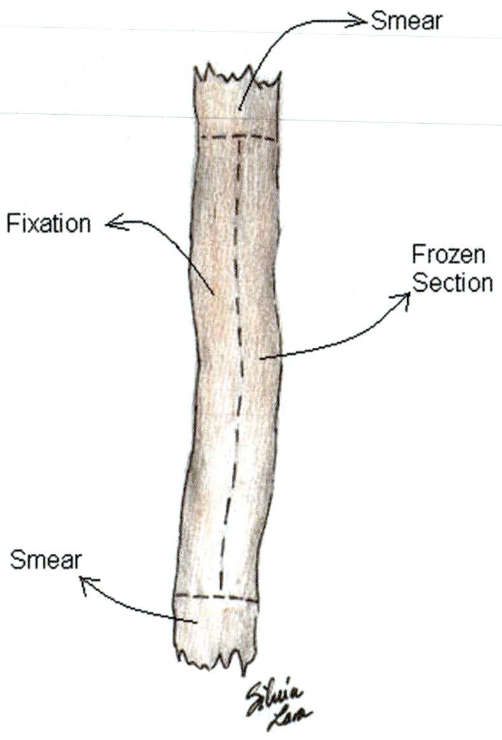

Figure 3-2

DIVISION OF STEREOTACTIC BIOPSY CORES DURING INTRAOPERATIVE CONSULTATION

A piece of each end is removed for smear preparation; these can be placed on the same slide (see fig. 3-1B) or, if the core is oriented by the neurosurgeon, on two separate slides. The remaining core is carefully bisected: half is frozen for intraoperative consultation, the other half is subsequently placed in formalin for standard processing if not needed for intraoperative consultation.

In some institutions, the neurosurgeon provides double cores for each target. This is helpful since it allows use of one core for frozen section, smear, and special studies and the other core for formalin fixation and paraffin embedding. Nonetheless, although from the "same" site, the variability of the targets and the variability of the underlying processes may mean that the two cores are not equally representative.

Open Biopsies

Open biopsies of the brain are undertaken for superficial lesions, for areas in which stereotactic approaches pose too great a risk of complications, and for processes in which a larger sampling may increase the likelihood of establishing a diagnosis. The latter issue arises since many non-neoplastic processes are topographically variable, being present for example in one region but not in an adjacent area; a good example of this is the spongiform change that attends prion diseases.

Open cerebral and cerebellar biopsy specimens vary in size, depending on the size of the lesion and the region involved, but are typically about 1 cm in maximum dimension. In the setting of suspected non-neoplastic diseases, they are often accompanied by meningeal sampling (see below). If possible, the cerebral specimens should be oriented; this is often possible without the neurosurgeon, simply by identifying the smooth pial surface of the cerebral cortex or the foliar arrangement of the cerebellum. These specimens should be divided into thin sections while fresh, perpendicular to the pial surface, in order to most optimally orient the subsequent blocked tissue and to identify any grossly visible lesions. The macroscopically abnormal areas can then be divided appropriately for any special studies.

The spinal cord is always sampled in an open manner. In the setting of suspected non-neoplastic disorders, however, these specimens tend to be exceedingly small because of the delicate nature of the cord. The approach to handling such specimens is the same as for cerebral stereotactic specimens, discussed above.

Resection/Lobectomy Specimens

Resections and lobectomies are performed for a number of non-neoplastic conditions of the cerebral and cerebellar hemispheres. These can be divided into three groups: lobectomies and resections for seizure control; resections of vascular malformations or other non-neoplastic mass lesions (e.g., cysts); and debulking procedures to reduce intracranial pressure, secondary to trauma or cerebral infarction.

Of these three types, the last two present no problems to the surgical pathologist. Resections of vascular malformations and non-neoplastic masses are processed like any other surgical pathology specimen. Margins are not of concern for such lesions and therefore it is not necessary to ink the edges. Standard representative samples can be submitted for histologic examination. For debulking procedures, diagnostic issues are not of prime importance and one or two representative sections usually suffice for histology.

Lobectomies and resections for seizure control, however, require careful orientation. Review of the specimen with the neurosurgeon is strongly encouraged and is mandatory for specimens for which anterior-posterior orientation is important. Unless otherwise specified, for example, if a rare metabolic disease is suspected for which frozen tissue may prove helpful for diagnosis, orientation can be more optimally done on formalin-fixed materials, even after a few hours of fixation. Precise orientation is necessary for two major reasons: to orient the cerebral cortex and underlying white matter, since many malformation can only be appreciated in well-oriented cortex; and to orient the hippocampus, if provided, since neuroanatomical considerations are important for assessment of hippocampal abnormalities.

For cerebral cortical samples, the goal for the surgical pathologist is to section the specimen perpendicular to the pial surface (fig. 3-3). This should allow identification of the tan-colored cerebral cortex and the underlying white matter. In some situations, for example in tubers, the cortex may be macroscopically abnormal; in other settings, the white matter may be gliotic and have a yellow or tan hue. Wide representative sampling of such specimens is usually important since dysplastic changes can be focal. With modern neuroimaging and neurophysiologic monitoring, the neurosurgeon may have a strong indication that a specific region of the sample is more likely to be abnormal, which again emphasizes the need for close interaction with the neurosurgeon in orienting the specimen. The amygdala, which is often included in anterior temporal lobectomies, should not be misinterpreted as abnormal cortex; if this occurs on gross inspection, the typical appearance of the amygdala on histology (see chapter 1) will correct the misinterpretation.

Hippocampal samples are usually orientable without help from the surgeon if careful attention is paid to sectioning in a coronal plane (fig. 3-4). The goal for the surgical pathologist is to provide sections that offer the typical "seahorse" appearance of the hippocampus and the

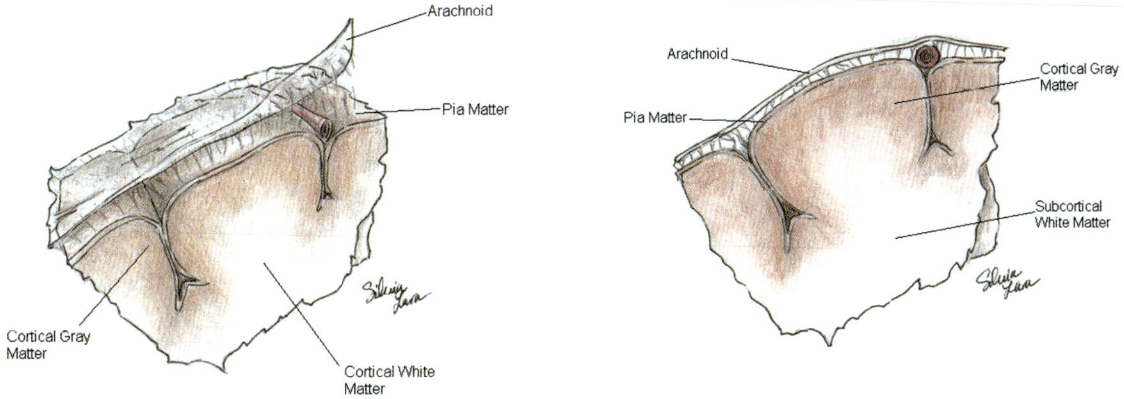

Figure 3-3

ORIENTATION OF CORTICAL BIOPSIES

Cortical biopsies should be frozen and/or placed into cassettes with an orientation perpendicular to the pial surface, allowing cross-sectional examination from the pia and arachnoid (if present) to the underlying white matter. The pial surface appears smooth and tan, whereas the other surface, having been cut by the surgeon, appears jagged and either tan or white (if subcortical white matter is also sampled). Arachnoid appears as an easily detachable, thin, translucent membrane.

adjacent entorhinal cortex. This orientation is important since certain pathologic changes are primarily present in particular subregions of the hippocampus, for example, hippocampal sclerosis in the cornu ammonis (CA)1 sector.

Meningeal Biopsies

As discussed above, meningeal biopsies typically encompass sampling of dura, arachnoid, and pia maters. As a result, meningeal biopsies are often a combination of a dural and a cerebral cortical sample, the latter having attached arachnoid and pia mater. The processing of the cerebral specimens is similar to that discussed for open brain biopsies above, with particular care directed to preserving the delicate arachnoid membrane. The dural specimens can be processed in standard manners, divided for frozen section and special studies if necessary; the tough nature of these specimens, however, make smears impossible.

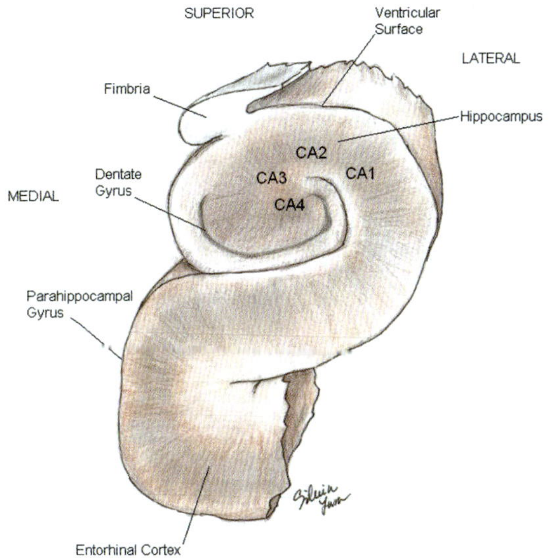

Figure 3-4

ORIENTATION OF THE HIPPOCAMPUS

Sections of the hippocampus should be placed into cassettes in the coronal orientation depicted, which enables microscopic examination of the key neuroanatomic structures. The medial surfaces of the hippocampus and adjacent entorhinal cortex should have smooth surfaces. The fimbria should be identifiable as a band along the superior surface, which is smooth and white. CA (cornu ammonis) fields 1 through 4 refer to the pyramidal layer (see chapter 1); CA1 is Sommer sector, the region most affected by ischemic and Alzheimer changes.

REFERENCES

1. Moss TH, Nicoll JAR, Ironside JW. Intra-operative diagnosis of CNS tumours. London: Arnold; 1997.
2. Dawson TP, Neal JW, Llewellyn L, Thomas C. Neuropathology techniques. London: Arnold; 2003.
3. Adams JH, Graham DI, Doyle D. Brain biopsy: the smear technique for surgical biopsies. London: Chapman & Hall; 1981.
4. Asa SL. Tumors of the pituitary gland. AFIP Atlas of Tumor Pathology, 3rd Series, Fascicle 22. Washington, DC: American Registry of Pathology; 1998.

4 DIAGNOSTIC APPROACH TO BRAIN BIOPSY INTERPRETATION

GENERAL COMMENTS

The approach to the differential diagnosis in surgical neuropathology has changed greatly with the radiologic and neurosurgical advances of the past two decades. Modern neuroimaging has provided the clinician with a markedly improved ability to narrow the differential diagnosis, i.e., to estimate which conditions are more or less likely responsible for a patient's illness with a reasonable degree of accuracy prior to biopsy diagnosis. As a result, the process of biopsy interpretation now begins at a different stage than it did in the era prior to modern neuroimaging. Indeed, today, in addition to clinical details, neuroimaging data are used by the pathologist to inform the tissue differential diagnosis.

Modern neurosurgery has also changed the face of surgical neuropathology by increasing the ability to sample deep-seated lesions safely, particularly through the use of stereotactic biopsy. While modern neuroimaging and laboratory medicine improvements have decreased the number of biopsies for certain conditions (e.g., herpes simplex encephalitis), the advent of stereotactic biopsies has increased the safety and the range of brain biopsies, thus increasing the biopsies taken from diagnostically challenging conditions. It seems likely that the combination of neuroradiologic, laboratory medicine, and neurosurgical improvements has skewed diagnostic biopsies of non-neoplastic conditions toward rarer entities, heightening the challenge to the diagnostic pathologist.

Given the above, the most practical differential diagnostic approach to biopsies of non-neoplastic conditions of the central nervous system (CNS) in the modern era is based on a few key principles. First, the vast majority of CNS biopsies are for neoplastic conditions. In other words, neoplasia must always be considered carefully in the differential diagnosis. Second, there are only a few common non-neoplastic conditions that closely mimic neoplastic diseases of the brain and result in biopsy. These are cerebral infarct, acute demyelinating disease, and brain abscess. As a result, these three possibilities need to be considered often; other non-neoplastic conditions that are biopsied are all uncommon diseases. Third, these non-neoplastic conditions represent the entire gamut of neurologic diseases, a bewilderingly wide spectrum to be considered in the differential diagnosis. This spectrum constitutes the remaining chapters of this book.

Close communication with clinicians and neuroradiologists is essential to narrow the differential diagnosis and to arrive at the correct diagnosis. The importance of close communication with other physicians involved in the patient's care cannot be overemphasized, and key clinical correlates are therefore stressed in the following chapters. In this way, it is hoped that knowledge of clinical correlates will aid the pathologist, particularly when the histologic findings are nonspecific.

"Blinded" review of histology slides is an important first step in any differential diagnostic approach. While, as discussed in chapter 3, the clinical and radiologic findings are important to consider prior to the final processing of the specimen, a review of the histologic features without clinical and radiologic information is often the most unbiased manner to *first* evaluate the biopsy. Clearly, however, as discussed in the next section, careful clinicopathologic correlation is essential prior to formulating a *final* diagnosis.

CLINICOPATHOLOGIC CORRELATION

No neurosurgical biopsy should be signed out in the absence of clinical and radiologic information. This is especially important for non-neoplastic diseases, for which close clinicopathologic correlation is crucial. Ideally, sufficient information would be provided with the surgical pathology requisition form. In reality, however, requisition forms essentially never contain all the relevant information and consultation with clinicians is required. Typically,

Table 4-1

CLINICOPATHOLOGIC FEATURES IN THE INTERPRETATION OF BIOPSIES OF THE CENTRAL NERVOUS SYSTEM FOR NON-NEOPLASTIC DISEASES

Location (see Tables 4-2 through 4-9)
Current clinical course and physical findings
Medications
Age and gender (see Table 4-10)
Past medical and family history
Past illnesses and therapies
Radiation and chemotherapy
Drug or alcohol use
Travel history
Laboratory findings
Neuroimaging features

this consultation involves the neurosurgeon, radiologist, neurologist, and sometimes, internist, particularly when infectious disease is suspected. The increasingly widespread availability of electronic medical records has facilitated access by the pathologist to important clinical information, but cannot serve as a substitute for close communication with the patient's physicians.

It is the responsibility of the pathologist to review the available medical records and discuss the case with the involved clinicians. Each of the clinical and radiologic variables discussed in this chapter should be addressed, since each may influence the differential diagnosis. In many situations, biopsies for non-neoplastic conditions of the brain show nonspecific findings; in these cases, the clinical and radiologic features may influence how the pathologist words the comments to weight one possible diagnosis over another.

For these reasons, the pathologist should consider the following clinicopathologic features in all biopsies: the location of the abnormality; the specific features of the clinical course, including its tempo; the patient's current physical examination findings and medications; the patient's past medical history, including prior drug or alcohol use, previous therapies, and travel history; family history; laboratory findings; and neuroimaging characteristics (Table 4-1). Each of these parameters is discussed below.

Location

The non-neoplastic diseases that affect the CNS sometimes show remarkable predilections for certain locations. Knowledge of the location of a lesion can greatly shorten the list of most likely diagnoses for a particular case. At the same time, it is important to remember that exceptions to the following predilections occur, and that some diseases affect the CNS in a global manner.

Table 4-2

NON-NEOPLASTIC DISEASES OF THE CENTRAL NERVOUS SYSTEM THAT AFFECT THE MENINGES

Infections (see chapter 7)
Viral
Bacterial
Tuberculosis/atypical mycobacteria
Fungal
Inflammatory processes (see chapter 8)
Sarcoidosis
Paraneoplastic processes
Rheumatoid diseases
Intracranial hypertension (see chapter 8)
Hematopoietic conditions (see chapter 8)
Erdheim-Chester disease
Rosai-Dorfman
Castleman disease
Plasma cell granuloma
Vascular diseases (see chapter 6)
Arteriovenous malformations
Aneurysms
Vasculitides
Cerebral amyloid angiopathy
Trauma (see chapter 11)
Seizure disorders (see chapter 13)
Meningioangiomatosis
Sturge-Weber syndrome
Heterotopias
Encephaloceles and myelomeningocele
Reaction to neoplasms and antineoplastic therapy (see chapter 14)

Meninges. Diseases with a tendency to affect the meninges are listed in Table 4-2. Many entities are distinct from those that preferentially affect the cerebral parenchyma. Of particular interest is the entire spectrum of viral, bacterial, mycobacterial, fungal, and parasitic infections. Some of these show a predilection for the meninges around the base of the brain (e.g., tuberculosis) whereas others favor the convexities (e.g., many bacterial meningitides). Inflammatory processes such as sarcoidosis and rheumatoid disease, and a host of hematopoietic conditions such as Rosai-Dorfman and Castleman diseases, affect the meninges more often than the brain parenchyma. Many

Table 4-3

NON-NEOPLASTIC DISEASES OF THE CENTRAL NERVOUS SYSTEM THAT AFFECT THE CEREBRAL CORTEX

- Ischemia and infarction (see chapter 5)
- Vascular diseases (see chapter 6)
  - Vascular malformations
  - Vasculitides
  - Cerebral amyloid angiopathy
- Infections (see chapter 7)
  - Viral encephalitis
    - Herpes simplex
  - Whipple disease
  - Syphilis
  - Toxoplasma
- Inflammatory processes (see chapter 8)
  - Paraneoplastic encephalitis
  - Rasmussen encephalitis
  - Subacute sclerosis panencephalitis (see chapter 10)
- Dementia and related disorders (see chapter 10)
  - Neurodegenerative diseases
  - Transmissible spongiform encephalopathies
- Trauma (see chapter 11)
  - Contusions
- Metabolic diseases (see chapter 12)
- Seizure disorders (see chapter 13)
  - Chaslin gliosis
  - Malformative lesions
  - Tubers
  - Neurofibromatosis 2: hamartomas and meningio-angiomatosis
  - Sturge-Weber syndrome
- Reaction to neoplasms and antineoplastic therapy (see chapter 14)

entities affect both the leptomeninges and the brain itself; for example, vasculitides often affect meningeal vessels in addition to parenchymal vessels, making leptomeningeal biopsy a method for diagnosing vasculitis. A variety of malformative lesions also affect the meninges in combination with the brain.

Cerebral Cortex. The cerebral cortex, usually with some underlying white matter, is the most commonly sampled portion of the CNS. Some diseases affect the cortex in specific places, requiring a biopsy to target those affected areas; other diseases, for example, many of the more common dementing illnesses, affect the cortex in a more diffuse manner. In the latter setting, the most commonly biopsied site is the nondominant frontal lobe, given that it is considered "noneloquent" and is readily accessible.

Table 4-4

NON-NEOPLASTIC DISEASES OF THE CENTRAL NERVOUS SYSTEM THAT AFFECT THE CEREBRAL WHITE MATTER

- Intracerebral hemorrhage (see chapter 5)
- Infections (see chapter 7)
  - Viral encephalitis
    - Progressive multifocal leukoencephalopathy
    - Human immunodeficiency virus
  - Brain abscess
- Demyelinating diseases (see chapter 9)
  - Multiple sclerosis
  - Acute disseminated encephalomyelitis
  - Weston Hurst disease (acute hemorrhagic leuko-encephalitis)
  - Hereditary demyelinating diseases (see chapter 12)
- Toxic encephalopathies (see chapter 10)
  - Solvent vapor inhalation
  - Chemotherapy associated (see chapter 14)
- Metabolic diseases (see chapter 12)
- Reaction to neoplasms and antineoplastic therapy (see chapter 14)

The spectrum of diseases preferentially affecting the cerebral cortex is broad (Table 4-3), and includes neurodegenerative diseases, infections (particularly viral and prion diseases), and inflammatory diseases (such as paraneoplastic encephalitis, Rasmussen encephalitis, and subacute sclerosing panencephalitis). Vascular diseases are common and include infarcts, vascular malformations, vasculitides, and cerebral amyloid angiopathy. Seizure disorders are usually associated with cortical pathology, including Chaslin gliosis and malformative lesions. The hippocampus and amygdala, superficial gray matter structures in the medial temporal lobe that include regions of cortex, are commonly included in temporal lobectomies performed for seizure control, and are affected by malformative processes as well as nonspecific gliosis.

Cerebral White Matter. The cerebral white matter is affected in many diseases, both as part of generalized processes that affect both gray and white matter and as part of specific disorders of the white matter (Table 4-4). Among the latter, demyelinating diseases figure prominently, as do some viral processes (such as progressive multifocal leukoencephalopathy and human immunodeficiency virus [HIV] encephalitis). The white matter is also differentially sensitive to some therapeutic and toxic

Table 4-5

NON-NEOPLASTIC DISEASES OF THE CENTRAL NERVOUS SYSTEM THAT AFFECT THE DEEP CEREBRAL GRAY MATTER

Ischemia, infarction, and intracerebral hemorrhage (see chapter 5)
Vascular diseases (see chapter 6)
Vascular malformations
Infections (see chapter 7)
Bacterial abscess
Some viral (e.g., flaviviruses)
Inflammatory processes (see chapter 8)
Sarcoidosis
Dementia and related disorders (see chapter 10)
Transmissible spongiform encephalopathies
Hypothalamic hamartoma (see chapter 14)
Reaction to neoplasms and antineoplastic therapy (see chapter 14)

Table 4-6

NON-NEOPLASTIC DISEASES OF THE CENTRAL NERVOUS SYSTEM THAT AFFECT THE CEREBRAL VENTRICLES

Intracerebral hemorrhage (see chapter 5)
Infections (see chapter 6)
Viral (e.g., cytomegalovirus)
Bacterial
Fungal (e.g., *Cryptococcus*)
Xanthogranuloma of the choroid plexus (see chapter 8)
Reaction to neoplasms and antineoplastic therapy (see chapter 14)

Table 4-7

NON-NEOPLASTIC DISEASES OF THE CENTRAL NERVOUS SYSTEM THAT AFFECT THE CEREBELLUM

Ischemia, infarction, and hemorrhage (see chapter 5)
Vascular malformations (see chapter 6)
Infections (see chapter 7)
Viral encephalitis
Abscess
Inflammatory processes (see chapter 8)
Paraneoplastic processes
Trauma (see chapter 11)
Reaction to neoplasms and antineoplastic therapy (see chapter 14)

agents, particularly antineoplastic treatments such as radiation and chemotherapies.

Deep Cerebral Gray Matter. The deep gray matter structures are less often sampled than the cerebral cortex and, when sampled, are targeted by stereotactic biopsies that yield small samples. The deep gray nuclei are affected by many processes (Table 4-5). Those that affect the deep gray matter more than the overlying white matter and cerebral cortex include hypertensive hemorrhage, some neurodegenerative diseases (primarily those related to movement disorders) and transmissible spongiform encephalopathies, as well as the rare hypothalamic hamartomas.

Ventricles. Few non-neoplastic CNS diseases are specific to the ventricles, their ependymal lining, and the choroid plexus (Table 4-6). Given the access of cerebrospinal fluid (CSF) between the subarachnoid space and ventricles, many processes, particularly infections, that produce meningitis may lead to ventricular inflammation. Indeed, one common autopsy sequela of remote meningitis is the presence of so-called granular ependymitis in which a focal stripping of the ependymal surface is accompanied by a mound-like proliferation of subependymal astrocytes (see chapter 2). Cytomegalovirus infection shows a striking tendency to affect the ependymal cells, yielding a true primary "ventriculitis"; however, diagnosing cytomegalovirus ventriculitis on surgical biopsy is rare. In addition, primary disorders of the choroid plexus affect the ventricles; the non-neoplastic choroid plexus lesions that are biopsied include xanthogranulomas (see chapter 8).

Cerebellum. In distinction to neoplastic diseases of the CNS, which show a distinct spectrum in the cerebellum, non-neoplastic diseases of the cerebellum are generally similar to those of the cerebrum (Table 4-7). Ischemic, hemorrhagic, and infectious diseases predominate. Of note are inflammatory conditions that display specificity, such as the paraneoplastic disorders that target Purkinje cells (see chapter 10), and the viral infections that affect the cerebellum more than other structures, such as rabies encephalitis (see chapter 7). The rhombic encephalitides of children, as their name suggests, preferentially affect posterior fossa structures, but these are a poorly defined group of entities pathologically.

Brain Stem. The brain stem per se is seldom biopsied because of the risk of damaging vital structures. Nonetheless, well-demarcated

Table 4-8

NON-NEOPLASTIC DISEASES OF THE CENTRAL NERVOUS SYSTEM THAT EFFECT THE BRAIN STEM

Infarction (see chapter 5)
Vascular diseases (see chapter 6)
Vascular malformations
Infections (see chapter 7)
Herpes zoster
Bacterial encephalitis (*Listeria*)
Demyelinating diseases (see chapter 9)
Multiple sclerosis
Acute disseminated encephalomyelitis
Reaction to neoplasms and antineoplastic therapy (see chapter 14)

processes affected the brain stem may be seen on biopsy specimens since diffuse processes may extend into the cerebellar peduncles, a site amenable to biopsy. As a result, those entities that more commonly affect the brain stem must be kept in mind (Table 4-8). Of primary importance are the acute demyelinating diseases, which commonly target brain stem structures. In addition, given the common use of radiation in the treatment of brain stem and base of skull neoplasms, consideration must be given to radiation damage in the setting of prior therapy. Finally, certain organisms (e.g., *Listeria*) may preferentially involve the brain stem and posterior fossa, as well as the leptomeninges surrounding the brain stem.

Spinal Cord. A wide variety of diseases demonstrate a predilection for the spinal cord (Table 4-9). In addition, paraspinal processes may impinge upon the coverings of the cord and must be considered in many diagnostic situations. The diagnosis of spinal cord conditions is difficult as many cord biopsies only yield minute specimens. Infarcts occur as a result of ischemic insults from causes as divergent as atherosclerotic emboli to embolic intervertebral disc material. Infections include those that arise from the cord itself, the meninges, the paraspinal soft tissues, and the vertebral bodies. Demyelinating diseases, such as the neuromyelitis optica (Devic) form of multiple sclerosis, also lead to biopsy. Pediatric lesions, such as neural tube closure abnormalities, may also come to the pathologist's attention as part of therapeutic procedures.

Table 4-9

NON-NEOPLASTIC DISEASES OF THE CENTRAL NERVOUS SYSTEM THAT AFFECT THE SPINAL CORD

Infarction, including embolic disk material (see chapter 5)
Vascular diseases (see chapter 6)
Vascular malformations
Infections (see chapter 7)
Abscess, spinal, and paraspinal
Herpes zoster
Schistosomiasis
Inflammatory processes (see chapter 8)
Sarcoidosis
Demyelinating diseases (see chapter 9)
Multiple sclerosis (neuromyelitis optica, Devic)
Adrenomyeloneuropathy (see chapter 12)
Trauma (see chapter 11)
Pediatric lesions (see chapter 14)
Neural tube closure abnormalities
Reaction to neoplasms and antineoplastic therapy (see chapter 14)

Current Clinical Course, Physical Findings, and Medications

The pathologist must have a clear idea of the patient's current clinical course and physical findings. The difference between an illness of acute or gradual onset, or of rapid or protracted course, can steer the pathologist and clinician to consider one diagnostic possibility over another. An association with specific neurologic signs or symptoms (e.g., myoclonus and sharp waves on electroencephalogram [EEG] in the setting of prion diseases) or with systemic conditions (e.g., liver failure, coagulopathy, or infectious diseases) can facilitate a correct diagnosis. In some situations, similar histologic findings are interpreted in different ways depending on the clinical course.

Current medications must also be considered since some may be responsible for the underlying neurologic condition, or produce histologic changes that overlay those of the primary neurologic condition. A full discussion of the neurologic effects of specific medicines is beyond the scope of this text, and the reader is referred to reference texts (1,2).

Age and Gender

Age is an important parameter to consider because some non-neoplastic diseases of the

CNS have a predilection for specific age groups, as shown in Table 4-10. For example, in biopsies from patients in the first 5 years of life, particular consideration should be given to the possibility of infectious, postinfectious, metabolic, and developmental conditions. In older children, in addition to these major categories, attention should be paid to the possibility of vascular diseases and toxic/drug-related causes. In adults, the major differential entities still include infections, particularly related to immunocompromise or travel, and toxic/drug-related conditions, but also expand to inflammatory and autoimmune diseases as well as reactions to neoplasms. In older adults, the most likely differential diagnostic entities shift considerably to include vascular diseases, from atherosclerosis-related infarcts to vasculitis to amyloid angiopathy, and neurodegenerative diseases.

Most non-neoplastic diseases of the CNS that are biopsied affect both sexes in roughly equal numbers. Biopsies of those non-neoplastic diseases that occur more often in men or women are rare, although some autoimmune diseases such as multiple sclerosis more commonly affect women. Certain variants of paraneoplastic disease (see chapter 10) occur in patients with breast or gynecological cancers, such as cerebellar degeneration from anti-Purkinje cell antibodies, but clinical features and laboratory tests usually suffice for diagnosis. Other examples of diseases that preferentially affect one gender include X-linked hereditary conditions, such as adrenoleukodystrophy, Pelizaeus-Merzbacher disease, and Fabry disease, but these rarely if ever come to the attention of the surgical pathologist (see chapter 12).

Table 4-10

NON-NEOPLASTIC DISEASES OF THE CENTRAL NERVOUS SYSTEM THAT AFFECT APPROXIMATE AGE GROUPS

Age Under 5 Years
Viral meningoencephalitis (see chapter 7)
Bacterial meningoencephalitis (see chapter 7)
Sequelae of fetal infections (see chapter 7)
Rasmussen encephalitis (see chapter 13)
Acute disseminated encephalomyelitis (ADEM)/acute hemorrhagic leukoencephalitis (AHL) (see chapter 9)
Subacute sclerosing panencephalitis (SSPE) (see chapter 10)
Metabolic diseases (see chapter 12)
Malformative lesions (see chapter 13)
Age 5 to 20 Years
Vascular malformations (see chapter 6)
Viral meningoencephalitis
Bacterial meningoencephalitis
Sequelae of fetal infections
Rasmussen encephalitis
ADEM/AHL
Toxic and drug-related conditions (see chapters 10 and 14)
SSPE
Metabolic diseases
Malformative lesions
Age 20 to 50 Years
Vascular malformations
Brain abscess (see chapter 7)
Infections in immunocompromised (see chapter 7)
Infections after travel (see chapter 7)
Inflammatory processes (see chapter 8)
Multiple sclerosing (see chapter 9)
Toxic and drug-related conditions
Malformative lesions (see chapter 13)
Reaction to neoplasms or antineoplastic therapies (see chapter 14)
Age over 50 Years
Ischemia, infarction, and intracerebral hemorrhage (see chapter 5)
Vasculitides, e.g., temporal arteritis (see chapter 6)
Cerebral amyloid angiopathy (see chapter 6)
Infections (see chapter 7)
Inflammatory diseases, e.g., paraneoplastic processes and rheumatoid arthritis
Neurodegenerative diseases (see chapter 10)
Transmissible spongiform encephalopathies (see chapter 10)
Medication-related conditions (see chapter 10)
Reaction to neoplasms or antineoplastic therapies

Past Medical and Family History

Attention to a number of aspects of the patient's past medical and family history is important. All coexisting medical conditions and all prior major medical issues must be known. Information about drug and alcohol use is crucial in older children and adults, since both may be related to specific conditions (e.g., vascular conditions in intravenous drug use or coagulopathy and history of falls in alcoholism).

The spectrum of diseases that affect the CNS is greatly altered in the immunocompromised state. In addition to lymphoid and smooth muscle neoplasms, non-neoplastic diseases, particularly infections, are found more frequently. Of particular importance are those infections occurring in the setting of medication-related immunosuppression for organ transplant or autoimmune disease, and those occurring in the setting of HIV infection. Toxoplasmosis ranks highest in the list of immunocompromise-related infections that result in biopsy, with fungal and mycobacterial infections following (see chapter 7).

An accurate travel history is important when assessing inflammatory lesions of unknown etiology that may prove to be infectious, as certain infectious conditions of the CNS are endemic to particular regions of the world (see chapter 7). In South and Central America, for example, cysticercosis is a common cause of intracranial masses; in India, tuberculoma is a frequent cerebral mass lesion.

Knowledge of prior therapies is relevant in many situations, particularly if the patient has been treated with radiation therapy or chemotherapy for a neoplasm in the past. Effects on the CNS may follow therapy for systemic neoplasms in addition to CNS neoplasms. For instance, chemotherapeutic agents such as 5-FU, used for the treatment of gastrointestinal cancers, can affect the white matter (see chapter 14).

A family history is important in some situations, particularly the metabolic conditions that most commonly affect children (see chapter 12) and early-onset neurodegenerative diseases (see chapter 10). Given the recent advances in understanding the genetic basis of coagulopathies and hypercoagulable states, a family history is also important in the evaluation of cerebral hemorrhages and infarcts.

Laboratory Findings

Many patients have had considerable laboratory workups prior to brain biopsy, since clinicians attempt to secure diagnoses in a less invasive manner than through a CNS biopsy. As a result, nearly all patients coming for brain biopsy lack a definitive diagnosis. Nonetheless, knowledge of laboratory test results can aid the pathologist in weighting entities in the differential diagnosis. Clearly, a list of neurologically relevant laboratory tests is beyond the scope of this book and the reader is referred to recent neurology and laboratory medicine textbooks for more complete information (1–4).

Neuroimaging Features

The pathologist must be generally aware of how neuroimaging information affects the differential diagnosis. At the same time, it must be recognized that neuroradiology is a complex discipline that is well beyond the scope of this book. The reader is referred to a number of practical neuroimaging texts for further details (5,6).

In general, neuroradiologic information breaks down into two sets of data: anatomic and functional. Anatomic information relates to the location of the abnormalities and their relationship to the adjacent CNS tissues. As discussed in the first part of this chapter, the precise localization of a process can narrow the differential diagnosis considerably. Functional data relates to the dynamic characteristics of the lesions with different imaging techniques. Again, the functional features of a process (e.g., whether it is metabolically active or whether the blood-brain barrier is intact) can narrow the differential diagnosis in important ways.

The major modalities used for evaluation of non-neoplastic neurologic conditions include magnetic resonance imaging (MRI), computerized tomography (CT) scanning, single photon/positron emission computerized tomography (SPECT/PET), and angiography. Each of these modalities has multiple variations that give different sets of information. For example, the type of labeled compound used in PET imaging determines what type of data is gathered, from glucose or oxygen utilization to blood flow. MRI, in particular, has burgeoned with the discovery of numerous imaging parameters. By "weighting" images, one can obtain T1-weighted and T2-weighted images that provide complementary information about processes: for instance, a cerebral infarct appears dark on T1 images and bright on T2, whereas an acute hemorrhage appears bright on both T1 and T2, and bright on CT scans. The use of contrast agents also provides important information, with contrast-enhancement favoring certain entities over others. Other useful MRI techniques include diffuse-weighted imaging, which is particularly helpful in the early phase of cerebral infarcts, and MRI spectroscopy, in which selected molecules are measured (e.g., N-acetylaspartate [NAA], a marker of neurons, and lactate, a marker of hypoxia).

As a result of these many incarnations of MRI and other imaging approaches, modern neuroradiologic evaluations typically narrow the differential diagnosis extensively prior to biopsy. In nearly all situations, however, the radiologic conclusion remains a differential diagnosis more than a definitive diagnosis of a specific entity. At the present time, none of these investigations is a substitute for biopsy and direct tissue examination. The neuroradiologist provides essential information to help guide a final diagnosis, but in most situations, a final diagnosis relies on the pathologist's interpretation of tissue.

Given the complexity of neuroradiology, the surgical pathologist must rely on close contact with neuroradiologists in evaluating cases. For major entities in this book, the basic neuroimaging features are given in the hope that it will help pathologists without immediate access to an expert neuroradiologist. The optimal workup of a case, however, requires consultation with a radiologist familiar with neurologic differential diagnoses.

REFERENCES

1. Ropper AH, Brown RH. Adams and Victor's principles of neurology. New York: McGraw-Hill; 2005.
2. Love S, Louis DN, Ellison DW, eds. Greenfield's neuropathology, 8th ed. London: Hodder Arnold; 2008.
3. Lewandrowski K. Clinical chemistry: laboratory management and clinical correlations. Philadelphia: Lippincot Williams & Wilkins; 2002.
4. Spencer PS, Schaumburg HH, Ludolph AC. Experimental and clinical neurotoxicology. New York: Oxford University Press; 2000.
5. Grossman RI, Yousem DM. Neuroradiology: the requisites. Philadelphia: C.V. Mosby; 2003.
6. Atlas SW, ed. Magnetic resonance imaging of the brain and spine, 3rd ed. Philadelphia: Lipincott Williams & Wilkins; 2002.

5 ISCHEMIA, INFARCT, AND INTRACEREBRAL HEMORRHAGE

Cerebrovascular disease is the second leading cause of death worldwide and a major cause of long-term disability. Despite the frequency of cerebrovascular disease, the development of a useful and comprehensive approach to its histopathologic classification has been a relatively slow process. Earlier classifications were largely based on animal studies that did not always accurately mirror the evolution of changes observed in human tissue. For those cases that come to autopsy, however, most pathologists can confidently render an accurate descriptive diagnosis and, in many cases, even determine an etiology. For patients who survive, the disease is largely managed medically and rarely comes to the attention of the pathologist. Given these observations, it is not surprising that few general pathologists accumulate significant experience with biopsy interpretation. The goal of this chapter is to present guidelines that will help the general pathologist to demystify the surgical pathologic diagnosis of the disorders encompassed by the term cerebrovascular disease. The key questions addressed are: "What is the differential diagnosis of an infarct and how do you work it up to establish the correct diagnosis?" and "What is the workup for a blood clot?"

CEREBRAL ISCHEMIA

Ischemia refers to a decrease in the cerebral blood flow (CBF) sufficient to impair cellular function. Ischemic disorders of the central nervous system (CNS) are common diseases, albeit with different pathogeneses and clinical manifestations, and signal derangements of basic pathophysiologic principles. The brain is highly dependent on adequate blood flow, and a consistent supply of oxygen and glucose is essential to maintain neuronal function. Under normal circumstances, the brain receives 15 percent of the resting cardiac output and accounts for 20 percent of oxygen consumption. In order to ensure an uninterrupted supply of vital nutrients, CBF is maintained at a constant value of 55 mL/100 g/min by the phenomenon known as autoregulation, which allows arteries and arterioles to adjust their resistance in response to changes in cerebral perfusion pressure (1). Autoregulation fails when the mean arterial pressure drops below 60 mm Hg in the normotensive individual (2). In patients with chronic hypertension, the curve of autoregulation is shifted upward. The consequence of this failure is inadequate CBF to maintain normal cellular function.

Ischemia is usually coupled with the lack of oxygen, or anoxia, in the region(s) involved. The severity of the ischemic process can be defined as moderate if the CBF is 15 mL/100 g/min and severe if the CBF is less than 10 mL/100 g/min (3). Moderate ischemia produces reversible or nonlethal injury to neurons with the possibility of functional recovery; severe ischemia results in irreversible or lethal injury and cellular death. The degree of neuronal injury after an ischemic event is modulated by key factors such as blood glucose levels, body temperature, and the duration and degree of ischemia. It is estimated that lethal or irreversible neuronal injury supervenes after 5 minutes of anoxia-ischemia (4).

For practical purposes, all lesions attributed to ischemia, anoxia, oligemia, hypoxia, and anoxia/ischemia are considered under the heading of ischemia. Ischemic lesions are classified according to their topography and their presumed etiology. In the following discussion, special attention is given to issues that might confront the surgical pathologist.

Ischemia, regardless of the cause, gives rise to a constant pattern of brain injury that is either generalized or localized. As the name implies, *global ischemia* refers to widespread neuronal injury caused by conditions such as hypotension and transient cardiac arrest in which a decrease in CBF affects all arterial territories in the brain and spinal cord. The other principal pattern of *focal ischemia* leads to a well-circumscribed area of infarct with irreversible central necrosis surrounded by an area of potentially reversible tissue injury known as the ischemic penumbra in the distribution of a specific arterial territory.

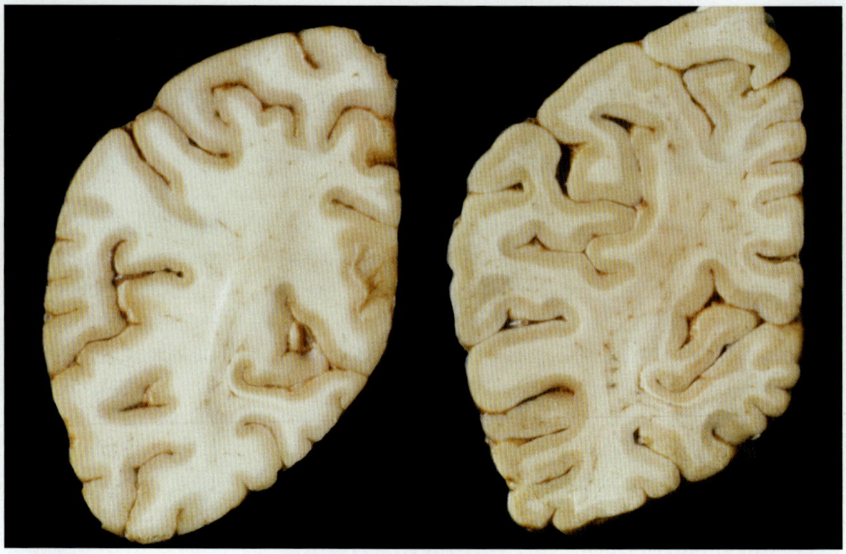

Figure 5-1

ACUTE ANOXIC-ISCHEMIC ENCEPHALOPATHY

Left: A coronal section of the left cerebral hemisphere through the posterior parietal lobe shows diffuse gray dusky discoloration of the cerebral cortex.

Right: Normal brain.

Atherosclerosis and embolic disease are major pathophysiologic mechanisms that predispose to the development of focal ischemia

Global Ischemia

Global ischemia is characterized by a decrease in the CBF that affects all arterial territories of the brain, and to some extent, the spinal cord, without vascular occlusion. The most common clinical conditions associated with episodes of global anoxia/ischemia are hypotension, transient cardiac arrest, respiratory arrest, prolonged status epilepticus, cranial trauma with associated increased intracranial pressure, subarachnoid hemorrhage, strangulation, and near drowning (3,5). The parenchymal lesions associated with these conditions vary from case to case, but tend to be bilateral and symmetric in distribution. The various patterns of CNS injury may be explained by the concept of selective vulnerability, which describes the susceptibility to the effects of ischemia of certain neuronal groups over others within the CNS.

The following classification lists the six major patterns of global anoxic-ischemic damage encountered in the adult brain.

1. *Global Irreversible Anoxic-Ischemic Encephalopathy ("Respirator or Nonperfused Brain")*. The initial phase associated with the arrest of blood flow to the brain is characterized by massive cerebral edema and intracranial hypertension. If the intracranial pressure increases and becomes greater than the systemic blood pressure, CBF ceases and the brain undergoes a process of "autolysis in vivo." Nonperfused brain is soft and friable, and has a dusky brown discoloration; the cerebellum tends to disintegrate easily during the gross examination. Herniation and hemorrhagic necrosis of the cerebellar tonsils are usually present. As a result, fragments of necrotic cerebellum may be present in the subdural or subarachnoid spaces of the spinal cord. The pituitary gland frequently shows similar changes.

Sectioning of nonperfused brain reveals blurring of the interface between the cortex and the subjacent white matter, accompanied by patchy or generalized dusky discoloration of the cerebral and cerebellar cortical ribbon, and deep gray and brain stem nuclei (fig. 5-1). Areas of hemorrhagic necrosis may be present (fig. 5-2). The ventricular system is often compressed and deeper portions of the centrum semiovale may appear pink due to resistance to fixation of edematous or necrotic brain.

Microscopic examination usually, although not invariably, discloses acute neuronal injury. Cells exhibit shrinkage, eosinophilic or vacuolated cytoplasm, and peripherally located hyperchromatic nuclei; vacuolation of the neuropil indicative of edema; mild gliosis; and vascular congestion (6). Macrophages or an inflammatory reaction is not present unless there is an associated infarct (fig. 5-3). Surprisingly, the macroscopic appearance of nonperfused brain is often far more dramatic than the microscopic picture. Brain tissue from individuals who have

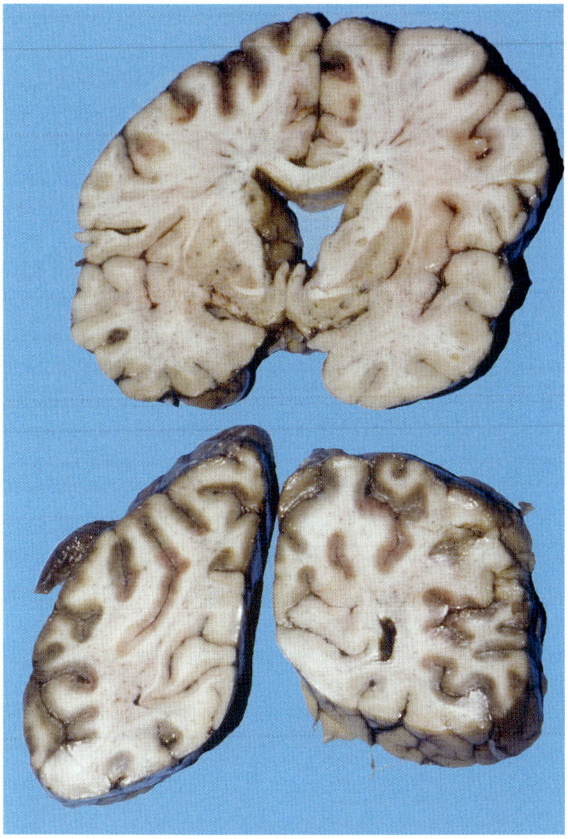

Figure 5-2

ACUTE ANOXIC-ISCHEMIC ENCEPHALOPATHY

Changes associated with hemorrhagic cortical necrosis and edema in the territories of the major cerebral arteries.

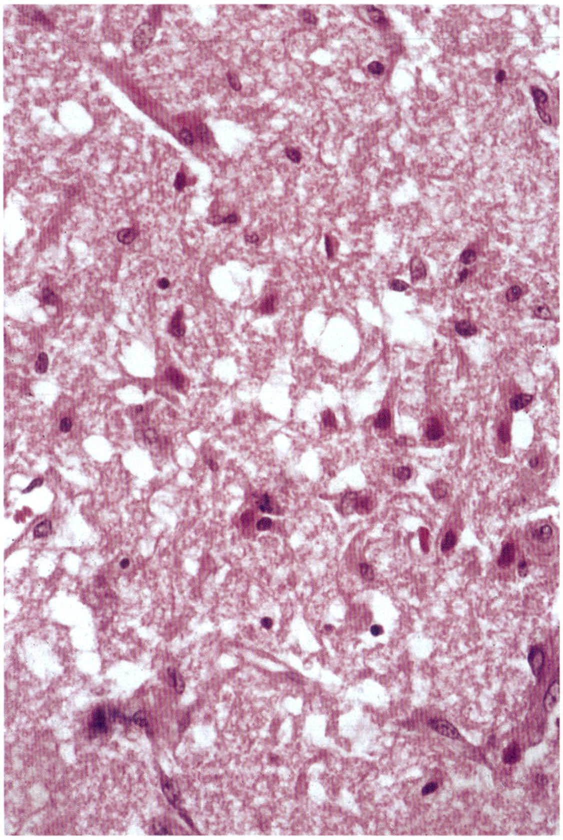

Figure 5-3

ACUTE ANOXIC-ISCHEMIC ENCEPHALOPATHY

The cerebral cortex exhibits eosinophilic neurons, vacuolation, and absence of inflammation and macrophages.

survived in a "vegetative state" for several weeks, months, or even years connected to a respirator demonstrates diffuse brain atrophy of variable severity (fig. 5-4). Microscopically, this atrophy correlates with extensive neuronal loss and gliosis involving all brain regions (fig. 5-5). Because of obvious environmental health concerns, the most important entity in the differential diagnosis of brain atrophy related to global anoxia-ischemia is prion disease in which the degree of gliosis mimics a spongiform encephalopathy (Creutzfeldt-Jakob disease; see chapter 10).

2. *Hippocampal Sclerosis*. Selective loss of large pyramidal neurons in the CA-1 field (Sommer sector) of the hippocampus is the hallmark of hippocampal sclerosis. More extensive lesions may involve the subiculum or the entire hippocampus (4). A delay in neuronal cell death in the hippocampus has been demonstrated in

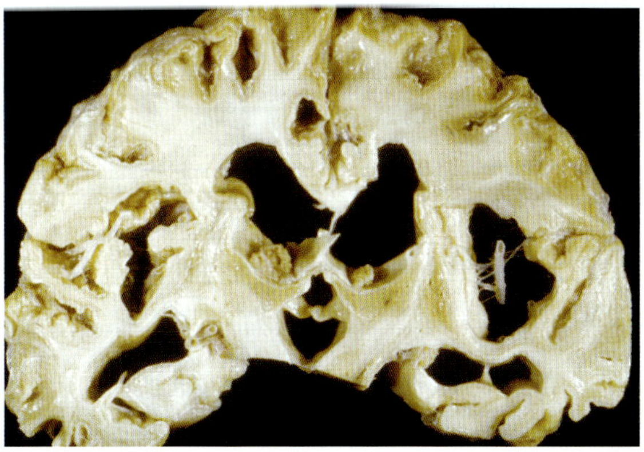

Figure 5-4

CHRONIC ANOXIC-ISCHEMIC ENCEPHALOPATHY

Marked, diffuse cerebral atrophy in a person who survived in a "vegetative state" for 2 years. (Figs. 5-4 and 5-5 are from the same patient.)

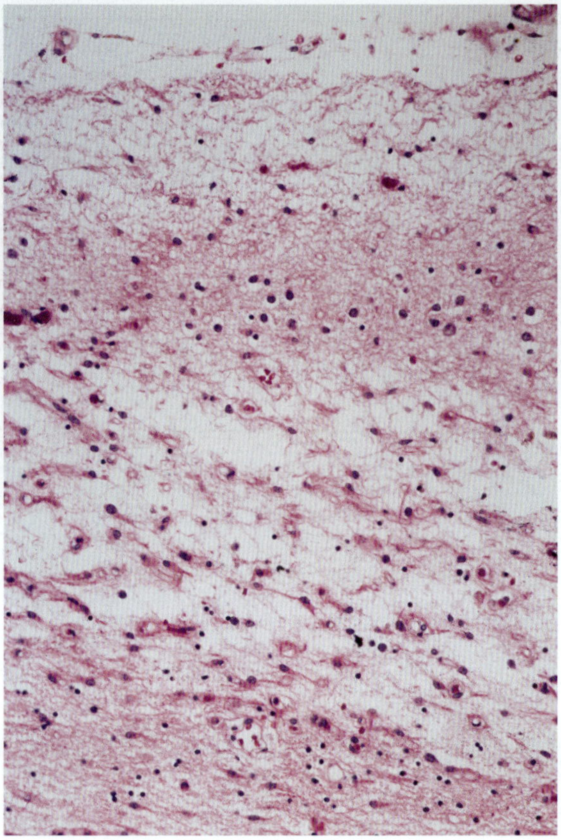

Figure 5-5

CHRONIC ANOXIC-ISCHEMIC ENCEPHALOPATHY

The marked atrophy of the cerebral cortex is related to the loss of neurons and glial cells, and the cavitation of deeper cortical layers.

humans who survived longer after the initial injury (7).

The initial stage of ischemic damage encompasses not only acute neuronal injury but also the presence of macrophages and reactive astrocytes. Gliosis is the predominant cellular reaction visible in later stages. The lesion may be observed grossly as an area of softening and gray discoloration within the hippocampal formation. Unilateral or bilateral atrophy may be prominent in some cases. Hippocampal sclerosis may accompany severe or repeated episodes of hypoglycemia and is the most common histopathologic finding in temporal lobectomy specimens from patients with intractable seizures (see chapter 13).

3. *Laminar Necrosis*. Selective neuronal loss caused by anoxic-ischemic injury occurs in certain layers of the cortex, especially layers 3 to 5, resulting in laminar necrosis. At gross examination, slit-like cavities are present in deep cortical areas (fig. 5-6). Initial microscopic examination shows coagulative necrosis and conspicuous loss of all cellular elements in these cortical layers (fig. 5-7). Later stages are characterized by extensive cellular loss, microcystic change, vascular proliferation, and gliosis, sometimes giving the cerebral cortex a macroscopically granular appearance (granular atrophy) (fig. 5-8).

4. *Isolated Purkinje Cell Loss*. Loss of Purkinje cells, characterized by acidophilic necrosis in the cerebellar cortex, may be focal or more

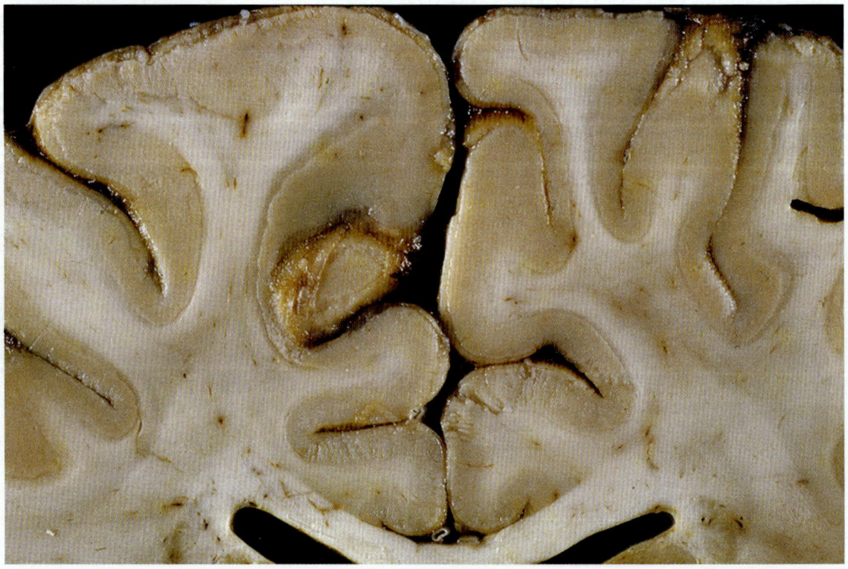

Figure 5-6

LAMINAR NECROSIS

The lesion is the linear cavity of the deep cortical layers in the left superior frontal gyrus.

widespread (8). Purkinje cell loss is a nonspecific finding associated with such conditions as global anoxia-ischemia, chronic alcoholism, mercury intoxication, and treatment with antiepileptic medications like phenytoin. Purkinje cell loss is followed by a characteristic proliferation of Bergmann astrocytes (a form of gliosis), and the presence of "torpedoes" and "empty baskets" (fig. 5-9). The term torpedo refers to localized swellings of Purkinje cell axons within the granular cell layer, whereas basket cells are interneurons with an inhibitory effect on Purkinje cells (fig. 5-10). As a result of Purkinje cell loss, the dendritic tree of the basket cells is devoid of neuronal contact and is known as an empty basket (fig. 5-11). Special stains for nerve fibers, such as the Bielschowsky silver impregnation method, and immunohistochemistry for neurofilament proteins are useful for accentuating torpedoes and empty baskets.

5. *Arterial Border Zone, or "Watershed," Infarcts.* The end zones of brain parenchyma, which are irrigated by the distal branches of the cerebral arteries, experience the most severe ischemia during global cerebral hypoperfusion. Arterial border zone, or watershed, infarcts tend to occur in the cerebrum, cerebellum, and spinal cord between the most distal territories supplied by two or more major arteries (9). In the cerebrum, these infarcts are easy to recognize as wedge-shaped areas of hemorrhagic cortical necrosis along the middle frontal and orbital gyri, corresponding

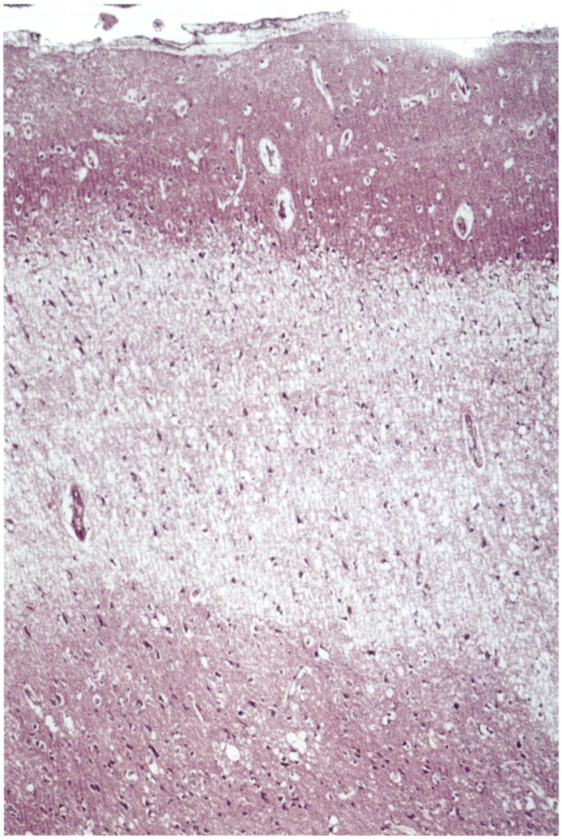

Figure 5-7

LAMINAR NECROSIS

Necrosis involves layers 3 to 5 of the cerebral cortex.

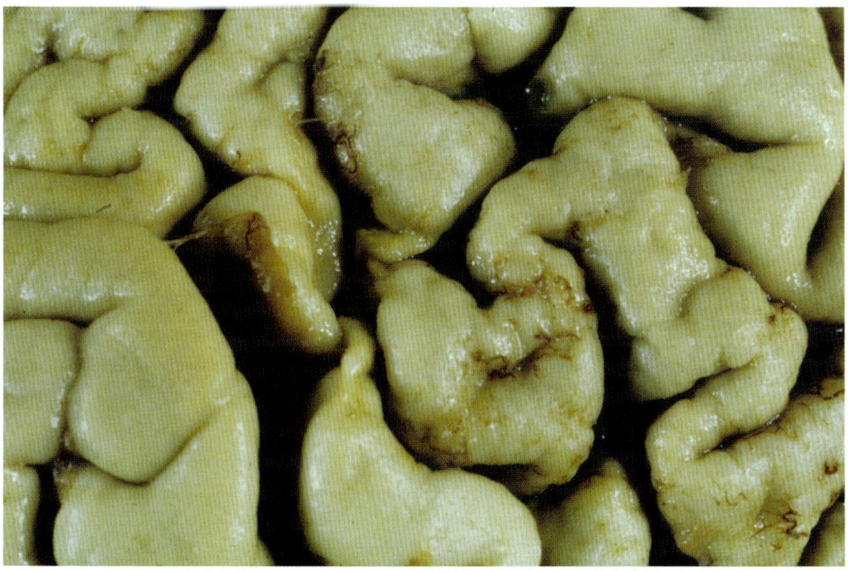

Figure 5-8

GRANULAR NECROSIS

Old laminar necrosis may be associated with cortical granular atrophy.

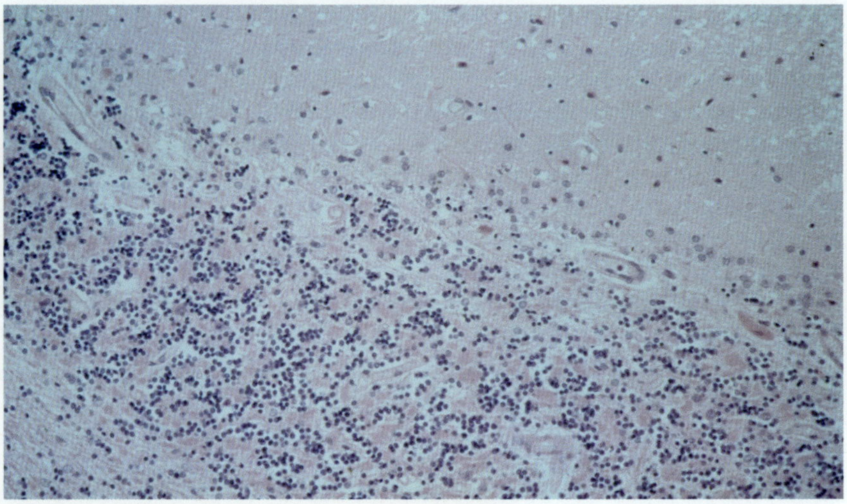

Figure 5-9

ISOLATED PURKINJE CELL LOSS

Selective loss of Purkinje cells in the cerebellar cortex is associated with Bergmann astrocytes. (Also see fig. 2-16.)

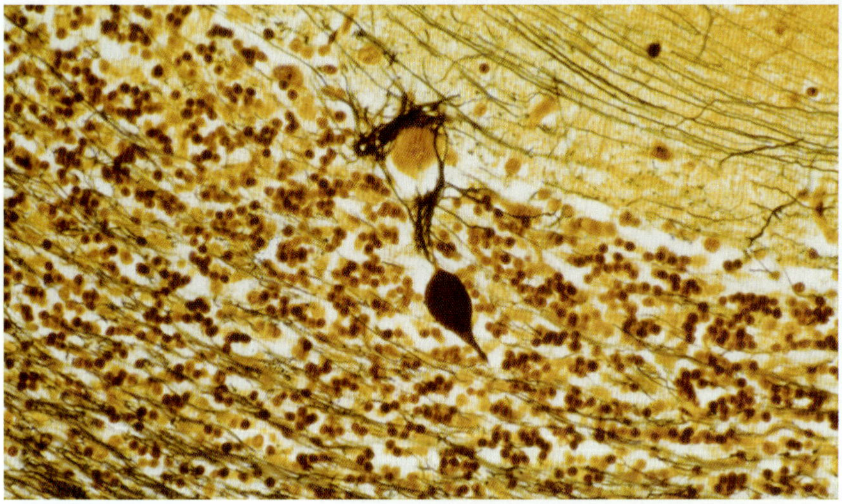

Figure 5-10

TORPEDO

The loss of Purkinje cells is associated with a dilated axon, or torpedo, within the granular cell layer (silver impregnation).

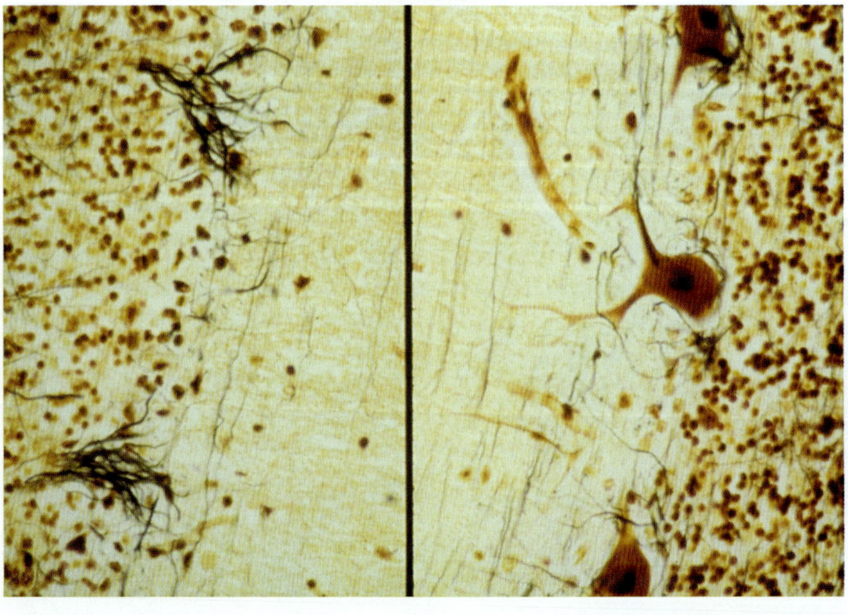

Figure 5-11

EMPTY BASKETS

Left: Purkinje cell loss in the cerebellar cortex is associated with preserved dendritic trees of basket cells lacking neuronal contacts.

Right: Preserved Purkinje cells (silver impregnation).

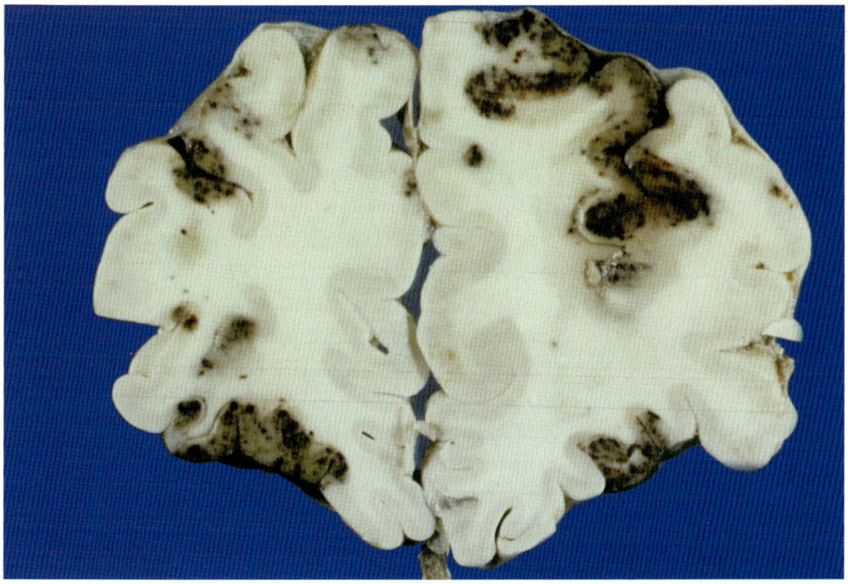

Figure 5-12

ARTERIAL BORDER ZONE INFARCTS

Bilateral hemorrhagic cortical infarcts in border zone areas between the anterior (ACA) and middle cerebral arteries (MCA). These lesions resulted from hypotension during heart surgery 9 days before the patient's death.

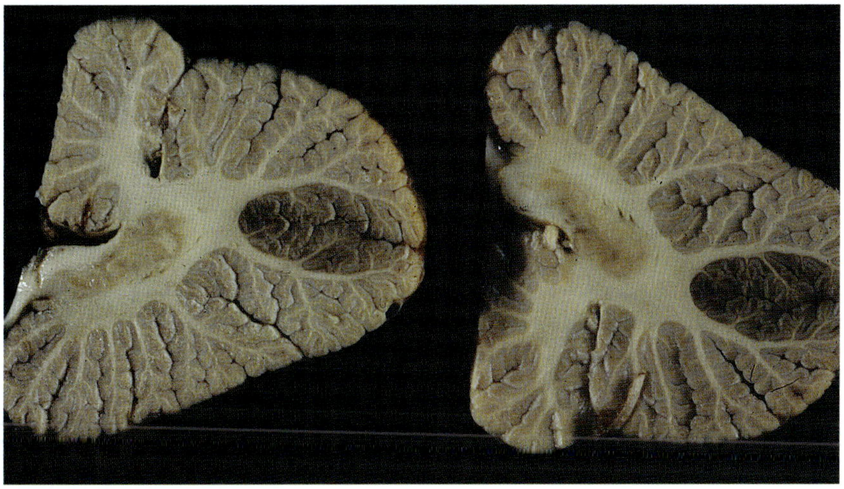

Figure 5-13

ARTERIAL BORDER ZONE INFARCT

The cerebellum shows a "watershed" infarct in the cortical area between the territories of the major arteries.

to the border zone territories between the anterior and middle cerebral arteries. They are also seen in the parietooccipital notch, or border zone of the territories of the three major cerebral arteries (fig. 5-12). Older lesions are recognized by the appearance of granular atrophy of the external surface of the cerebral cortex. In the cerebellum, the border zone between the superior and the anterior inferior/posterior inferior cerebellar arteries is located between the superior and inferior cerebellum (fig. 5-13). In the spinal cord, the most vulnerable region is in the thoracic cord at the border zone between the anterior spinal artery and the radicular artery of Adamkiewicz.

6. *Subcortical Leukoencephalopathy.* Cerebral white matter is also susceptible to anoxic/ischemic injury, although to a lesser degree than gray matter. Ischemic white matter lesions may occur in subcortical areas that are supplied by the long penetrating terminal small arteries and arterioles. White matter deprived of adequate circulation is identified as infarcts or as ischemic foci that can have a gray discoloration (fig. 5-14) (10,11). In the case of infarcts, microscopic examination shows necrosis, accompanied by variable inflammatory infiltrates, depending on the age of the lesion. The more subtle lesions associated with leukoencephalopathy are characterized by patchy myelin loss, the presence of macrophages, and swollen

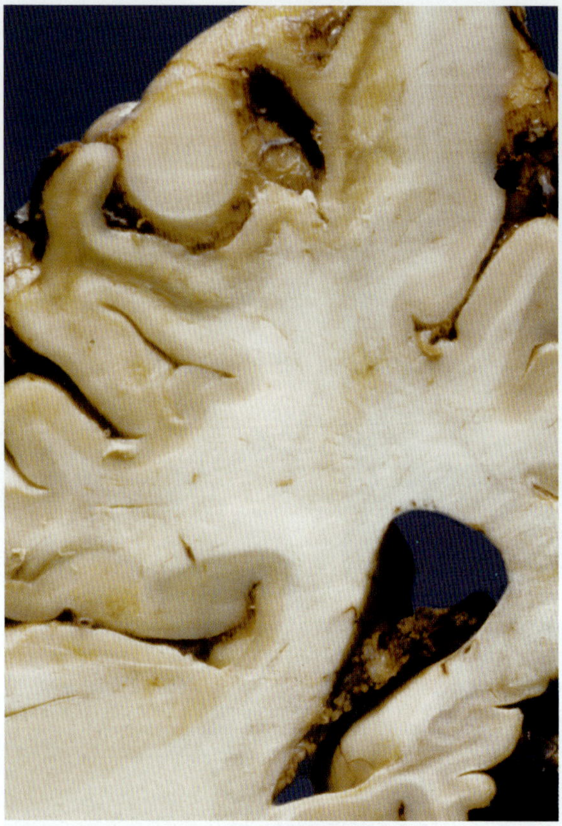

Figure 5-14

SUBCORTICAL LEUKOENCEPHALOPATHY

The parietal subcortical white matter appears gray and cavitated.

axons with relative preservation of the axonal population.

Cerebral Infarct

Definition. *Infarcts* are areas of coagulative necrosis that develop in the brain and spinal cord as a result of severe ischemia, usually secondary to an arterial or venous occlusion.

General Comments. Arterial infarcts commonly result from the occlusion of either a large or small artery supplying the brain. Most infarcts are located in the territory of the middle cerebral artery (MCA). In *MCA infarcts*, the occlusion may be either in the main trunk, between its origin at the internal carotid artery and its bifurcation, or at the trifurcation, with the resulting lesion affecting the basal ganglia, white matter, and various cortical areas (12). If the occlusion is located in a peripheral cortical branch, the ischemic lesion is found in the territory supplied by the respective artery. Occlusion of a lenticulostriate artery produces a lesion described as a *lacunar infarct,* or *lacune,* with a diameter typically less than 1 cm in the basal ganglia.

Arterial occlusion is caused by complicated atherosclerosis, various sources of embolism, vasculopathies, coagulopathies, vasospasm associated with subarachnoid hemorrhage, and extrinsic compression due to herniation of brain tissue. The size and appearance of an infarct depend on several factors including the caliber and type of the blood vessel occluded, the mode and duration of the luminal occlusion, and the adequacy of collateral circulation.

Clinical Features. In clinical parlance, the term *stroke* (ischemic or hemorrhagic) is a cardinal manifestation of underlying cerebrovascular disease and refers to the abrupt onset of a focal or global neurologic deficit or altered level of consciousness. For the most part, there are no telltale clinical features that reliably distinguish ischemic from hemorrhagic stroke, although ischemia is by far the leading cause. Common clinical signs include abrupt onset of hemiparesis, monoparesis, or quadriparesis; visual field deficits; diplopia; dysarthria; ataxia; vertigo; aphasia; and a sudden decrease in the level of consciousness. There is a plethora of clinical syndromes associated with occlusion of specific arteries. Familiarity with individual syndromes not only helps the clinician to localize the lesion and guide appropriate management, but in many instances, points to whether the deficit is of vascular origin or of an alternate etiology. Although uncommon, the signs/symptoms caused by a mass lesion such as a neoplasm can mimic a stroke, although the location rarely conforms to a specific vascular territory. Given the obvious therapeutic and prognostic consequences, it is the latter scenario for which the pathologist needs to be particularly vigilant. As a result, it is especially helpful for those tasked with rendering a tissue diagnosis to be acquainted with the clinical and anatomic hallmarks of the principal stroke syndromes.

There are four major syndromes caused by the disruption of blood supply to respective cerebrovascular distributions, as well as the small lacunar infarcts: 1) *Anterior cerebral artery (ACA) occlusion*, although rarely isolated, affects medial frontal lobe function, producing altered mental status, impaired judgment, contralateral lower extremity weakness, hypesthesia, and gait apraxia. 2) *MCA occlusion* causes a clinical syndrome that produces contralateral hemiparesis, contralateral hypesthesia, ipsilateral hemianopsia, and gaze preference toward the side of the lesion. Agnosia is another common manifestation. Receptive or expressive aphasia may result if the lesion occurs in the dominant hemisphere. 3) *Posterior cerebral artery (PCA) occlusion* causes occipital lobe infarction, and therefore, contralateral visual field loss. This type of occlusion may also cause contralateral hemiparesis, altered mental status, and impaired memory. 4) *Vertebrobasilar artery occlusions* are notoriously challenging to diagnose because of the complex mixture of cranial nerve, cerebellar, and brain stem deficits at presentation. The clinical manifestations depend on the level and extent of the infarction in the brain.

A brief review of the pertinent neuroanatomy may aid in localizing and identifying the source of the occlusion. The two major branches of the vertebral arteries are arteries to the spinal cord and the posterior inferior cerebellar artery that supplies the inferior cerebellum and lateral medulla. The two vertebral arteries unite to form the basilar artery. The major branches of the basilar artery are the anterior inferior cerebellar artery and the superior cerebellar artery. The basilar artery terminates by bifurcating into the two posterior cerebral arteries that supply the medial temporal lobe, occipital lobe, and portions of the thalamus. Oculomotor deficits and/or ataxia with crossed sensory/motor deficits are the cardinal features of basilar artery infarction. Lower cranial nerve deficits and/or ataxia with crossed sensory deficits point to occlusion of the vertebral artery.

Lacunar infarcts, which result from small vessel occlusive disease, usually occur in patients with longstanding hypertension or diabetes mellitus. Recurrent stereotyped episodes of pure motor or sensory dysfunction, often waxing and waning, are known harbingers of imminent lacunar infarction, with permanent deficits resembling those of the premonitory symptoms. Small infarcts in the basal ganglia or the pons, close to central motor pathways, appear to be the primary lesions in these cases. Specific syndromes associated with lacunar infarcts include hemiparesis without sensory loss, pure sensory or pure motor loss, and ataxia-crural paresis, among others. The pathophysiology is disputed, but has been ascribed to an in situ process called lipohyalinosis (arteriolar sclerosis), or alternatively, to emboli lodging in the terminal branches of larger vessels. Recent research suggests that genetic factors may play an important role (13). The final common denominator is thought to be hemodynamic compromise of small penetrating arterial territories. Clinically, the diagnosis rests on the presentation and exclusion of other causes.

The distinguishing features of embolic infarcts include a documented source of embolism, maximal neurologic deficit at onset, involvement of multiple cerebrovascular territories, tendency toward hemorrhagic transformation, an enhanced risk of syncope or seizure associated with presentation, and a lower likelihood of premonitory transient ischemic attacks.

Radiologic Findings. Although traditional clinical diagnostic skills are still essential, neuroimaging strategies are assuming an increasingly important role in the initial evaluation and management of patients with cerebrovascular disease. Given that the first few hours of an ischemic event are the most critical for attempts to salvage brain tissue, accurate and rapid diagnosis is crucial in determining clinical outcome. Unequivocal imaging evidence of an ischemic lesion confirms the clinical suspicion of an ischemic event and rules out other differential diagnoses. The pattern of damage may even be indicative of stroke origin (e.g., a multiplicity of acute lesions in different vascular territories would favor an embolic origin). Since most infarcts that are biopsied resemble neoplastic or infectious processes, it is advantageous for the pathologist to be familiar with the basic radiologic findings.

Radiographically, a cortical infarct is notable for its wedge-shaped configuration that involves both gray and white matter, with its base in prominent relation to the cortical surface (fig. 5-15). The infarcted zone has sharp edges that conform to a specific vascular territory or territories. The size of the infarct depends on the vessel occluded and the extent of the collateral circulation. Peripheral contrast enhancement may appear after 7 to 10 days and simulate a glioblastoma. For the most part,

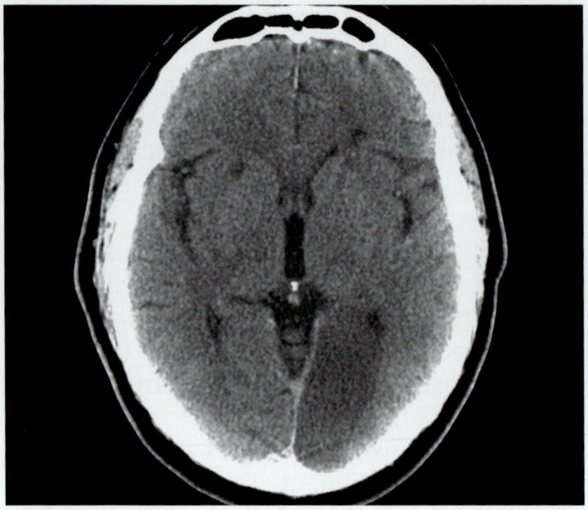

Figure 5-15

CEREBRAL INFARCT

A noncontrast axial computerized tomography (CT) scan demonstrates an asymmetric hypodensity within the medial aspect of the right occipital lobe.

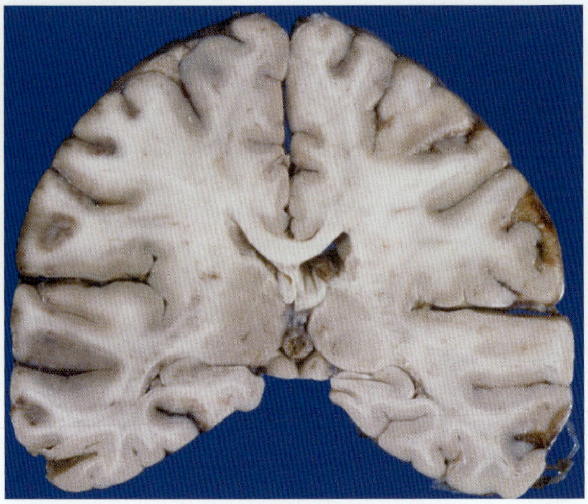

Figure 5-16

EARLY STAGE OF ISCHEMIC INFARCT

An infarct in the territory supplied by the left MCA is associated with blurring of the white-gray matter junction and dusky cortical discoloration. Survival was 4 days poststroke.

the shape of the lesion and its cortical location combine to alert the radiologist and pathologist to the greater likelihood of an ischemic lesion and minimize that of a glioblastoma (14).

A computerized tomography (CT) scan may be negative for the first 24 to 48 hours. The magnetic resonance imaging (MRI) scan is usually positive within 3 to 4 hours following a stroke. Increased hypointensity and thickening of the gray matter with concomitant effacement of the adjacent sulci are considered diagnostic signs of a cortical infarct on T1-weighted images. The affected tissue becomes hyperintense on T2-weighted images. Embolic infarcts are more frequently hemorrhagic and limited to a smaller arterial branch. Gyriform hyperintensity on T1-weighted imaging is considered a reliable sign of petechial hemorrhage in the infarcted cortex. If an infarct is due to systemic hypotension or hypoxia, the area of infarction is commonly found in the watershed areas between the major vascular territories (14).

Infarcts in the deep gray matter (basal ganglia/thalamus) often assume a spherical configuration. Lacunar infarcts are typically small, multiple lesions up to 1 cm in size, with a predilection for the basal ganglia, thalamus, and brain stem. On T2-weighted images, lacunar infarcts are visible as foci of increased signal intensity.

Laboratory Findings. General laboratory studies that are essential and may shed additional light on the etiology of the cerebrovascular accident include a complete blood count (to rule out polycythemia or leukemia), a chemistry panel (metabolic disorders that may mimic cerebrovascular or underlying causes, such as diabetes), and cardiac biomarkers because of the association of cerebral vascular disease with coronary artery disease.

Gross Findings. Based on their gross appearance, brain infarcts are classified as ischemic, hemorrhagic, lacunar, or incomplete, although these features can be difficult to assess in piecemeal biopsy specimens. Both gross and microscopic features evolve over time in a predictable pattern that often correlates with the clinical course.

Ischemic Infarct. Ischemic infarcts are also known as *pale infarcts* due to the absence of a hemorrhagic component. Grossly, they show the following stages of evolution (3). The early stage (3 to 4 days) is characterized by a blurring of the junction of white-gray matter and a softening of the tissue involved, described as encephalomalacia (fig. 5-16). The intermediate stage (4 to 7 days) is characterized by swelling (edema) associated with increased brain weight, flattening and widening of cortical gyri, narrowing of sulci, and sometimes herniation (fig.

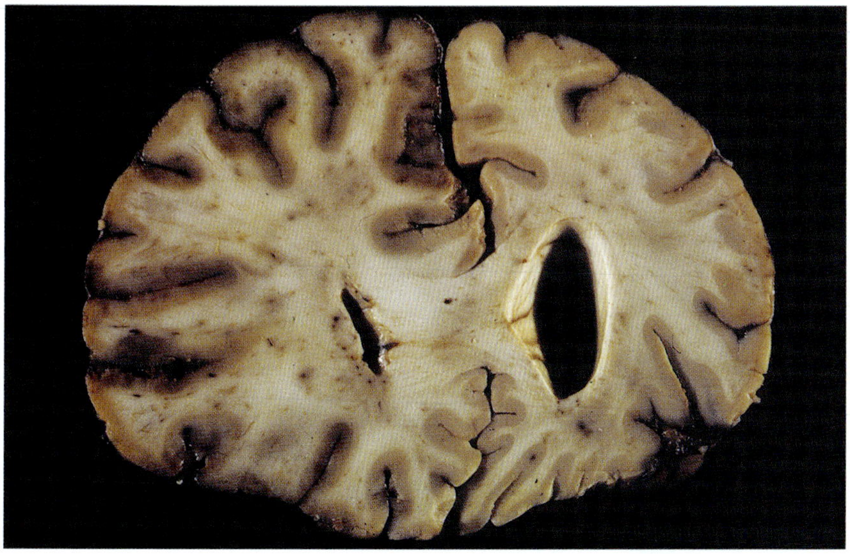

Figure 5-17

INTERMEDIATE STAGE OF ISCHEMIC INFARCT

An infarct in the distribution of the left MCA and ACA is associated with edema, shift of the midline structures from left to right, and herniation of the left cingulate gyrus.

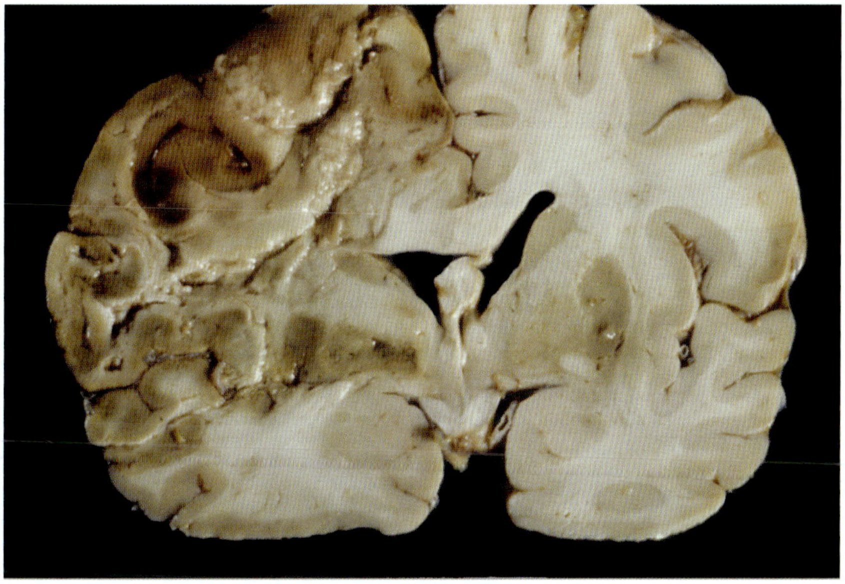

Figure 5-18

LATE STAGE OF ISCHEMIC INFARCT

An infarct in the area of distribution of the left ACA and MCA shows sharp demarcation and cavitation.

5-17). The edema may be unilateral to a cerebral hemisphere or localized to the infarcted area. The late stage (7 to 14 days) is notable for demarcation of the necrotic area with early cavitation and disappearance of swelling (fig. 5-18). The terminal stage (after 14 days) represents the formation of a cavity filled with clear fluid (fig. 5-19). A list of macroscopic and microscopic findings of human brain infarct is presented in Table 5-1.

Hemorrhagic Infarct. The designation hemorrhagic infarct should be reserved for ischemic lesions that have a hemorrhagic component and appear red on macroscopic examination of the brain. Two types are recognized: infarcts with a hemorrhagic component limited to the gray matter, usually cortical petechial hemorrhages (fig. 5-20), and lesions associated with the formation of a hematoma within the necrotic area (fig. 5-21). Hemorrhagic infarcts are thought to result from hemorrhage into a previously anemic or pale infarct as a consequence of reperfusion after patency is restored to the occluded artery. This occurs in up to 40 percent of initially anemic infarcts. Hemorrhagic transformation of an infarct with hematoma formation is also

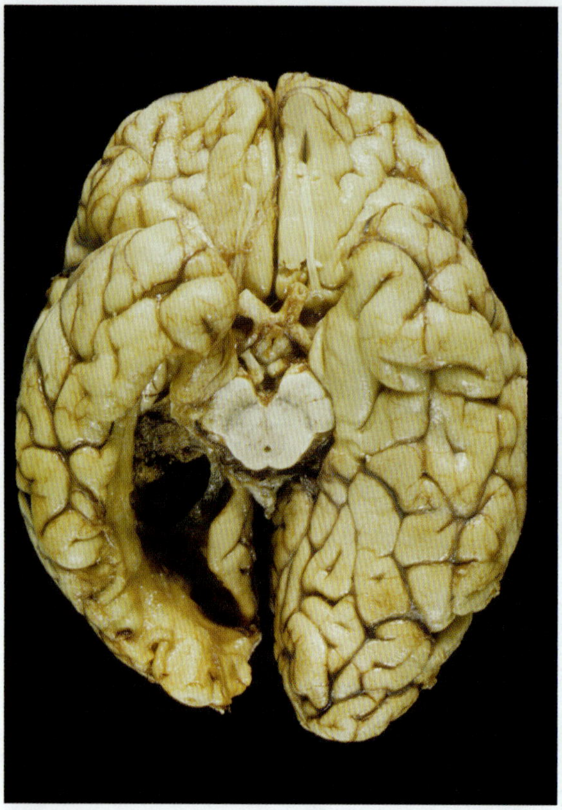

Figure 5-19

TERMINAL STATE OF ISCHEMIC INFARCT

Cavitated infarct in the distribution of the right posterior cerebral artery (PCA) is associated with communication between the right lateral ventricle and the subarachnoid space.

Table 5-1

COMPARATIVE GROSS AND MICROSCOPIC FEATURES OF HUMAN CEREBRAL INFARCT

Macroscopic Findings	Microscopic Findings
Early stage (3-4 days) Blurring of white-gray matter junction, encephalomalacia	Red neurons[a] (1-35 days) Cytoplasmic vacuolation[a] (1-60 days) Ghost neurons[a] (1-60 days)
Intermediate stage (4-7 days) Brain edema	Vacuolation of neuropil[a] (1 day and older)
Late stage (7-14 days) Demarcation of necrotic area, early cavitation, no edema	Spheroids (1 day and older) Gliosis (2 days and older) Necrosis[b] (1 day-5 years) Neutrophils[b,c,d] (1-37 days) Chronic inflammation[d] (3 days-53 years) Macrophages (3 days-53 years) Neovascularization (3 days and older) Neuronal ferrugination (3 days and older)
Terminal stage (>14 days) Cavity filled with clear fluid	Cavitation (12 days and older)

[a]Required for phase of acute neuronal injury (1-2 days of evolution).
[b]Required for phase of organization with acute inflammation (3-37 days).
[c]Absent in phase of organization with chronic inflammation (10 days-53 years).
[d]Absent in phase of resorption (26 days-53 years).

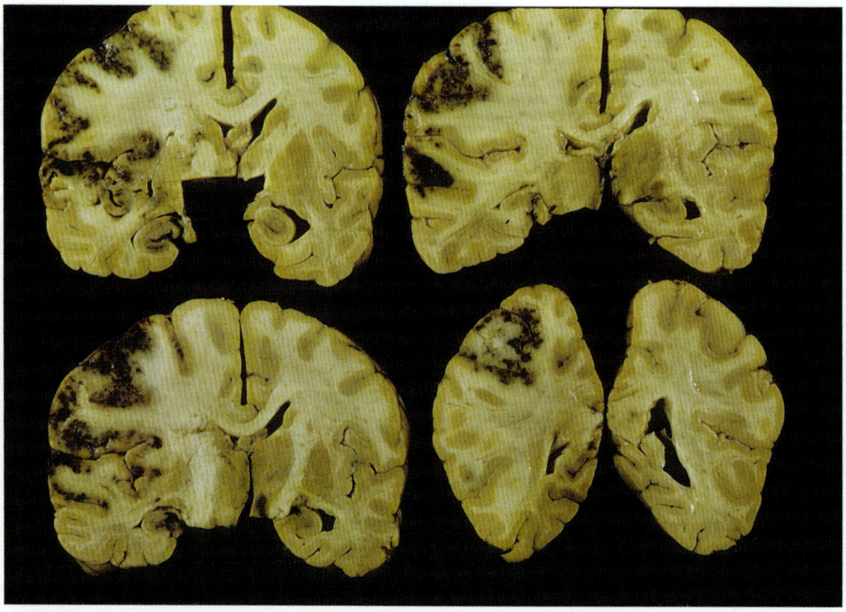

Figure 5-20

HEMORRHAGIC INFARCT

The lesion is associated with petechial cortical hemorrhages in the area of distribution of the left MCA.

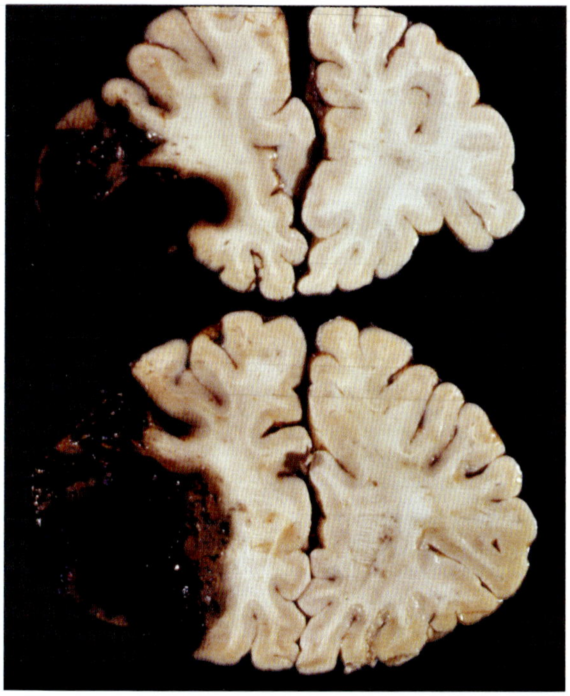

Figure 5-21

HEMORRHAGIC INFARCT

The lesion is associated with hematoma formation in the territory supplied by the left MCA.

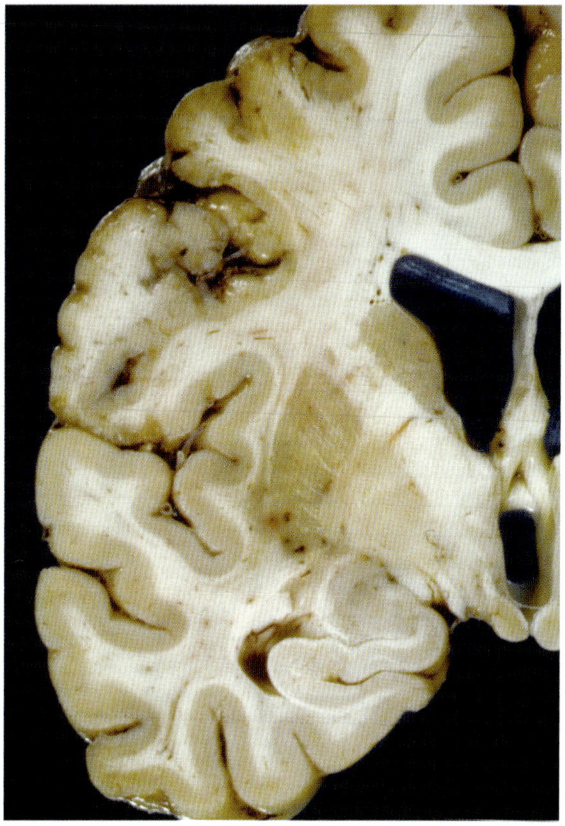

Figure 5-22

INCOMPLETE INFARCT

Lesion without cavitation or necrosis involves cortex and white matter after an embolic occlusion of a peripheral branch of the left MCA. 3. (Fig. 7.6 from Garcia J, Mena H. Injuries to the brain and spinal cord associated with ischemia. In: Nelson J, Mena H, Parisi J, Schochett S Jr, eds. Principles and practice of neuropathology, 2nd ed. New York: Oxford University Press; 2003:119.)

linked to the administration of thrombolytic agents, with subsequent rapid deterioration of the patient's neurologic condition. Infarcts related to the partial occlusion of arteries due to compression by herniated brain tissue are also prone to hemorrhage.

Incomplete Infarct. Incomplete infarct refers to an ischemic lesion devoid of coagulative necrosis (fig. 5-22) (2). These occur in areas subjected to ischemia of short duration and moderate intensity. Similar areas may be present near areas of complete infarction when the development of the collateral circulation is sufficient to prevent complete tissue necrosis. The area surrounding the necrotic core, the ischemic penumbra, contains viable neurons that are electrically unexcitable (15). Over time, gliosis becomes evident.

Lacunar Infarct. Lacunar infarcts are related to the occlusion of small terminal parenchymal arteries, especially the lenticulostriate and thalamoperforating arteries. They typically are found at autopsy as small (less than 1 cm), irregular cavities in the basal ganglia, thalamus, deep white matter, and pons (figs. 5-23, 5-24). Hypertensive change (arteriolar sclerosis), small emboli, and an in situ process called lipohyalinosis are the most common causes. Other uncommon causes include fat embolism and embolic atherosclerotic material (16).

Microscopic Findings. Properly performed morphologic interpretation of a biopsy is the critical first step in the diagnosis of an ischemic infarct and the exclusion of other causes that may require a different treatment approach. It cannot be overemphasized that knowledge of the clinical and radiographic findings can help frame the differential diagnosis and provide critical information for the pathologist.

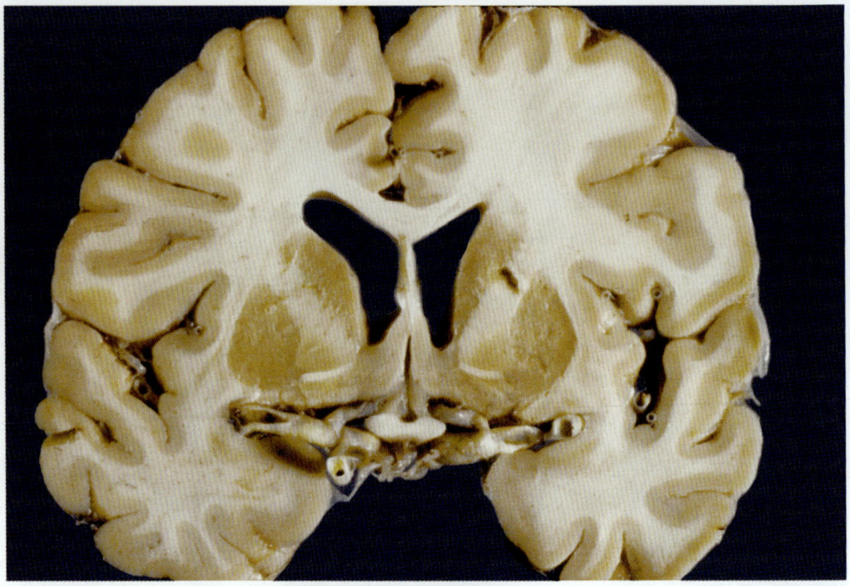

Figure 5-23

LACUNAR INFARCT

A lacunar infarct in the right internal capsule. (Figs. 5-23 and 5-24 are from the same patient.)

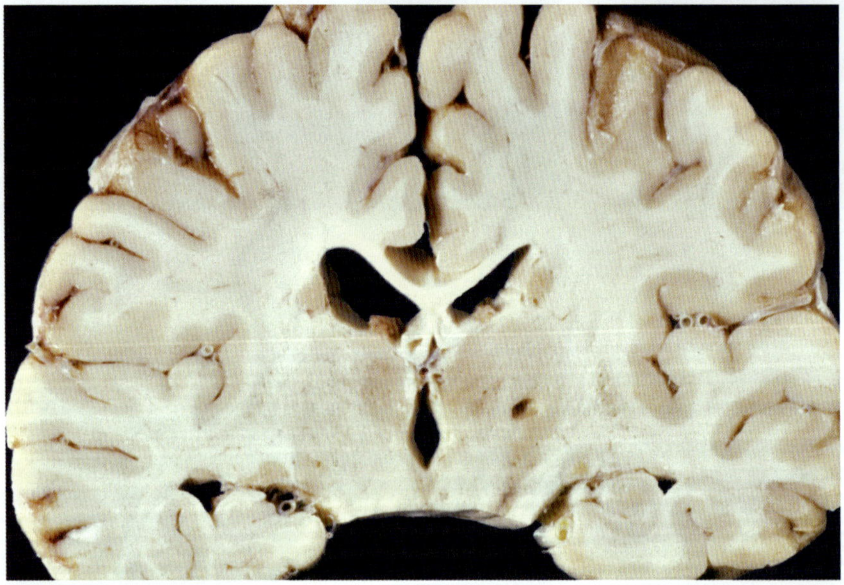

Figure 5-24

LACUNAR INFARCT

A lacunar infarct in the right thalamus.

Except for the hemorrhagic component of an infarct, the cellular reactions that participate in the organization of an infarct are similar regardless of the size of the occluded vessel. This process involves cellular elements intrinsic to the CNS (neurons, glial cells, and endothelial cells) and the accompanying inflammatory reaction. The microscopic features that should be noted in a biopsy specimen include evidence of acute neuronal injury such as eosinophilic neurons ("red neuron" change), neurons with vacuolated cytoplasm, neurons with karyolysis ("ghost" cells), and dead neurons with mineralized cytoplasmic deposits (ferrugination); swollen axons; coagulative necrosis; acute and chronic inflammation; macrophages; tissue vacuolation indicative of edema in recent lesions or loss of cellular elements in older infarcts; gliosis; vascular proliferation; cavitation; and recent or old hemorrhage in hemorrhagic infarcts. The systematic evaluation of each of these components should provide sufficient data to determine the approximate age of the lesion. Overlapping histologic features are frequent and a definite conclusion about the temporal progression of the lesion is not always possible, especially in small biopsy specimens.

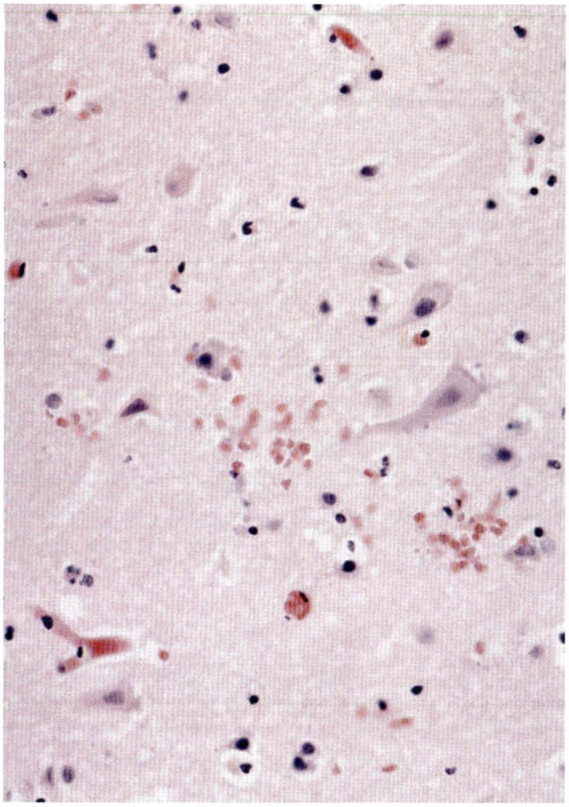

Figure 5-25

PHASE OF ACUTE NEURONAL INJURY OF CEREBRAL INFARCT

On day 2 of infarct evolution, the cerebral cortex is pale and shows eosinophilic neurons, neurons with karyolysis, and extravasated erythrocytes.

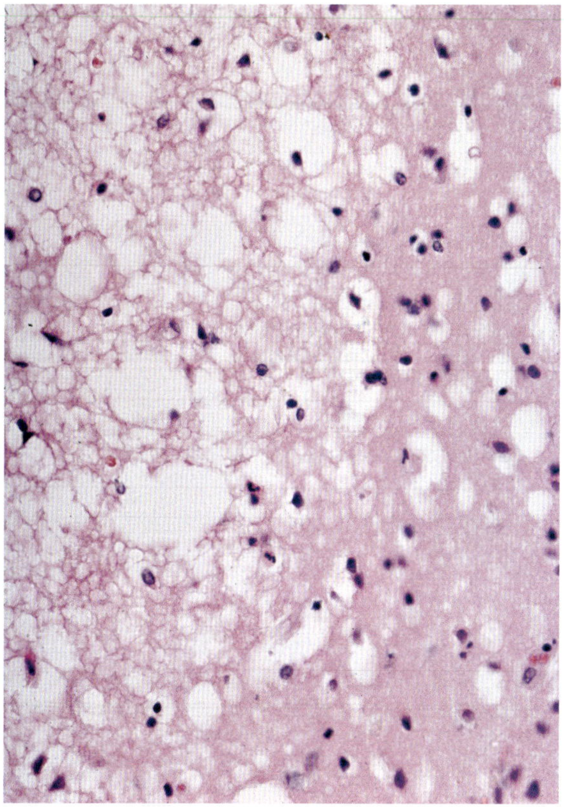

Figure 5-26

PHASE OF ACUTE NEURONAL INJURY OF CEREBRAL INFARCT

Vacuolation of the neuropil and cells with enlarged clear cytoplasm are probably due to accumulation of edema fluid.

Based on experience with autopsy and surgical material, the following evolutionary phases of cerebral infarcts, which are not influenced by the size or location of the lesion, have been proposed (17).

Phase of Acute Neuronal Injury with a Duration of 1 to 2 Days. Features of acute neuronal injury and vacuolation of the neuropil herald this phase (figs. 5-25, 5-26). Other variable microscopic findings include coagulative necrosis, neutrophils, reactive astrocytes, and swollen axons. Neuronal ferrugination, chronic inflammation, macrophages, vascular proliferation, and cavitation are not encountered during this phase.

Phase of Organization in which the Predominant Inflammatory Reaction Is Acute or Chronic. The phase of organization with acute inflammation has an evolution of 3 to 37 days and is characterized by coagulative necrosis that in the majority of the cases is associated by infiltration with neutrophils (fig. 5-27). Other histopathologic features include acute neuronal injury and ferrugination, macrophages, gliosis, vascular proliferation, and cavitation. The phase of organization with chronic inflammation occurs from 10 days to 53 years and may show all the histologic findings with the exception of neutrophils (figs. 5-28–5-30).

Phase of Resorption. This phase ranges from 26 days to greater than 50 years. The salient feature is the absence of inflammation. Cavitation, spongiosis related to the loss of cellular elements and processes, and swollen axons are the most notable of the remaining microscopic features (figs. 5-31, 5-32). In our experience, 64 (47 percent) of 139

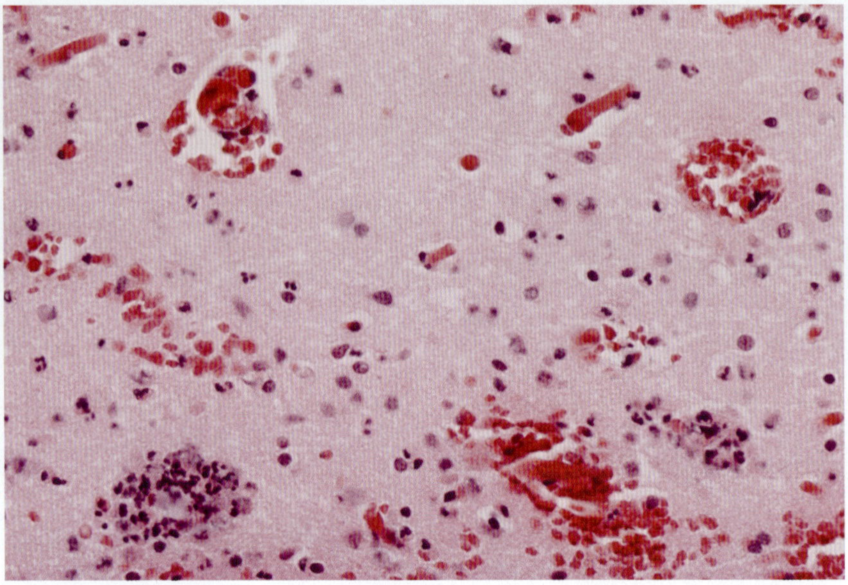

Figure 5-27

PHASE OF ORGANIZATION OF CEREBRAL INFARCT WITH ACUTE INFLAMMATION

At 8 days of infarct evolution, the necrotic cerebral tissue shows petechial hemorrhages and infiltration by neutrophils.

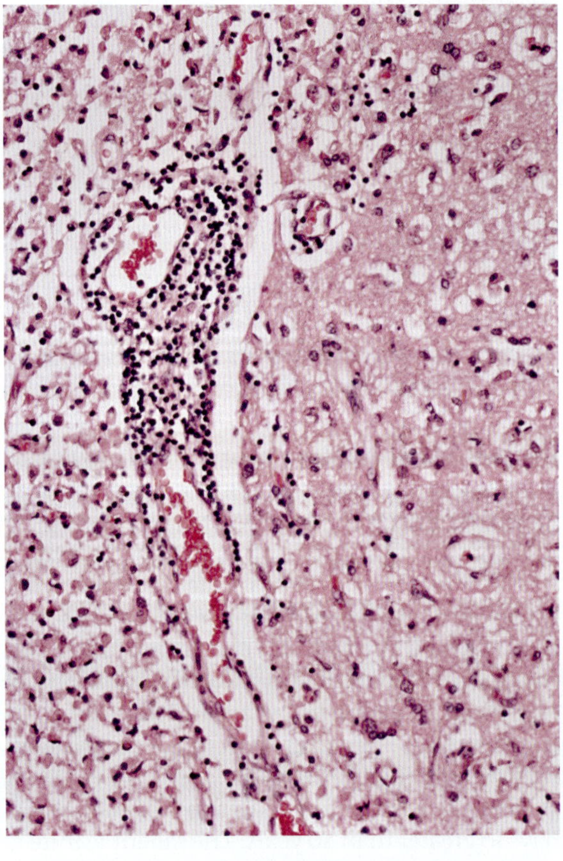

Figure 5-28

PHASE OF ORGANIZATION OF CEREBRAL INFARCT

At 37 days of evolution, the necrotic cerebral tissue is infiltrated by macrophages and chronic perivascular inflammation.

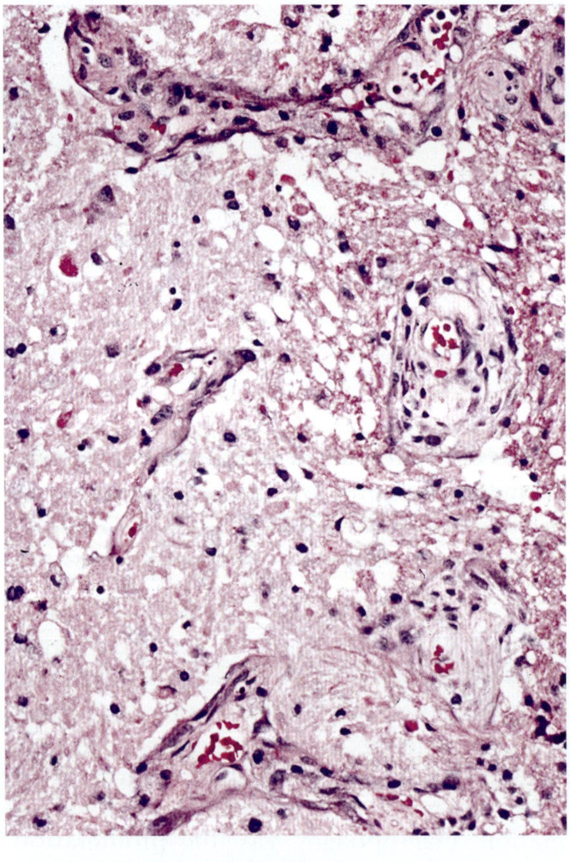

Figure 5-29

PHASE OF ORGANIZATION OF CEREBRAL INFARCT

The interface between the necrotic and preserved white matter demonstrates vascular proliferation with prominent endothelial cells.

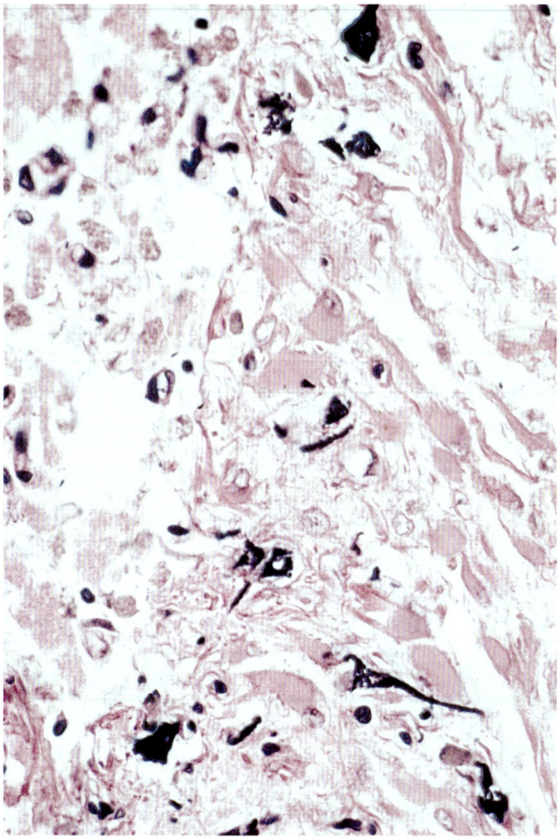

Figure 5-30

PHASE OF RESORPTION OF CEREBRAL INFARCT

The periphery of a partially cavitated infarct demonstrates reactive astrocytes and mineralized neurons.

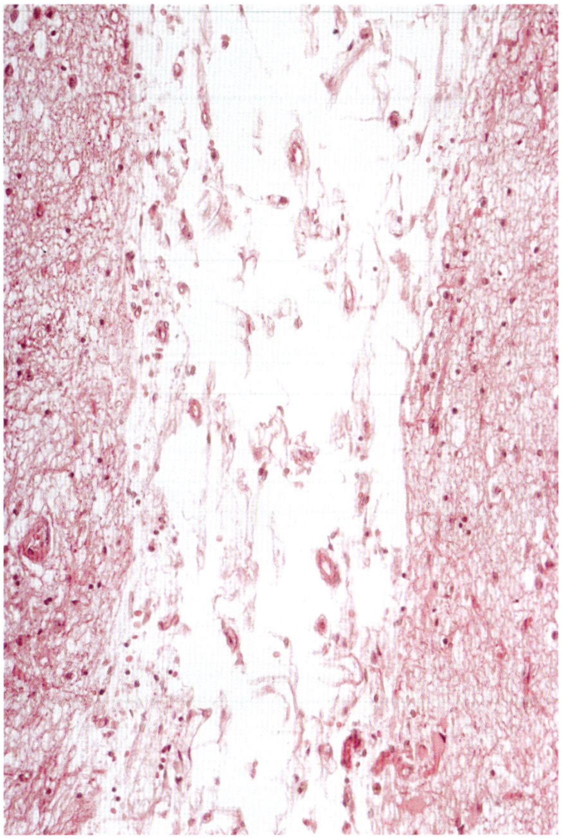

Figure 5-31

PHASE OF RESORPTION OF CEREBRAL INFARCT

At 6 years of evolution, the necrotic cerebral tissue is replaced by a cavity partially filled with blood vessels and strands of glial tissue.

infarct cases showed a hemorrhagic component with hemosiderin-laden macrophages.

Immunohistochemical Findings. The use of immunohistochemistry in the study of cerebrovascular disease is largely restricted to the study of experimental models and the exclusion of other entities that masquerade as cerebrovascular disease. Immunohistochemical stains that are useful to support the diagnosis of infarcted tissue include glial fibrillary acidic protein (GFAP), CD68 and lectins (*Ulex europaeus*), as well as amyloid precursor protein for swollen axons.

It is now generally accepted that apoptosis plays a pivotal role in cell death after hypoxia. Recently, caspase activation has emerged as the central molecular event leading to apoptosis, preceding DNA degradation and the development of apoptotic morphology. Although considered largely a research tool, activated caspase-3 immunohistochemistry is available for the study of cerebral ischemia (18). In addition, research studies have used terminal deoxynucleotidyltransferase-mediated dUTP-biotin nick-end labeling (TUNEL) to document apoptosis, but this assay appears to have greater variability than immunohistochemistry for activated caspases.

Ultrastructural Findings. Ultrastructural examination is not necessary for the surgical pathologic diagnosis of cerebral infarcts. The reader is referred to other sources for discussions of the ultrastructural changes that attend experimental ischemic lesions (3,19).

Differential Diagnosis. The relative frequency with which a cerebral infarct is mistaken for other lesions underscores the need for the pathologist to be aware of this potential pitfall.

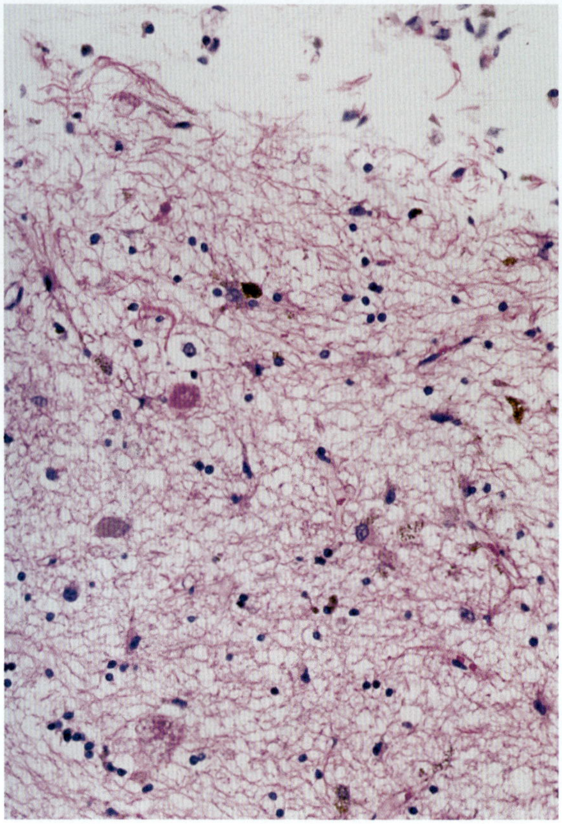

Figure 5-32

PHASE OF RESORPTION OF CEREBRAL INFARCT

At 6 years of evolution, tissue spongiosis, a few swollen axons, and reactive astrocytes are seen at the periphery of a cavitated infarct.

This confusion is particularly hazardous in the setting of subacute infarcts for a number of clinical, neuroradiologic, and histopathologic reasons. Subacute infarcts that result in biopsy are often clinically unusual cases that are diagnostically suspicious of other entities; that have neuroimaging findings, such as enhancement, that mimic neoplasms; and that have numerous macrophages and sometimes feature vascular proliferation. These features may lead the pathologist to consider neoplasia in the differential diagnosis. Indeed, it is critical to realize that infarcts, because of their deceptive hypercellularity, which is sometimes accompanied by vascular proliferation, can microscopically resemble neoplastic processes. Perhaps the essential diagnostic step is the recognition of macrophages, which are less likely to be found in a neoplasm and serve to caution the pathologist to the need for closer scrutiny.

The primary entities in the differential diagnosis are primary gliomas, particularly high-grade diffuse gliomas such as high-grade oligodendrogliomas, because of the resemblance of the macrophages to the "fried-egg" appearance of oligodendroglioma cells. Attention to the cytologic features of the macrophages is key and is relatively easy on smear preparations. As opposed to glial tumor cells, macrophages have less hyperchromatic nuclei, but most importantly, have well-defined, often granular or bubbly cytoplasm (fig. 5-33). Immunohistochemistry for macrophage markers, such as CD68, is confirmatory (fig. 5-34). As mentioned above, the presence of sheets of macrophages is rare in untreated malignant gliomas, although oligodendrogliomas do rarely feature perivascular macrophages. In the setting of prior surgery and radiation treatment of gliomas, macrophages are not uncommon and this differential diagnosis can be more challenging (see chapter 15). Finally, it is important to note that microvascular proliferation attends organizing infarcts, and it is these infarcts that present the greatest challenge in the clinical and radiologic distinction from glioblastoma. Nonetheless, the vascular proliferation that accompanies cerebral infarction does not attain the "glomeruloid" appearance of glioma-associated microvascular proliferation. The vessels have plump, activated endothelial cells, but multilayering is not prominent (fig. 5-35).

In addition to neoplasms, the differential diagnosis of brain infarct includes radiation-induced changes, demyelinating lesions presenting as space-occupying masses, and other necrotizing infectious or inflammatory processes. Histologically, radionecrosis is a form of coagulation necrosis usually found in white matter, although deeper cortical laminae may be affected. In addition to cytologic atypia and microcalcification, radionecrosis often shows thickened vessels with striking mural hyalinization, sometimes accompanied by fibrinoid necrosis (see chapter 15).

Demyelinating lesions are defined by loss of myelin with relative sparing of axons (see chapter 9). Their often discrete borders can be accentuated by stains for myelin, such as

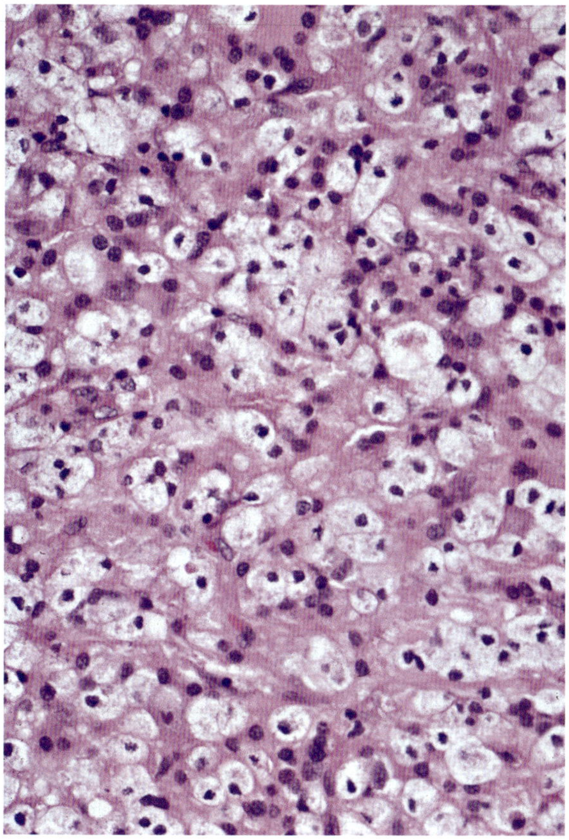

Figure 5-33

CHALLENGING MICROSCOPIC FEATURES OF CEREBRAL INFARCT

Macrophages with finely granular cytoplasm are seen. (Figs. 5-33 to 5-35 are from the same patient.)

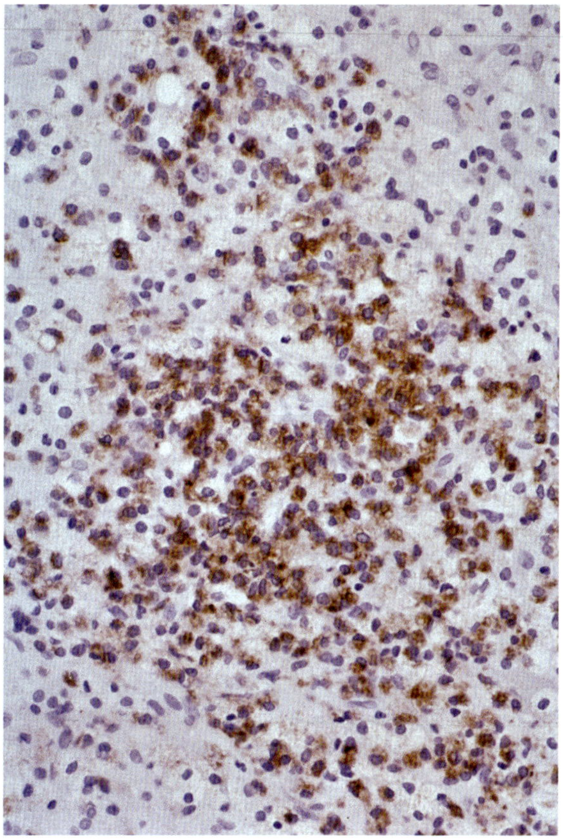

Figure 5-34

CHALLENGING MICROSCOPIC FEATURES OF CEREBRAL INFARCT

CD68 is expressed by the macrophages (immunoperoxidase stain).

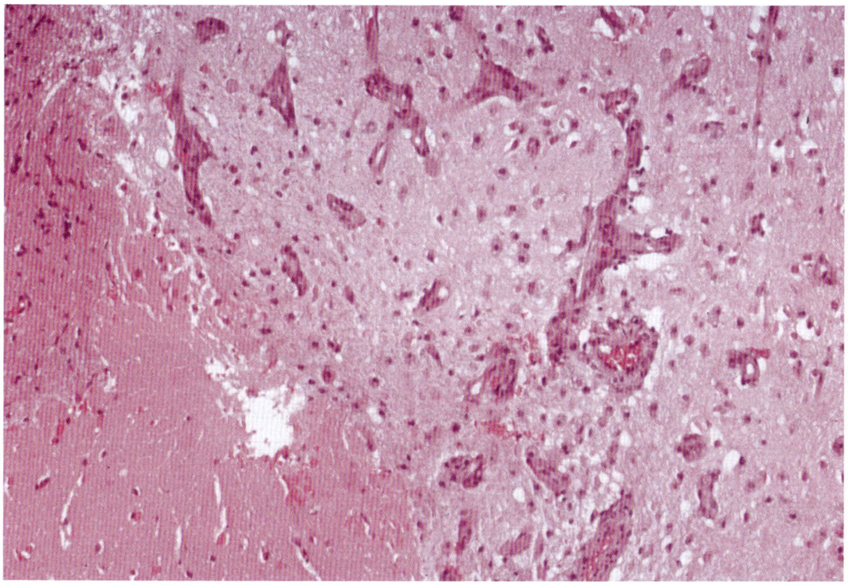

Figure 5-35

CHALLENGING MICROSCOPIC FEATURES OF CEREBRAL INFARCT

Necrotic zone associated with vascular proliferation which may be mistaken for glioblastoma.

Luxol fast blue. Unequivocal confirmation of a demyelinating lesion is accomplished by a concomitant stain for neurofilaments. In contrast to a demyelinating lesion, the distinguishing feature of an infarct is the loss of both myelin and axons. Other demyelinating diseases, such as progressive multifocal leukoencephalopathy (see chapter 7), are less commonly confused with infarcts, since they have other diagnostic features and less often have sheets of macrophages. A practical approach for differentiating demyelinating and other lesions is presented in Table 9-1, chapter 9.

Treatment and Prognosis. The two basic approaches to treatment are surgical and medical. If administered within the first 48 hours of stroke onset, antiplatelet therapy with aspirin has been shown to significantly reduce the risk of recurrence during the first 2 weeks and, possibly, improve outcome at 6 months. Carotid endarterectomy has been the mainstay of surgical therapy for most patients with carotid occlusive disease. Recently, less invasive endovascular techniques such as combined thrombolysis and carotid artery stenting have been proposed as alternatives to carotid endarterectomy in cerebral revascularization. Thrombolysis is aimed at recanalization of occluded arteries and reperfusion of the ischemic penumbra, a region of critically hypoperfused, functionally impaired, but potentially viable brain. The placement of an intraarterial stent has emerged as a complimentary technique aimed at maintaining the patency of the diseased vessel. Neurointerventional therapy is centered on treating occlusions of the MCA or basilar artery. Unfortunately, the procedure itself is not risk free, and a diagnostic angiogram may cause an embolic event in a small percentage of patients (20).

For patients at risk for cerebral embolism, it is well established that prophylactic anticoagulant therapy represents the most effective treatment modality. The major concern is intracranial hemorrhage as a complication of treatment (see below, Intracerebral Hemorrhage). Predisposing factors for anticoagulant-related intracranial hemorrhage include advanced age, intensity of the anticoagulation, prior ischemic stroke, and hypertension (20,21).

Despite diagnostic and therapeutic progress, the majority of stroke survivors have residual neurologic dysfunction. Maximum recovery occurs in the first 3 months after stroke. Prognosis hinges on the type of event (hemorrhagic or ischemic), the anatomic location, and the underlying pathogenetic mechanism. In general, larger infarcts are associated with a worse prognosis than smaller lesions. Cerebral edema and elevated intracranial pressure peak at 2 to 5 days and may complicate the clinical course of an expanding infarction. Consequently, secondary infarctions occur in some patients with large MCA infarcts due to the compression of the ACA and PCA by edematous infarcted tissue. Similarly, cerebellar infarction may lead to basilar artery compression and brain stem ischemia (20,21).

INTRACEREBRAL HEMORRHAGE

Definition. Brain hemorrhage refers to the extravasation of blood, which may be parenchymal, localized to one of the extraparenchymal compartments, or both parenchymal and extraparenchymal.

General Comments. Blood clots removed from the intracranial compartment, whether intracerebral or related to the dura, are common neurosurgical specimens. They are removed in acute, often emergent settings, typically to relieve symptoms and signs of acutely increased intracranial pressure. The pathologist most often receives moderate amounts of fresh blood clot and sometimes portions of adjacent brain. Because of the emergent nature of many of these neurosurgical procedures, patient information provided initially to the pathologist may be somewhat incomplete, and further patient workup may be needed over the following days to weeks to pinpoint the cause of the hemorrhage. The pathologist can play a significant role in this workup through careful examination of the clots.

Traumatic brain injuries account for a significant number of cases associated with parenchymal, subarachnoid, subdural, and epidural hemorrhages. In fact, cranial trauma is the leading cause of subarachnoid hemorrhage. (Details concerning subdural and epidural hemorrhages are considered in chapter 11). The rupture of a saccular aneurysm of one of the intracranial arteries is the primary cause of nontraumatic subarachnoid hemorrhage (fig. 5-36). Other causes of subarachnoid hemorrhage

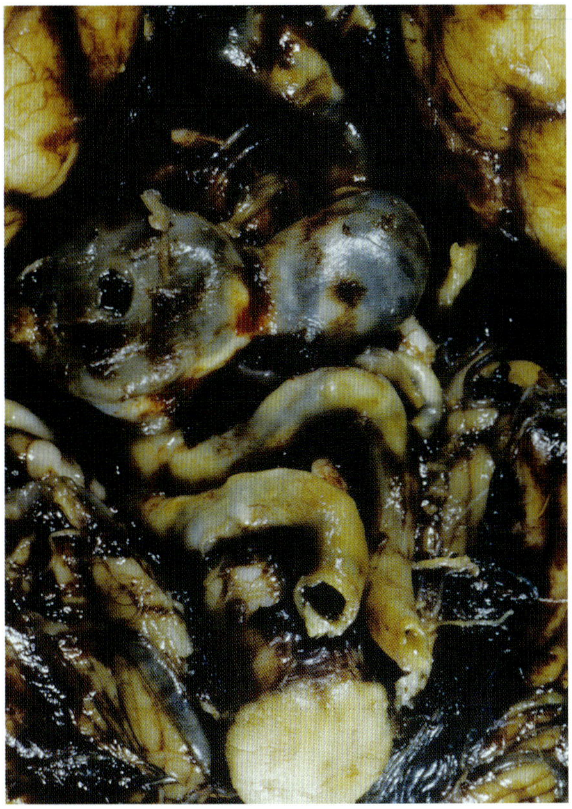

Figure 5-36

SUBARACHNOID HEMORRHAGE

Ruptured saccular aneurysm of the basilar artery with subarachnoid hemorrhage.

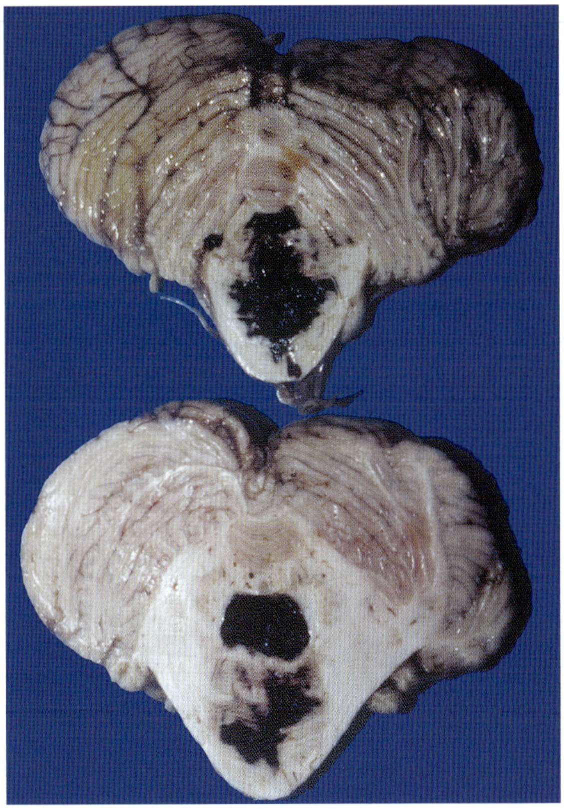

Figure 5-37

HYPERTENSIVE HEMORRHAGE

A pontine hemorrhage was the cause of death in a hypertensive patient.

include vascular malformations, arterial dissections, infectious causes, and rarely, metastatic neoplasms. Leukemic infiltrates of the meninges may be associated with subarachnoid, subdural, and epidural hemorrhages. More thorough discussions of topics other than hypertensive hemorrhage are found in respective chapters, particularly chapter 6.

Intracerebral hemorrhage (ICH) is characterized by parenchymal hematoma formation, with surrounding inflammation and edema. Spontaneous ICH is most often attributed to rupture of the small perforating vessels of the cerebral arteries caused by chronic hypertension, which induces pathologic changes in small vessels. These hemorrhagic lesions are usually deeply situated in the cerebral hemispheres (basal ganglia and thalamus) and brain stem (pons); less common sites are in the subcortical white matter and cerebellum (fig. 5-37) (22).

Major causes of nonhypertensive hemorrhage include hemorrhagic infarction (see above), vascular malformations, amyloid angiopathy, the use of anticoagulant and antifibrinolytic agents (fig. 5-38), coagulopathies, sympathomimetic substance abuse (fig. 5-39), infections including mycotic aneurysms, and neoplasms. Oligodendroglioma and glioblastoma are primary brain tumors with a predilection to bleed. Metastatic tumors that may be hemorrhagic include choriocarcinoma, melanoma, and renal cell carcinoma, among others. Single or multiple parenchymal hemorrhages may be a fatal complication of acute leukemia. Certain fungal organisms, e.g., *Aspergillus,* have a propensity to invade blood vessels and cause hemorrhage. Overall, these conditions usually produce hemorrhages in the subcortical white matter (lobar), some predominantly in the elderly (cerebral amyloid angiopathy) and others mainly in the

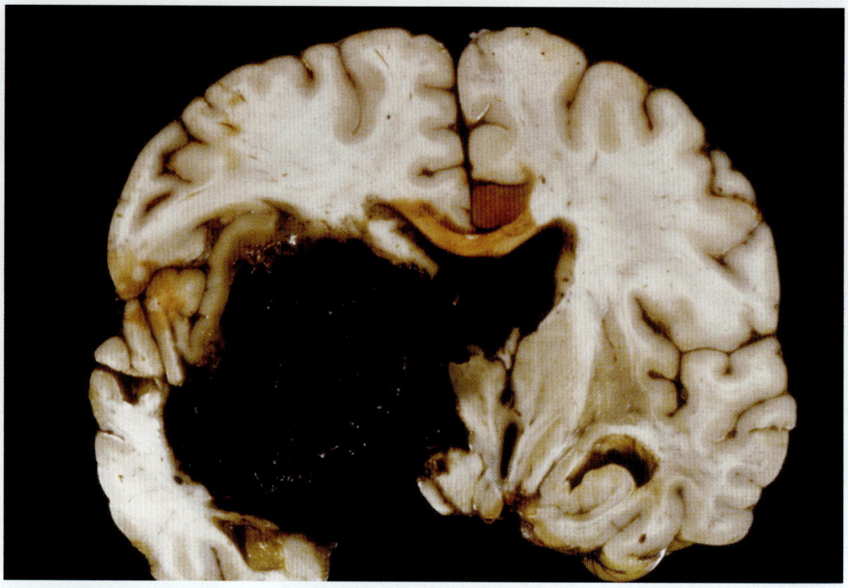

Figure 5-38

INTRACEREBRAL HEMORRHAGE

Acute intracerebral hemorrhage related to coumadin therapy.

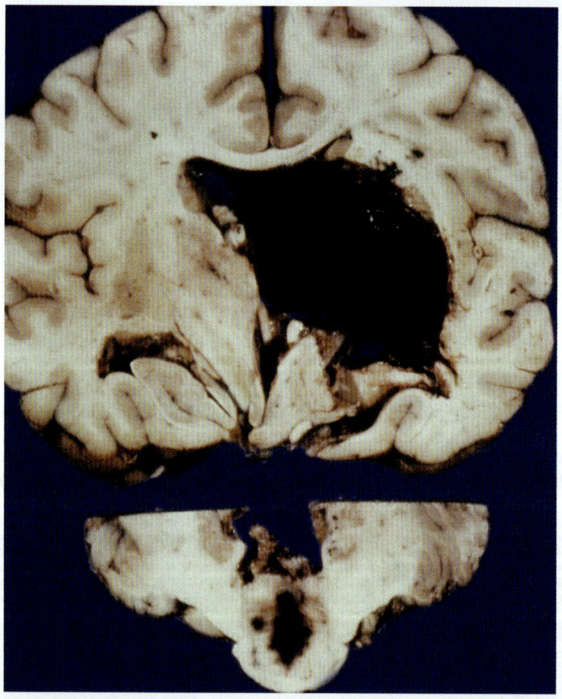

Figure 5-39

HEMORRHAGE AND SUBSTANCE ABUSE

Thalamic and basal ganglia hemorrhage due to cocaine abuse.

young (vascular malformations and sympathomimetic drugs).

Clinical Features. Patients with hemorrhagic stroke present with similar neurologic deficits as those with ischemic stroke, but tend to be more acutely ill. Hemorrhagic stroke victims are more likely to exhibit symptoms of increased intracranial pressure resulting in headache, altered mental status, seizures, nausea and vomiting, and marked hypertension. None of these findings, however, reliably distinguish hemorrhagic and ischemic strokes (23).

Radiologic Findings. Neuroimaging modalities such as MRI and CT angiography have made major contributions to the diagnosis and management of stroke patients (14). Acute hemorrhage, regardless of etiology, has a high density and appears hyperdense on CT when compared with the surrounding brain tissue. ICH has a dynamic appearance on MRI, changing in signal intensity over time. Acute blood, in the form of oxyhemoglobin, is isointense with the brain parenchyma. Hemosiderin produces a characteristic black ring around the hematoma on T2-weighted images.

Gross Findings. The location of the hemorrhage sometimes provides important clues regarding the underlying pathophysiology. Hemorrhages due to chronic hypertension are discrete masses commonly situated in the putamen, caudate, thalamus, pons, cerebellum, and subcortical white matter/gray-white junction. Since they are deep and near ventricular surfaces, ventricular rupture is common. Brain edema and herniation are often present. Cerebral amyloid angiopathy-related hemorrhage is almost always found in

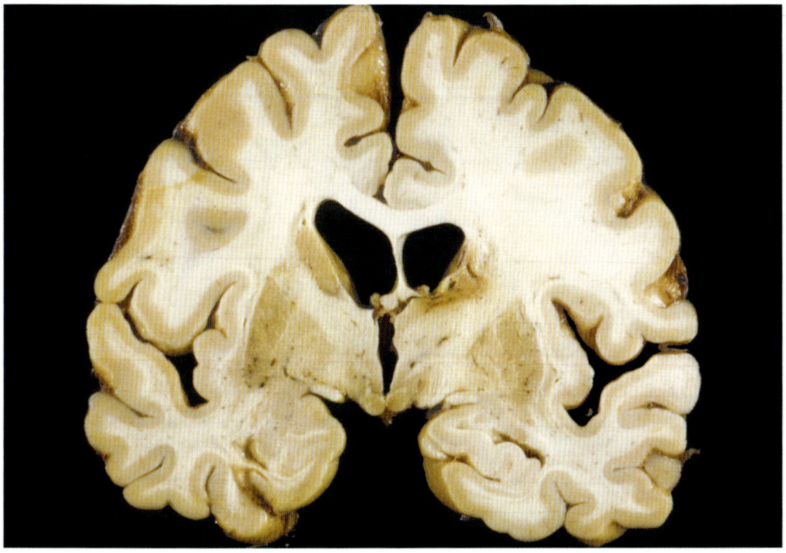

Figure 5-40

ORGANIZING HYPERTENSIVE HEMORRHAGE

Hemorrhage of right caudate nucleus undergoing organization, which includes cavitation and brown-yellow discoloration.

the supratentorial white matter, in a so-called lobar location. Unlike hemorrhagic infarcts, lesions due to hypertensive brain hemorrhage do not correspond to a specific vascular territory.

As a hematoma matures, the surrounding uninvolved parenchyma retracts and leaves a slit-like cystic cavity that is orange-brown as a result of staining by residual altered blood pigment (fig. 5-40). Traces of altered blood pigment often remain in remote lesions for many years and further distinguish them from their ischemic counterparts.

Microscopic Findings. Studies related to the organization of an intraparenchymal hematoma describe sequential microscopic changes in lesions associated with hypertension. Brain swelling in tissue adjacent to the hematoma becomes evident a few hours or days after the initial event. Sections of the acute hematoma reveal fresh blood with intact erythrocytes. At approximately 4 to 10 days, erythrocytes lyse and there is infiltration of the blood clot by inflammatory cells, initially neutrophils and later, macrophages (fig. 5-41). During this phase, hemosiderin and hematoidin pigments can be recognized. A limiting membrane, comprised initially of granulation tissue and reactive astrocytes and later of a fibrous capsule and gliosis, appears between 5 and 6 weeks. In the final stages, the hematoma becomes a fluid-filled cavity or a fibrous scar with scattered, residual hemosiderin-laden macrophages and possible eosinophilic granular, or cytoid, bodies.

The microvascular pathology is especially prominent surrounding the hemorrhagic core. The walls of arterioles often show onion-skin type thickening as well as lipohyalinosis, which results in luminal constriction. Although not essential for diagnostic purposes, the patient pathologist may sometimes by rewarded by finding ectatic ballooning of small vessels, known as *Charcot-Bouchard microaneurysms*, which are of putative pathogenetic importance in hypertensive hemorrhage.

Immunohistochemical Findings. In general, immunohistochemical approaches to the study of ICH are mostly confined to the use of keratins or other differentiation markers (GFAP, melanoma markers, and others) to evaluate the possibility of a primary or metastatic neoplasm concealed by hematoma, or to the use of Congo red and beta amyloid stains to evaluate the possibility of cerebral amyloid angiopathy.

Differential Diagnosis. Although the clinical and neuroimaging characteristics of a common hypertensive hemorrhage usually permit ready microscopic confirmation, the differential diagnosis of a spontaneous parenchymal "blood clot" should be systematically explored in every case. Difficulties arise primarily in cases in which the hematoma obscures features of an underlying pathologic process. The following nine categories comprise the broad range of diagnostic possibilities: hypertension, cerebral amyloid angiopathy, vascular malformation, hemorrhagic infarct, coagulopathy due to systemic disease

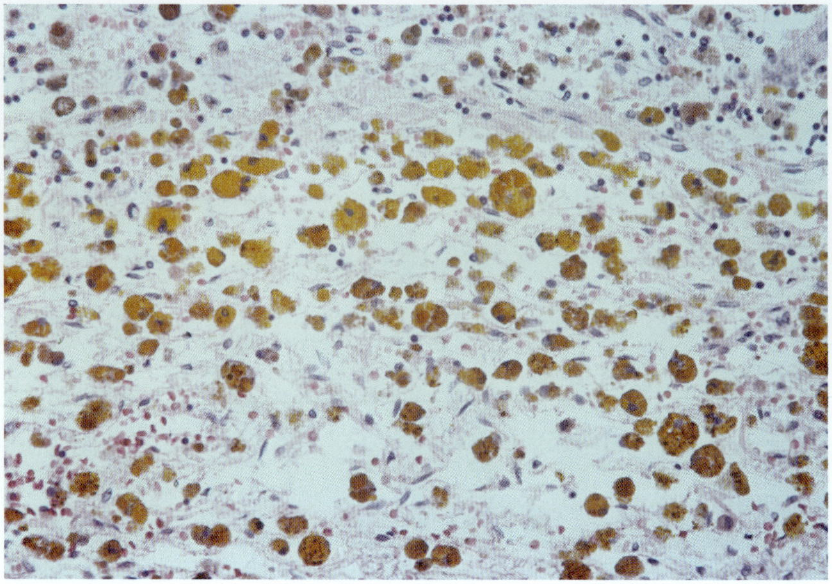

Figure 5-41

ORGANIZING HYPERTENSIVE HEMORRHAGE

Many of the macrophages are laden with hemosiderin and hematoidin blood pigments.

or anticoagulant therapy, sympathomimetic drugs, infection including mycotic aneurysms, neoplasm, and acute demyelinating disease. With the exception of neoplasms and drugs, the reader is referred to the respective chapters for a more detailed discussion.

Amyloid angiopathy is a frequent cause of lobar hemorrhage in the elderly. In order to exclude the various forms of amyloid angiopathy, histopathologic sections should be stained with a Congo red or beta-amyloid immunohistochemical preparation.

Occult vascular malformations with the greatest tendency to deep hemorrhage are cavernous hemangiomas and arteriovenous malformations. Aneurysmal rupture rarely results in an isolated deep, intraparenchymal hematoma; nevertheless, careful inspection of the basilar vasculature is still advised. A trichrome stain accompanied by an elastic stain (alternatively, a Movat pentachrome stain) accentuates disrupted fragments of a vascular malformation that may be hidden by a clot.

Bleeding diathesis can accompany a variety of systemic illnesses, ranging from congenital (hemophilia, von Willebrand disease) to acquired (vitamin K deficiency, liver disease, systemic lupus erythematosus with circulating anticoagulants). In patients with solid tumors, low-grade activated coagulation can result in systemic and cerebral arterial or venous thrombosis, predisposing to hemorrhagic infarcts. Cancer treatment can further contribute to coagulopathy. These considerations can be established by awareness of the clinical setting and examination of the peripheral smear, the platelet count, and tests of coagulation function. Iatrogenic bleeding occurs in patients receiving anticoagulation or thrombolytic agents.

Pathologists should pay particular attention to areas with increased cellularity to detect a neoplasm, either primary or metastatic. Primary brain tumors that have the greatest propensity to hemorrhage are glioblastoma (figs. 5-42, 5-43) and oligodendroglioma, but vascular neoplasms such as meningioma, hemangiopericytoma, and hemangioblastoma share this presentation, although less commonly. The leading metastatic suspects, which may present even before the primary neoplasm is evident, include pulmonary adenocarcinoma, melanoma, renal cell carcinoma (figs. 5-44, 5-45), and choriocarcinoma. Adequate sampling of the clot and adjacent tissue helps avert potential diagnostic missteps. In these cases, immunohistochemistry is decisive in that metastatic carcinomas generally are S-100 protein and GFAP immunonegative, whereas glial neoplasms are strongly GFAP positive. Metastatic melanoma is typically S-100 protein, HMB45, and Melan-A positive. Other tissue-specific markers should be used when tumors of germ cell or other derivation are suspected.

Disorders involving capillaries, small veins, and venules may be associated with petechial

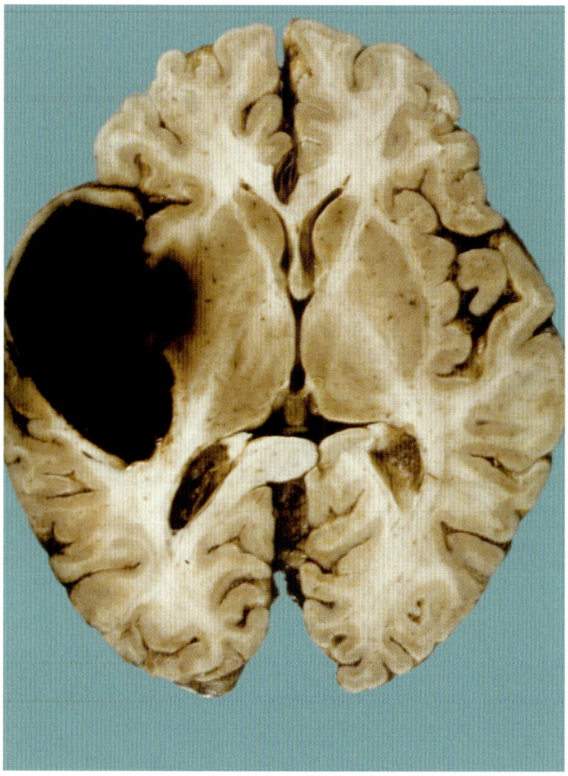

Figure 5-42

GLIOBLASTOMA WITH CEREBRAL HEMORRHAGE

A 70-year-old male with glioblastoma presented with a left temporal lobe hematoma. (Figs. 5-42 and 5-43 are from the same patient.)

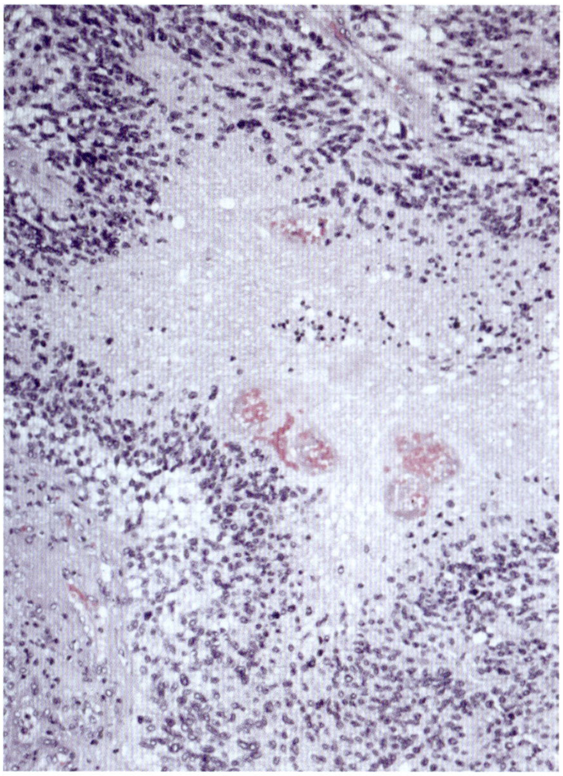

Figure 5-43

GLIOBLASTOMA WITH CEREBRAL HEMORRHAGE

Tissue from the periphery of the hematoma demonstrates features of glioblastoma, including nuclear palisades (H&E stain).

hemorrhages and the brain may show the characteristic pattern of brain purpura. White matter petechiae are commonly found in cases of cerebral malaria, fat embolism, disseminated intravascular coagulopathy, air embolism, and lead and arsenic poisoning. Gray matter petechiae are more characteristic of thrombotic thrombocytopenic purpura. While it may be difficult to distinguish between these entities on hematoxylin and eosin (H&E)-stained specimens, it is easy to identify the causal agent with special histochemical stains such as Sudan black for fat globules, Giemsa stain for malarial protozoa, iron stain for hemosiderin pigment, and Mallory phosphotungstic acid hematoxylin method for fibrin.

Entertaining the diagnosis of an infectious etiology is essential (see chapter 7). Clinical and radiographic features may be suggestive of infection. Infective aneurysms result from bacterial or fungal colonization of the vessel wall. Despite the older nomenclature of "mycotic" aneurysm, bacterial endocarditis is the most common underlying condition (figs. 5-46–5-48). Aneurysms associated with infective endocarditis are most often located on distal branches of the MCA. Septic aneurysms in patients with aspergillosis are usually located on the proximal segment of the basilar or carotid artery. Rhinocerebral mucormycosis typically features hemorrhagic necrosis in the orbital portion of the frontal lobe. Herpes encephalitis is a fulminating infection that exhibits a similar predilection for hemorrhagic necrosis of the orbitofrontal and temporal regions. Malaria is another infectious cause that enters into the differential diagnosis in the appropriate clinical setting. Careful examination of clot specimens

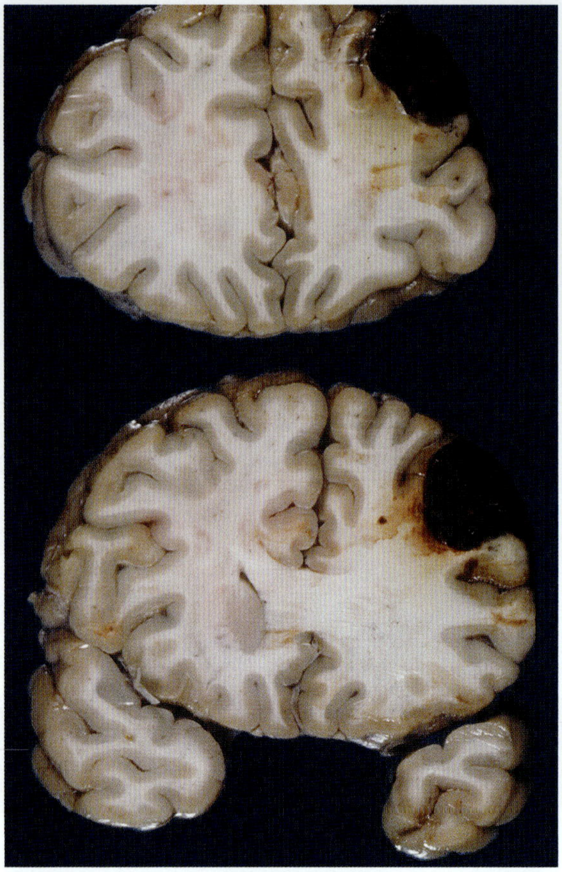

Figure 5-44

HEMORRHAGIC METASTATIC RENAL CELL CARCINOMA

A sharply demarcated hemorrhage is associated with metastatic renal cell carcinoma. (Figs. 5-44 and 5-45 are from the same patient.)

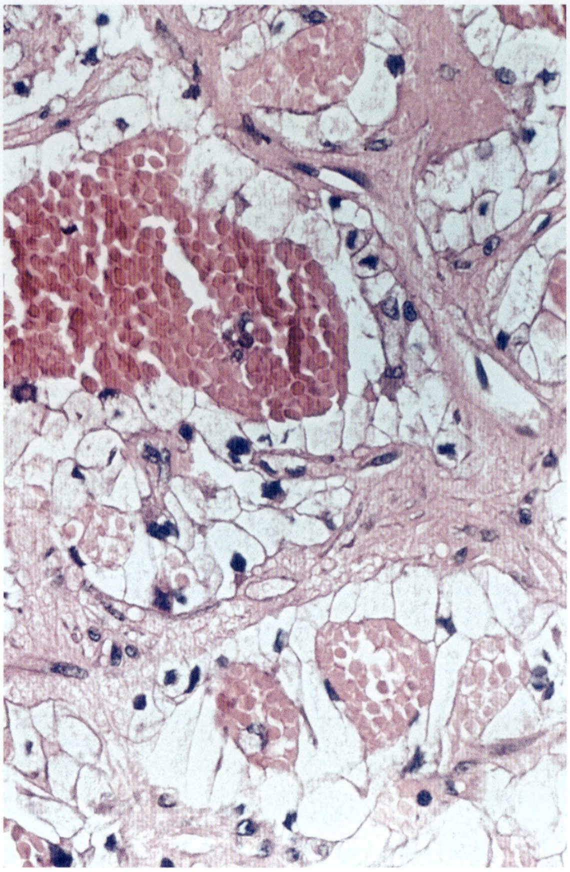

Figure 5-45

HEMORRHAGIC METASTATIC RENAL CELL CARCINOMA

The neoplasm is composed of clear cells arranged in tubular structures.

for microorganisms and viral inclusions and the application of special stains can assist in excluding these diseases.

An extremely rare cause of brain purpura is Weston Hurst acute hemorrhagic leukoencephalitis (see chapter 9), a form of acute disseminated encephalomyelitis characterized microscopically by classic "ring and ball" hemorrhages around a zone of fibrinoid necrosis. Mononuclear inflammatory infiltrates often accompany foci of demyelination. Preparations for myelin and silver impregnation to confirm relative axonal sparing should help distinguish these lesions.

Treatment and Prognosis. ICH is less common than ischemic stroke and is associated with a worse prognosis. The volume of the hemorrhage and the level of consciousness are the two most powerful predictors of outcome. Of particular concern is the observation that early hematoma expansion is common even in patients with normal coagulation profiles. Not surprisingly, hematoma enlargement is associated with the worse outcome. Furthermore, ICH often coexists with other serious medical problems that adversely affect prognosis, such as hypertension, diabetes, and obesity. Specific therapeutic options other than control of intracranial pressure and addressing the above risk factors are limited and of uncertain benefit. Only in life-threatening lobar and cerebellar hematomas, are surgical remedies of clear benefit. A novel medical therapy in which patients are administered the hemostatic agent, recombinant activated factor VII, holds promise but further investigation is needed (24,25).

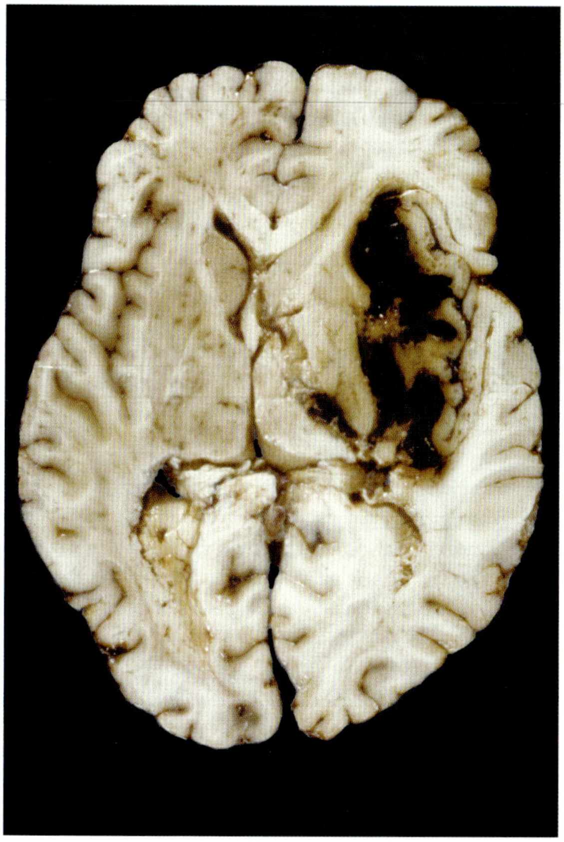

Figure 5-46

"MYCOTIC" ANEURYSM AND CEREBRAL HEMORRHAGE

A 26-year-old male with gonococcal septicemia developed a right temporal lobe hematoma. (Figs. 5-46 to 5-48 are from the same patient.)

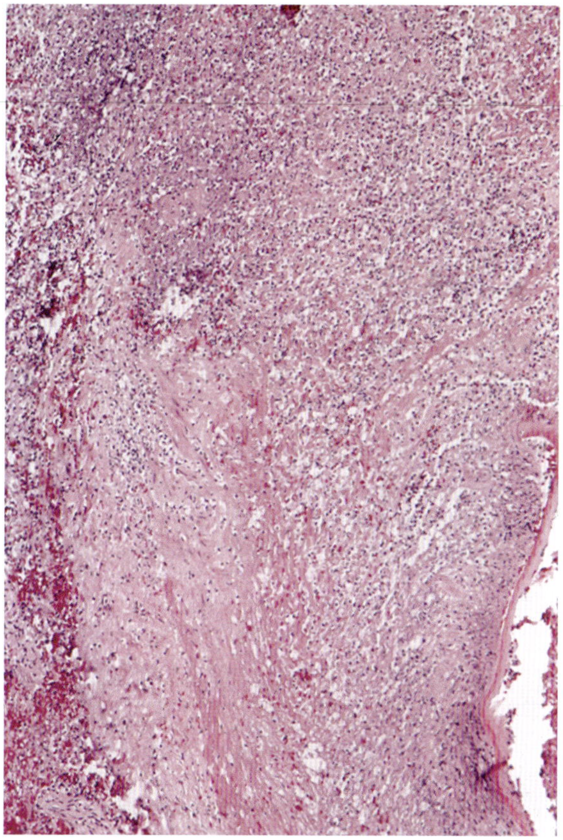

Figure 5-47

"MYCOTIC" ANEURYSM AND CEREBRAL HEMORRHAGE

The right MCA shows panarteritis and necrosis of its wall.

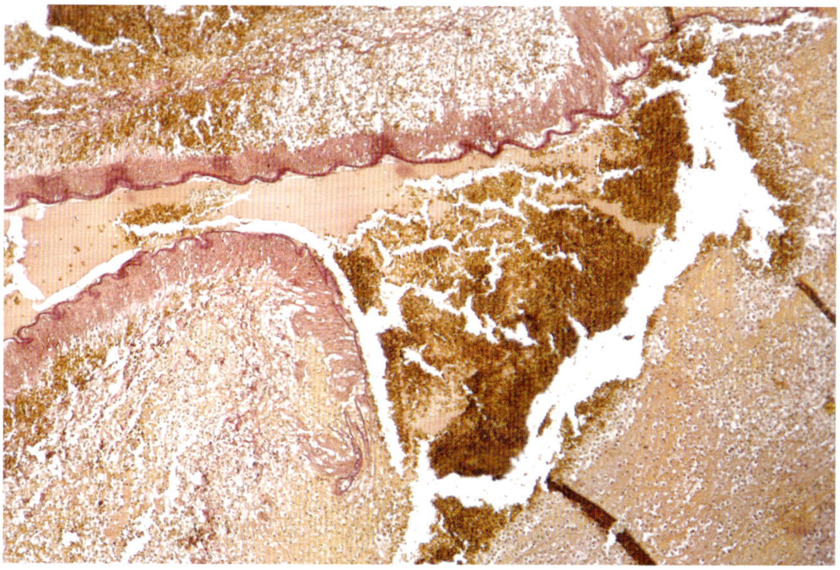

Figure 5-48

"MYCOTIC" ANEURYSM AND CEREBRAL HEMORRHAGE

The internal elastic lamina is disrupted by the necrotizing panarteritis in the right MCA (elastic stain).

REFERENCES

1. Sundt TM. Blood flow regulation in normal and ischemic brain. In: Current concepts. Kalamazoo, Michigan: Upjohn Co; 1979:1-32.
2. Lassen NA. Incomplete cerebral infarction-focal incomplete ischemic tissue necrosis not leading to embolism. Stroke 1982;13:522-523.
3. Garcia JH, Mena H. Injuries to the brain and spinal cord associated with ischemia. In: Nelson JS, Mena H, Parisi JE, Schochett SS Jr, eds. Principles and practice of neuropathology, 2nd ed. New York: Oxford University Press; 2003:112-121.
4. Collins RC, Dobkin BH, Choi DW. Selective vulnerability of the brain: new insights into the pathophysiology of stroke. Ann Intern Med 1989;110:992-1000.
5. Ellison D, Love S, Chimelli L, et al. Neuropathology, a reference text of CNS pathology, 2nd ed. Edinburgh: Mosby; 2004:163-206
6. Garcia JH. Morphology of global cerebral ischemia. Crit Care Med 1988;16:979-987.
7. Petito CK, Feldman NE, Pulsinelli WA, Plum F. Delayed hippocampal damage in humans following cardiorespiratory arrest. Neurology 1987;37:1281-1286.
8. Cole G, Cowie VA. Long survival after cardiac arrest: case report and neuropathological findings. Clin Neuropathol 1987;6:104-109.
9. Lindenberg R. The pathology of the arterial border zones of the brain. J Neuropathol Exp Neurol 1959;18:348-349.
10. De Reuck JL, Eecken HM. Periventricular leukomalacia in adults. Clinicopathological study of four cases. Arch Neurol 1978;35:517-521.
11. Ginsberg MD, Hedley-Whyte ET, Richardson EP Jr. Hypoxic-ischemic leukoencephalopathy in man. Arch Neurol 1976;33:5-14.
12. Warlow C. Disorders of the cerebral circulation. In: Walton J, ed. Brain's disease of the nervous system, 10th ed. Oxford: Oxford Medical Publications; 1993:197-268
13. Ringelstein EB, Nabavi DG. Cerebral small vessel diseases: cerebral microangiopathies. Curr Opin Neurol 2005;18:179-188.
14. Yuh WT, Crain MR. Magnetic resonance imaging of acute cerebral ischemia. Neuroimaging Clin N Am 1992;2:421-440.
15. Siesjo BK. Pathophysiology and treatment of focal cerebral ischemia. Part II: Mechanisms of damage and treatment. J Neurosurg 1992;77:1337-1354.
16. Millikan C, Futrell N. The fallacy of the lacune hypothesis. Stroke 1990;21:1251-1257.
17. Mena H, Cadavid D, Rushing EJ. Human cerebral infarct: a proposed histopathologic classification based on 137 cases. Acta Neuropathol 2004;108:524-530.
18. Chan PH. Mitochondria and neuronal death/survival signaling pathways in cerebral ischemia. Neurochem Res 2004;29:1943-1949.
19. Garcia JH, Yoshida Y, Chen H, Li Y, Zhang ZG, Lian J. Progression from ischemic injury to infarct following middle cerebral artery occlusion in the rat. Am J Pathol 1993;142:623-635.
20. Zweifler RM. Management of acute stroke. South Med J 2003;96:380-385.
21. Albers GW, Alberts MJ, Broderick JP, Lynden PD, Sacco RL. Recent advances in stroke management. J Stroke Cerebrovasc Dis 2000;9:95-105.
22. Lammie GW. Hypertensive cerebral small vessel disease and stroke. Brain Pathol 2002;12:358-370.
23. Quereshi S, Tuhrim J, Broderick H, et al. Spontaneous intracerebral hemorrhage. N Engl J Med 2001;344:1450-1460.
24. Mayer SA, Brun NC, Begtrup K, et al. Recombinant activated factor VII for acute intracerebral hemorrhage. N Engl J Med 2005;352:777-785.
25. Aronowski J, Hall CE. New horizons for primary intracerebral hemorrhage treatment: experience from preclinical studies. Neurol Res 2005; 27:268-279.

6 VASCULAR DISORDERS

The normal development of the central nervous system (CNS) is accompanied by the formation of a complex vascular system that is necessary to support cerebral function. The formation of the CNS vasculature occurs during intrauterine life, from the early differentiation of precursor cells into angioblasts through the development of the circle of Willis. There are variations, however, in CNS vasculogenesis; for example, only 40 percent of the population have the classic adult pattern of the circle of Willis, with paired symmetrical posterior communicating arteries joining the internal carotid and vertebrobasilar systems. Most such cerebrovascular abnormalities do not come to the attention of the surgical pathologist, but are of considerable interest at autopsy. On the other hand, advances in cross-sectional brain and spinal cord imaging have played a pivotal role in the early detection and surgical management of some cerebrovascular abnormalities, notably arteriovenous malformations and cavernous angiomas. Moreover, inflammatory, hereditary, and degenerative conditions of the CNS vasculature are often biopsied in order to establish a diagnosis. While these are often rare conditions, a cerebral or meningeal biopsy may be a mainstay of diagnosis. For this reason, the surgical pathologist needs to be familiar with malformative and other diseases of the CNS vasculature. The present chapter discusses vascular malformations, primarily those that are surgically resected, as well as the differential diagnosis of CNS vasculitides and noninflammatory vasculopathies.

VASCULAR MALFORMATIONS

Cerebral vascular malformations are common, found in 3 percent of the population (1). They comprise a variety of clinicopathologic entities that are associated with variable clinical presentations. The natural history of a vascular malformation depends on the lesion type, location, size, and overall hemodynamics. Cerebrovascular malformations occur throughout the entire CNS and involve the parenchyma, meninges, or both. Although the majority are solitary lesions restricted to the CNS, some may be a component of a systemic disorder such as hereditary hemorrhagic telangiectasia (Osler-Weber-Rendu disease) (1). Most cerebrovascular malformations are probably congenital. Although initially congenital, however, vascular malformations typically only become symptomatic in later childhood or young adulthood, following expansion of the original nidus and attendant hemorrhages. CNS vascular malformations include arteriovenous malformation, cavernous angioma (cavernous malformation), venous angioma, capillary telangiectasia, and mixed vascular malformation.

Arteriovenous Malformation

Definition. *Arteriovenous malformation* (AVM) is a vascular malformation composed of a conglomerate of abnormal arteries and veins, without an intervening capillary bed.

General Comments. AVMs may be parenchymal or meningeal or, perhaps most commonly, meningocerebral, and can affect the cerebral hemispheres, posterior fossa structures, or spinal cord. The majority are related to the cerebral gray and white matter, mainly in the frontal lobe. Most AVMs remain asymptomatic during life. Saccular aneurysms and AVMs are the most common CNS vascular abnormalities, and their frequencies appear related to geographic or ethnic factors: in Singapore, AVMs are four times more common than aneurysms, whereas aneurysms are five times more common than AVMs in the United States (2). Most AVMs are solitary; however, multiple lesions may occur.

Clinical Features. AVMs occur with equal frequency in males and females, and have a tendency to become symptomatic during the second and third decades of life. The clinical presentation may include intracranial hemorrhage, seizures, focal neurologic deficits, impairment of higher cortical functions, headache, or

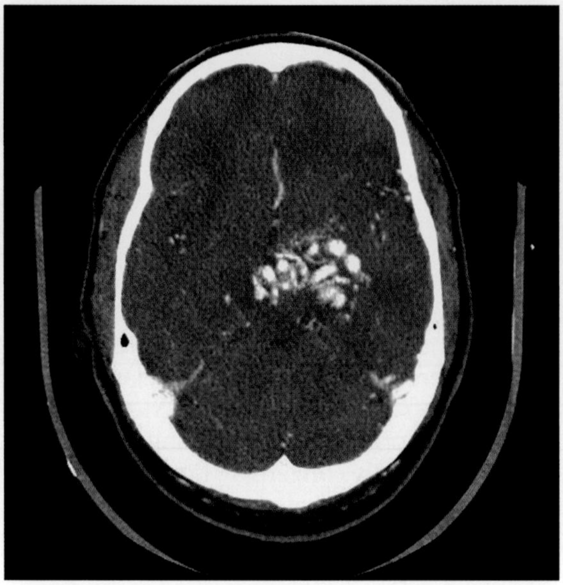

Figure 6-1

ARTERIOVENOUS MALFORMATION

The postcontrast computerized tomography (CT) image shows intensely enhancing tubular structures, vessels of different diameters, throughout the lesion.

a vascular bruit. Intracranial hemorrhage is the most common presentation, and is typically associated with sudden, severe headache. AVM-associated hemorrhage is usually intraparenchymal, with preference for infratentorial structures, but may also present as an intraventricular or subarachnoid bleed. Hemorrhage may result from rupture of dilated veins or microaneurysms within the AVM nidus (3). Mortality from the first hemorrhage varies between 6 and 14 percent. The likelihood of rebleeding is approximately 6 percent during the first year and 4 percent for subsequent years. The risk factors for intracranial hemorrhage associated with an AVM include hypertension, small size of the lesion, location in the basal ganglia or thalamus, and presence of an aneurysm within the nidus.

Seizure is the presenting symptom in 28 to 67 percent of patients with AVMs, particularly for those with large lesions, and is the most common initial symptom in patients between 11 and 20 years of age (4). Some large AVMs are associated with high blood flow and a steal phenomenon in certain regions of the brain, which become susceptible to ischemia and resulting focal neurologic deficits. Aneurysms from the vein of Galen may result from AVMs located in the third ventricle or pons (5); such aneurysms present with cardiomegaly and cardiac failure in the neonatal period or as obstructive hydrocephalus secondary to aqueduct compression in older children.

Radiologic Findings. Modern neuroimaging studies, including computerized tomography (CT) scan, CT angiography, magnetic resonance imaging (MRI), MR angiography, and standard angiography, are essential to characterize AVMs and define treatment approaches (4). Noncontrast CT scans may suggest an AVM by demonstrating intraparenchymal hemorrhage. The presence of serpentine enhancement after contrast administration is highly suspicious for an AVM. High-resolution dynamic contrast-enhanced CT can delineate the size of the nidus (fig. 6-1). Standard sequences such as T1- and T2-weighted MRIs provide precise information on the size and location of an AVM. MR angiography provides information on the relationship of the feeding arteries and draining veins. Three-dimensional time-of-flight techniques are helpful for visualizing arterial flow, and two-dimensional time-of-flight is best for showing the slower flow in the venous drainage. Functional imaging, including xenon CT scanning after administration of acetazolamide, is useful in determining the effects of an AVM on the cerebral blood flow and the regulatory capacity of the surrounding brain. The presence of a steal phenomenon may indicate loss of autoregulation in the brain adjacent to an AVM. Functional MRI may show the relationship of an AVM to vital cortical areas.

The vascular pattern of an AVM is well delineated by conventional angiography. The blood supply may arise from one or several intracranial arteries. The venous drainage may be through the superficial or deep venous systems, dural sinuses, or a combination of these.

Gross Findings. The size of an AVM varies from a microscopic lesion to a grossly identifiable vascular abnormality several centimeters in diameter that occupies a large area of the brain. The most classic appearance is that of a triangular mass, with a broad base affecting the leptomeninges and cortex and the apex of the triangle in the underlying white matter (fig. 6-2). Some are identified as a well-demarcated

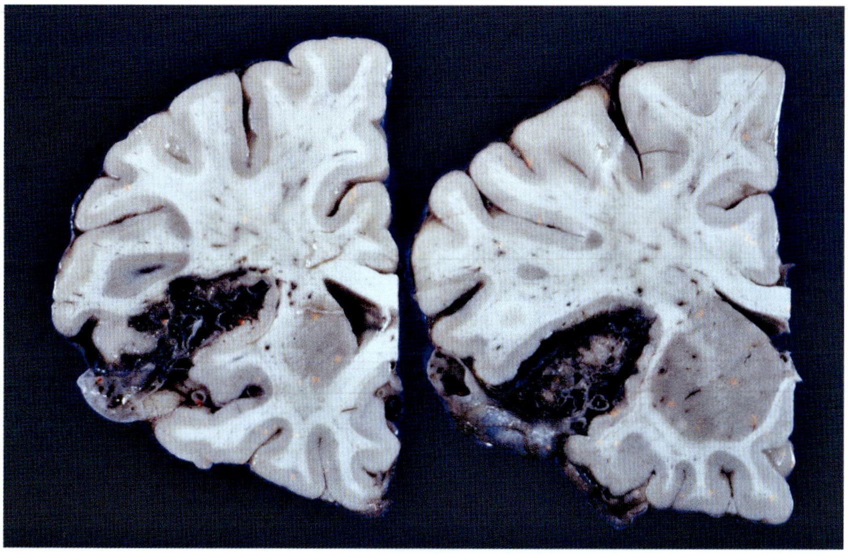

Figure 6-2

ARTERIOVENOUS MALFORMATION

The focally hemorrhagic arteriovenous malformation (AVM) involves the leptomeninges and cerebral cortex.

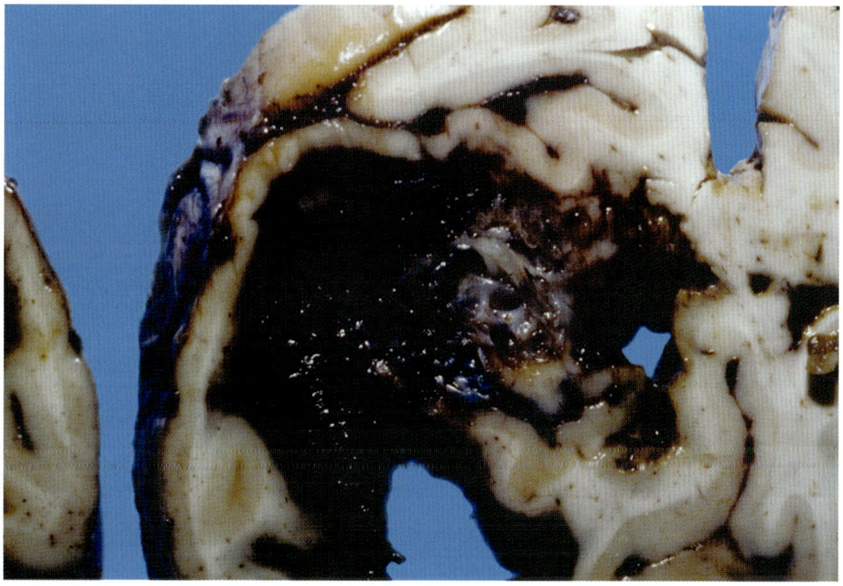

Figure 6-3

ARTERIOVENOUS MALFORMATION

The AVM is partially obscured by a parenchymal hematoma.

conglomerate of vascular channels without intervening hemorrhage. Others are obscured by focal or large areas of recent and old hemorrhage (figs. 6-3, 6-4). The caliber and wall thickness of the individual blood vessels are variable and their lumens may be patent or occluded (fig. 6-5). The intervening tissue may show yellow discoloration due to old hemorrhage or cystic change related to ischemic infarction, and may be firm and gritty as a result of fibrosis, calcification, and sometimes ossification. AVMs related to the vein of Galen are associated with massive dilation of the vein with compression of adjacent neural structures (fig. 6-6).

Microscopic Findings. An AVM is composed of a tangle of arteries, veins, and other vascular channels that entrap brain parenchyma between them (fig. 6-7). The arteries usually have thick walls with a muscular layer and a continuous or discontinuous elastic lamina. Many malformative arteries display marked variation in wall thickness, which can be seen in cross sections of individual vessels; a single vessel can change from a thick, muscularized wall to a thin, collagenous wall in a short distance. Veins show thinner walls than arteries, with few smooth muscle cells and an absence of elastic lamina. Some veins, referred as "arterialized,"

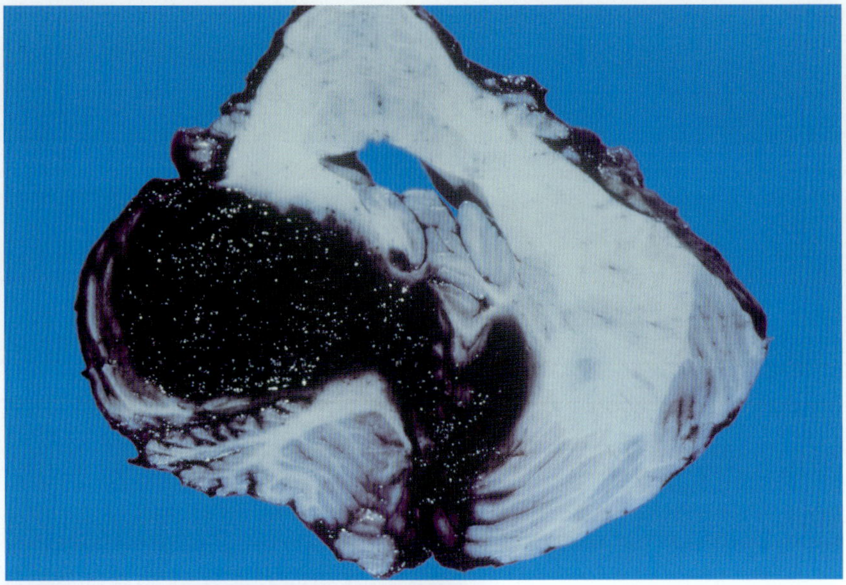

Figure 6-4

ARTERIOVENOUS MALFORMATION

This AVM is associated with hemorrhage centered in the middle cerebellar peduncle and subarachnoid extension. This may be the case for hemorrhages in locations not usual for hemorrhage associated with hypertension or cerebral amyloid angiopathy (CAA).

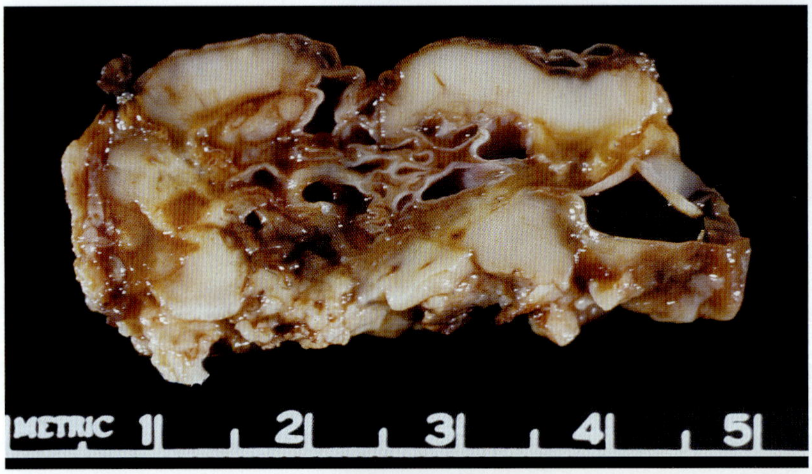

Figure 6-5

ARTERIOVENOUS MALFORMATION

The AVM is composed of dilated vascular channels in the cortex and white matter.

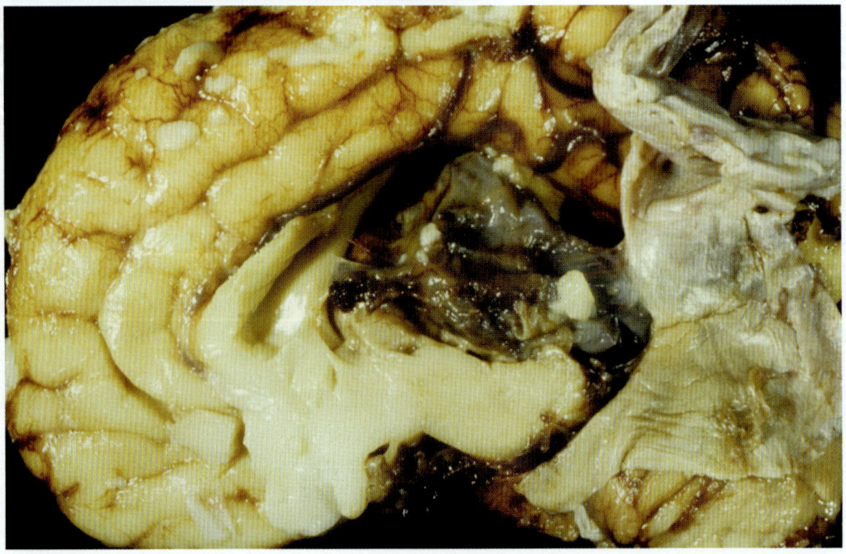

Figure 6-6

ANEURYSM OF VEIN OF GALEN

Aneurysm in the vein of Galen is related to an AVM in the posterior fossa. It presents as a space-occupying mass.

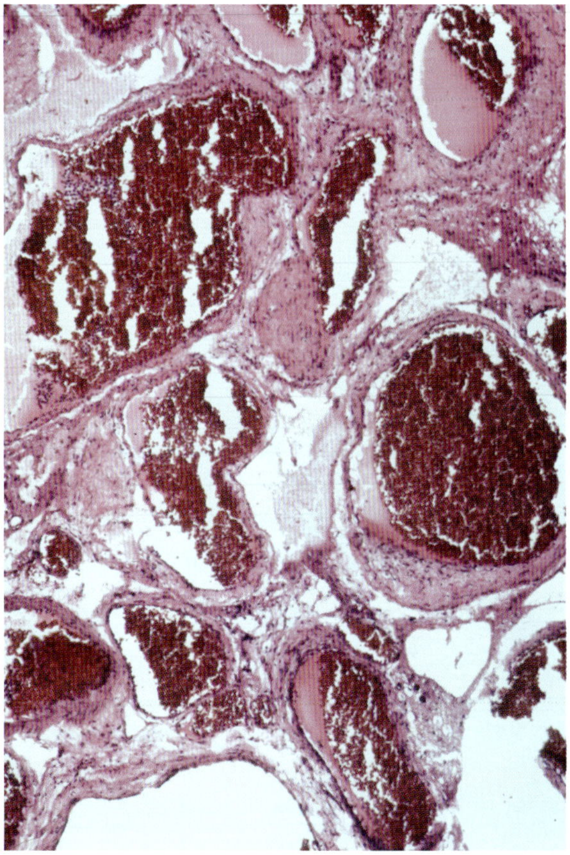

Figure 6-7

ARTERIOVENOUS MALFORMATION

The AVM is composed of vascular channels of variable thickness and intervening brain tissue.

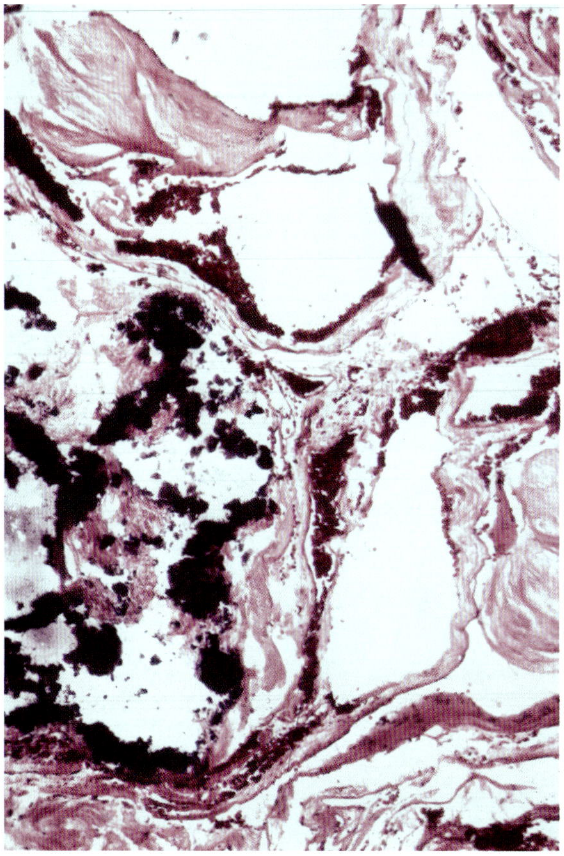

Figure 6-8

ARTERIOVENOUS MALFORMATION

The vascular channels show recanalized thromboemboli and calcification.

contain a more organized smooth muscle layer. Capillaries are absent.

The lumens of the various vascular channels may be patent or occluded by recent or organized thromboemboli (fig. 6-8). AVMs that were embolized before surgery may show embolization material associated with foreign body granulomas within the vascular lumens or adjacent tissues. Elastic and Masson trichrome stains help characterize the vascular walls, but are only required for diagnosis in challenging cases (figs. 6-9, 6-10).

The brain parenchyma, which is typically prominent between the abnormal vessels, shows evidence of remote hemorrhage, with hemosiderin-laden macrophages, gliosis with variable numbers of reactive astrocytes, focal fibrosis, calcification, and ossification. Foci of inflammatory mononuclear cells may be present. On occasion, amyloid is identified within the vascular walls. Treatment of AVMs with radiation-based approaches may lead to the formation of scar tissue rich in myofibroblasts and collagen fibrils.

Immunohistochemical Findings. Immunohistochemistry is not of diagnostic value. Endothelial cells express factor VIII and other endothelial markers. Laminin expression is associated with the elastic lamina (1). The basal lamina of the endothelial cells expresses type IV collagen and smooth muscle cells in the media express myosin heavy chain, actin, and smoothelin, a novel marker for contractile vascular smooth muscle cell phenotype. Expression of smoothelin is less prevalent in large AVM vessels, which may reflect the loss of contractile property associated with hemodynamic stress (6).

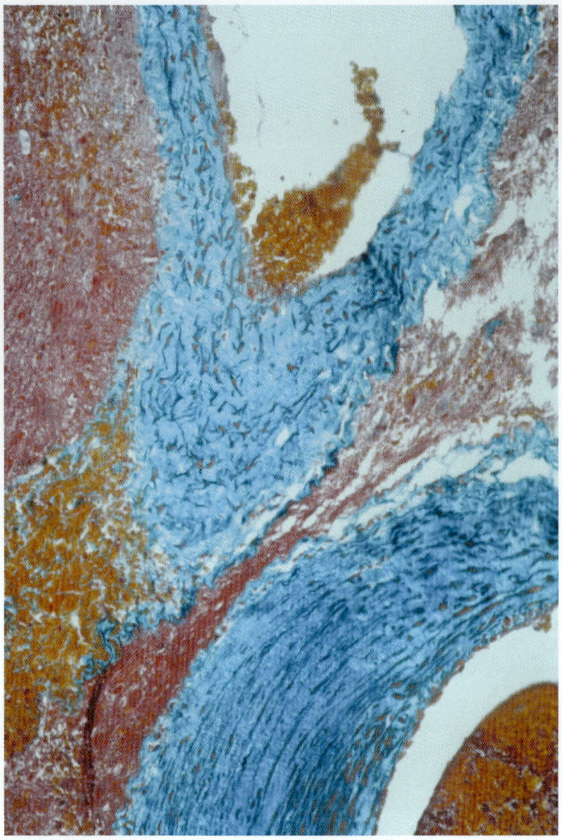

Figure 6-9

ARTERIOVENOUS MALFORMATION

The arterial vascular channels have thick muscular layers (trichrome stain).

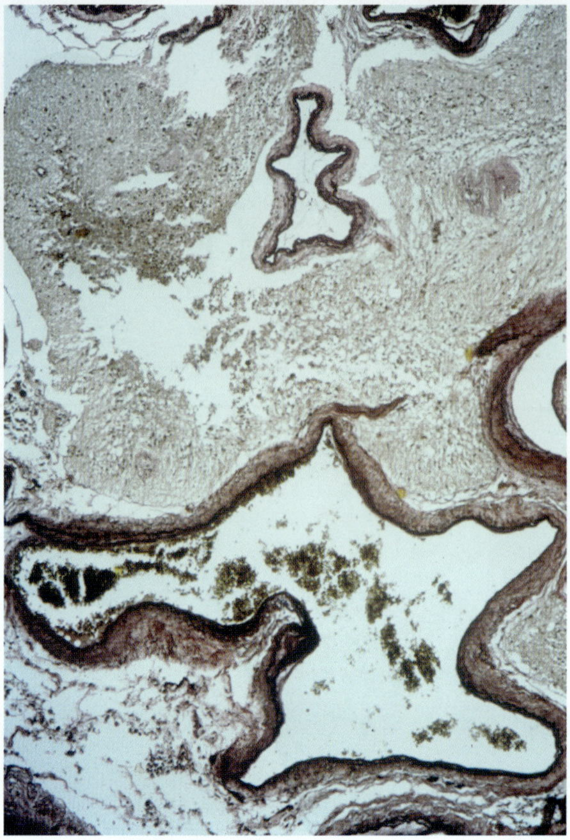

Figure 6-10

ARTERIOVENOUS MALFORMATION

The vascular channels show continuous elastic lamina (elastic stain).

Ultrastructural Findings. Electron microscopic studies are not needed in the diagnosis of AVMs. The cellular constituents of the vascular walls appear normal at the ultrastructural level. Endothelial cells contain pinocytotic vesicles and Weibel-Palade bodies, are in contact with a basal membrane, and have intercellular tight junctions (7). Smooth muscle cells display abundant actin microfilaments related to plasmalemmal attachment plaques, and thicker myofilaments. They are invested by a thin basal membrane and joined together by small junctional complexes. Fibroblasts show prominent cisternae of rough endoplasmic reticulum and a close relationship with collagen fibrils.

Differential Diagnosis. The main entities in the differential diagnosis of AVM are cavernous angioma, saccular aneurysm, glioma, and artifactually condensed leptomeningeal vessels. Cavernous angiomas (see below) are composed of vascular channels with fibrous walls that lack the smooth muscle cells and elastic lamina characteristic of the arterial vessels of AVMs. Cavernous angiomas generally lack intervening neural tissue, except sometimes at their edges, and have dense hemosiderin deposits forming a halo around the lesion. This contrasts with AVMs, in which the interstitial neural tissue is prominent and demonstrates astrocytosis often accompanied by hemosiderin-laden macrophages.

Exclusion of a saccular aneurysm is important in the microscopic examination of tissue fragments obtained piecemeal during surgical procedures. The wall of a saccular aneurysm is composed of fibrous tissue and endothelium, without smooth muscle cells and elastic fibers (fig. 6-11). Some AVMs are associated with

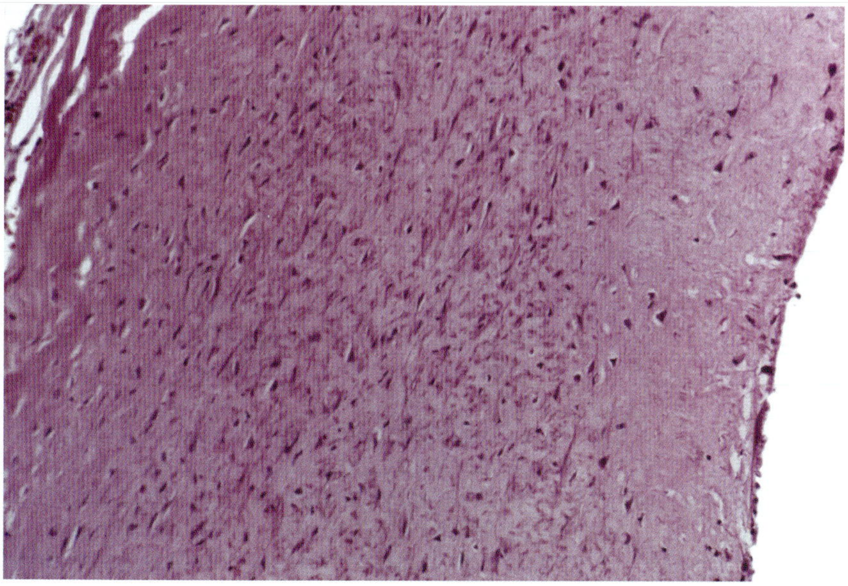

Figure 6-11

SACCULAR ANEURYSM

The wall of the aneurysm is composed of an endothelial cell layer and a thickened fibrous layer. Elastic lamina and smooth muscle cells are absent.

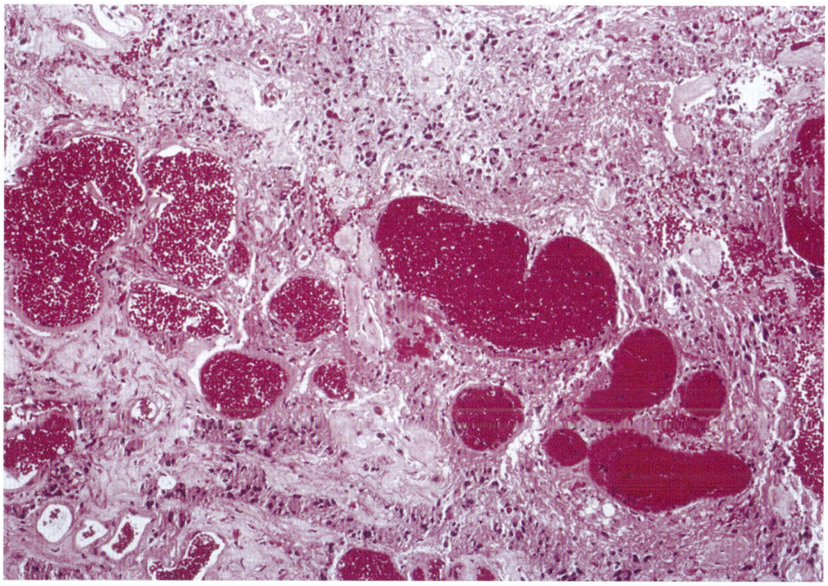

Figure 6-12

PILOCYTIC ASTROCYTOMA

The prominent vascular component of a pilocytic astrocytoma mimics an AVM intermixed with neoplastic astrocytes.

aneurysmal dilatation of vascular channels. Typically, however, the clinical and radiologic findings readily distinguish these two entities.

The vascular component of some gliomas, including pilocytic astrocytoma and malignant gliomas, may be so prominent as to suggest the possibility of an AVM (fig. 6-12). In such situations, thorough examination of the entire specimen for features of glioma readily ensures a correct diagnosis. More problematic, however, is the concern over the cellularity of the intervening and surrounding brain tissue associated with an AVM. In many AVMs, the reactive gliosis becomes moderately hypercellular and is associated with some cellular pleomorphism, raising the concern for a coexisting glioma. Caution should be exercised in making such a diagnosis, given the sometimes marked gliosis associated with AVMs. Nonetheless, rare cases of coexisting AVM and glioma have been reported (8). Some AVMs have associated increases of surrounding oligodendroglial cells that can suggest a coexisting oligodendroglioma; in most cases, this is a reactive phenomenon, but occasional cases of oligodendroglioma have been reported in association with AVM (9).

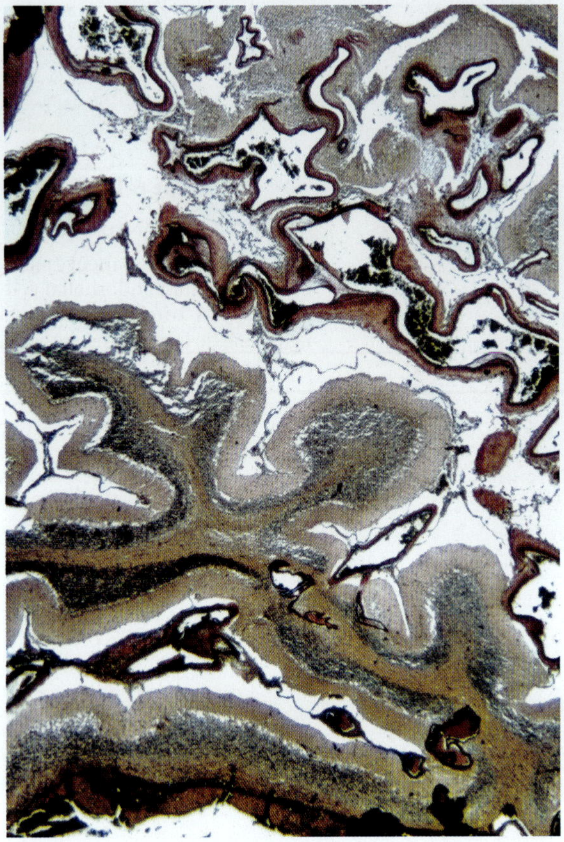

Figure 6-13

CEREBELLAR LEPTOMENINGES

The blood vessels are artifactually compressed, resembling an AVM (elastic stain).

The leptomeninges in some areas of the brain, mainly the cerebellum, are highly vascularized and the vessels may be artifactually compacted in surgical specimens, simulating an AVM (fig. 6-13). A misdiagnosis is easily avoided if one is aware of this artifact and if attention is paid to the correlation between the microscopic absence of morphologically abnormal vessel walls and the radiologic features.

Treatment and Prognosis. Hemorrhage is the main factor associated with the morbidity and mortality of a patient with an AVM. The risk of hemorrhage is eliminated by the surgical excision of the lesion. The factors that mitigate the use or extent of surgical procedures include the size of the lesion, number of feeding arteries, amount of blood flow through the lesion, degree of steal from surrounding brain, location of the lesion, functional importance of adjacent brain, and path of venous drainage (4).

To facilitate surgical decisions, grading systems are used to predict the operative risks for patients with AVMs. For this, the Spetzler-Martin scale, which focuses on size and location of the AVM and the deep venous drainage, is commonly used (10). Large lesions may be managed by a combination of preoperative embolization and staged resection. Preoperative embolization is often carried out to produce thrombosis of the vascular channels and to decrease the number of feeding arteries.

Nonoperative therapy has been advocated for AVMs, with radiosurgery being an accepted modality for the treatment of AVMs of the basal ganglia, internal capsule, and thalamus since it significantly decreases the risk of hemorrhage. Treatment of AVMs with gamma knife surgery may be successful, with complete or incomplete obliteration of the nidus; however, long-term complications may develop including delayed cyst formation, hemorrhage, increased seizure frequency, middle cerebral artery stenosis, and white matter lesions (11).

Cavernous Angioma (Cavernous Malformation)

Definition. *Cavernous angioma*, also known as *cavernous malformation*, or less commonly, *cavernoma*, is a vascular malformation composed of vascular channels with closely opposed fibrous walls.

General Comments. Cavernous angiomas occur throughout the entire CNS, including the meninges, cerebrum, cerebellum, brain stem, and spinal cord. The most common location is the cerebral white matter. Most cavernous angiomas occur as single lesions, however, multiple lesions may be present in both sporadic and familial cases. Cavernous angiomas are the most common component of mixed vascular malformations.

Clinical Features. Most cavernous angiomas remain asymptomatic during life. Clinical symptoms related to hemorrhage, seizures, and focal neurologic deficits occur most often during the second to fourth decades of life, with seizures being the most common clinical manifestation. Progressive neurologic deficits occur with lesions of the brain stem. The risk for hemorrhage is higher in children than in adults.

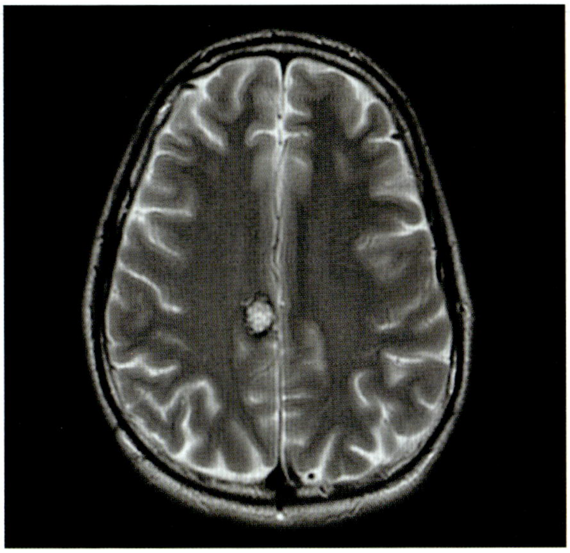

Figure 6-14

CAVERNOUS ANGIOMA

Within the right cingulated gyrus is a focus of abnormal signal which, on coronal T2-weighted fluid-attenuated inversion recovery (FLAIR) images demonstrates a heterogeneous bright signal within, but a dark rim.

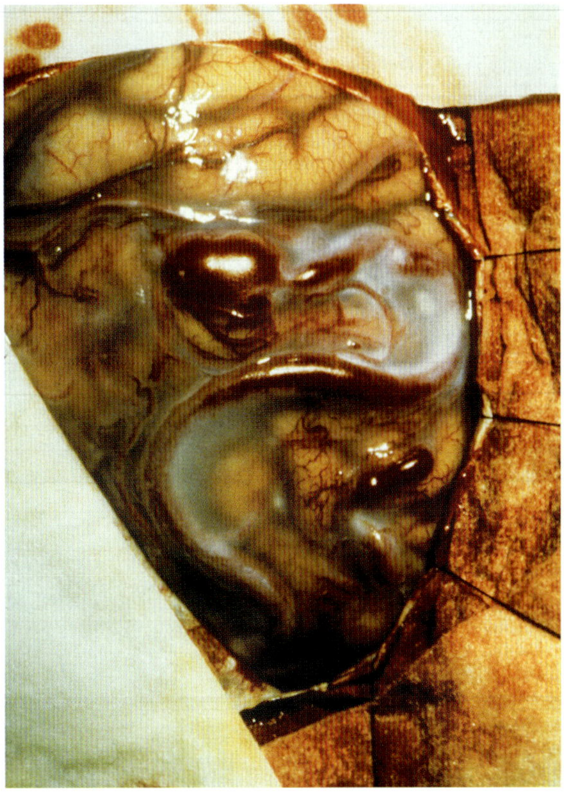

Figure 6-15

CAVERNOUS ANGIOMA

The lesion in the cerebral leptomeninges is composed of dilated, tortuous and congested vascular channels.

Cavernous angiomas have been reported to develop in children after radiation therapy for brain tumors (12), but the major predisposing factor is genetic. Individuals of Hispanic, Italian, and French descent, among others, show a familial predisposition to develop cavernous angiomas and these patients may harbor multiple lesions. Indeed, a hereditary predisposition should be considered in a patient with more than one cavernous angioma. Familial cavernous angiomas are inherited in an autosomal dominant manner secondary to alterations at the *CCM1*, *CCM2*, and *CCM3* loci (1). Linkage in Hispanic families is to the *CCM1* locus on chromosome 7q21-q22, with mutations in the *KRIT1* gene (13). Loci for non-Hispanic patients are found on chromosomes 7p15-13 (*CMM2*) and 3q25.2-27 (*CCM3*) (14). The *CCM3* gene has been identified as *PDCD10* (15).

Radiologic Findings. Cavernous angiomas usually show nearly diagnostic features on MRI. The MRI pattern includes a central core of increased intensity surrounded by a rim of decreased intensity on T2-weighted sequences, or multiloculated areas of increased signal on T1-weighted sequences (fig. 6-14) (4). Multiple lesions raise the possibility of being familial. Cavernous angiomas are rarely visualized on angiography because they lack detectable communication with the arterial system, have thrombosis of vascular channels, and display slow intralesional blood flow.

Laboratory findings. The cerebrospinal fluid (CSF) is usually unremarkable. A xanthochromic CSF may be present if subarachnoid hemorrhage has occurred.

Gross Findings. A cavernous angioma is usually identified as a well-demarcated mass of compacted blood vessels, resulting in a "mulberry-like" lesion (figs. 6-15, 6-16). Associated hemorrhage is typically present in the surrounding brain parenchyma.

Microscopic Findings. Cavernous angiomas are composed of vascular channels with thick, fibrous, hyalinized walls lacking features of either veins or arteries. The channels are usually

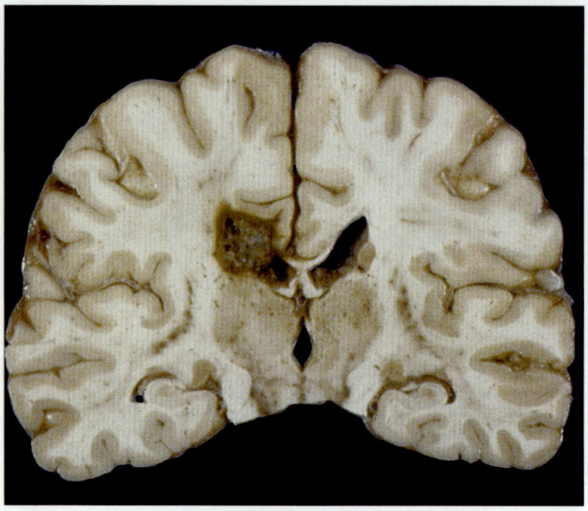

Figure 6-16

CAVERNOUS ANGIOMA

The cavernous angioma of the left caudate nucleus is composed of compacted blood vessels in a "mulberry-like" pattern.

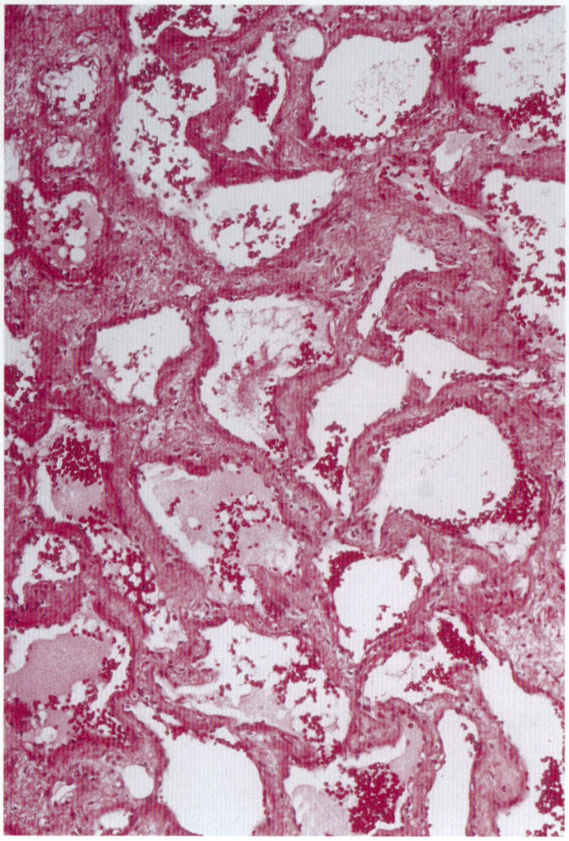

Figure 6-17

CAVERNOUS ANGIOMA

The vascular channels are apposed, with an absence of intervening neural tissue.

back-to-back without intervening neural tissue, but entrapped parenchyma is commonly found toward the edge of the malformation (fig. 6-17). Some lesions feature foci of closely arranged, small vessels, the size of larger capillaries, which may serve as a nidus for further growth (16). Vascular lumens may be occluded by recent or recanalized thrombi and the walls may demonstrate calcification or ossification. Some lesions, particularly in the temporal lobe, may become densely mineralized and are referred to as *hemangioma calcificans*. Neural tissue at the periphery of the lesion exhibits gliosis and old hemorrhage, with dense collections of hemosiderin-laden macrophages.

Immunohistochemical Findings. The endothelial cells express factor VIII and other endothelial markers (fig. 6-18). Fibronectin is present in the basal lamina (1) and cells of the subendothelial layer express actin. Expression of myosin heavy chain is found in 20 percent of cases.

Ultrastructural Findings. Vascular channels show endothelial cells with few tight junctions associated with amorphous material lacking organized collagen (7). Smooth muscle cells are few. At the periphery, capillaries are often associated with hemosiderin.

Differential Diagnosis. In most situations, the preoperative radiologic findings strongly suggest a cavernous angioma. Sometimes, however, cavernous angioma occurs in the setting of an isolated cerebral hemorrhage, without a definite radiologically detectable malformation. Such isolated parenchymal hemorrhages may occur secondary to a diverse group of lesions, including primary and metastatic neoplasms, ruptured saccular or infectious (mycotic) aneurysms, and vascular malformations. For this reason, sections for microscopic examination should sample not only the hematoma but also the interface between the hemorrhage and neural tissue. The vascular channels of cavernous angiomas lack the characteristic features of arteries, veins, and capillaries that are present in AVMs, venous angiomas, and telangiectasias, respectively. Stains for elastic and trichrome and immunohistochemistry for smooth muscle cells differentiate between the various vascular

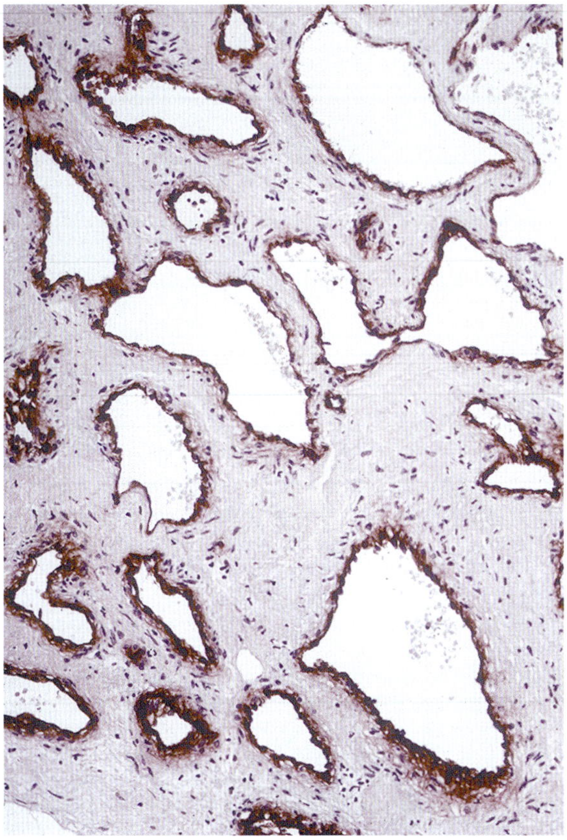

Figure 6-18

CAVERNOUS ANGIOMA

Factor VIII is expressed by the endothelial cells (immunoperoxidase method).

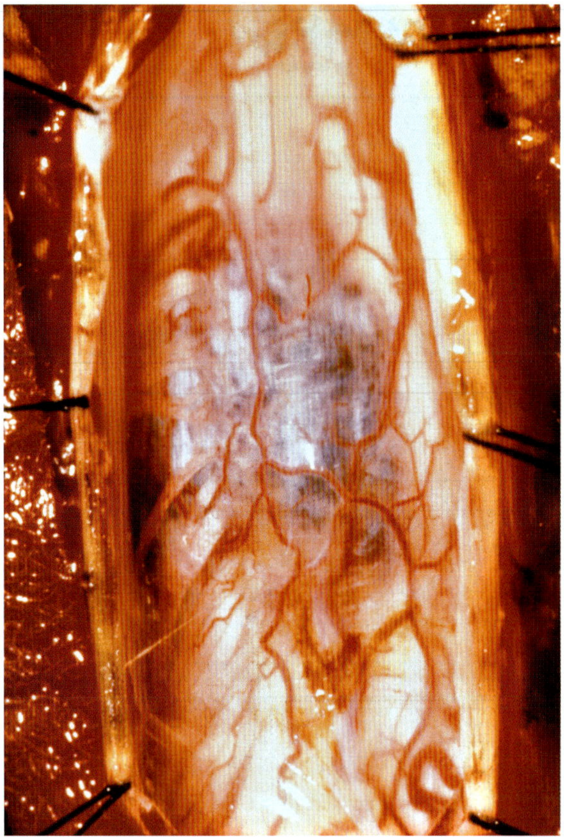

Figure 6-19

VENOUS ANGIOMA

The venous angioma of the spinal cord is composed of dilated superficial veins.

malformations and aneurysms. Smooth muscle cells are present in the walls of vascular channels in AVMs and venous angiomas. An infectious aneurysm usually shows localized necrotizing panarteritis in an otherwise unremarkable arterial wall.

Treatment and Prognosis. The prognosis after surgical excision is excellent. Seizures resolve in 92 percent of cases. The risk for hemorrhage has been estimated at 2 percent for incidental cavernous angiomas and 7 percent for symptomatic lesions (17). Hemorrhage associated with a cavernous angioma is usually self-limited and patients have a good or fair outcome. Recurrent hemorrhage after an initial episode of bleeding has been estimated to occur in 20 to 85 percent of cases. Cavernous angiomas of the brain stem carry a higher risk of rebleeding and significant morbidity (17).

Venous Angioma

The *venous angioma*, more recently referred to in the radiologic literature as *developmental venous anomaly*, is a vascular malformation composed of dilated veins and lined by a single layer of endothelial cells associated with a thin wall of smooth muscle cells, fibroblasts, and collagen fibers. The intervening neural tissue is histologically unremarkable. Venous angiomas are the most common vascular malformations of the CNS with a preference for the preventricular cerebral white matter and thoracic spinal cord (fig. 6-19) (18).

Although the majority are asymptomatic lesions, some may be clinically significant if associated with cavernous angiomas (19). Otherwise, these lesions do not come to the attention of surgical pathologists. The diagnosis is

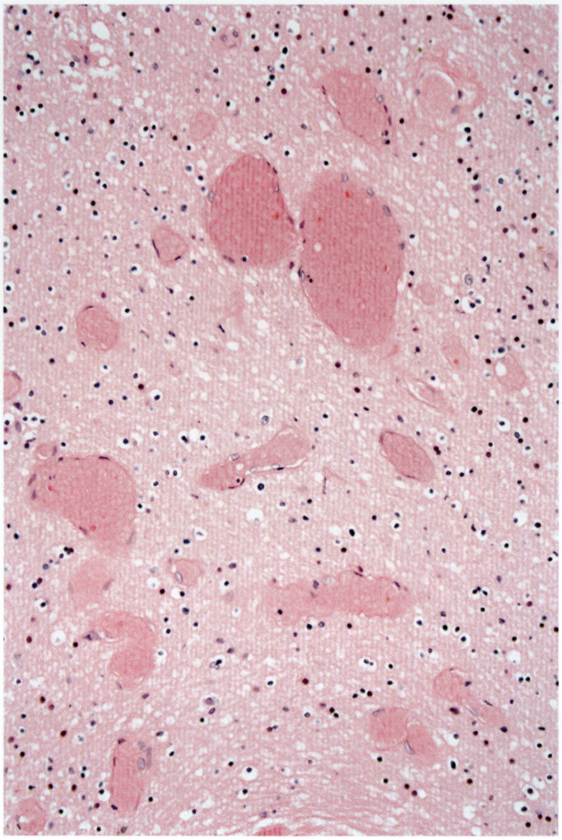

Figure 6-20

CAPILLARY TELANGIECTASIA

An incidental capillary telangiectasia of the cerebral white matter is composed of dilated capillaries.

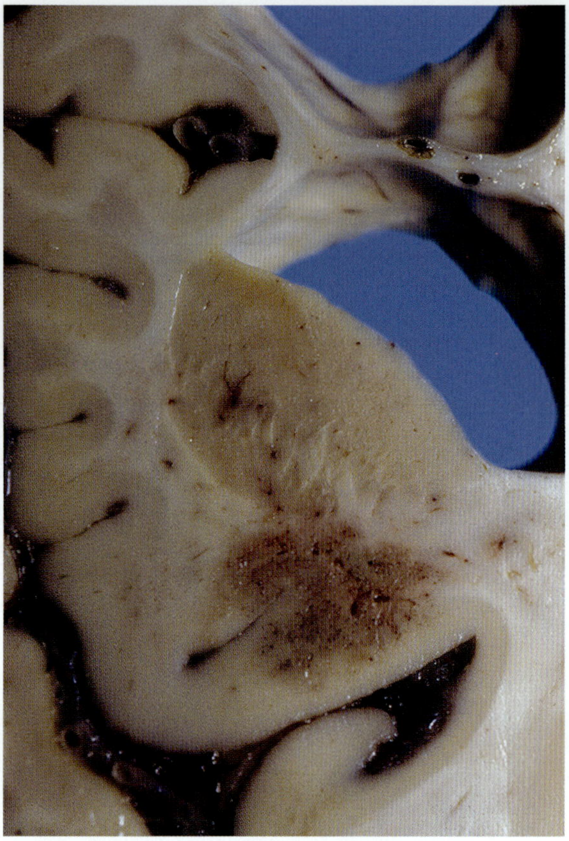

Figure 6-21

CAPILLARY TELANGIECTASIA

Asymptomatic capillary telangiectasia involves the cortex and white matter of the right lateral orbital gyri at the level of the caudate nucleus.

suggested by characteristic findings on contrast-enhanced CT and MRI, including the presence of a large dilated enhancing vein and several small tributary feeding veins with a radial configuration. Angiography is seldom needed for confirmation.

Capillary Telangiectasia

Capillary telangiectasias are composed of dilated capillaries with unremarkable intervening brain tissue (5). Individual vascular channels are lined by a single layer of endothelial cells resting on a delicate wall composed of reticulin fibers (fig. 6-20). Smooth muscle cells are absent.

Capillary telangiectasias are usually solitary lesions found incidentally as small, dark red spots within the CNS parenchyma at the time of the postmortem examination (fig. 6-21). In the pons, a common site, capillary telangiectasia may be detected as a nebulous blush on angiography and may show contrast enhancement on MRI. Although typically regarded as quiescent lesions, capillary telangiectasias may be associated with hemorrhage, including the syndrome of perimesencephalic hemorrhage (20). Rarely, slowly progressive neurologic symptoms herald the presence of diffuse capillary telangiectasias (21). In surgical neuropathology, these are usually encountered as incidental findings in resections for other conditions.

Dural Arteriovenous Fistula (Foix-Alajouanine Syndrome)

Dural arteriovenous fistula (*Foix-Alajouanine syndrome*) predominantly affects the lower spinal cord. It is rarely encountered as a surgical specimen in the setting of lower spinal cord

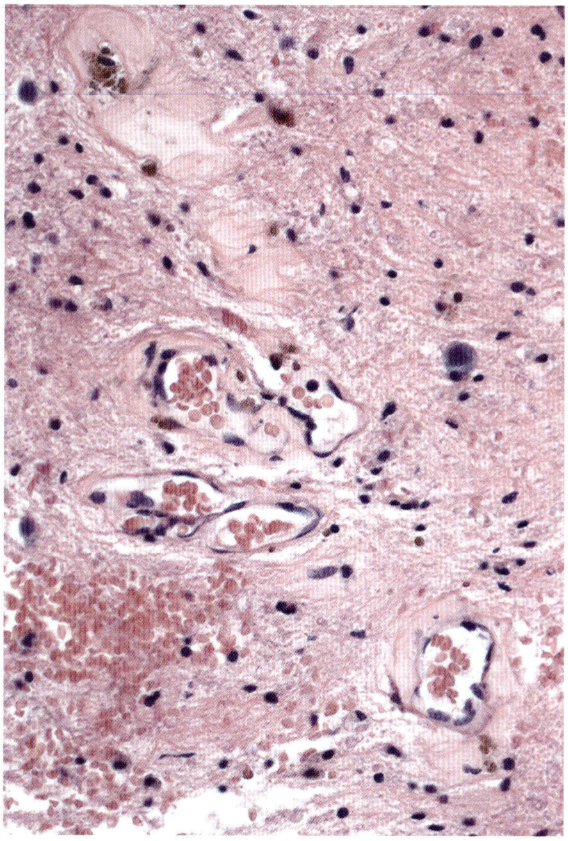

Figure 6-22

DURAL ARTERIOVENOUS FISTULA

Small caliber vessels in a spinal cord biopsy show thickened, collagenous walls with evidence of prior hemorrhage.

dysfunction. The histopathologic findings include necrosis of the affected cord regions. Gray matter structures are more severely involved. These features are accompanied by small blood vessels with thickened fibrotic walls in the affected spinal cord segments; enlarged, tortuous, and thick-walled subarachnoid veins may be observed overlying the surface of the cord (fig. 6-22).

VASCULITIDES

A wide variety of vasculitides affect the CNS, but few are restricted to the CNS. Most notably, giant cell arteritis and primary angiitis of the nervous system are conditions that remain isolated to the brain and that come to the attention of surgical pathologists. The remaining vasculitides are usually part of a systemic illness and a correct diagnosis is more often based on the clinical and laboratory features than on biopsy (Table 6-1).

Table 6-1

PATHOLOGIC FINDINGS IN SELECTIVE CENTRAL NERVOUS SYSTEM (CNS) VASCULOPATHIES

Granulomatous Vasculitis
Giant cell arteritis
Primary angiitis of CNS
Takayasu arteritis
Inflammatory cerebral amyloid angiopathy
Necrotizing Nongranulomatous Vasculitis
Polyarteritis nodosa
Wegener granulomatosis
Kawasaki disease
Churg-Strauss syndrome
Hypersensitivity angiitis
Inflammatory bowel disease
Sjögren syndrome
Behcet syndrome
Cogan syndrome
Systemic lupus erythematosus (rare)
Rheumatoid arthritis
Mixed connective tissue disease
Noninflammatory Vasculopathy
Sneddon syndrome
Malignant atrophic papulosis (Kohlmeier-Degos)
Susac syndrome
Systemic lupus erythematosus
Scleroderma
Cerebral amyloid angiopathy
CADASIL[a]
Arteriolar sclerosis secondary to hypertension, diabetes

[a]CADASIL = cerebral autosomal dominant arteriopathy with subcortical infarcts and leukoencephalopathy.

Findings from laboratory studies, including cerebral vasculature imaging, aid in the diagnosis of vasculitis and often obviate the need for brain biopsy. Nonetheless, meningeal and brain biopsy is sometimes performed to establish a diagnosis prior to the use of immunosuppressive therapies. Since physicians caring for the patient are often waiting for brain biopsy results to initiate therapy, frozen sections are often requested. Vascular wall damage with associated inflammation can be detected on frozen section; however, the patchy nature of the disease process may result in a false negative result because of limited sampling. There is, therefore, a trade-off between a rapid return of information and the introduction of artifact at tissue freezing. One solution is the use of rapid processing of fixed tissue to provide evaluation of paraffin-embedded sections in a timely manner. Given the sometimes patchy nature of the vasculitic process, it is often useful to place individual tissue fragments into separate cassettes. Although this results in a slight increase in the time of laboratory processing, there is the strong advantage of being able to perform step sectioning to search for vasculitis independently on each tissue fragment.

Giant Cell Arteritis

Definition. *Giant cell arteritis* is a systemic vasculitis characterized by granulomatous inflammation and a preference for arteries of the head, including the eye. Giant cell arteritis is also known as *temporal arteritis, cranial arteritis,* and *Horton disease.*

General Comments. Giant cell arteritis is a systemic vasculitis that affects the aorta and its main branches, including elastic and muscular arteries. The involvement of medium and small arteries of the head and eye, mainly temporal, ophthalmic, and posterior ciliary arteries, explains the neurologic and ocular symptoms. The etiology is unknown, but may be related to an immune reaction activating T cells that produce interferon gamma in the adventitial vasa vasorum of the arterial wall. Proinflammatory S-100A8, S-100A9, and S-100A12 proteins released by neutrophils and CD68-positive monocytes have been demonstrated in serum and temporal artery specimens (22). Giant cell arteritis is associated with a heterogeneous group of disorders including malignancies and autoimmune disease. Risk factors include human leukocyte antigen (HLA)-DR4, polymyalgia rheumatica, and preexisting degenerative vascular disease.

Clinical Features. Giant cell arteritis is seldom seen before the age of 50 years and is more common in women. The clinical presentation is related to the vessels involved. Compromise of the superficial temporal artery may be associated with polymyalgia rheumatica and ophthalmologic complications. At palpation, the artery may be firm, nodular, and pulseless. Patients with temporal arteritis may experience gradual or sudden onset of headache, jaw claudication, and visual disturbances. Nonspecific constitutional manifestations such as fever, malaise, fatigue, anemia, sore throat, and hepatic dysfunction are common. Ocular symptoms include visual loss of varying severity, amaurosis fugax, diplopia, and pain. Visual loss, the most dramatic complication, is related to anterior ischemic optic neuropathy from occlusion of the posterior ciliary arteries. Blindness may be unilateral or bilateral. The clinical syndrome of polymyalgia rheumatica is characterized by pain and stiffness of muscles of the shoulder and pelvic girdles associated with nonspecific constitutional symptoms and an elevated erythrocyte sedimentation rate (ESR). Polymyalgia rheumatica is not exclusively associated with giant cell arteritis; only about half of the patients who present with polymyalgia rheumatica develop giant cell temporal arteritis.

Involvement of the CNS may manifest as stroke or transient ischemic attacks. In particular, stroke is a complication of giant cell arteritis when the internal carotid or vertebral arteries are involved (23). In such cases, the inflammatory lesion is localized to the extradural segment of the artery. Occasionally, the intradural segment of one or several arteries is involved. The mechanism responsible for the clinical presentation of stroke results from critical luminal stenosis induced by intimal proliferation or thrombotic occlusion of the lumen secondary to inflammation of the arterial wall. Embolic phenomena may also occur distal to regions of vascular inflammation.

Radiologic Findings. Angiography may show areas of dilation and constriction along the length of the involved artery, but the artery may be unremarkable or the changes nonspecific. Color duplex sonography may show a characteristic hypoechoic halo around the temporal artery.

Laboratory Findings. Patients with giant cell arteritis usually show a markedly increased ESR and may have normochromic or hypochromic anemia as well as normal or increased white blood cell counts. Abnormalities in the CSF are present if the intracranial arteries are involved. CSF pressure and glucose levels are usually normal, but there may be pleocytosis with lymphocytes and polymorphonuclear leucocytes as well as increased protein. Elevated levels of immunoglobulin (Ig)G and the presence of oligoclonal bands, indicative of an immune-mediated response, may be seen in association with giant cell arteritis and other vasculitides. Some patients have elevated liver enzymes.

Gross Findings. The artery may be thickened and nodular in the areas involved by arteritis. If

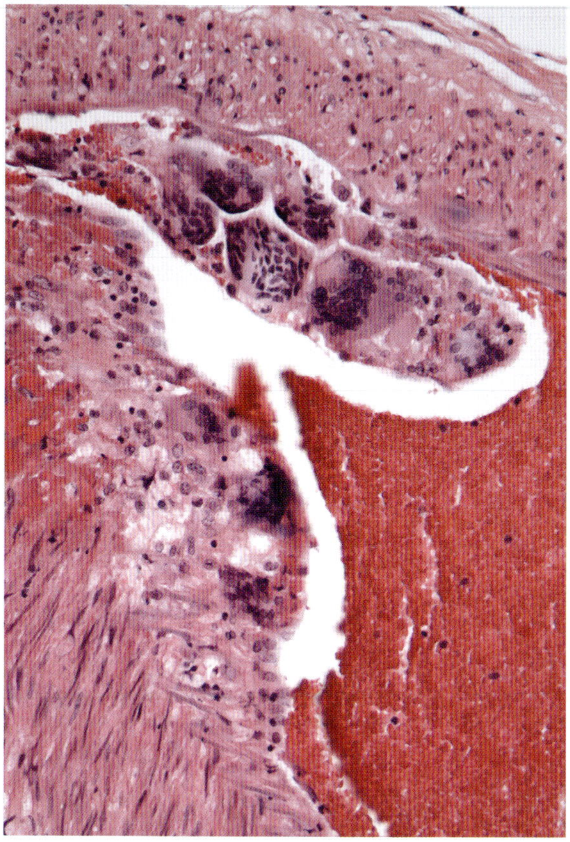

Figure 6-23

GIANT CELL ARTERITIS

Granulomatous inflammation with multinucleated giant cells.

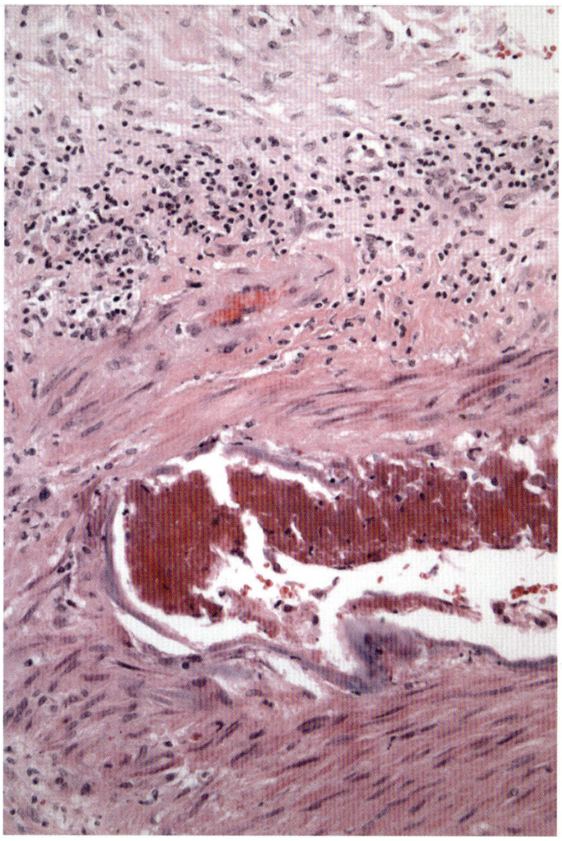

Figure 6-24

GIANT CELL ARTERITIS

Active nongranulomatous vaculitis.

the artery is abnormal at palpation, a biopsy of a 2-cm segment should be sufficient for diagnosis. If the artery is grossly unremarkable, a longer 4-cm segment should be excised. The pathologic findings tend to be focal. Examination of the entire specimen using serial cross sections is controversial (24,25), but may yield diagnostic insights. If the first temporal artery biopsy is negative for arteritis, the opposite artery may be biopsied; a second biopsy is positive in 5 percent of cases after an initial negative biopsy (26).

Microscopic Findings. Microscopic examination may yield active or healed vasculitis. In cases showing active arteritis, the inflammatory process is transmural, but may be granulomatous or nongranulomatous, and shows evidence of both acute and chronic inflammation. Granulomatous inflammation with multinucleated giant cells is present in less than 50 percent of positive temporal artery biopsies. In these cases, the giant cells are more frequently found at the interface between the endothelial cell layer and the tunica muscularis (fig. 6-23). Giant cells are variable in number and are in close association with fragments of the internal elastic lamina. Other inflammatory cells include lymphocytes, plasma cells, eosinophils, and polymorphonuclear leukocytes (figs. 6-23, 6-24). Foci of medial necrosis may be identified. Arterial atrophy and calcification of the internal elastic lamina may play a role in the evolution of the inflammatory reaction (27). The intima shows subendothelial thickening with proliferation of smooth muscle cells (myofibroblasts) in a myxoid background. Intimal thickening may be associated with luminal narrowing, stenosis, or thrombotic occlusion. Chronic inflammation may be present in the adventitia.

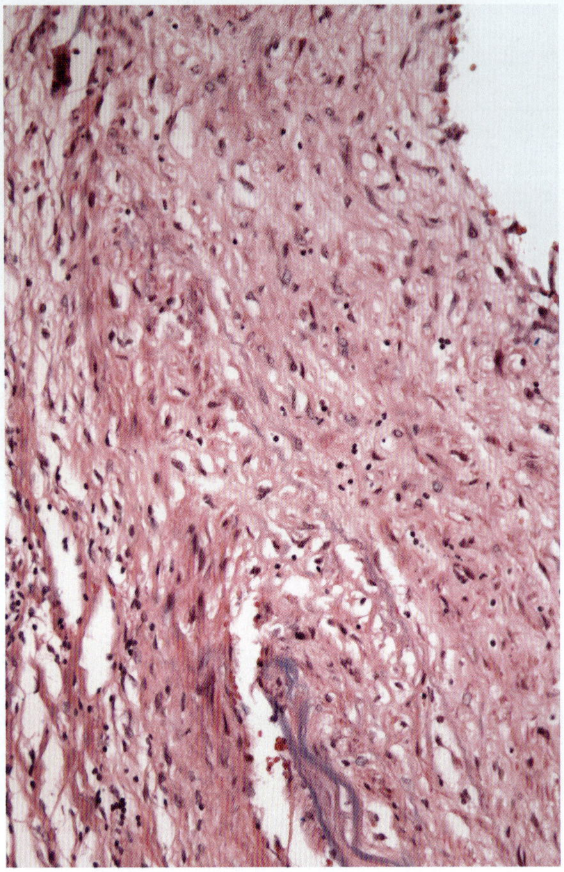

Figure 6-25

GIANT CELL ARTERITIS

Loss of the elastic lamina (remaining only in bottom center) and isolated remaining giant cell (top left).

Healed arteritis shows changes involving the endothelial cell layer, internal elastic lamina, and muscular layer. The tunica media exhibits irregular fibrosis and scarring, foci of lymphocytes and macrophages, and neovascularization. There is marked fragmentation of the internal elastic membrane and irregular intimal fibrosis (fig. 6-25). Steroid treatment–induced microscopic findings are similar to those of healed arteritis.

Immunohistochemical Findings. Immunohistochemical stains show a polyclonal inflammatory cellular infiltrate, including interferon-gamma–producing T cells (CD4+) and macrophages (CD68+). Deposits of immunoglobulins have been demonstrated in the arterial walls.

Ultrastructural Findings. Electron microscopic studies are not necessary for the diagnosis of giant cell arteritis. Electron microscopy of granulomas may differentiate between multinucleated foreign body giant cells and Langhans giant cells: the latter are rich in lysosomes.

Differential Diagnosis. Giant cell arteritis showing active inflammation should be differentiated from polyarteritis nodosa, which rarely involves the temporal arteries. A biopsy of an artery involved by polyarteritis nodosa usually shows focal lesions in different stages of development, alternating with areas of an unremarkable arterial wall. The pathologic features of polyarteritis nodosa include focal necrosis with microaneurysm formation, necrotizing vasculitis with fibrinoid necrosis, and proliferative endarteritis.

Healed arteritis may be confused with atherosclerotic changes. In atherosclerosis, the tunica media shows hyalinization and there is concentric fibrosis of the muscular layer and adventitia. Other features include fragmentation of internal elastic lamina without long breaks, absence of inflammation, and focal calcification along the internal elastic lamina.

Treatment and Prognosis. Giant cell temporal arteritis responds to steroid therapy. The disease appears to be self-limited, but relapses occur. Giant cell arteritis may be fatal because of the complications of stroke, myocardial infarct, or aortic rupture.

Primary Angiitis of the Central Nervous System

Definition. *Primary angiitis of the CNS* (PACNS) is a vasculitis limited to small leptomeningeal and superficial parenchymal arteries and veins of the brain and spinal cord. PACNS is also known as *granulomatous angiitis of the CNS* as well as *isolated angiitis*.

General Comments. Controversy still exists regarding the proper classification of PACNS since its clinical manifestations, laboratory findings, radiologic features, and pathologic changes are nonspecific and its diagnosis is a matter of exclusion. The etiology is unknown. Diagnostic queries arise from the association of PACNS with such diverse entities as Hodgkin lymphoma, varicella zoster infection, cerebral amyloid angiopathy, acquired immunodeficiency syndrome, sarcoidosis, and myelodysplastic syndromes (28–31).

Clinical Features. PACNS may affect individuals of any age, including children and the elderly; the majority of patients are men in the fourth decade of life. Initial symptoms include headache, focal neurologic deficits, seizures, and alterations of consciousness. Many patients develop hemiplegia, extensor plantar responses, and papilledema. Patients with spinal cord involvement may develop evidence of progressive or acute myelopathy, with paraplegia and incontinence. Systemic symptoms are uncommon.

Radiologic Findings. Although angiography in PACNS may show alternating areas of dilation and constriction of small and medium-sized arteries, a pattern described as "beading," this feature is nonspecific (32) since it is observed in other vasculitides and noninflammatory conditions such as atherosclerosis. Furthermore, angiography may be normal in some patients. Features on neuroimaging studies are equally nonspecific and heterogeneous. CT scan findings include single or multiple infarcts or hemorrhages; hemorrhagic lesions mimicking tumors; and ring-enhancing lesions suggestive of multifocal gliomas, metastatic neoplasms, and abscesses. Brain MRI may show multiple enhancing abnormalities with high signal intensity on T2-weighted images of the deep and subcortical white matter. These abnormalities may also be present in infratentorial structures and spinal cord.

Laboratory Findings. The CSF profile may mimic chronic meningitis, with an increase in protein and immunoglobulins, and a moderate lymphocytic pleocytosis. The ESR is usually normal and no laboratory tests are diagnostic. Drug and toxicology screens are negative.

Gross Findings. PACNS tends to involve small arteries, arterioles, veins, and venules within the leptomeninges and parenchyma. For this reason, biopsy material should include the meninges and CNS tissue. Macroscopic examination may show opacification of the leptomeninges. Involved blood vessels may be occluded by thrombus. The brain may show ischemic or hemorrhagic infarction.

Microscopic Findings. Like giant cell temporal arteritis, the microscopic features in PACNS tend to be segmental in distribution. The inflammatory infiltrate is that of necrotizing, granulomatous, or lymphocytic arteritis (33–35). In cases of necrotizing arteritis, the necrotic vascular wall exhibits a mixed cellular infiltrate comprised mainly of lymphocytes and a variable number of plasma cells, histiocytes, eosinophils, and polymorphonuclear leukocytes. Multinucleated giant cells are absent. In granulomatous vasculitis, the inflammatory lesions include multinucleated giant cells, either of Langhans or foreign body type. Fibrointimal proliferation and thrombosis may be additional features. Some cases show an associated chronic leptomeningitis and areas of organizing ischemic or hemorrhagic infarcts in the brain parenchyma (35). Occasionally, a combination of PACNS and amyloid angiopathy is present, but this more likely represents inflammation secondary to amyloid angiopathy (see below).

Immunohistochemical Findings. Immunohistochemistry is of little value in the diagnosis of PACNS, but will demonstrate a mixed population of B and T lymphocytes. It is also helpful in ruling out angiocentric immunoproliferative lesions.

Differential Diagnosis. Since PACNS is somewhat a diagnosis of exclusion and, by definition, restricted to the CNS, a variety of disorders characterized by inflammatory reactions of intracranial blood vessels must be included in the differential diagnosis. The majority correspond to systemic disorders, drug-related processes, infectious diseases, and neoplasms. The major entities are discussed in the following section.

Treatment and Prognosis. The duration and course of the illness are variable. While PACNS may be fatal, it may respond to immunosuppressive therapies.

Systemic Vasculitides Involving the Central Nervous System

Many systemic vasculitides affect the CNS, either via direct inflammatory involvement of cerebral blood vessels or via secondary effects from inflammation of systemic vessels. Most of these conditions are diagnosed on the basis of clinical and laboratory findings and therefore only rarely are biopsied. Even when biopsied, the variability of findings—from nonspecific perivascular chronic inflammation to frank vasculitis to healed vasculopathy—often do not allow for a specific diagnosis on the basis of tissue examination alone. The vasculitides that have

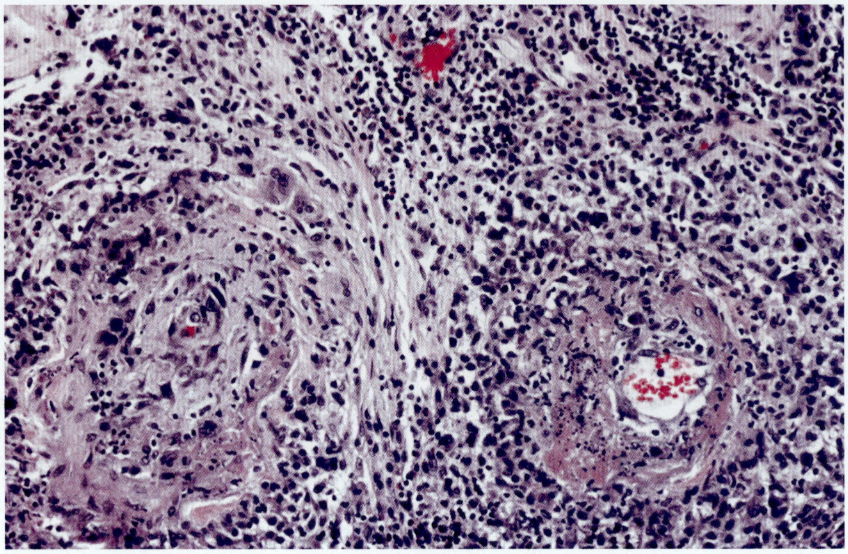

Figure 6-26

WEGENER GRANULOMATOSIS

The choroid plexus arteries are involved by active vasculitis associated with luminal occlusion.

been reported to affect the CNS, and that could conceivably be diagnosed on brain biopsy, are reviewed in the following sections.

Wegener Granulomatosis. *Wegener granulomatosis* is a rare systemic disorder characterized by necrotizing granulomas of the upper and lower respiratory tract, glomerulonephritis, and systemic vasculitis. Diagnosis is supported by the presence of circulating antineutrophil cytoplasmic antibodies (C-ANCA) (36). The CNS is involved in 4 to 8 percent of patients. Neurologic complications are usually present in patients with evidence of systemic disease and include peripheral neuropathies, mononeuritis multiplex, cranial nerve palsies, and CNS vasculitis (fig. 6-26). CNS parenchymal involvement is rare (36). Dural vasculitis may be present.

Churg-Strauss Syndrome. This disorder, also called *allergic angiitis and granulomatosis*, features peripheral eosinophilia, systemic vasculitis, and asthma (37). Along with Wegener granulomatosis and hypersensitivity angiitis, it is included within the group of ANCA-associated vasculitides (36). The organs more frequently involved are the paranasal sinuses, skin, peripheral nerves, and lung. Mononeuritis multiplex occurs in up to 78 percent of patients (36). The diagnosis is confirmed by a muscle or peripheral nerve biopsy that shows necrotizing vasculitis with abundant eosinophils and extravascular eosinophilic granulomas.

Hypersensitivity Angiitis. *Hypersensitivity angiitis* is also known as *microscopic polyangiitis, microscopic polyarteritis,* and *leukocytoclastic angiitis*. It is a hypersensitivity vasculitis that is related to the deposit of immune complexes (Arthus reaction) in the vascular walls after exposure to particular infections, toxins, and drugs. Other cases are associated with anaphylactoid purpura (Henoch-Schonlein purpura), essential mixed cryoglobulinemia, mixed connective tissue disorders, and malignant neoplasms. The lesions consist of necrotizing vasculitis characterized by transmural infiltration of the vascular wall by neutrophils with prominent karyorrhexis ("nuclear dust"). The blood vessels involved are arterioles, capillaries, and venules, as well as small and medium-sized arteries. The organs most commonly involved are lung, heart, kidney, eye, and peripheral nerves (36). Occasionally, the brain is affected by hemorrhage (38). Perinuclear (P)-ANCA has been demonstrated in 70 percent of affected patients (36).

Polyarteritis Nodosa. *Polyarteritis,* or *panarteritis, nodosa* is a necrotizing vasculitis that may affect all organs except lung and spleen. Currently, two forms of the disease are recognized. In systemic polyarteritis nodosa, visceral organs such as heart, kidney, and gastrointestinal tract are more frequently involved. The localized form, on the other hand, tends to affect skeletal muscle and the nervous system, primarily the peripheral nerves. CNS involvement is only seen in patients with advanced disease. The affected blood vessels are medium and small arteries, which on angiography may show aneurysmatic dilations. The acute phase of the disease is characterized by necrotizing vasculitis with fibrinoid necrosis and an inflammatory infiltrate, with predominance of polymorphonuclear leucocytes. The chronic and healing phase shows mononuclear cell inflammation and vascular fibrosis. In cases affecting the CNS, these changes may affect the large arteries of the circle of Willis and smaller leptomeningeal arteries, and may be associated with occlusion of the lumen and infarcts (39).

The pathogenesis of polyarteritis nodosa is controversial. Although attributed to an immune complex deposition, many patients are seropositive for hepatitis B and C viruses.

Kawasaki Disease. *Kawasaki disease (mucocutaneous lymph node syndrome)* is a rare systemic vasculitis that predominantly affects infants and children. The clinical manifestations are mucocutaneous lesions, lymph node enlargement, and fever. The most common complications are coronary and peripheral arterial aneurysms. The pathologic changes are similar to those of polyarteritis nodosa. Cerebral vascular manifestations are usually restricted to the compromise of carotid arteries. Involvement of intracranial arteries may be associated with stroke or encephalopathy.

Inflammatory Bowel Disease. Neurologic complications have been described in a variety of inflammatory bowel diseases, including *celiac disease, Whipple disease, Crohn disease,* and *ulcerative colitis*. Patients with regional enteritis and ulcerative colitis may develop peripheral neuropathies and cerebrovascular disease. In these cases, the radiologic and pathologic changes of vasculitis have been described (40).

Sjögren Syndrome. *Sjögren syndrome* is an autoimmune disorder characterized by keratoconjunctivitis sicca and xerostomia, which result from involvement of the lacrimal and salivary glands, respectively. Sjögren syndrome may be primary or secondary. Secondary Sjögren syndrome is related to autoimmune disorders such as rheumatoid arthritis, systemic lupus erythematosus, mixed connective tissue disease, polymyositis, scleroderma, vasculitis, and thyroiditis. The neurologic manifestations include distal sensory or sensorimotor axonal neuropathy, cognitive dysfunction, psychiatric manifestations, acute myelitis, and progressive myelopathy. The CNS manifestations in both the primary and secondary forms are related to the vasculitis, but the histologic features are not specific.

Behcet Syndrome. *Behcet syndrome* is a systemic vasculitis with clinical manifestations centering on the triad of uveitis, skin lesions, and oral aphthous or genital mucous membrane ulcers. Additional clinical manifestations include cutaneous angiitis, thrombophlebitis colitis, and CNS vasculitis. Meningoencephalitis is the most common presentation in the brain. Neuroimaging may show large lesions in the brain stem or basal ganglia, with extension into the diencephalon. Microscopic examination of CNS lesions discloses vasculitis of small vessels (mainly venules), meningoencephalitis, gliosis, and demyelination (41). Children with repeated strokes may have HLA-B51 (42).

Cogan Syndrome. *Cogan syndrome* is defined by nonsyphilitic interstitial keratitis and vestibuloauditory dysfunction. A mortality rate of 10 percent is attributed to the vasculitis, with stroke as the major neurologic complication.

Sneddon Syndrome. *Sneddon syndrome* features livedo reticularis and recurrent strokes. It may be primary or secondary to systemic lupus erythematosus or the antiphospholipid syndrome. Familial occurrence has been reported. Patients with Sneddon syndrome may have dementia and antiphospholipid syndrome (43). Hyperplasia and fibrotic occlusion of blood vessels results in multiple cortical infarcts (44). Occasionally, intracerebral hemorrhage with vasculitis is observed (45). It is possible that the initial vascular event corresponds to inflammatory or immune-related injury of small arteries, followed by proliferation of smooth muscle cells and subsequent luminal occlusion or stenosis (46).

Malignant Atrophic Papulosis. *Malignant atrophic papulosis*, also known as *Degos disease* or *Kohlmeier-Degos disease*, is a generalized vasculopathy affecting the skin, gastrointestinal tract, and CNS. The skin lesions are erythematous, umbilicated, raised papules that develop a central area of necrosis to leave a porcelain-like scar. The neurologic complications are varied and include transient ischemic attacks and progressive focal or multifocal deficits from microinfarcts. The parenchymal lesions include hemorrhagic infarcts, including in the spinal cord (47). The vascular lesions, which affect medium and small arteries and veins throughout the body, show prominent fibrointimal proliferation associated with thrombosis in the absence of inflammation (48).

Susac Syndrome. *Susac syndrome* (*retinocochleocerebral vasculopathy*) is a rare disease of young women characterized by encephalopathy, fluctuating hearing loss, and visual loss. The condition is a vasculopathy of the retina, cochlea, and brain. MRI of the brain usually shows multifocal white matter lesions that can affect the corpus callosum, deep gray matter nuclei, and posterior fossa. Parenchymal and leptomeningeal enhancement is also present. Brain biopsy has demonstrated sclerosis of small blood vessels or healed arteritis, gliosis, and microinfarcts (49). Similar vascular changes may be present in skeletal muscle, suggesting a generalized vasculopathy.

Systemic Lupus Erythematosus. Neurologic manifestations occur in about 13.6 percent of patients with *systemic lupus erythematosus* (SLE) (50). The most common are seizures, encephalopathy, and behavioral changes. Despite the term "lupus cerebritis," inflammatory changes are rare. The pathologic findings are usually nonspecific: frank vasculitis is rare, but perivascular lymphocytic inflammation is common (51,52). Infarcts result from embolic vascular occlusions from marantic endocarditis, thrombotic thrombocytopenic purpura, hypercoagulability states related to circulating antiphospholipid antibodies, and infections. Although SLE is common, the CNS manifestations typically arise in patients with well-documented disease and therefore biopsy is uncommon.

Rheumatoid Arthritis. Neurologic complications of *rheumatoid arthritis* are rare and usually occur in patients with longstanding, clinically active disease. These neurologic manifestations may be related to rheumatoid nodules, vasculitis, or compromise of the cervical vertebrae by arthritis (53–55). The vasculitis usually involves small leptomeningeal blood vessels and may be responsible for subdural and subarachnoid hemorrhages, as well as for parenchymal hematomas. The synovitis of the cervical spine that is caused by rheumatoid arthritis may be associated with atlantoaxial subluxation, basilar invagination, and subaxial subluxation, which produce compressive myelopathy or ischemic necrosis. With the exception of rheumatoid nodules that affect the meninges, these manifestations do not lead to biopsy.

Scleroderma. *Scleroderma* rarely involves the central and peripheral nervous systems or the skeletal muscle. *Scleroderma en coup de saber* is a descriptive term denoting linear scleroderma of the frontoparietal area of the face and scalp that is associated with epilepsy. The pathologic findings include sclerosis of the leptomeninges and blood vessels, intraparenchymal calcifications, and anomalous ectatic vessels (56).

NONINFLAMMATORY VASCULOPATHIES

Noninflammatory vasculopathies are a heterogeneous group of clinically underrecognized and underdiagnosed disorders that selectively involve small parenchymal arteries, arterioles, veins, and venules and are primarily noninflammatory in nature. Most entities are systemic vasculopathies with evidence of involvement in other organs, but others are restricted to the CNS. The latter include cerebral amyloid angiopathy, cerebral autosomal dominant arteriopathy with subcortical infarcts and leukoencephalopathy (CADASIL), and arteriolar sclerosis/hypertensive cerebrovascular disease.

Cerebral Amyloid Angiopathy

Definition. *Cerebral amyloid angiopathy* (CAA) is a localized vasculopathy that results from the deposition of an amyloid protein in the walls of small arteries and arterioles, and sometimes capillaries and veins, of the leptomeninges and brain (57–59). In the majority of cases, it is not associated with systemic amyloidosis.

General Comments. Most cases of CAA are sporadic and characterized by restricted amyloid deposition in the superficial brain and leptomeninges. The amyloid is the beta-amyloid fragment of amyloid precursor protein, the same amyloid deposited in cases of Alzheimer disease.

CAA has been linked to mutations in a variety of genes whose mutant protein products are amyloidogenic (58,59). Mutant cystatin C in hereditary cerebral hemorrhage with amyloidosis of Icelandic type (HCHWA-I) is inherited in an autosomal dominant manner and is characterized by the deposition of cystatin C as amyloid in the brain and other organs and tissues. Patients present with their first episode of intracerebral hemorrhage in the third or fourth decade, but sometimes as early as 15 years of age. Hereditary cerebral hemorrhage with amyloidosis Dutch type and familial Alzheimer disease with deposition of either beta-amyloid variants or wild-type beta-amyloid (HCHWA-D) is autosomal dominant with complete penetrance, related to mutations of the *APP* gene, and features deposits of beta-amyloid. The age of onset is in the sixth decade and the majority of those affected have intracerebral hemorrhage. Variant transthyretins (ATTR) are associated with meningovascular amyloidosis, which produces dementia, ataxia, and spasticity. Mutated gelsolin (AGel) is associated with familial amyloidosis of Finnish type; disease-associated prion protein (PrP[SC]) is associated with a variant of Gerstman-Straussler-Scheinker syndrome; and ABri and ADan in CAAs are described in *BRI2* gene-related dementias, familial British dementia, and familial Danish dementia.

Clinical Features. Although frequently asymptomatic, CAA comes to clinical attention as one of several clinicopathologic entities. It is an important cause of cerebral hemorrhage, stroke, and dementia (60). CAA is recognized during life with high accuracy (61). Presenting signs and symptoms include headache, epilepsy, and dementia. Intracerebral bleeding is the most common clinical presentation in both the sporadic and familial forms. Most patients with the sporadic form present with cerebral bleeding after 60 years of age, whereas those with the hereditary form may develop fatal cerebral bleeding during early adulthood. The region most frequently affected by CAA corresponds to the frontal and occipital cortex and subcortical white matter, but some patients have diffuse encephalopathy.

Radiologic Findings. CT of the brain usually shows a single, large, lobar hemorrhage that extends through the cortex into the subarachnoid space or into the ventricles (fig. 6-27). Multiple, recurrent lesions may be present in patients who survived the initial episode. MRI may show a stippled appearance of the cerebral cortex, which corresponds to microinfarcts and microhemorrhages. Serial gradient-echo MRI may detect new small hemorrhages in patients with previous CAA-related lobar hemorrhage (62). Gradient-echo T2-weighted MRI may show small areas of signal loss associated with intracerebral hemorrhage, which may indicate remnants of previous microscopic bleeds (63).

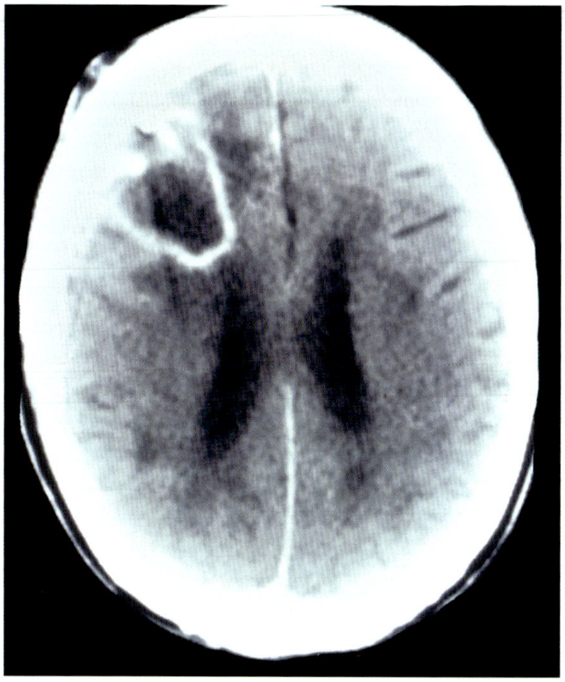

Figure 6-27

CEREBRAL AMYLOID ANGIOPATHY

CT scan revealed a frontal lobe hematoma with peripheral enhancement in an 81-year-old man with headaches. He underwent craniotomy for evacuation of bleeding. (Figs. 6-27 and 6-28 are from the same patient.)

Laboratory Findings. Low levels of beta-amyloid 42 have been found in the CSF at autopsy in individuals affected with amyloid-related pathologies (64). The enzyme cysteine protease inhibitor cystatin C (L68Q-cystatin C) and wildtype cystatin C have been demonstrated in plasma, and cystatin C dimers and monomers have been found in the CSF, of individuals affected with HCHWA-I (65).

Gross Findings. Macroscopic examination reveals single or multiple parenchymal hemorrhages, which may be well circumscribed. Surgical specimens often show small microhemorrhages and infarcts in the cerebral cortex. Autopsy cases may show larger white matter hematomas that extend into the cerebral cortex, deep gray matter nuclei, subarachnoid space, or ventricular system. A yellow color at the periphery may indicate some degree of organization. The white matter may exhibit prominent vascular markings.

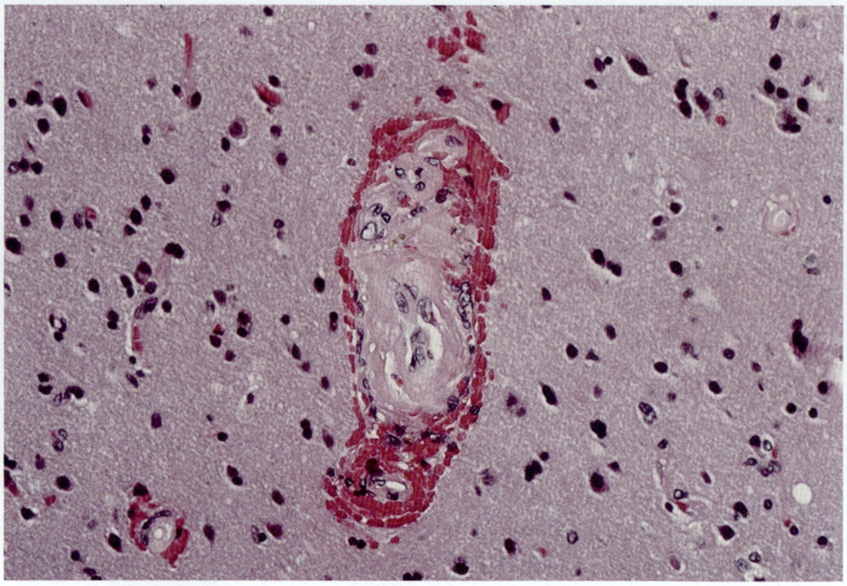

Figure 6-28

CEREBRAL AMYLOID ANGIOPATHY

Small cortical artery with thickened wall and perivascular hemorrhage.

Microscopic Findings. Hematoxylin and eosin (H&E)-stained sections of the leptomeninges and superficial cerebral cortex show small, strikingly rounded arteries and arterioles with walls thickened by eosinophilic material (fig. 6-28) (66,67). The lumens also have a strikingly rounded appearance but may be narrowed. Sometimes the small involved vessels have the nearly pathognomonic appearance of a "double barrel." Congo red stains identify the amyloid by its salmon red appearance and its characteristic apple green birefringence under polarized light. The hemorrhagic lesions in the surrounding cortex may be recent or organizing, but usually have perivascular hemosiderin-laden macrophages and gliosis; in many cases, microinfarcts are also present. The microhemorrhages and microinfarcts correspond to the stippled appearance of the cortex noted on MRI. The underlying white matter is often unaffected, and the affected blood vessels stop fairly abruptly near the gray-white junction. Some cases, however, have diffuse, ill-defined regions of white matter degeneration, characterized by axonal and myelin loss that may be ischemic.

The most common situation in surgical pathology to find CAA is during the evacuation of an intracerebral hematoma in a patient 60 years of age or older. Typically, an acute hemorrhage has occasional blood vessels with the markedly rounded profile and hyalinized walls typical of CAA (67). Careful examination of all intracerebral hematomas for such vessels is warranted, followed by Congo red staining or beta-amyloid immunohistochemistry if indicated. If a diagnosis of CAA is suspected on clinical grounds, submission of the entire hematoma for histologic examination may be warranted. The documentation of CAA is of substantial clinical importance since it may affect subsequent patient management.

Perhaps the most important feature to recognize in the setting of CAA is inflammation (28,68), since patients with inflammatory CAA may respond, sometimes dramatically, to antiinflammatory therapies. Vascular wall inflammation occurs as multinucleated giant cells with intracellular amyloid, as well as less specific chronic inflammatory cells. Such giant cell reactions account for reports of CAA coexisting with PACNS (69,70). Careful examination of all biopsied vessels for giant cell changes is warranted in all cases.

Immunohistochemical Findings. Immunohistochemistry for beta-amyloid (or cystatin C) is helpful for documenting the deposition of specific proteins. Immunoreactivity for beta-amyloid is usually present in leptomeningeal and parenchymal blood vessels in the cortex and in the multinucleated cells in inflammatory cases (fig. 6-29). The vascular deposition may be diffuse or focal (71).

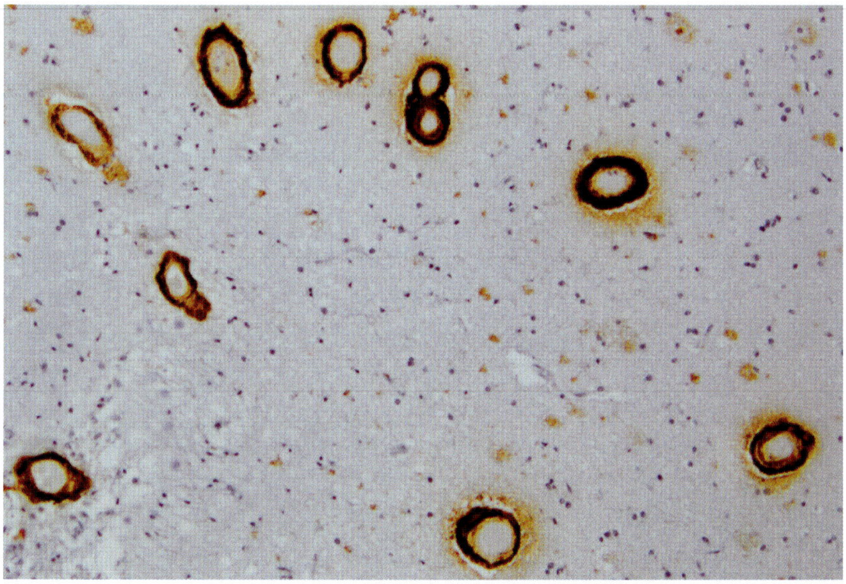

Figure 6-29

CEREBRAL AMYLOID ANGIOPATHY

Expression of beta-amyloid in walls of small cortical arteries and arterioles (immunoperoxidase method).

Ultrastructural Findings. Electron microscopic examination of involved blood vessels shows deposits of nonbranching, 5-nm amyloid filaments, but is not required for diagnosis.

Differential Diagnosis. The diagnosis of CAA is usually straightforward, given the characteristic light microscopic appearance and the diagnostic use of Congo red stains and immunohistochemistry. The differential diagnosis includes CADASIL (see below) and arteriolar sclerosis, as well as some of the rare vasculopathies discussed elsewhere in this chapter. Periodic acid–Schiff (PAS) stains and immunohistochemistry for beta-amyloid are of substantial help in this differential diagnosis, since CAA is positive on both PAS and beta-amyloid immunohistochemistry, whereas CADASIL is PAS positive only and arteriolar sclerosis is negative for PAS and amyloid stains.

Treatment and Prognosis. There is no treatment for primary CAA, although, as mentioned, antiinflammatory approaches are often useful in treating those CAA cases with superimposed inflammatory changes. In the future, the treatment of CAA may be improved through the use of drugs that interfere with amyloid formation or that facilitate amyloid degradation. Neurosurgical procedures may control intracranial bleeding, but must be tempered by knowledge that brains affected by CAA are more prone to bleeding during neurosurgery. The prognosis may depend on the extent of bleeding and associated secondary effects.

Cerebral Autosomal Dominant Arteriopathy with Subcortical Infarcts and Leukoencephalopathy

Definition. *Cerebral autosomal dominant arteriopathy with subcortical infarcts and leukoencephalopathy* (CADASIL) is an underdiagnosed hereditary systemic vasculopathy that involves small arteries in the central and peripheral nervous systems as well as in other organs (72). It occurs because of mutations in the *NOTCH3* gene on chromosome 19q12 (73).

General Comments. The diagnosis of CADASIL relies on clinicopathologic correlations, including family history and ultrastructural findings. In many cases, the diagnosis is confirmed by mutation analysis (73).

Clinical Features. The CNS manifestations include stroke, transient ischemic attacks, migraine, dementia, cognitive impairment, gait disturbance, urinary incontinence, pseudobulbar palsy, and psychiatric disorders. An autosomal dominant family history of migraine, early-onset stroke, or dementia may be found. Japanese with familial CADASIL present with recurrent strokes, progressive motor disturbances of the extremities, and pseudobulbar palsy (74). Even in the absence of a family history, the disease should be considered in individuals younger than 60 years of age who present with recurrent subcortical ischemic strokes, migraine with atypical or prolonged aura, and early cognitive decline or subcortical dementia (75).

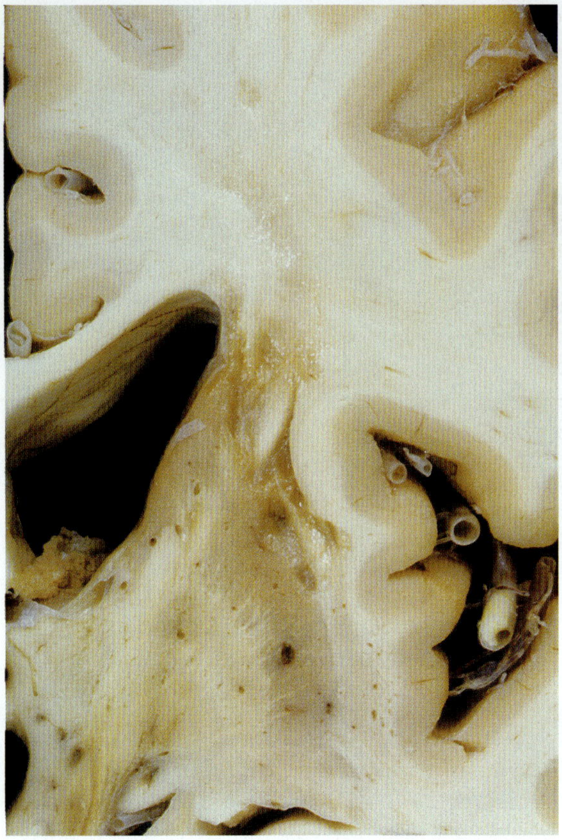

Figure 6-30

CEREBRAL AUTOSOMAL DOMINANT ARTERIOPATHY WITH SUBCORTICAL INFARCTS AND LEUKOENCEPHALOPATHY (CADASIL)

Gray discoloration and cavitation of a large lesion in the parietal white matter. (Figs. 6-30 to 6-32 are from the same patient.)

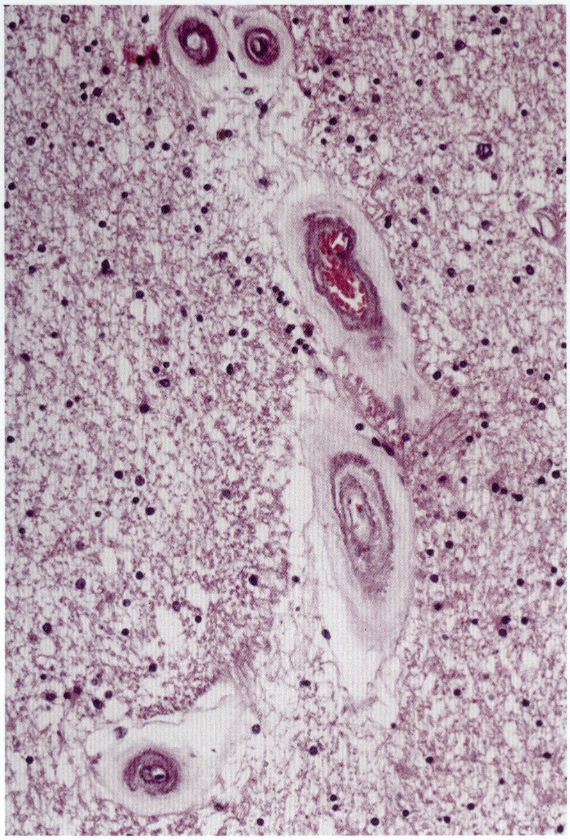

Figure 6-31

CADASIL

Small arteries in the white matter are thickened due to deposits of hyaline granular material in the tunica muscularis.

Radiologic Findings. MRI scans in older individuals usually show subcortical white matter abnormalities in the frontal and temporal lobes. On T1-weighted images, the lesions may be well demarcated or poorly defined. Sagittal T2-weighted images may show involvement of the corpus callosum. Other abnormalities include lacunar infarcts; areas of hyperintensity involving the external capsule, basal ganglia, and brain stem; and microhemorrhages. Microhemorrhages are more frequently found in the cortical-subcortical regions, white matter, thalamus, and brain stem. Fluid-attenuated inversion recovery (FLAIR) sequences may show multiple, small, punctuate hyperintensities in the deep or periventricular white matter.

Gross Findings. The main gross pathologic findings are leukoencephalopathy and lacunar infarcts. The leukoencephalopathy is characterized by areas of gray discoloration involving the cerebral subcortical white matter and sparing of the U fibers (fig. 6-30). Lacunar infarcts are present in the white matter, basal ganglia, thalami, and brain stem.

Microscopic Findings. H&E-stained sections of the organs involved, including brain, peripheral nerves, and skin, show deposits of basophilic, slightly granular PAS-positive (but Congo red-negative) material within the extracellular matrix and muscular layer of the involved arteries (figs. 6-31, 6-32) (72,76,77). In these regions, the smooth muscle cells are destroyed and replaced by the granular material, a process that is followed by fibrosis and

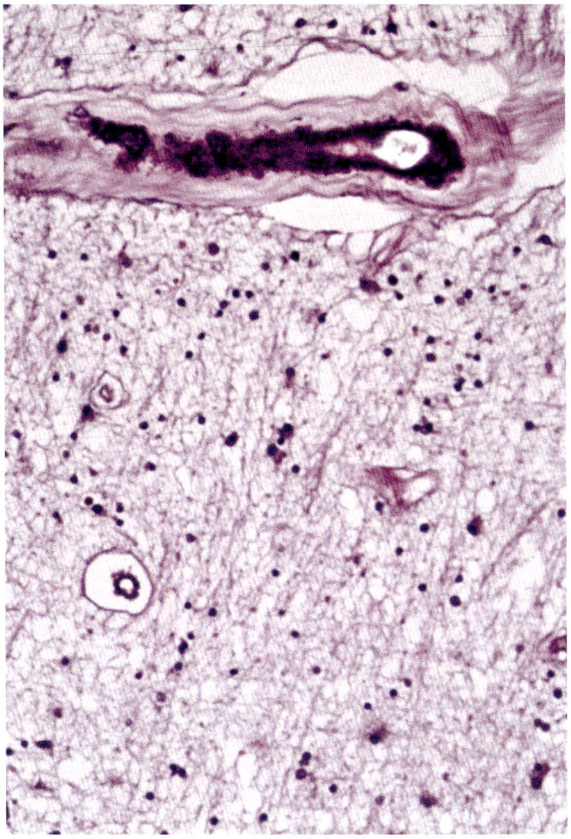

Figure 6-32

CADASIL

The granular material in the tunica media is periodic acid–Schiff (PAS) positive.

thickening of the arterial wall (78). Fragmentation of the elastic lamina may be demonstrated with elastic stains. These morphologic changes sometimes resemble periarteritis nodosa and manifest as fibrinoid necrosis of the tunica media and perivascular inflammatory infiltrates found in arteries not only in the CNS but also in internal organs. The central artery of the retina and its branches, as well as the microvasculature of the heart, may also be affected.

Immunohistochemical Findings. Studies claim that immunostaining of skin biopsy material with antibodies for NOTCH3 is sensitive and specific for diagnosis (79). Some studies, however, have reported variable results that do not always correlate with the clinical and radiologic findings of CADASIL. Immunohistochemistry for amyloid protein is negative.

Ultrastructural Findings. Electron microscopy plays an important role in the examination of specimens submitted to the pathology laboratory with a suspicion of CADASIL. Confirmation is made by the presence of granular osmiophilic material within cells of the muscular layer of small and medium-sized arteries of the brain, peripheral nerves, skeletal muscle, or skin (fig. 6-33) (78,80,81). Vascular changes in the skin may be focal, requiring examination of serially prepared sections (82). The nature of this material has not been elucidated, but its ultrastructural appearance and location are pathognomonic.

Differential Diagnosis. As discussed above in the section on CAA, differentiation of CADASIL, CAA, and arteriolar sclerosis is facilitated with the PAS stain, immunohistochemistry for beta-amyloid, and electron microscopy. Further discussion of arteriolar sclerosis is found below.

Treatment and Prognosis. No specific treatment is available, but genetic counseling may be of use in familial cases. The clinical course is variable and includes periods of acute worsening, chronic progression, stabilization, and improvement. The mean duration of the disease is 20 years. Women may survive longer than men.

Arteriolar Sclerosis

Hyaline change involving the small parenchymal arteries and arterioles is frequently seen in adults at postmortem examination. It may be associated with aging, diabetes mellitus, or chronic systemic hypertension. Vascular hypertensive changes may result from injury to the blood brain barrier and increased vascular permeability. The pathologic findings include hyalinosis, lipohyalinosis, microatheroma, fibrinoid necrosis, and miliary (Charcot-Bouchard) aneurysms. Since these lesions are similar to those in the kidneys, we use the designation of *arteriolar sclerosis* (fig. 6-34). These vascular changes may be associated with parenchymal lesions, including lacunar infarcts and hypertensive hemorrhages, as well as myelin pallor in the subcortical white matter. It has been proposed that luminal occlusion is responsible for lacunar infarcts, while rupture of the vascular wall affected by fibrinoid necrosis or microaneurysm is the cause of the bleeding. The cause of subcortical leukoencephalopathy has not been elucidated. Although these changes do not

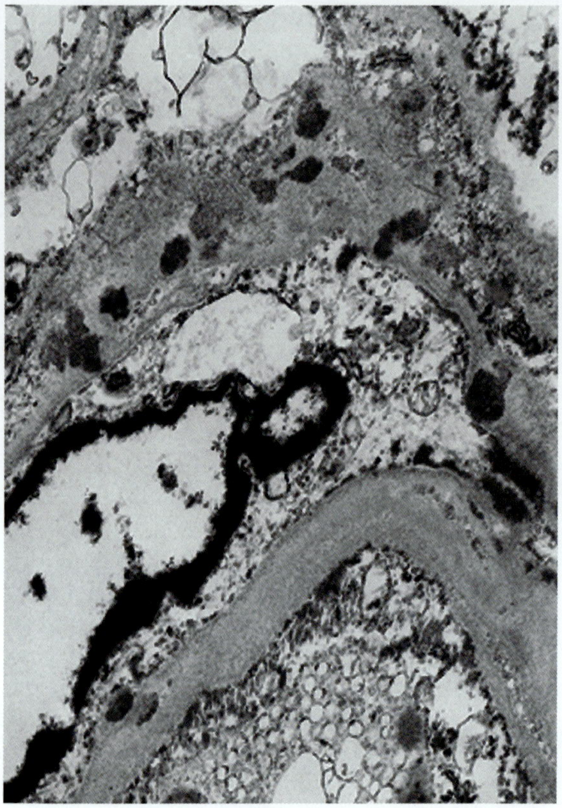

Figure 6-33

CADASIL

Electron-dense granular material surrounds myocytes within a blood vessel in the affected white matter.

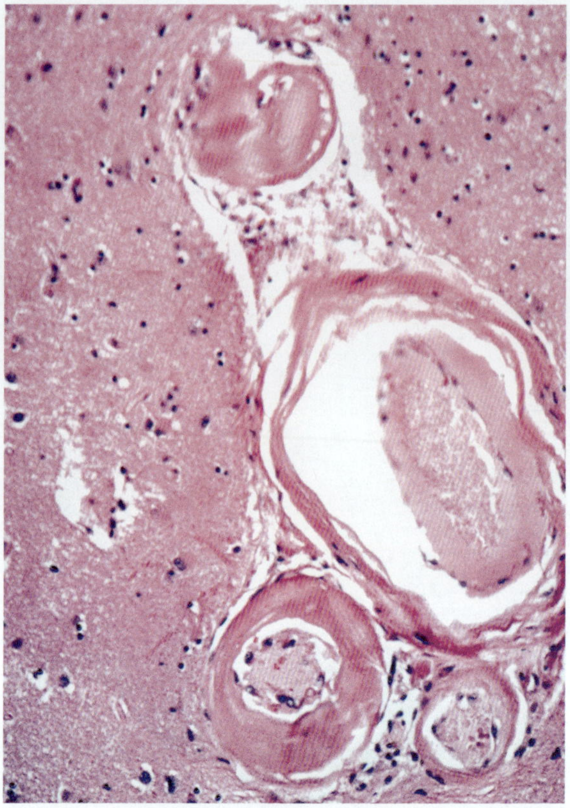

Figure 6-34

ARTERIOLAR SCLEROSIS

The small parenchymal arteries show hypertensive changes, including thickening and hyalinization as well as focal fibrinoid necrosis.

lead to biopsy, one must be aware of the pathologic findings of arteriolar sclerosis in order to differentiate them from the vascular disorders described elsewhere in this chapter.

Brain Embolism and Thrombosis

Embolism to the brain from cardiac or vascular sources may result in occlusion of intracranial and parenchymal blood vessels of variable caliber. In situ *thrombosis* may occur in the setting of hypercoagulable states. Thrombotic or embolic occlusion of a large artery may result in an infarct in the distribution of that blood vessel, but such scenarios do not often lead to cerebral biopsy. Thromboembolic occlusion of small parenchymal blood vessels, however, may result in biopsy since diffuse encephalopathy may result and defy a ready clinical or radiologic diagnosis. Typically, this occurs as a manifestation of a systemic disease in which the brain is predominantly affected. Parenchymal lesions usually correspond to multiple petechial hemorrhages and microinfarcts (fig. 6-35). This may be the result of fat embolism, disseminated intravascular coagulation, or other conditions such as thrombotic thrombocytopenic purpura (fig. 6-36). The identification of the pathology may require the use of special stains including Sudan black for fat or phosphotungstic acid-hematoxylin (PTAH) for fibrin. In the spinal cord, careful examination for fibrocartilaginous disc material may be diagnostic.

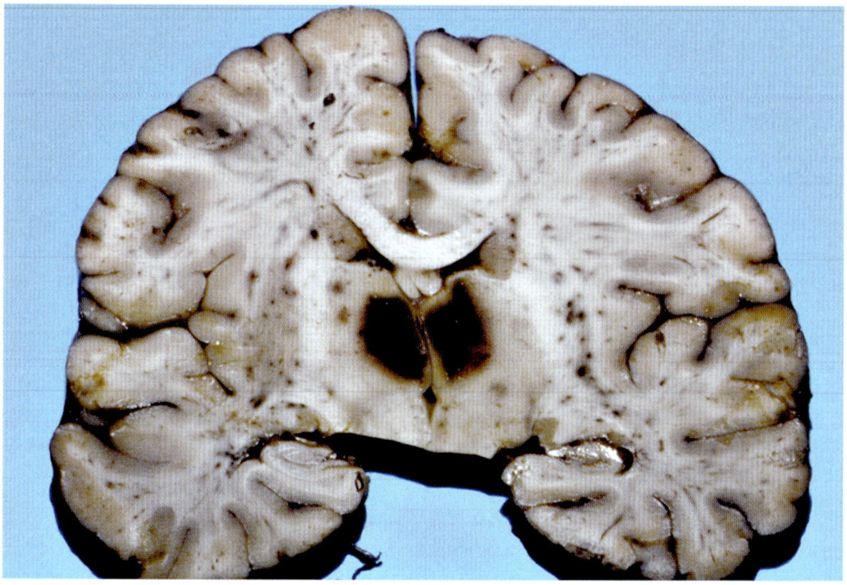

Figure 6-35

FIBRIN EMBOLI

Disseminated intravascular coagulation with fibrin emboli is associated with white matter petechial hemorrhages and hemorrhagic necrosis of the thalami.

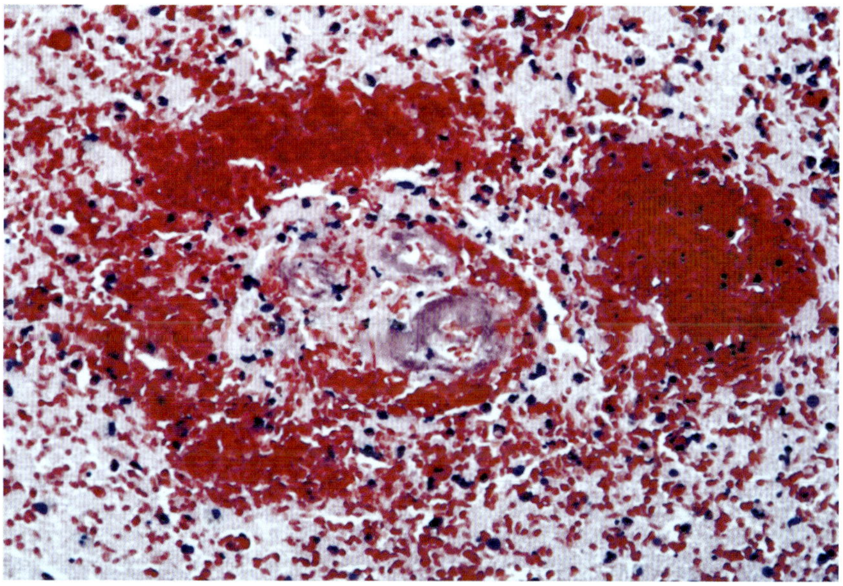

Figure 6-36

FIBRIN EMBOLI

Disseminated intravascular coagulation with occlusion of a small parenchymal artery by fibrin emboli.

REFERENCES

1. Gault J, Sarin H, Awadallah NA, Shenkar R, Awad IA. Pathobiology of human cerebrovascular malformations: basic mechanisms and clinical relevance. Neurosurgery 2004;55:1-16; discussion 16-17.
2. Ohaegbulam SC. The epidemiology of brain arteriovenous malformations. Neurosurgery 2001;49:226-228.
3. Meng JS, Okeda R. Histopathological structure of the pial arteriovenous malformation in adults: observation by reconstruction of serial sections of four surgical specimens. Acta Neuropathol (Berl) 2001;102:63-68.
4. Selman WR, Tarr RW, Sunshine JL, Ratcheson RA. Vascular diseases of the nervous system. In: Bradley WG, Daroff RB, Fenichel GM, Jankovic J, eds. Neurology in clinical practice. Philadelphia: Butterworth Heinemann; 2004:1197-1323.
5. Challa VR, Moody DM, Brown WR. Vascular malformations of the central nervous system. J Neuropathol Exp Neurol 1995;54:609-621.
6. Uranishi R, Baev NI, Kim JH, Awad IA. Vascular smooth muscle cell differentiation in human cerebral vascular malformations. Neurosurgery 2001;49:671-679; discussion 679-680.
7. Wong JH, Awad IA, Kim JH. Ultrastructural pathological features of cerebrovascular malformations: a preliminary report. Neurosurgery 2000;46:1454-1459.
8. Ziyal IM, Ece K, Bilginer B, Tezel GG, Ozcan OE. A glioma with an arteriovenous malformation: an association or a different entity? Acta Neurochir (Wien) 2004;146:83-86; discussion 86.
9. Paydarfar D, de la Monte SM. Case Records of the Massachusetts General Hospital. Weekly clinicopathological exercises. Case 12-1997. A 50-year-old woman with multiple sclerosis and enlarging front-lobe mass. N Engl J Med 1997;336:1163-1171.
10. Spetzler RF, Martin NA. A proposed grading system for arteriovenous malformations. J Neurosurg 1986;65:476-483.
11. Izawa M, Hayashi M, Chernov M, et al. Long-term complications after gamma knife surgery for arteriovenous malformations. J Neurosurg 2005;102(Suppl):34-37.
12. Baumgartner JE, Ater JL, Ha CS, et al. Pathologically proven cavernous angiomas of the brain following radiation therapy for pediatric brain tumors. Pediatr Neurosurg 2003;39:201-207.
13. Denier C, Labauge P, Brunereau L, et al. Clinical features of cerebral cavernous malformations patients with KRIT1 mutations. Ann Neurol 2004;55:213-220.
14. Craig HD, Gunel M, Cepeda O, et al. Multilocus linkage identifies two new loci for a mendelian form of stroke, cerebral cavernous malformation, at 7p15-13 and 3q25.2-27. Hum Mol Genet 1998;7:1851-1858.
15. Bergametti F, Denier C, Labauge P, et al. Mutations within the programmed cell death 10 gene cause cerebral cavernous malformations. Am J Hum Genet 2005;76:42-51.
16. Ogilvy CS, Louis DN, Ojemann RG. Intramedullary cavernous angiomas of the spinal cord: clinical presentation, pathological features, and surgical management. Neurosurgery 1992;31:219-229; discussion 229-230.
17. Mathiesen T, Edner G, Kihlstrom L. Deep and brainstem cavernomas: a consecutive 8-year series. J Neurosurg 2003;99:31-37.
18. Garner TB, Del Curling O Jr, Kelly DL Jr, Laster DW. The natural history of intracranial venous angiomas. J Neurosurg 1991;75:715-722.
19. Abdulrauf SI, Kaynar MY, Awad IA. A comparison of the clinical profile of cavernous malformations with and without associated venous malformations. Neurosurgery 1999;44:41-46; discussion 46-47.
20. Farrell DF, Forno LS. Symptomatic capillary telangiectasis of the brainstem without hemorrhage. Report of an unusual case. Neurology 1970;20:341-346.
21. Tang SC, Jeng JS, Liu HM, Yip PK. Diffuse capillary telangiectasia of the brain manifested as a slowly progressive course. Cerebrovasc Dis 2003;15:140-142.
22. Foell D, Hernandez-Rodriguez J, Sanchez M, Vogl T, Cid MC, Roth J. Early recruitment of phagocytes contributes to the vascular inflammation of giant cell arteritis. J Pathol 2004;204:311-316.
23. Wilkinson IM, Russell RW. Arteries of the head and neck in giant cell arteritis. A pathological study to show the pattern of arterial involvement. Arch Neurol 1972;27:378-391.
24. Nordborg E, Nordborg C. Giant cell arteritis: strategies in diagnosis and treatment. Curr Opin Rheumatol 2004;16:25-30.
25. Chakrabarty A, Franks AJ. Temporal artery biopsy: is there any value in examining biopsies at multiple levels? J Clin Pathol 2000;53:131-136.
26. Pless M, Rizzo JF 3rd, Lamkin JC, Lessell S. Concordance of bilateral temporal artery biopsy in giant cell arteritis. J Neuroophthalmol 2000;20:216-218.
27. Nordborg C, Nordborg E, Petursdottir V. The pathogenesis of giant cell arteritis: morphological aspects. Clin Exp Rheumatol 200018:(Suppl):S18-21.
28. Scolding NJ, Joseph F, Kirby PA, et al. Abeta-related angiitis: primary angiitis of the central nervous system associated with cerebral amyloid angiopathy. Brain 2005;128:500-515.

29. Incalzi RA, Arena V, Capelli A, Gambassi G. Isolated PACNS-like presentation of a systemic vasculitis complicating a myelodysplastic syndrome. J Intern Med 2004;255:674-679.
30. Nogueras C, Sala M, Sasal M, et al. Recurrent stroke as a manifestation of primary angiitis of the central nervous system in a patient infected with human immunodeficiency virus. Arch Neurol 2002;59:468-473.
31. Rosen CL, DePalma L, Morita A. Primary angiitis of the central nervous system as a first presentation in Hodgkin's disease: a case report and review of the literature. Neurosurgery 2000;46:1504-1508; discussion 1508-1510.
32. Kadkhodayan Y, Alreshaid A, Moran CJ, Cross DT 3rd, Powers WJ, Derdeyn CP. Primary angiitis of the central nervous system at conventional angiography. Radiology 2004;233:878-882.
33. Kolodny EH, Rebeiz JJ, Caviness VS Jr, Richardson EP Jr. Granulomatous angiitis of the central nervous system. Arch Neurol 1968;19:510-524.
34. Lie JT. Primary (granulomatous) angiitis of the central nervous system: a clinicopathologic analysis of 15 new cases and a review of the literature. Hum Pathol 1992;23:164-171.
35. Volcy M, Toro ME, Uribe CS, Toro G. Primary angiitis of the central nervous system: report of five biopsy-confirmed cases from Colombia. J Neurol Sci 2004;227:85-89.
36. Seo P, Stone JH. The antineutrophil cytoplasmic antibody-associated vasculitides. Am J Med 2004;117:39-50.
37. Abril A, Calamia KT, Cohen MD. The Churg-Strauss syndrome (allergic granulomatous angiitis): review and update. Semin Arthritis Rheum 2003;33:106-114.
38. Paolini S, Ciappetta P, Piattella MC, Domenicucci M. Henoch-Schonlein syndrome and cerebellar hemorrhage: report of an adolescent case and literature review. Surg Neurol 2003;60:339-342.
39. Provenzale JM, Allen NB. Wegener granulomatosis: CT and MR findings. AJNR Am J Neuroradiol 1996;17:785-792.
40. Ghezzi A, Zaffaroni M. Neurological manifestations of gastrointestinal disorders, with particular reference to the differential diagnosis of multiple sclerosis. Neurol Sci 2001;22(Suppl 2):S117-122.
41. Rubinstein LJ, Urich H. Meningo-encephalitis of Behcet's disease: case report with pathological findings. Brain 1963;86:151-160.
42. Arayssi T, Hamdan A. New insights into the pathogenesis and therapy of Behcet's disease. Curr Opin Pharmacol 2004;4:183-188.
43. Gomez-Puerta JA, Cervera R, Calvo LM, et al. Dementia associated with the antiphospholipid syndrome: clinical and radiological characteristics of 30 patients. Rheumatology (Oxford) 2005;44:95-99.
44. Hilton DA, Footitt D. Neuropathological findings in Sneddon's syndrome. Neurology 2003;60:1181-1182.
45. Aquino Gondim Fde A, Leacock RO, Subramanian TA, Cruz-Flores S. Intracerebral hemorrhage associated with Sneddon's syndrome: is ischemia-related angiogenesis the cause? Case report and review of the literature. Neuroradiology 2003;45:368-372.
46. Sepp N, Zelger B, Schuler G, Romani N, Fritsch P. Sneddon's syndrome—an inflammatory disorder of small arteries followed by smooth muscle proliferation. Immunohistochemical and ultrastructural evidence. Am J Surg Pathol 1995;19:448-453.
47. Dastur DK, Singhal BS, Shroff HJ. CNS involvement in malignant atrophic papulosis (Kohlmeier-Degos disease): vasculopathy and coagulopathy. J Neurol Neurosurg Psychiatry 1981;44:156-160.
48. Molenaar WM, Rosman JB, Donker AJ, Houthoff HJ. The pathology and pathogenesis of malignant atrophic papulosis (Degos' disease). A case study with reference to other vascular disorders. Pathol Res Pract 1987;182:98-106.
49. Susac JO, Hardman JM, Selhorst JB. Microangiopathy of the brain and retina. Neurology 1979;29:313-316.
50. Cervera R, Khamashta MA, Font J, et al. Morbidity and mortality in systemic lupus erythematosus during a 5-year period. A multicenter prospective study of 1,000 patients. European Working Party on Systemic Lupus Erythematosus. Medicine (Baltimore) 1999;78:167-175.
51. Johnson RT, Richardson EP. The neurological manifestations of systemic lupus erythematosus. Medicine (Baltimore) 1968;47:337-369.
52. Gibson T, Myers AR. Nervous system involvement in systemic lupus erythematosus. Ann Rheum Dis 1975;35:398-406.
53. Jackson CG, Chess RL, Ward JR. A case of rheumatoid nodule formation within the central nervous system and review of the literature. J Rheumatol 1984;11:237-240.
54. Bathon JM, Moreland LW, DiBartolomeo AG. Inflammatory central nervous system involvement in rheumatoid arthritis. Semin Arthritis Rheum 1989;18:258-266.
55. Kraus E, Klinge H, Rautenberg M. Intradural manifestation of rheumatoid arthritis causing spinal cord compression. Neurochirurgia (Stuttg) 1990;33(Suppl 1):56-57.
56. Chung MH, Sum J, Morrell MJ, Horoupian DS. Intracerebral involvement in scleroderma en coup de sabre: report of a case with neuropathologic findings. Ann Neurol 1995;37:679-681.
57. Rensink AA, de Waal RM, Kremer B, Verbeek MM. Pathogenesis of cerebral amyloid angiopathy. Brain Res Brain Res Rev 2003;43:207-223.
58. Revesz T, Ghiso J, Lashley T, et al. Cerebral amyloid angiopathies: a pathologic, biochemical, and genetic view. J Neuropathol Exp Neurol 2003;62:885-898.

59. Revesz T, Holton JL, Lashley T, et al. Sporadic and familial cerebral amyloid angiopathies. Brain Pathol 2002;12:343-357.
60. Ghiso J, Frangione B. Cerebral amyloidosis, amyloid angiopathy, and their relationship to stroke and dementia. J Alzheimers Dis 2001;3:65-73.
61. Knudsen KA, Rosand J, Karluk D, Greenberg SM. Clinical diagnosis of cerebral amyloid angiopathy: validation of the Boston criteria. Neurology 2001;56:537-539.
62. Greenberg SM, O'Donnell HC, Schaefer PW, Kraft E. MRI detection of new hemorrhages: potential marker of progression in cerebral amyloid angiopathy. Neurology 1999;53:1135-1138.
63. Fazekas F, Kleinert R, Roob G, et al. Histopathologic analysis of foci of signal loss on gradient-echo T2*-weighted MR images in patients with spontaneous intracerebral hemorrhage: evidence of microangiopathy-related microbleeds. AJNR Am J Neuroradiol 1999;20:637-642.
64. Strozyk D, Blennow K, White LR, Launer LJ. CSF Abeta 42 levels correlate with amyloid-neuropathology in a population-based autopsy study. Neurology 2003;60:652-656.
65. Bjarnadottir M, Nilsson C, Lindstrom V, et al. The cerebral hemorrhage-producing cystatin C variant (L68Q) in extracellular fluids. Amyloid 2001;8:1-10.
66. Vonsattel JP, Myers RH, Hedley-Whyte ET, Ropper AH, Bird ED, Richardson EP Jr. Cerebral amyloid angiopathy without and with cerebral hemorrhages: a comparative histological study. Ann Neurol 1991;30:637-649.
67. Greenberg SM, Vonsattel JP. Diagnosis of cerebral amyloid angiopathy. Sensitivity and specificity of cortical biopsy. Stroke 1997;28:1418-1422.
68. Eng JA, Frosch MP, Choi K, Rebeck GW, Greenberg SM. Clinical manifestations of cerebral amyloid angiopathy-related inflammation. Ann Neurol 2004;55:250-256.
69. Streichenberger N, Girard-Madoux P, Verejan I, Pialat J, Vital C, Kopp N. Giant cell angiitis of the central nervous system with amyloid angiopathy. A case report and review of the literature. Clin Exp Pathol 1999;47:311-317.
70. Anders KH, Wang ZZ, Kornfeld M, et al. Giant cell arteritis in association with cerebral amyloid angiopathy: immunohistochemical and molecular studies. Hum Pathol 1997;28:1237-1246.
71. Izumihara A, Ishihara T, Hoshii Y, Ito H. Cerebral amyloid angiopathy associated with hemorrhage: immunohistochemical study of 41 biopsy cases. Neurol Med Chir (Tokyo) 2001;41:471-477; discussion 477-478.
72. Ruchoux MM, Maurage CA. CADASIL: cerebral autosomal dominant arteriopathy with subcortical infarcts and leukoencephalopathy. J Neuropathol Exp Neurol 1997;56:947-964.
73. Kalaria RN, Viitanen M, Kalimo H, Dichgans M, Tabira T, CADASIL Group of Vas-Cog. The pathogenesis of CADASIL: an update. J Neurol Sci 2004;226:35-39.
74. Abe K, Murakami T, Matsubara E, Manabe Y, Nagano I, Shoji M. Clinical features of CADASIL. Ann N Y Acad Sci 2002;977:266-272.
75. Vahedi K, Chabriat H, Levy C, Joutel A, Tournier-Lasserve E, Bousser MG. Migraine with aura and brain magnetic resonance imaging abnormalities in patients with CADASIL. Arch Neurol 2004;61:1237-1240.
76. Arima K, Yanagawa S, Ito N, Ikeda S. Cerebral arterial pathology of CADASIL and CARASIL (Maeda syndrome). Neuropathology 2003;23:327-334.
77. Rafalowska J, Dziewulska D, Fidzianska A. CADASIL: what component of the vessel wall is really a target for Notch 3 gene mutations? Neurol Res 2004;26:558-562.
78. Miao Q, Paloneva T, Tuominen S, et al. Fibrosis and stenosis of the long penetrating cerebral arteries: the cause of the white matter pathology in cerebral autosomal dominant arteriopathy with subcortical infarcts and leukoencephalopathy. Brain Pathol 2004;14:358-364.
79. Joutel A, Favrole P, Labauge P, et al. Skin biopsy immunostaining with a Notch3 monoclonal antibody for CADASIL diagnosis. Lancet 2001;358:2049-2051.
80. Schroder JM, Sellhaus B, Jorg J. Identification of the characteristic vascular changes in a sural nerve biopsy of a case with cerebral autosomal dominant arteriopathy with subcortical infarcts and leukoencephalopathy (CADASIL). Acta Neuropathol (Berl) 1995;89:116-121.
81. Okeda R, Arima K, Kawai M. Arterial changes in cerebral autosomal dominant arteriopathy with subcortical infarcts and leukoencephalopathy (CADASIL) in relation to pathogenesis of diffuse myelin loss of cerebral white matter: examination of cerebral medullary arteries by reconstruction of serial sections of an autopsy case. Stroke 2002;33:2565-2569.
82. Schultz A, Santoianni R, Hewan-Lowe K. Vasculopathic changes of CADASIL can be focal in skin biopsies. Ultrastruct Pathol 1999;23:241-247.

7 INFECTIOUS DISEASES

Infections of the central nervous system (CNS) are surprisingly common, and at times, serious medical conditions. Infectious diseases overall are now the leading cause of death worldwide and are ranked third among the causes of death in the United States (1). Epidemiologic studies implicate the acquired immunodeficiency disease (AIDS) pandemic as partially responsible for this chilling statistic (2). As is now all too familiar, CNS infectious diseases figure prominently in patients with AIDS, and thus AIDS-related diagnoses occasionally confront the pathologist. Another factor contributing to the prevalence of infectious diseases is a shift in immigration patterns, which has extended the geographic distribution of certain infectious diseases, such as West Nile virus, to include regions in which they were considered merely a curiosity (1,3). This entity and other emerging infectious diseases pose new challenges, reflecting the changing roles that biologic reservoirs and vectors play in human-pathogen interactions.

Despite modern antimicrobial chemotherapy, the incidence of severe neurologic sequelae associated with selected pathogens remains high. Early and accurate diagnosis, in which the surgical pathologist often plays a pivotal role, remains the cornerstone of effective management of both the more familiar and less well-known entities. Unlike the bulk of neoplastic diseases of the CNS, in the case of infectious diseases, the diligent pathologist is sometimes rewarded with the gratifying diagnosis of a treatable illness. First and foremost, prompt diagnosis mandates a systematic approach and comprehensive awareness of both familiar and unexpected pathogens that threaten the nervous system.

This chapter focuses on those infections that affect the CNS and that may come under the purview of the surgical pathologist. The reader is referred to other texts for more information on aspects of these infections that relate to other clinical situations and other infections not covered in this chapter.

BASIC DEFINITIONS

Traditionally, infections that involve the CNS are divided into two broad categories based on location: those that mainly involve the meninges and those that are primarily confined to the parenchyma. These categories can be further subdivided according to the specific location of the inflammatory process, which is often influenced by the infectious agent. *Pachymeningitis*, which refers to inflammation of the dura mater, usually results from the contiguous spread of bacterial infection within the epidural space or from cranial and spinal osteomyelitis. The more restricted term *(lepto)meningitis* is reserved for an infectious or inflammatory process that selectively involves the leptomeninges (arachnoid and pia mater), although the exudate may extend into the brain along the Virchow-Robin perivascular spaces without actually violating the parenchyma. The pia mater appears to be an effective barrier against parenchymal spread. In addition to infectious etiologies, numerous noninfectious causes can mimic meningitis and must be considered in the differential diagnosis of leptomeningeal infiltrates. Examples of important noninfectious causes include medications (nonsteroidal antiinflammatory drugs, antibiotics) and carcinomatosis.

An infection confined to the brain parenchyma is designated *encephalitis*, or if restricted to the spinal cord, is called *myelitis*. Usually a feature of viral and not bacterial or fungal infection, more than one anatomic area or compartment may be involved, such as *meningoencephalitis;* if the meninges, parenchyma, and spinal cord are involved, the infection is classified as *meningoencephalomyelitis*.

Either bacterial or fungal infections can cause *abscess* formation, a discrete, loculated, multilayered lesion with a necrotic core that is accompanied by an inflammatory exudate and surrounded by a fibrous capsule. Abscesses may be found within the brain parenchyma, or less commonly, within the epidural compartment.

In contrast to the subdural location, suture lines provide an effective barrier to the spread of *epidural abscesses*. In the initial phase, prior to lamination or organization of the abscess, there is focal, poorly delimited inflammation, or *cerebritis* within the brain parenchyma. Pyogenic infection within the subdural space spreads too rapidly for effective organization; this poorly circumscribed accumulation is known as *empyema*.

The temporal evolution of CNS infections has profound clinical and pathologic consequences. Under the heading of meningeal infections, there are three basic categories: *acute bacterial meningitis, acute viral meningitis,* and *chronic meningitis*. These categories represent different types of cellular inflammatory response and provide a logical framework for relating pathologic findings to the causative organism. Acute meningitis denotes the evolution of symptoms within hours to several days, while chronic meningitis has an onset of weeks to months. In many instances, however, these syndromes overlap because of variables that govern the host-pathogen interaction.

As a final point of clarification, *aseptic meningitis* is a broad term that denotes an inflammation devoid of organisms, which may be caused by many different etiologic agents. In many cases, a specific cause is not apparent after initial evaluation. Patients characteristically have an acute onset of meningeal symptoms, fever, and cerebrospinal pleocytosis that is prominently lymphocytic. After an extensive workup, many of these cases are later found to have a viral etiology and then can be reclassified as acute viral meningitis. While viruses cause most cases of aseptic meningitis, it can also be caused by bacterial, fungal, mycobacterial, and parasitic agents. For the most part, these entities remain in the bailiwick of the clinician and clinical pathologist.

In this chapter, in addition to the brief introductory definitions, general observations, and basic diagnostic approaches, the topic of CNS infection is organized according to time course (i.e., acute or chronic) and dominant location, recognizing that infections may involve more than one compartment. In the case of CNS infections caused by selected organisms, a more detailed description follows.

Table 7-1

STEP-BY-STEP APPROACH TO THE INTRAOPERATIVE DIAGNOSIS OF SUSPECTED CENTRAL NERVOUS SYSTEM (CNS) INFECTION

Preliminary measures
Review patient records for relevant history of foreign travel, systemic infections, immunosuppressive therapy, antecedent trauma, etc.
Review neuroimaging studies and/or radiographic reports for clues to an infectious etiology
Specimen transport precautions
Laboratory personnel should be notified prior to each specimen delivery
Tissue should be transported to the frozen section room in well-sealed, labeled containers
Precautions for handling the specimen within the frozen section room
Specimen should be handled within a well-ventilated hood
Appropriate protective garments including masks and gloves should be worn
Disposable equipment, when available, is helpful
Once the diagnosis of infection is either established or not excluded, the surgeon should be advised to obtain intraoperative cultures

GENERAL APPROACH TO CNS INFECTIONS

The surgical pathologist is the frontline in the rapid diagnosis or exclusion of an infectious disease. Table 7-1 provides a step-by-step approach to intraoperative diagnosis of potential CNS infections. Accurate interpretation relies heavily on the knowledge of the clinical circumstances and an open communication with the team of medical providers. Demographic data, details of the patient travel history, and the presence of a predisposing illness or systemic infection can help the pathologist draw up a short list of diagnostic possibilities. Knowledge of the radiologic signal characteristics and location of the lesion on imaging studies, complemented by the surgeon's intraoperative observations, helps maximize the yield of the microscopic findings.

It is essential for the pathologist and laboratory personnel to respect potentially infectious tissue. Although every tissue specimen should be treated as if it were potentially hazardous material, biopsy materials from cases of suspected Creutzfeldt-Jacob disease and other prion diseases, human immunodeficiency virus (HIV), and tuberculosis require special preparations. Prior to delivery from the operating room, the specimen needs to be properly sealed in a well-labeled, tightly closed container and laboratory personnel should receive advance warning of each specimen. Tissue samples should be handled only while wearing disposable gloves and masks within ventilated safety hoods and preferably using disposable instruments. The reader is referred to additional resources for detailed guidelines on handling both fresh and fixed tissue from suspected cases of prion diseases (4).

As a key initial step, the interpretation of cytologic preparations and frozen section biopsies allows for the identification of a wide variety of infectious diseases. Smear cytology has increasingly become the mainstay for the rapid diagnosis of infection and sometimes obviates the need for cryostat sections. This is especially relevant in cases in which contamination of equipment, e.g., the cryostat, may be a concern. In many instances, however, it is helpful to check the frozen section to localize the infectious process and identify additional morphologic features. Various staining methods have relative advantages and disadvantages, but hematoxylin and eosin (H&E) staining of both smears and frozen sections provides a good screening method for most microorganisms.

An infectious case may be suspected when the basic cellular response is dominated by acute, chronic, or granulomatous inflammation or necrosis. In addition to the type and location of the inflammatory response, attention should focus on identifying the microorganisms or viral-associated cytopathic effects. Once the pathologist has determined that a disease is likely to be due to an infection, the neurosurgeon should be alerted promptly to obtain intraoperative cultures to avoid the increased risk of contamination of cultures performed within the frozen section environment.

Although many microorganisms or their cytopathic effects are clearly visible on routine H&E-stained sections, additional histochemical stains are often needed for their complete characterization (Table 7-2). Highly specific techniques, such as immunohistochemistry, in situ hybridization, and nucleic acid amplification and detection with the polymerase chain reaction (PCR), are used in certain instances to establish the diagnosis of infection. PCR assays detect rapidly and accurately the presence of fastidious and slow-growing microorganisms, such as mycobacteria, herpesviruses, and enteroviruses, directly from clinical specimens (5–9).

Table 7-2

PRINCIPAL HISTOLOGIC STAINING METHODS FOR MICROORGANISMS

Stain	Microorganism
Hematoxylin and eosin (H&E)	Bacteria appear as blue rods or cocci regardless of Gram reaction; colonies appear as fuzzy blue clusters; fungi are blue
Periodic acid–Schiff (PAS)	Fungal organisms except *Cryptococcus* are red; also outlines tissue structures such as blood vessels, basement membranes
Gomori or Grocott methenamine silver method (GMS)	Fungi including *Histoplasma, Candida, Blastomyces, Cryptococcus* appear black
Ziehl-Neelsen	Acid-fast organisms including *Mycobacterium tuberculi* and *M. lepri* and *Cryptosporidium* appear bright red
Modified Fite, GMS, Gram	*Nocardia* appears red with modified Fite, black with GMS, and purple Gram methods
Warthin-Starry	Spirochetes; organisms are black
Brown-Hopps or Brown-Brenn modified Gram stain	Gram-positive bacilli are blue; gram-negative are red; background is yellow
Giemsa	Leishmania or malaria; organisms are blue

The pathologist needs to be aware of the potential for false negative as well as false positive diagnoses of infection. For example, the germ cell component of a germinoma may be obscured by an exuberant inflammatory infiltrate that masquerades as an infectious disease. Other non-neoplastic conditions, such as demyelinating diseases, are often characterized by brisk inflammation during the active phase of the disease, thus raising the question of an infectious etiology. In other instances, artifacts can mimic the appearance of microorganisms, for example, branching parenchymal blood vessels against an inflammatory background may resemble hyphal elements or nuclear or other necrotic debris may mimic bacteria. Careful study, sometimes aided by special stains for microorganisms, usually rescues the pathologist from these potential pitfalls. In the case of fraudulent "bacteria," close inspection usually reveals that the necrotic fragments are, in fact, too large and irregular to be confused with bacteria.

MENINGEAL INFECTIONS

Acute Bacterial Meningitis

General Comments. In the early part of the 20th century, the prognosis for patients with most forms of bacterial meningitis was bleak. Scientific advances led to early diagnosis and the introduction of successive generations of antimicrobial therapy that dramatically improved clinical outcome. The relative frequency of the various causes of bacterial meningitis has changed over the decades and varies according to the age of the patient and whether the infection is acquired in the community or is nosocomial (Table 7-3) (10). In general, hospital-acquired infections are more likely to be produced by gram-negative or multiple organisms. Over the past decade, widespread infant vaccination (e.g., *Haemophilus influenzae* type B), coupled with the emergence of bacterial resistance (especially penicillin-resistant *Streptococcus pneumoniae*) have altered the relative frequencies of infection (11–13). As a consequence, bacterial meningitis is becoming more common in adults. Those at the extremes of life remain particularly vulnerable to infection, depending on the integrity of the host immune system and the innate virulence of the organism.

The diagnosis of isolated acute meningitis is more likely to be handled by the cytopathologist or the pathologist entrusted with the examination of the cerebrospinal fluid (CSF). It is only when other conditions are entertained that this entity crosses into the domain of the surgical pathologist.

Clinical Features. The most common clinical features of bacterial meningitis are fever, nuchal rigidity, and altered mental status. Seizures, either focal or generalized, and other focal neurologic findings are reported less frequently (14–16).

Radiologic Findings. Radiologic evaluation has gained importance in the diagnosis, treatment planning, and monitoring of all forms of CNS infections. Although of limited use in the early detection of bacterial meningitis, computerized tomography (CT) or magnetic resonance imaging (MRI) is usually performed prior to lumbar puncture to detect brain swelling and mass lesions that might enhance the risk of herniation. MRI is the most sensitive, specific, and accurate diagnostic method. The salient imaging findings are usually limited to thickening and enhancement of the meninges (fig. 7-1A). The gold standard in diagnosing meningitis is the contrast-enhanced T1-weighted image. Enhancement of the underlying cerebral cortex may indicate brain infarction secondary to the occlusion of inflamed meningeal vessels.

Table 7-3

THE MOST COMMON BACTERIAL PATHOGENS BASED ON AGE

Age	Major Pathogens
Less than 3 months	Group B *Streptococcus* *Listeria monocytogenes* *Escherichia coli* *Streptococcus pneumoniae*
3 months to 18 years	*Neisseria meningitiditis* *Streptococcus pneumoniae* *Haemophilus influenzae*
18 years to 50 years	*Streptococcus pneumoniae* *Neisseria meningitiditis* *Haemophilus influenzae*
Greater than 50 years	*Streptococcus pneumoniae* *Listeria monocytogenes* Gram-negative bacilli

Microbiology. In infants less than 1 month of age, encapsulated group B *Streptococcus* is the most common cause of meningitis. Transmission of group B *Streptococcus* to the neonate occurs orally through amniotic fluid contaminated from the flora of the maternal genital tract or from the hands of nursery workers. Two clinical syndromes are recognized. In infants less than 5 days old, the "early-onset acute syndrome" is characterized by sepsis with respiratory distress and pneumonia; meningitis is usually not present. In cases with delayed onset in infants older than 10 days, septicemia and meningitis dominate the clinical picture. Risk factors include low birth weight infants, maternal premature rupture of amniotic membranes, and fever. In adults, group B streptococcal infection is often nosocomial and targets mainly the infirm or elderly (13,16).

Escherichia coli is second only to group B streptococci as a cause of neonatal meningitis. Low birth weight and a positive result from CSF cultures are predictors of poor outcome.

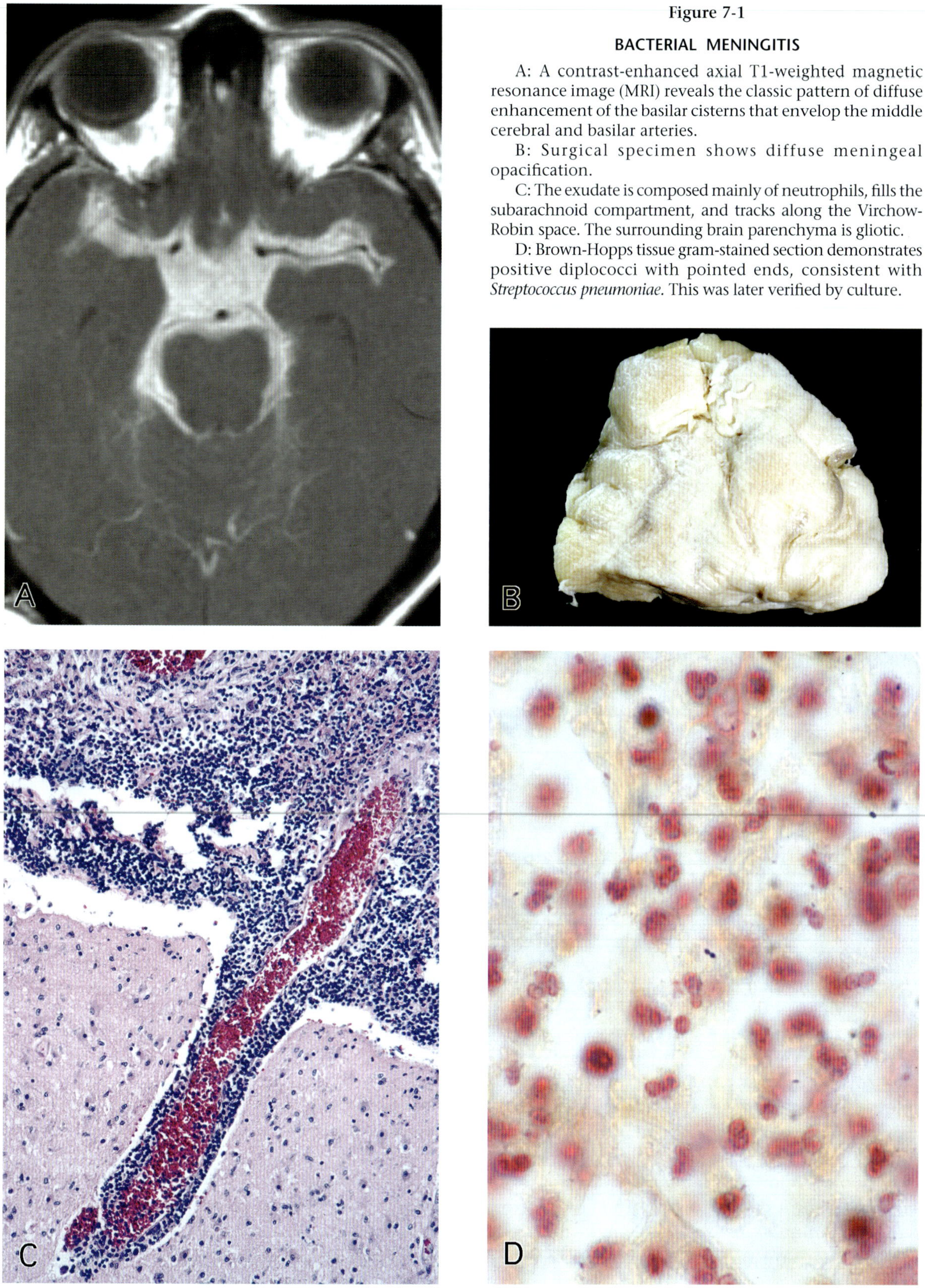

Figure 7-1

BACTERIAL MENINGITIS

A: A contrast-enhanced axial T1-weighted magnetic resonance image (MRI) reveals the classic pattern of diffuse enhancement of the basilar cisterns that envelop the middle cerebral and basilar arteries.

B: Surgical specimen shows diffuse meningeal opacification.

C: The exudate is composed mainly of neutrophils, fills the subarachnoid compartment, and tracks along the Virchow-Robin space. The surrounding brain parenchyma is gliotic.

D: Brown-Hopps tissue gram-stained section demonstrates positive diplococci with pointed ends, consistent with *Streptococcus pneumoniae*. This was later verified by culture.

In adults, *E. coli* meningitis is rare but has been reported following neurosurgical trauma/procedures (13,16).

Listeria monocytogenes is a small anaerobic gram-positive rod that causes meningitis in infants less than 1 month old and the elderly (17,18). Most cases are sporadic and food-borne. Clinically, *L. monocytogenes* meningitis may be difficult to diagnose because the meningeal signs are less frequent, there is a lower CSF white blood cell count with less neutrophilic predominance, and a lower protein level. Predisposing factors include pregnancy, alcoholism, conditions associated with iron overload (transfusion-induced and hemochromatosis), and immunosuppression (14,18,19). Similar to group B streptococci, early-onset and late-onset patterns of infection are recognized. The term *granulomatosis infantiseptica* refers to the triad of *Listeria*-associated hepatosplenomegaly, myocarditis, and meningoencephalitis (16). Isolated infection of the brain stem (*rhomboencephalitis*) accompanied by cranial nerve dysfunction occurs. Unlike other forms of CNS *Listeria* infection, isolated brain stem infection usually occurs in otherwise healthy adults. Cerebritis and abscess formation are uncommon but recognized sequelae (17–19).

Streptococcus pneumoniae (pneumococcus) now accounts for most cases of bacterial meningitis in all age groups except newborns. It is the most common etiologic agent in patients between 6 and 18 months of age, and often causes meningitis in infants in the 4- to 12-week-old range (13,15). This gram-positive coccus occurs in pairs and has an external polysaccharide capsule that determines its serotype. The nasopharynx is the primary site of pneumococcal colonization. Spread to the meninges occurs through local extension of infection in a contiguous structure (sinuses or middle ear). Particularly severe or unusual pneumococcal infections can be seen in HIV-positive patients. Other major risk factors for meningitis with this organism include splenectomy; ear, nose, and throat procedures; chronic CSF leak; diabetes mellitus; multiple myeloma; liver disease; alcoholism; hypogammaglobulinemia; complement deficiency (C1-4); and pneumococcal pneumonia (13,15,16).

Haemophilus influenzae is a small, often encapsulated gram-negative coccobacillus that colonizes the upper respiratory tract of humans who are its only natural host (15,16). Type B, which produces an endotoxin important for virulence, is responsible for most cases. Among children older than 6 months of age, this pathogen formerly accounted for most cases of purulent meningitis. Its frequency has declined dramatically in recent years after the introduction of an effective vaccine. Spread occurs through respiratory droplets or by direct contact with respiratory secretions. Factors that potentiate the risk of infection include head trauma, neurosurgery, paranasal sinusitis, otitis media, and CSF leak (15).

Neisseria meningitidis, an encapsulated gram-negative organism that appears in pairs, leads the causes of epidemic meningitis. Children and young adults are the typical victims. The capsular polysaccharide enhances virulence and endotoxin release. Five (A, B, C, W, and Y) of at least 13 serogroups are known to cause meningococcal meningitis. Groups A and C usually cause epidemic meningitis, whereas B, W, and Y cause endemic meningitis (13,15). Epidemics are documented among persons living in close quarters like dormitories, chronic care facilities, or barracks. As with other encapsulated organisms, asplenia is a risk factor for infection. Invasion of the CNS is thought to occur through the choroid plexus and other sites with fenestrated capillaries.

As a group, gram-negative meningitis (other than *H. influenza*) is increasing in incidence. In adults, the most common pathogens causing gram-negative meningitis are *Pseudomonas aeruginosa, Escherichia coli, Enterobacter aerogenes, Proteus morganii*, and *Klebsiella pneumoniae*. The clinical manifestations are protean and require a high index of suspicion for prompt diagnosis. The risk factors include compromised immunity, disruption of normal barriers that occurs after recent brain or spinal surgery, and recent trauma. Similarly, spinal abnormalities, urinary tract abnormalities, and a local or urinary tract infection elevate the risk for this type of meningitis (13,15).

Staphylococcus aureus meningitis targets those compromised by antecedent neurosurgery, head trauma, or overwhelming bacteremia. Methicillin-resistant *S. epidermidis* is reported in nosocomial meningitis due to prosthetic devices (13,15).

Laboratory Findings. The most important diagnostic procedure in cases of suspected bacterial meningitis is a lumbar puncture. It is performed to obtain CSF to determine the white blood cell count and differential, to measure protein and glucose levels, and for culture and Gram stain. In bacterial meningitis, the CSF protein level is elevated and the glucose level is low. The white blood cell count is elevated and neutrophils nearly always predominate (8,20). Gram stains and CSF cultures are positive in the majority of cases. PCR is another technique that has facilitated the rapid diagnosis of bacterial infections, especially meningococcal meningitis (7).

Gross Findings. The gross appearance of the leptomeninges from biopsies of pyogenic meningitis is often striking. Sampling should reflect the sites of predilection for specific organisms. In surgical specimens that include underlying brain, a creamy, purulent exudate fills the meninges over the surface of the brain and travels along the Virchow-Robin spaces into the superficial cortex (fig. 7-1B). The spinal cord may show similar changes. In pneumococcal meningitis, copious exudates often have a greenish tinge. *Neisseria* meningitis is marked by massive cerebral edema and congestion with minimal exudates. Localization of the exudate may provide further clues regarding the identity of the organism: in *H. influenzae* meningitis, the exudate is usually basal, whereas in pneumococcal meningitis, the accumulation localizes over the cerebral convexities adjacent to the sagittal sinus. *H. influenza* meningitis is notable for early endothelial and adventitial vascular proliferation and ensuing extensive necrosis of the cerebral cortex and subcortical white matter, and intense gliosis.

In neonatal meningitis, exudates predominate over the base of the brain in half of the cases and are more evenly distributed in the remainder. Venous thrombosis and occlusion of penetrating arteries may result in hemorrhagic infarcts, another feature commonly encountered in this population.

Microscopic Findings. In the acute phase of the infection, the microscopic picture is dominated by intense leptomeningeal congestion and large numbers of neutrophils and necrotic debris within the subarachnoid space and tracking along the perivascular spaces into the cerebral cortex (fig. 7-1C). Purulent exudates often permeate the walls of meningeal and cortical vessels, leading to thrombosis and infarction of the underlying brain. Although routine H&E-stained sections are useful for evaluating many of the pathologic features, ancillary methods such as special stains (Brown-Hopps, Brown-Brenn) and immunohistochemical preparations are indispensable for accurately identifying extracellular and intracellular (within polymorphonuclear leucocytes and macrophages) bacteria.

As the acute inflammation subsides during the second and third weeks of infection, variable numbers of chronic inflammatory cells are recruited and eventually predominate, with the dominant cells being mononuclear, mainly macrophages. Lymphocytes and small numbers of plasma cells may also be present, although these elements are usually inconspicuous in neonatal meningitis. After approximately 3 weeks, the inflammation diminishes and consists of scattered mononuclear cells accompanied by an arachnoidal fibroblast proliferation.

In neonatal group B streptococcal meningitis associated with prematurity, the leptomeningeal inflammatory infiltrates may be sparse (16). This observation may reflect an immaturity of host response to infection. Meningitis in this population is often marked by the presence of ventriculitis and inflammatory exudates within the choroid plexus, although these sites are rarely biopsied.

A critical piece of information is whether the patient received antibiotic therapy. Prior therapy may modify the histologic picture by causing significant diminution of the acute inflammatory reaction and reducing the likelihood of finding microorganisms.

Acute Viral Meningitis

General Comments. Viruses are the most important cause of *aseptic meningitis*, a syndrome defined by the absence of an identifiable bacterial pathogen (Table 7-4). Many viral pathogens (Table 7-5) are also capable of producing encephalitis. Certain viruses preferentially cause either one or the other form of the disease. Enteroviruses lead the causative agents for aseptic meningitis in children. Subgroups of this family include coxsackievirus, echovirus, and nonparalytic poliovirus; immunization programs in developed countries have largely controlled

Table 7-4

CAUSES OF ASEPTIC MENINGITIS

Partially treated bacterial, fungal, protozoan meningitis
Viral meningitis
Parameningeal infection (e.g., spinal or intracranial abscess, occult paranasal sinus infection)
Endocarditis
Cancer-related meningitis (e.g., carcinoma, lymphoma, leukemia)
Subarachnoid hemorrhage
Chemical meningitis
Sarcoidosis
Drugs (e.g., intrathecal contrast agents, chemotherapy)
Other inflammatory diseases

Table 7-5

SELECTED CAUSES OF VIRAL MENINGITIS

Enteroviruses (echo, polio, coxsackie)
Arboviruses (St. Louis encephalitis virus, West Nile virus)
Herpes simplex virus (usually type 2)
Human immunodeficiency virus
Lymphocytic choriomeningitis
Varicella zoster, Epstein-Barr virus, cytomegalovirus
Mumps virus
Adenovirus

paralytic polioviruses. The infection rate varies widely according to the age and socioeconomic circumstances of the population.

Other important viruses causing acute aseptic meningitis include HIV (meningitis is a common presenting feature of the illness), adenovirus, and mumps virus. Because most cases of aseptic meningitis resolve before the etiologic agent is identified, it is difficult to assess the ongoing epidemiologic role of many of these viruses. Within the herpesvirus family, herpes simplex virus (HSV)-2 is known to cause acute meningitis. Epstein-Barr virus (EBV), varicella-zoster virus (VZV), and cytomegalovirus (CMV) are encountered in immunosuppressed hosts, especially in patients with AIDS and transplant recipients (3,20). Occasional outbreaks of meningitis due to lymphocytic choriomeningitis (LCM) virus occur worldwide, especially among young individuals exposed to rodents (20).

Although encephalitis is the most commonly recognized manifestation of the arthropod-borne viruses, certain pathogens may cause acute aseptic meningitis during the summer and fall months. St. Louis encephalitis virus is reported to be the most common vector-transmitted cause of aseptic meningitis (27).

Clinical Features. Viral meningitis produces the same signs and symptoms as bacterial meningitis, although usually of less severity. Most patients report fever, headache, stiff neck, or photophobia. Younger children may simply be irritable and infants may present with nonspecific findings of poor feeding and lethargy. One of the key features of enteroviral meningitis is a macular or maculopapular rash.

Radiologic Findings. Imaging in patients with suspected viral meningitis is usually performed to rule out possible encephalitis. An enhancement in contrast-enhanced scans signals parenchymal involvement (17,27).

Laboratory Findings. The diagnosis of viral meningitis is supported by the typical CSF profile and is confirmed by the isolation of the virus, detection of viral nucleic acid, and/or serologic studies. The CSF appears clear and features a lymphocytic pleocytosis accompanied by a mild to moderately elevated protein concentration. Although mononuclear cell predominance is the rule, neutrophils may comprise the majority of cells in the first 12 to 24 hours; afterwards, the cell count is usually dominated by lymphocytes. The CSF protein level is usually only slightly elevated, but it may be high or normal. The glucose level is normal in most cases, but severe hypoglycorrhachia has been reported, especially with lymphocytic choriomeningitis or mumps. These viruses also elicit a brisk CSF lymphocytosis.

The methods available for identifying a specific virus include CSF culture and PCR to detect viral DNA or RNA. Acute and convalescent sera should be sent for antiviral immunoglobulin (Ig)G antibody detection, especially for coxsackievirus, echovirus, and enterovirus (27).

Microscopic Findings. Given the benign, self-limited nature of most of these infections, pathologic observations are scarce. In the rare case that is biopsied, usually due to unrelated systemic causes, the morphologic features are mild. Subtle leptomeningeal clouding appears

Table 7-6

PRINCIPAL CAUSES OF CHRONIC MENINGITIS

Category	Agent
Bacteria	*Mycobacterium tuberculosis* *Borrelia burgdorferi* *Treponema pallidum* *Brucella* species *Nocardia* species *Actinomyces* species
Fungi	*Cryptococcus neoformans* *Coccidioides immitis* *Blastomyces dermatitidis* *Histoplasma capsulatum* *Candida albicans* *Sporothrix schenckii* Paracoccidioidomycosis
Parasites	*Acanthamoeba* species *Naegleria fowleri* *Acanthamoeba cantonensis*

microscopically as a scanty mononuclear inflammatory infiltrate of the pia-arachnoid. Florid lymphocytic inflammation has been reported in the choroid plexus, as has necrosis of the ependymal lining. Parenchymal sequelae are usually limited to mild periventricular gliosis, although some cases of "granular ependymitis" seen at autopsy may reflect the effects of remote viral meningitis.

Treatment. In general, viral meningitis is treated symptomatically and rarely requires specific antiviral therapy.

Chronic Bacterial Meningitis

The principal bacterial, fungal, and parasitic agents responsible for chronic meningitis (classified as chronic if it persists for 4 weeks or more) are listed in Table 7-6. In this section, the discussion is restricted to cases of bacterial etiology; the sections on specific fungal and parasitic microorganisms below contain discussions of those entities. Treatment and prognosis vary with the nature of the causative agent. Specific therapy is available for infections caused by mycobacteria, fungi, and syphilis.

Chronic meningitis usually has an insidious onset that elicits complaints of headache, stiff neck, and fever. Alterations of mental status may also be noted.

Radiologic studies are helpful in guiding meningeal biopsies. MRI with gadolinium contrast is the most useful diagnostic imaging technique, demonstrating meningeal enhancement. Areas of enhancement provide the greatest diagnostic yield (21).

Examination of the CSF is the most important diagnostic test. Successful diagnosis requires adequate amounts for culture (bacterial and fungal). Additional CSF studies often include tests for syphilis (VDRL), cryptococcal antigen, fungal serologies, and cytology.

Tuberculosis

General Comments. *Tuberculosis,* the prototype for chronic bacterial meningitis, remains a major public health issue. The etiologic agent is *Mycobacterium tuberculosis,* a 1- to 3-µm acid-fast bacillus. The AIDS epidemic, immigration of people from the developing world, and inner city poverty are linked to the reemergence of classic neurotuberculosis. In developing countries, tuberculous meningitis often complicates primary infection, especially in children (22).

In the population with impaired cell-mediated immunity, the disease is rapidly progressive and more likely to involve extrapulmonary sites, including the meninges. Immunosuppression also predisposes to disease with the less virulent, atypical mycobacteria (*M. avium-intracellulare, M. africanus,* and rarely, *M. bovis* [16,23]), and disseminated infection after exposure to vaccination with attenuated bacilli Calmette-Guerin (BCG).

After the initial droplet-acquired pulmonary infection, mycobacteria multiply in alveolar spaces or macrophages. Within 2 to 4 weeks, hematogenous seeding of extrapulmonary sites occurs. At this point, tubercles may develop in the brain, spinal cord, cranial or spinal nerves, meninges, cranium, or vertebral column. Months to years later, these initial lesions may rupture into the subarachnoid space or ventricular system. In children, neurotuberculosis more commonly presents as a parenchymal tuberculoma. In patients with AIDS, another pattern of infection, the tuberculous abscess, is recognized (2).

Clinical Features. Tuberculosis presents as an acute, subacute, or chronic meningitic illness. Despite the "chronic" designation, tuberculous meningitis can manifest as the most rapidly progressive form of tuberculosis, sometimes mimicking pyogenic meningitis. Over half of the patients are ill for less than 2 weeks before diagnosis. Without appropriate therapy, the illness progresses from headache, fever, and meningismus to cranial nerve palsies or focal deficits, alterations of sensorium, seizures, coma, and eventually death. In less acute cases, focal manifestations caused by vasculitis may give rise to brain infarction before or concurrent with meningitic signs and symptoms. In such cases, seizures, hemiparesis, isolated cranial nerve palsies, and various spinal cord and root syndromes occur early in the course of the disease (22).

Radiologic Findings. CT scans of patients with tuberculous meningitis may be normal or may depict characteristic features of contrast enhancement in the subarachnoid cisterns, sulci, and brain parenchyma. Scans may show ventricular enlargement with prominent basal and sylvian fissure enhancement after intravenous contrast medium injection (23–25). As the disease progresses, T1-weighted images with contrast typically show abnormal meningeal enhancement, most commonly in the basal cisterns. None of the available techniques can reliably differentiate between neoplastic meningeal infiltrates and infectious agents (23–25).

Laboratory Findings. Examination of the CSF is the only way to make the diagnosis. CSF pressure may be normal or elevated. The CSF glucose level is depressed in almost all patients. The protein level is usually moderately elevated, but is occasionally very high. A modest pleocytosis occurs in virtually all patients, mostly composed of lymphocytes. PCR is a reliable technique for rapid diagnosis (8).

Gross Findings. Biopsies obtained from the basal aspects of the brain or spinal cord may be encased by thick gelatinous exudates (fig. 7-2A). Tubercles can be found within the meninges, superficial parenchyma, and ventricular lining. Infarcts may be identified in the branches of the middle cerebral artery. Tuberculomas develop anywhere along the neuraxis, especially in the cerebral hemispheres, cerebellum, and pontine tegmentum (16,21). These lesions appear as relatively circumscribed spherical masses with central necrosis and can be easily shelled out from the surrounding parenchyma.

Microscopic Findings. The histologic hallmark of active tuberculous meningitis is the "tubercle," which consists of a central core of homogeneous caseous necrosis, surrounded by layers of mononuclear cells, histiocytes, epithelioid cells, and often Langhans giant cells (fig. 7-2B). These multinucleated giant cells, 40 to 50 µm in diameter, are derived from the fusion of up to 20 macrophages. Central caseation is not always found in tuberculous lesions, but it is far more frequent than in granulomas of nontuberculous origin. Blood vessels in the subarachnoid space and perforating branches of the middle cerebral artery often develop exuberant proliferative changes (obliterative endarteritis) in response to the inflammatory infiltrates (fig. 7-2C). These changes cause infarcts in the underlying parenchyma. Brain parenchyma adjacent to the lesions shows reactive gliosis and microglial proliferation.

Mycobacteria require special stains for optimal visualization (fig. 7-2D). The microorganisms have a high content of complex lipids that bind the Ziehl-Neelsen (carbol fuchsin) stain and subsequently resist decolorization, hence the "acid-fast"designation. The auramine-rhodamine fluorescent technique is an especially sensitive, although more time-consuming, method of visualization. When more conventional methods fail, PCR is a useful tool for detecting organisms in tissue sections.

A *tuberculoma* is a tumor-like laminated lesion composed of a core of caseous necrosis surrounded by collections of lymphocytes, epithelioid cells, and Langhans type giant cells, and enclosed by an outer rind of fibroblasts and collagen. Similar in appearance to a pyogenic abscess, *tuberculous abscesses* contain numerous acid-fast bacilli; however, they typically lack epithelioid cells and giant cells.

In the immunosuppressed, mycobacteria do not elicit a vigorous granulomatous reaction; instead, sheets of foamy macrophages are packed with organisms demonstrable by acid-fast stains (16,27). Atypical mycobacterial infections are characterized by diffuse perivascular periodic acid–Schiff (PAS)-positive macrophage infiltrates accompanied by acid-fast microorganisms. Other infections, such as cryptococcal meningitis and CMV encephalitis, often coexist with atypical mycobacterial infections (2,26).

VIRAL INFECTIONS

Viral encephalitis occurs in epidemic settings or is sporadic. The herpesvirus family represents the most important cause of sporadic encephalitis and is most likely to be the subject of a brain

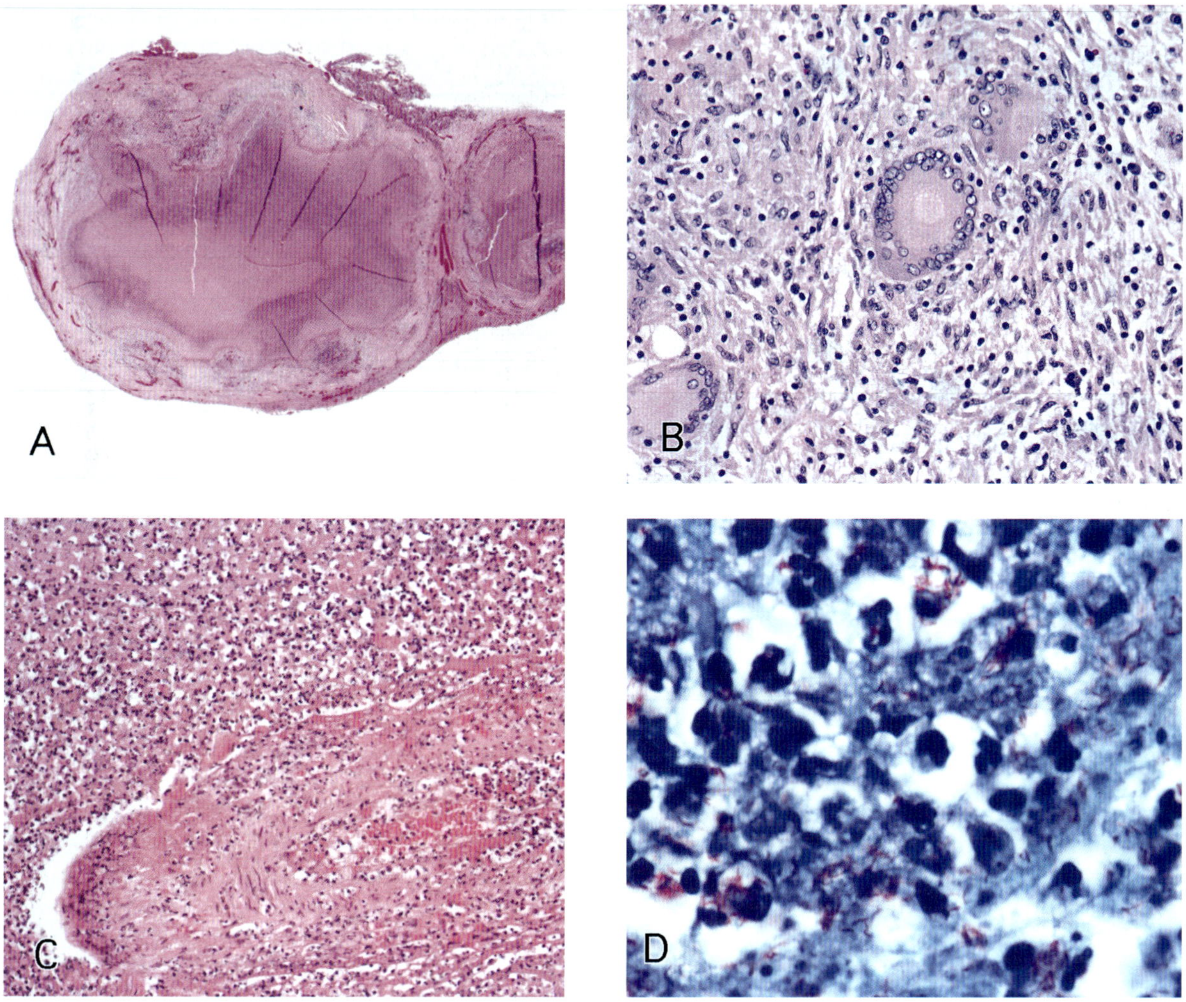

Figure 7-2

TUBERCULOSIS

A: Whole mount of surgical specimen shows ill-defined concentric zones of caseating granulomas.

B: The characteristic chronic inflammatory infiltrate is composed of lymphocytes, epithelioid histiocytes, and Langhans multinucleated giant cells.

C: The meningeal artery shows proliferation of the intimal connective tissue and extension of the inflammation through the adventitia and media.

D: Tubercle bacilli are optimally visualized with the Ziehl-Neelsen acid-fast stain.

biopsy. West Nile virus encephalitis has recently emerged as an important pathogen responsible for epidemics in the Western hemisphere after the apparent translocation of this mosquito-borne virus to a distant geographic region with immunologically naive avian and human hosts. Human herpesvirus-6 is a ubiquitous but typically benign herpesvirus that causes encephalitis in immunosuppressed human hosts. Other arbovirus pathogens (St. Louis encephalitis, Western equine, Eastern equine, and LaCrosse viruses) appear to be waning in importance in the United States. Globally, Japanese encephalitis virus is the most important emerging viral encephalitis (3,27,28).

The herpesviruses are a large family of DNA viruses that have a common nucleocapsid structure and the ability to cause lifelong latent infections in their hosts, from which they are periodically reactivated. Four human herpesviruses are associated with infectious neurologic disease: HSV types 1 and 2, VZV, CMV, and less commonly, EBV. Briefly, EBV CNS infections are further divided into two groups: CNS syndromes associated with primary or reactivated EBV infection and those associated with chronic EBV infection. In the former, diverse CNS syndromes including acute disseminated encephalomyelitis (ADEM) occur, whereas in the latter, chronic or recurrent CNS syndromes are produced (29–35). The EBV-driven lymphoproliferative disorders are more akin to neoplasms and are beyond the scope of this Fascicle.

Herpes Simplex Encephalitis

General Comments. HSV causes the most common form of sporadic acute encephalitis (*herpes simplex encephalitis* [HSE]). HSV-1 (herpes labialis) is the most common pathogen in adults, with only a minority of cases caused by HSV-2 (genital herpes). HSV-2 is the leading agent in neonates, who are infected by passing through the mother's infected birth canal. The neonatal form of this disease is typically a diffuse, nonfocal infectious process.

Clinical and Radiologic Findings. Primary HSV-1 virus establishes a latent, usually asymptomatic, infection in the trigeminal ganglion. Encephalitis may occur either during the primary infection or during reactivation of a latent infection. Brain infection is thought to occur by direct neuronal transmission of the virus from a peripheral site to the brain via the trigeminal or olfactory nerve. The clinical evolution is relatively short and in adults is associated with a triad of symptoms: fever, personality change, and seizures. *Neonatal herpes encephalitis* is characterized by seizure, fever, and lethargy. Mortality rates are high in the absence of therapy and only a minority of individuals returns to normal function. Neuroimaging studies of the brain typically show unilateral or bilateral changes in the medial temporal and inferior frontal areas. The characteristic expansile zones of brightness on MRI scan are best observed on T2-weighted images in the medial and inferior temporal lobe extending up into the insula (fig. 7-3A). Contrast enhancement and the changes of subacute hemorrhages may be seen.

Recurrent aseptic meningitis is now thought to be caused by HSV-2 infection, and is characterized by self-limited episodes of fever, meningismus, and severe headache. Many cases are indistinguishable from cases previously classified as *Mollaret meningitis*, a term that should be reserved for idiopathic cases of recurrent aseptic meningitis. A rare, often fatal form of necrotizing myelopathy has been ascribed to both HSV-1 and HSV-2 (31).

Laboratory Findings. Within the past decade, the rapid diagnosis of acute HSV-1 encephalitis has improved dramatically by the advent of PCR, a method that has become the gold standard of diagnosis avoiding, in many cases, invasive brain biopsy (6). HSV DNA cannot be detected in the CSF from latently infected individuals (9). CSF analysis typically reveals a mononuclear pleocytosis with mildly elevated protein levels and normal or mildly reduced glucose levels.

Gross Findings. The brain in classic adult cases is profoundly edematous. One or both temporal lobes, the insular cortices, and the orbital surfaces of the frontal lobes bear the brunt of the infection. The involved regions, which are the source of biopsy specimens, appear as an expanding mass of intensely congested, hemorrhagic and necrotic parenchyma (fig. 7-3B). In patients with protracted survival, involved areas show atrophy, yellow-brown discoloration, and cavitation.

Neonatal herpes, which is rarely biopsied, usually involves the periventricular white matter and spares the medial temporal and inferior frontal lobes. Grossly, the softened brain shows marked, diffuse edema and variable hemorrhage and necrosis. The disease may cause a wide range of CNS sequelae, from failure of brain growth and microcephaly to extensive destructive lesions resulting in multicystic encephalomalacia or even hydrencephaly (20).

Microscopic Findings. In the acute phase of the illness, microscopic examination discloses moderate leptomeningeal, and sparse perivascular and parenchymal mononuclear infiltrates composed of macrophages and lymphocytes. In full-blown cases, the degree of necrosis often overshadows the inflammatory response. Macrophages and perivascular lymphocytes are abundant. Intranuclear Cowdry A viral inclusions are (rarely) found within neurons, glia, and endothelial cells (30,31). Affected cells are heralded by their eosinophilic cytoplasm and nuclei containing homogenous, "ground glass," purple inclusions framed by an irregular rim of condensed chromatin (fig. 7-3C). During

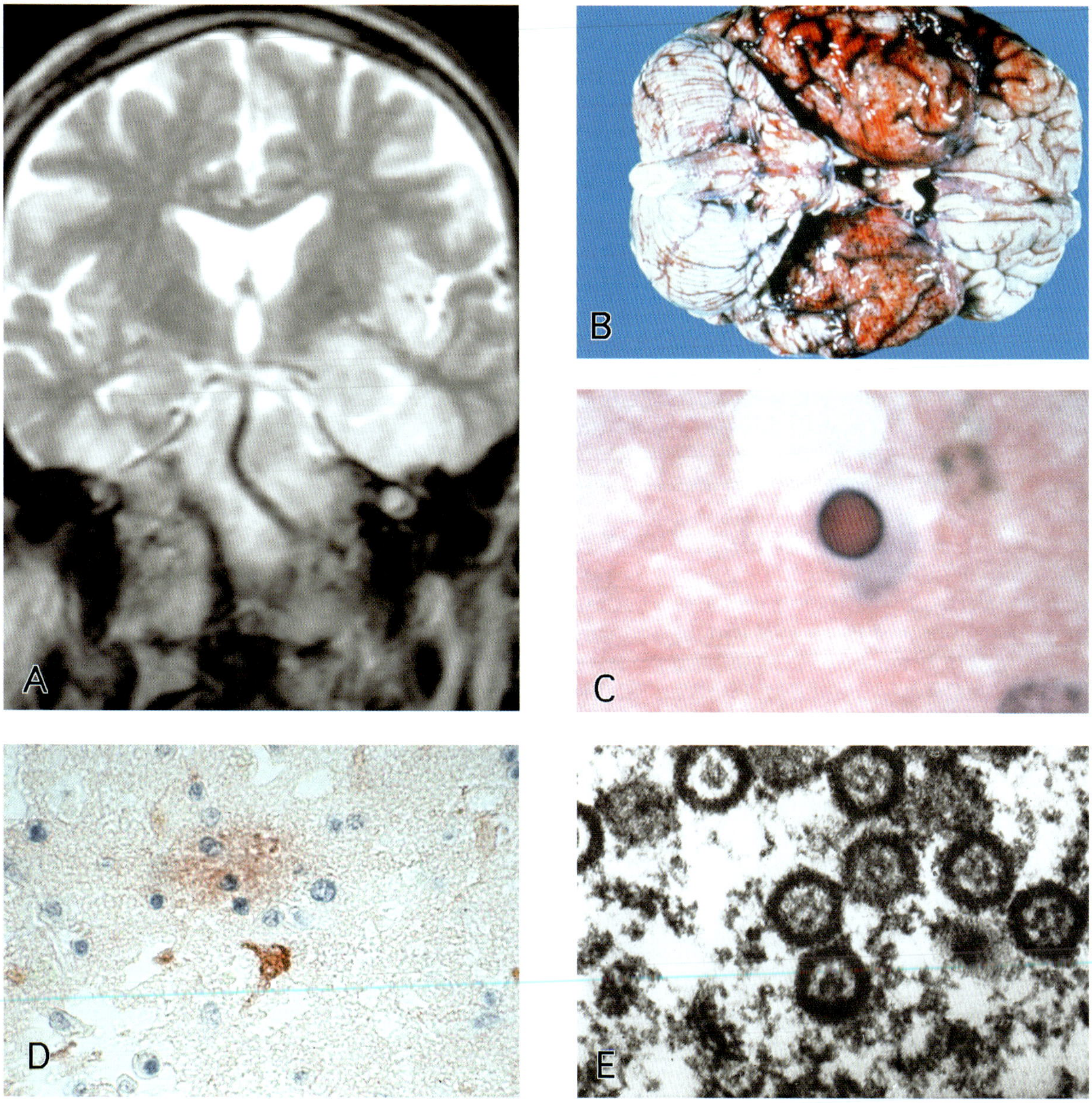

Figure 7-3

HERPES SIMPLEX ENCEPHALITIS

A: Coronal T2-weighted MRI shows the characteristic hyperintensity of the medial portion of the left temporal lobe.

B: Hemorrhagic necrosis of the inferior temporal lobe from a classic case of herpes encephalitis.

C: Microscopic section shows a necrotic background harboring an isolated cell with an eosinophilic intranuclear viral inclusion.

D: Immunohistochemical confirmation of herpes simplex virus antigen.

E: Electron micrograph discloses intranuclear herpesvirus nucleocapsid particles (180-200 nm).

later stages of the disease, large necrotic fields are accompanied by hemorrhage and intense inflammation (30,31). Viral inclusions are more difficult to find, and are usually restricted to the periphery of the necrotic lesions. Neuronophagia and microglial nodules, especially in less affected tissues, may be apparent at this stage.

HSV-1 antigen can be detected by immunohistochemistry (fig. 7-3D), HSV-1 DNA by in situ hybridization, and HSV nucleocapsids by electron microscopy. Ultrastructurally, infected cells are crowded with viral particles, appearing as hexagonal 90- to 100-nm capsids containing central nucleoids (fig. 7-3E). In "burned-out" cases, herpes viral DNA can usually be recovered in paraffin-embedded material by using highly sensitive PCR techniques (6).

Neonatal meningoencephalitis is characterized by macrophages and lymphocytic inflammatory infiltrates in the leptomeninges, multifocal parenchymal necrosis, and perivascular inflammation. Viral Cowdry A intranuclear inclusions are found in neuronal and glial, and especially oligodendroglial, cells. The infected nucleus is distorted and smudged, with clumped chromatin and irregular nuclear membranes (20).

Varicella Zoster

General Comments. *Varicella zoster virus* (VZV) is a neurotropic virus that causes chicken pox (varicella), after which it remains dormant in the dorsal root or trigeminal ganglia and can subsequently reactivate to cause herpes zoster (shingles). Although reactivation occurs in apparently normal individuals, the risk factors include immunosuppression due to a variety of factors, including HIV, waning cell-specific immunity, cancer, and radiation.

CNS complications follow both primary infection and reactivation of VZV. *Varicella cerebellitis* and *meningoencephalitis* may complicate primary infection (32). Acute cerebellitis is usually a self-limited illness that affects children under the age of 10 years. *Zoster encephalitis, myeloradiculitis,* and *vasculopathy/vasculitis* are features of reactivation and usually occur in adults (33,34). Manifestations that are more serious arise when VZV invades the spinal cord or cerebral arteries after reactivation of the virus, causing myelitis and focal vasculopathies. Large vessel disease is most common in immunocompetent individuals, whereas small vessel disease usually develops in immunocompromised patients. In some patients, both large and small vessels are involved (34,35).

Clinical Features. Subclinical infections are rare and primary infection is heralded by generalized cutaneous eruptions followed by a prodrome of fever, generalized malaise, and headache. Although varicella encephalitis is rare, it can occur at any age and take several forms. The presenting feature of one form is hyperexcitability that progresses to coma or cerebellar ataxia (35).

Herpes zoster attacks are often preceded by pain, which persists for several days before the classic skin lesions appear. The vesicular eruption is usually unilateral and most often appears on the thorax, limited to one or more dermatomes. A relatively common complication is postherpetic neuralgia, which may persist for months and be refractory to treatment (33).

VZV large vessel (granulomatous) vasculitis is characterized by acute, focal deficits that occur weeks after zoster of the contralateral trigeminal nerve. Small vessel vasculitis is characterized by headache, fever, mental status changes, seizures, and focal deficits.

Radiologic Findings. The pattern of abnormality on neuroimaging depends on the morphologic pattern of disease. With large vessel vasculopathy, neuroimaging may demonstrate ischemic and hemorrhagic infarcts of varying sizes. Angiography shows segmental narrowing, primarily in the internal carotid and middle or anterior cerebral arteries. In small vessel vasculopathy with ischemic and demyelinating lesions, neuroimaging may reveal multifocal subcortical lesions with the characteristic appearance of ischemic or hemorrhagic infarcts of gray and white matter. There may be spherical lesions scattered throughout the white matter and more than one pattern in a given patient (35).

Laboratory Findings. CSF examination discloses mild lymphocytic pleocytosis, a slight to moderate increase in the protein level, and a normal glucose level. PCR is used to detect VZV DNA in the CSF. A negative CSF PCR for VZV DNA, however, does not rule out VZV encephalitis (34).

Microscopic Findings. VZV meningoencephalitis features scattered petechial hemorrhages and perivenous demyelination. Cowdry type A intranuclear inclusions impart a ground glass appearance to the nucleus and are associated with margination of the chromatin (fig. 7-4). These viral inclusions can be found in cells of all types: glial, neuronal, and vascular. Variable amounts of inflammation and necrosis accompany the above findings. Ultrastructural study may be indicated to identify the viral particles (33,34).

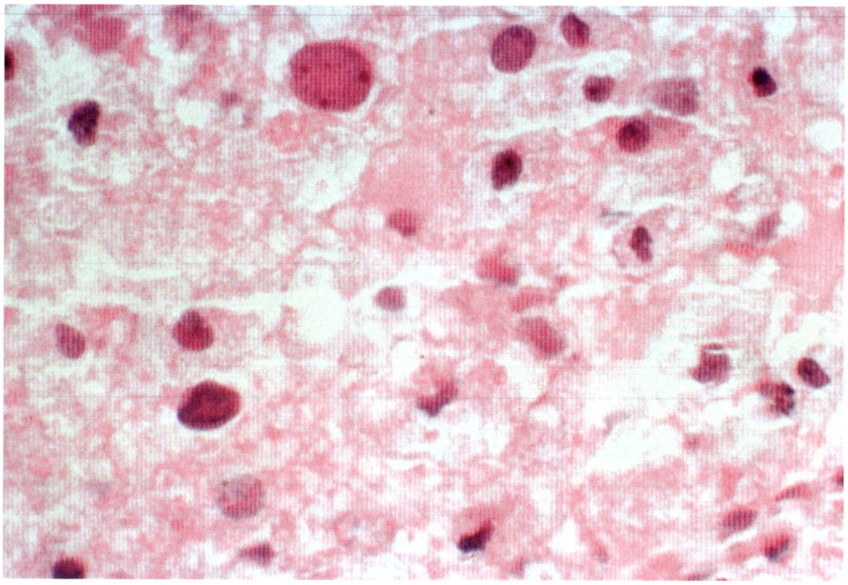

Figure 7-4

VARICELLA ZOSTER VIRUS MENINGOENCEPHALITIS

Cowdry type A intranuclear inclusions are seen.

A variety of other morphologic patterns are associated with viral reactivation, including multifocal white matter lesions that appear "punched out," ventriculitis, encephalitis involving the visual system, brain stem encephalitis, and myeloradiculitis, although these lesions are rarely biopsied (20,34).

Although uncommon, congenital VZV occurs. Examination of the brain reveals destructive and inflammatory lesions of the cerebral cortex and white matter, thalamus, brain stem, and spinal cord. Cerebellar heterotopias and bilateral polymicrogyric malformations of the insular cortex are sometimes present in surgical specimens from patients with intractable epilepsy (20,35).

Progressive Multifocal Leukoencephalopathy

Definition. *Progressive multifocal leukoencephalopathy* (PML) is a uniformly fatal, sometimes slowly evolving demyelinating disease of the CNS caused by a member of the papovavirus family, the JC virus.

General Comments. PML occurs in immunocompromised individuals. Papovavirus-induced CNS pathology supervenes after reactivation of the latent virus. Demyelinating lesions are a consequence of virus-induced killing of oligodendrocytes. Recently, the availability of highly active antiretroviral therapy has reduced the mortality in HIV-infected individuals, although the incidence has not diminished (2). Inflammatory forms of the disease and cases negative for the JC virus in the CSF after PCR analysis are also becoming more frequent (36). HIV infection often coexists with PML and may mimic some of the histopathologic features, e.g., demyelination, spongiform change, and gliosis.

Clinical and Radiologic Findings. The clinical features usually include headache, motor dysfunction, and visual loss. On CT, PML appears as one or more hypodense, nonenhancing white matter regions without mass effect (fig. 7-5A). MRI is more sensitive than CT scan in the detection of these lesions, which are hypodense to normal white matter on T1-weighted images and hyperintense on T2-weighted images. Contrast enhancement or mass effect is not typically seen (36).

Gross Findings. Small, discrete, rather round gelatinous lesions or pits, particularly along the gray-white junction, are typical features of cut sections, especially within the parietal and occipital lobes (fig. 7-5B). In more advanced cases, larger confluent areas of sunken, discolored parenchyma are found in the deep white matter, although they may also involve the cerebral cortex, deep gray matter, and brain stem.

Microscopic Findings. The cardinal features are patchy demyelination with sparing of axis cylinders and neuronal cell bodies; enlarged, pleomorphic bizarre-appearing astrocytes (fig. 7-5C), which may stain strongly on immunohistochemistry for p53, and can mimic neoplastic cells; and oligodendrocytes with enlarged,

Figure 7-5

PROGRESSIVE MULTIFOCAL LEUKOENCEPHALOPATHY

A: Contrast-enhanced coronal T1-weighted MRI demonstrates diffuse hypointensity primarily confined to the white matter within the left cerebral hemisphere. The adjacent cortical gray matter is not involved and there is a lack of enhancement.

B: Multiple small cavitary lesions within the white matter impart a granular appearance to the involved brain parenchyma.

C: Large, pleomorphic, reactive astrocytes are commonly observed in demyelinated areas.

D: Enlarged oligodendroglial nuclei harboring viral particles are often found along the edge of a focus of demyelination.

E: The virus can be detected by in situ hybridization with the JC probe.

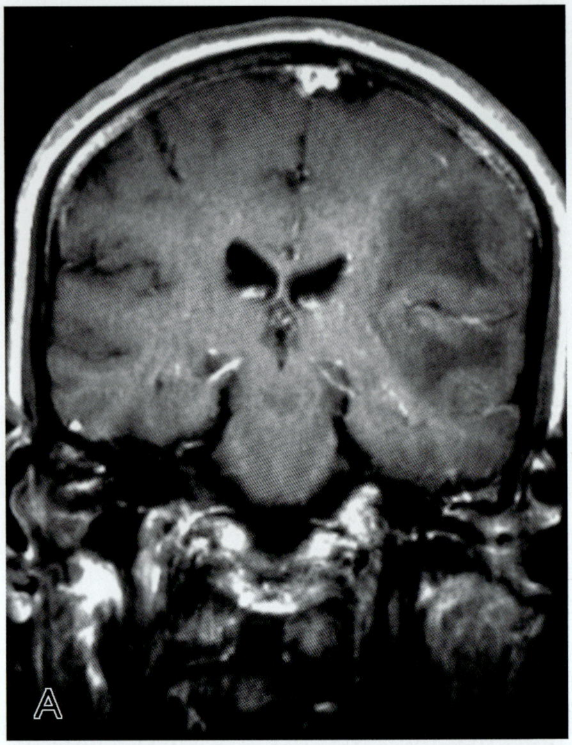

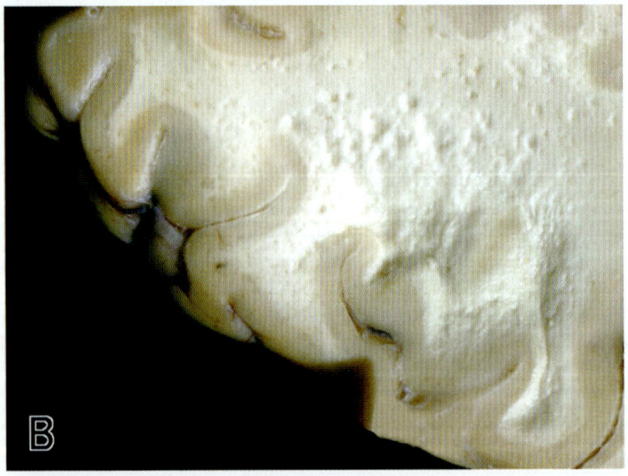

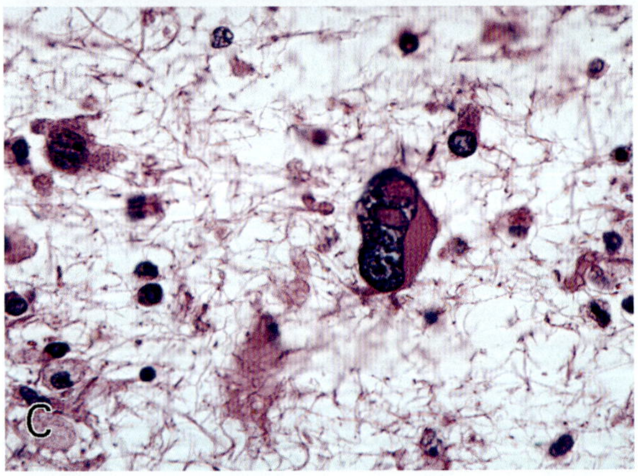

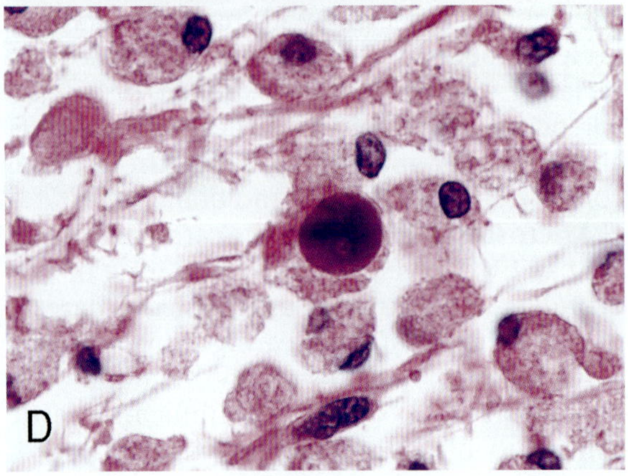

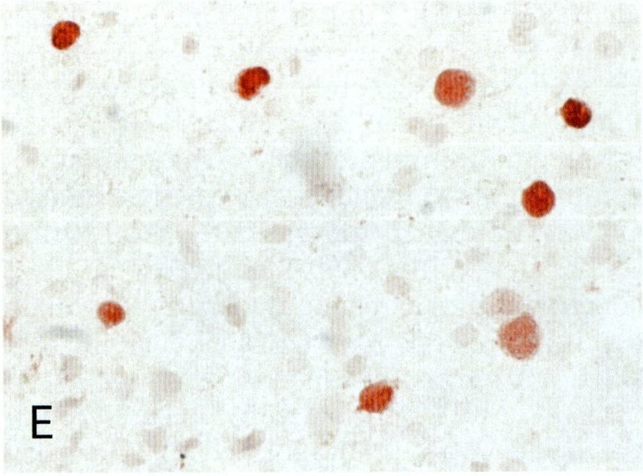

purple, ground glass–appearing nuclei packed with papovavirus particles (fig. 7-5D). Viral inclusions are best observed along the periphery of the lesion. Special stains for myelin (e.g., Luxol fast blue) highlight areas of myelin loss (fig. 7-5E). Corresponding adjacent sections should be stained for axons (Bielschowsky silver impregnation or neurofilament immunohistochemistry) to confirm relative axonal preservation. Noteworthy is the relative absence of inflammation. Lesions may contain moderate numbers of macrophages, but only sparse perivascular collections of lymphocytes (20).

Immunohistochemistry for JC virus reliably identifies infected cells (fig. 7-5F). Both infected oligodendrocytes and astrocytes are positive on in situ DNA hybridization, and p53 protein may accumulate in both cell types. Ultrastructural study may reveal infected oligodendrocytes filled with 30- to 40-nm spheres, often associated with 15- to 25-nm filamentous forms. Viral particles are not apparent within the bizarre astrocytes.

Human Immunodeficiency Virus

General Comments. The nervous system is a major target for *HIV infection* (Table 7-7). In addition to the increased susceptibility to opportunistic infections, many of which represent recrudescent latent or persistent infection, HIV is also capable of directly eliciting a plethora of effects on the central and peripheral nervous systems. With the advent of novel and effective retroviral therapy, the overall incidence of opportunistic infections has declined, and survival after such an AIDS-defining event has improved.

Alternatively, some HIV-infected patients experience clinical deterioration following highly active, antiretroviral therapy (HAART) therapy, usually within a few months of treatment (36a). This phenomenon is referred to as *immune reconstitution inflammatory syndrome* (IRIS). HAART-induced restoration of a pathogen-specific immune response contributes to the pathologic recognition of antigens associated with a known replicating infectious agent or persistent nonreplicating antigens from a prior IRIS infection. In most patients, immune reconstitution is beneficial, with only rare examples of fatal outcome. Although histopathologic criteria have not been codified, IRIS is usually dominated by inflammation, especially CD8-positive T lymphocytes. In some instances, exuberant angiocentric inflammation may masquerade as lymphoma or conceal underlying infectious agents, resulting in delayed diagnosis and inappropriate treatment. Awareness of this entity by pathologists is imperative to avoid diagnostic pitfalls.

Table 7-7

PRINCIPAL HUMAN IMMUNODEFICIENCY VIRUS (HIV)-RELATED INFECTIOUS DISEASES

Central Nervous System
Bacterial infections
Tuberculosis
Mycobacterium avium-intracellulare
Syphilis
Fungal infections
Cryptococcus neoformans meningitis
Candida sp.
Coccidioides immitis
Parasitic infections
Toxoplasmosis
Non-HIV–related viral encephalitis
Cytomegalovirus
Primary HIV encephalopathies
Multinucleate giant cell encephalitis (HIV encephalitis)
HIV-associated white matter disease (HIV leukodystrophy)
Neocortical/gray matter disease (HIV poliodystrophy)
Mixed patterns
Vacuolar myelopathy
Lymphocytic meningitis
Acute monophasic meningitis
Peripheral Nervous System
Progressive polyradiculopathy
Mononeuritis multiplex
Cytomegalovirus

HIV-infected adults are more susceptible to opportunistic infection, whereas children are more likely to manifest direct HIV infection of the brain (37). Other indirect consequences of HIV infection include primary and metastatic neoplasms, metabolic and nutritional abnormalities, drug toxicities, and cerebrovascular complications (38). The following descriptions are limited to direct HIV-related disorders. Brain biopsy is not generally indicated for diagnosis, but biopsy material may be obtained for other reasons and can confirm the diagnosis.

Clinical Features. In the initial phase of the illness, shortly after seroconversion, a minority of infected individuals develops self-limited aseptic meningitis. Many patients develop a progressive, devastating neurologic disease designated as *HIV-1 encephalitis* or *AIDS-dementia complex,* now the most common cause of dementia in young adults (39).

Radiologic Findings. Imaging studies support the diagnosis and rule out other opportunistic infections or neoplasms. CT or MRI may reveal cortical and subcortical atrophy. Although nonspecific, hyperintense lesions are noted in the periventricular white matter and centrum semiovale on T2-weighted images.

Laboratory Findings. CSF examination typically reveals nonspecific alterations consisting of elevated protein and immunoglobulin (Ig) G levels. The CSF is usually acellular, but mild pleocytosis may be present. HIV antibodies are present and the virus may be cultured from CSF or detected by PCR.

Gross Findings. Surgical specimens from HIV-infected brain may appear normal or show atrophy, especially in the frontotemporal regions. Sections from the basal ganglia and white matter may be discolored.

Microscopic Findings. Microscopic examination shows variable degrees of cortical and subcortical neuronal loss, myelin pallor, and gliosis associated with the presence of macrophages, scanty perivascular mononuclear inflammation, and microglial nodules (fig. 7-6, left). In some cases, the white matter is spared and there are loose aggregates of microglial cells or more diffuse patterns of microgliosis. Multinucleate giant cells (containing HIV-specific nucleic acid sequences, virus core protein, and glycoprotein [gp]-41), characterized by dark, angular nuclei, are derived from the fusion of HIV-infected macrophages clustering around blood vessels and are considered convincing evidence of direct HIV infection (fig. 7-6, right). Patchy myelin pallor (*HIV leukoencephalopathy*) or *microglial nodule encephalitis* (MGNE), composed of activated microglial lymphocytes and reactive astrocytes, may present as the dominant pattern of involvement. Immunohistochemical confirmation is possible with antibodies to gp41 or p24 (2).

Although typically not a source of biopsy material, vacuolar myelopathy frequently accompanies HIV-1 encephalopathy. Myelin pallor in the distribution of the dorsal and lateral columns of the thoracic spinal cord characterizes this condition, which closely resembles subacute combined degeneration associated with vitamin B12 deficiency (2).

Cytomegalovirus

General Comments. *Cytomegalovirus* (CMV) infection reaches the brain through viremic spread and causes different patterns of disease in infants and adults. *CMV encephalitis* is rare in normal adults but is common among neonates. Congenital CMV results from transplacental spread during maternal viremia, with most cases arising during primary maternal infection. The frequency of CMV encephalitis has increased in recent years in immunosuppressed adults, especially in HIV-infected individuals with advanced AIDS and recipients of allogenic organ transplants. The viral pathogen probably establishes a latent infection in peripheral blood mononuclear cells. Active CNS infection in adults may affect the brain (encephalitis, ventriculoencephalitis, cerebral mass lesions) or the spinal cord (transverse myelitis, myeloradiculitis) (20).

Clinical Features. Patients with CMV encephalitis typically have a chronic course of cortical dysfunction leading to confusion, disorientation, altered mental status, and occasionally, seizures. Brain stem lesions may result in focal deficits. In patients with AIDS, CMV encephalitis may be clinically indistinguishable from HIV encephalitis and is often not diagnosed until autopsy. The clinical features of neonatal CMV infection consist of hemolytic anemia, hyperbilirubinemia, hepatosplenomegaly with jaundice, and thrombocytopenia with petechiae or purpura. Various neurologic deficits, sensorineural hearing loss, chorioretinitis, and subsequent mental retardation complete the syndrome.

Radiologic Findings. The presence of bilateral periventricular calcifications is strongly suggestive of neonatal CMV infection. Neuroimaging may also demonstrate dilated lateral ventricles, enlarged subarachnoid space, oligogyria/pachygyria/polymicrogyria, abnormal myelination, and periventricular cysts. The differential diagnosis includes other infectious and noninfectious causes of encephalitis. The calcifications in neonatal toxoplasmosis are typically more widely distributed. The subependymal calcifications of tuberous sclerosis are not usually seen until childhood (20).

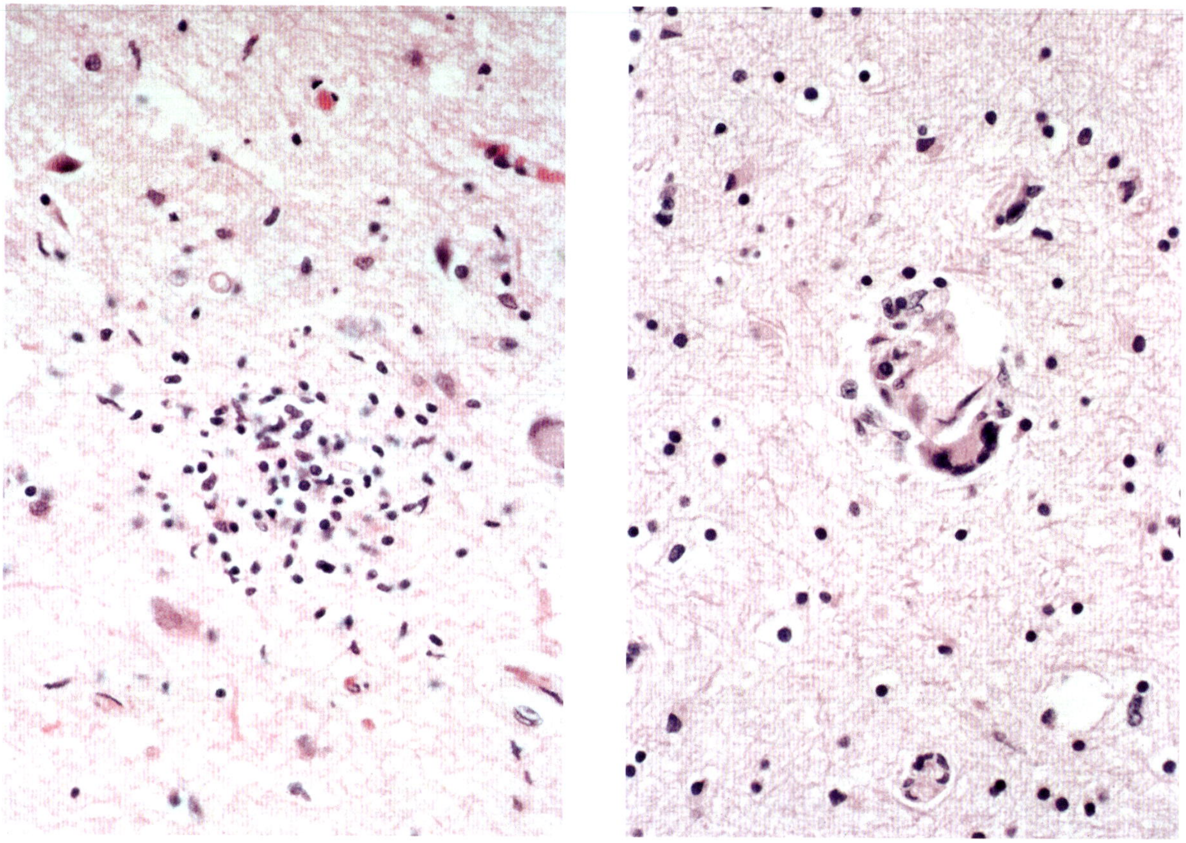

Figure 7-6

MICROGLIAL NODULE ENCEPHALITIS

Left: The microglial nodule is composed of activated microglia, lymphocytes, and reactive astrocytes in a patient with human immunodeficiency virus (HIV) infection of the brain.

Right: Multinucleated giant cells, considered evidence of direct HIV infection, typically cluster around blood vessels.

Laboratory Findings. PCR is the most sensitive diagnostic method of identifying the organism and can be used in conjunction with virus culture to determine suspected cases of CMV myelitis. CSF analysis typically reveals elevated protein and polymorphonuclear leukocytosis.

Gross Findings. CMV may infect any portion of the brain or spinal cord, including spinal nerve roots and cranial nerves. In a significant number of cases, it also causes ependymitis. In neonates, gross examination may reveal periventricular calcifications, microcephaly, scattered areas of focal softening, and hemorrhages.

Microscopic Findings. Microscopically, several distinct parenchymal patterns are documented in adults: 1) necrotizing encephalitis, 2) smoldering encephalitis with microglial nodules and CMV inclusions, with a predilection for the brain stem, 3) ventriculitis with sloughing of affected ependyma, and 4) lumbosacral myeloradiculitis. The virus typically evokes chronic perivascular and microglial nodule inflammation accompanied by enlarged cells bearing well-defined intranuclear and occasional smaller cytoplasmic inclusions. Affected cells of all types (ependymal, astrocytic, neuronal, and vascular) contain eye-catching, basophilic intranuclear inclusions that span half the nuclear diameter and are set off by a clear halo, imparting the classic "owl's eye" appearance (fig. 7-7). Immunohistochemical methods are available to highlight infected cells. PCR can detect genomic material in the absence of inclusions and inflammation (20).

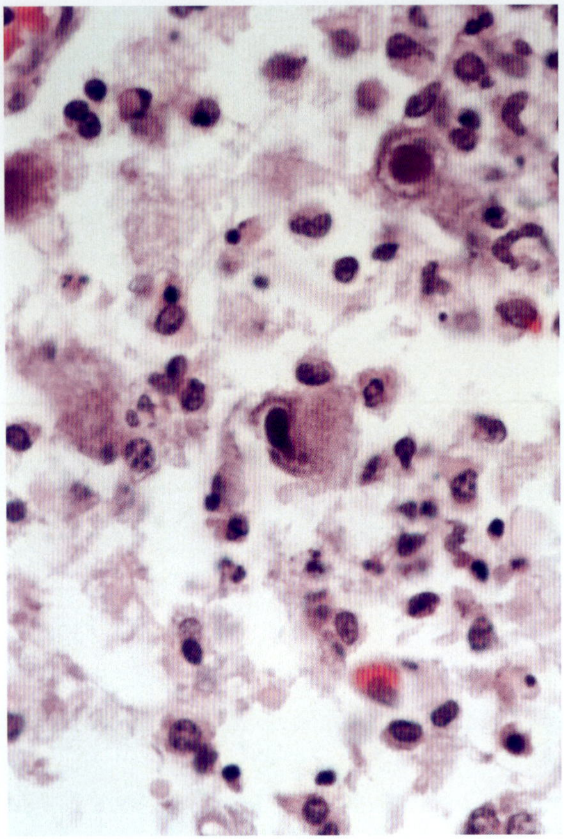

Figure 7-7

CYTOMEGALOVIRUS INFECTION

Classic "owl's eye" cytomegalovirus (CMV) inclusions in a patient with acquired immunodeficiency syndrome (AIDS) necrotizing encephalitis.

West Nile Virus

General Comments. *West Nile virus* (WNV) is an arbovirus that causes encephalitis in humans. The recent surge in cases of WNV in the United States reaffirms that typical geographic boundaries for the arboviruses and other pathogens are often breached in the era of frequent international travel. The infectious agent is transmitted from viremic birds, the natural host, to humans by *Culex* mosquitoes. WNV is also transmitted by blood transfusion, by organ transplantation, by breast feeding, placental transmission, or exposure of laboratory workers to infected sera or animals (40).

Clinical Features. After inoculation, the viral incubation period is 2 to 15 days. Most patients have asymptomatic infection, but a significant percentage develop fever, headache, backache, myalgia, and anorexia, lasting 3 to 6 days. About 1 in 150 infections results in a severe illness with meningoencephalitis. Age appears to be a strong predictor, with the greatest risk among the elderly. The range of reported symptoms includes flaccid weakness from involvement of anterior horn cells, to less commonly, parkinsonism, ataxia, polyradiculopathy, seizures, and cranial neuropathy. Mortality from the neurologic illness is about 10 percent, and recovery can be limited in nonfatal cases (39–41).

Gross Findings. Although biopsy specimens are unlikely, gross sections of the brain are unremarkable or may show mild, patchy leptomeningeal opacification.

Microscopic Findings. Microscopic examination demonstrates a non-necrotizing, subacute myelomeningoencephalitis. While both gray and white matter show mononuclear inflammation, gray matter is more severely involved. The deep gray matter nuclei are reported to show severe neuronal loss, with residual dying neurons surrounded by activated microglia (41). In some cases, there are perivascular lymphocytic infiltrates, microglial nodules, and loss of neurons in the brain stem and anterior horns of the spinal cord (fig. 7-8). Spinal nerve roots show patchy mononuclear infiltrates (42).

Other Arbovirides

General Comments. After WNV, the most common arboviruses causing encephalitic diseases in the United States are LaCrosse virus and St. Louis encephalitis (SLE) virus. Mosquitoes transmit the pathogens and infections flare up during late summer and early fall. No satisfactory treatment exists for arbovirus encephalitis. The deadliest and least common agent is the eastern equine encephalitis (EEE) virus, encountered in New England and surrounding states. The milder western equine encephalitis (WEE) virus is more common in rural communities west of the Mississippi (20). In Asia, the leading cause of viral encephalitis is the mosquito-borne Japanese encephalitis virus (Japanese B). This viral agent is closely related to WNV and SLE (21).

Clinical and Radiologic Findings. Symptoms are those of a flu-like illness, with variable evidence of brain involvement indicated

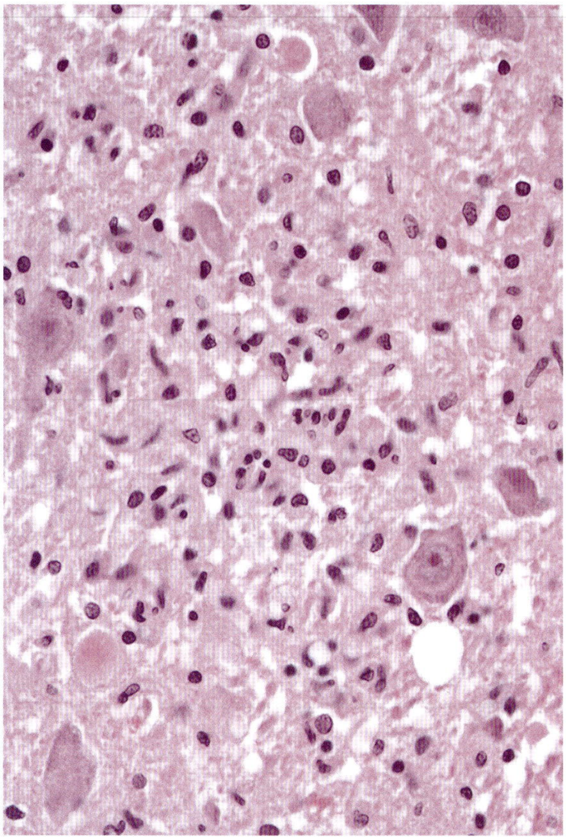

Figure 7-8

WEST NILE VIRUS MENINGOENCEPHALITIS

Perivascular mononuclear infiltrates (not shown) and microglial nodules, often within the deep gray nuclei, are nonspecific but common findings.

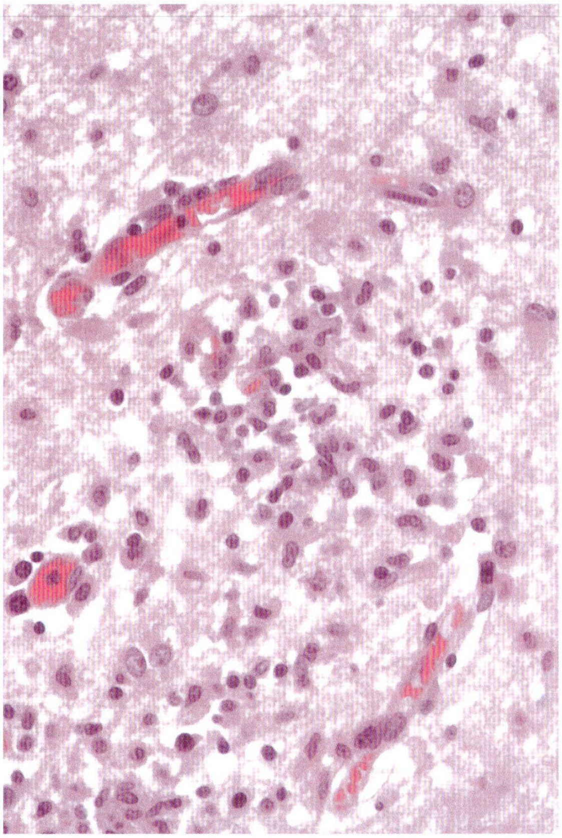

Figure 7-9

ARBOVIRUS ENCEPHALITIS

A microglial nodule surrounds degenerated neuronal cell bodies (neuronophagia) in a patient with eastern equine encephalitis (EEE).

by lethargy, confusion, irritability, tremors, or seizures. LaCrosse virus may produce focal neurologic signs, whereas SLE virus is associated with syndrome of inappropriate secretion of antidiuretic hormone (SIADH)-induced hyponatremia. Movement disorders have been described in SLE, EEE, and WEE. In general, neuroimaging is either normal or nonspecific in arboviral encephalitis. Focal lesions in the basal ganglia and thalamus are present on CT scan and MRI in EEE (43,44).

Laboratory Findings. CSF examination shows a lymphocytic pleocytosis. The diagnosis can be confirmed by several less invasive methods, including a four-fold rise in CSF antibody titer between acute and convalescent sera, viral isolation from CSF, or demonstration of IgM antibody in CSF (44).

Microscopic Findings. In rare cases in which the pathologist is called upon to consider the diagnosis, the lesions of arbovirus infection exhibit all the features expected in viral encephalitis, with minor differences according to the etiologic agent. The gross appearance is usually not helpful. Histologically, the essential features consist of variable numbers of microglial nodules and perivascular chronic inflammation (fig. 7-9). Inclusion bodies are not a feature of arbovirus infection. WEE and EEE are characterized by early involvement of the basal ganglia, brain stem, and thalami (28,44). In an autopsied case of SLE, lesions were found in the substantia nigra and thalamus. In cases of Japanese encephalitis, the lesions favor the thalamus, substantia nigra, Ammon horn, brain stem, and spinal cord (20).

BACTERIAL INFECTIONS

Acute Meningoencephalitis

The majority of pathogens already mentioned in the section on acute bacterial meningitis have the potential to invade the brain parenchyma. Other pathogens not alluded to can occasionally cause bacterial meningitis. The major neurologic symptom complex of infection caused by *Bacillus anthracis* results in fulminant and rapidly fatal hemorrhagic meningoencephalitis (16).

Brain Abscess

General Comments. *Intracerebral abscess* continues to be associated with high rates of neurologic impairment and death. Patients with this localized collection of purulent material often present with focal neurologic deficits or seizures. The most common sources of brain abscess are direct or indirect cranial infection arising from the paranasal sinuses, middle ear (otitis and mastoiditis), and teeth. Other routes for the infecting organisms include hematogenous seeding from distant sites of infection in the body (endocarditis or bronchiectasis) and penetrating head trauma. No age group is spared; however, risk factors tend to vary according to age. Specific risk factors include congenital heart disease with right to left shunt, bacterial endocarditis, lung abscess or bronchiectasis, and paranasal sinusitis (14,45).

The leading etiologic agents are various streptococcal strains and *Staphylococcus aureus*, although many other organisms have been reported. In some series, *Streptococcus viridans* is considered the most commonly isolated organism, but many abscesses are polymicrobial, and *S. aureus*, hemolytic *Streptococcus*, Enterobacteriaceae, *Bacteroides*, and other gram-negative anaerobes are also common. Immunosuppression and the emergence of multidrug-resistant strains of bacteria have contributed to the resurgence of intracerebral abscesses. Fungal or *Toxoplasma gondii* abscesses are diagnosed with greater frequency in immunocompromised patients. In the nursery, *Citrobacter* meningitis is a known antecedent infection. Low birth weight infants are particularly susceptible to certain fungi, especially *Candida,* which has been implicated as a cause of multiple abscesses (45).

Subdural empyema refers to another localized collection of pus that is found within the subdural space, usually arising through direct spread from a contiguous intracranial infection such as sinusitis. In the pediatric population, subdural empyema may complicate meningitis, especially when caused by either *Haemophilus influenza* or *Streptococcus pneumoniae*. For the most part, the range of responsible microorganisms parallels that of cerebral abscesses. In adults, especially immunocompromised individuals, *S. milleri* is a frequently isolated pathogen. Clinical signs and symptoms are like those of brain abscess, but seizures are especially common; treatment essentially always requires surgical drainage. Spinal epidural abscess typically produces a rapid-onset spinal cord syndrome. The most common cause is hematogenous spread of *S. aureus* infection.

Clinical Features. Patients present with signs and symptoms of increased intracranial pressure, such as headache, low-grade fever, focal neurologic deficits, and seizures. Mental status alterations may also be encountered. Symptoms vary depending on the size and location of the abscess, immune status of the host, and organism(s) involved.

Radiologic Findings. Imaging studies are extremely useful for evaluating the possibility of brain abscess. Early in the course, abscesses appear as irregular zones of hypodensity that do not show contrast enhancement. As the disease progresses, the distinctive ring enhancement becomes evident as the abscess wall thickens (fig. 7-10A). In contrast to neoplastic ring enhancement, the rim or capsule is thinner and more uniform than the irregular, shaggy ring of enhancement seen in glioblastoma; the rim may be thinner on its internal side, with occasional "daughter" abscesses forming toward the ventricle. MRI has the advantage over CT for evaluating the brain stem and the early cerebritis stage of brain abscesses. Since imaging studies still lack the specificity for definitive diagnosis and determination of causative organisms, stereotactic biopsy is usually performed to obtain diagnostic material and drain abscess contents.

Laboratory Findings. Lumbar puncture is rarely warranted and is contraindicated if increased intracranial pressure is present.

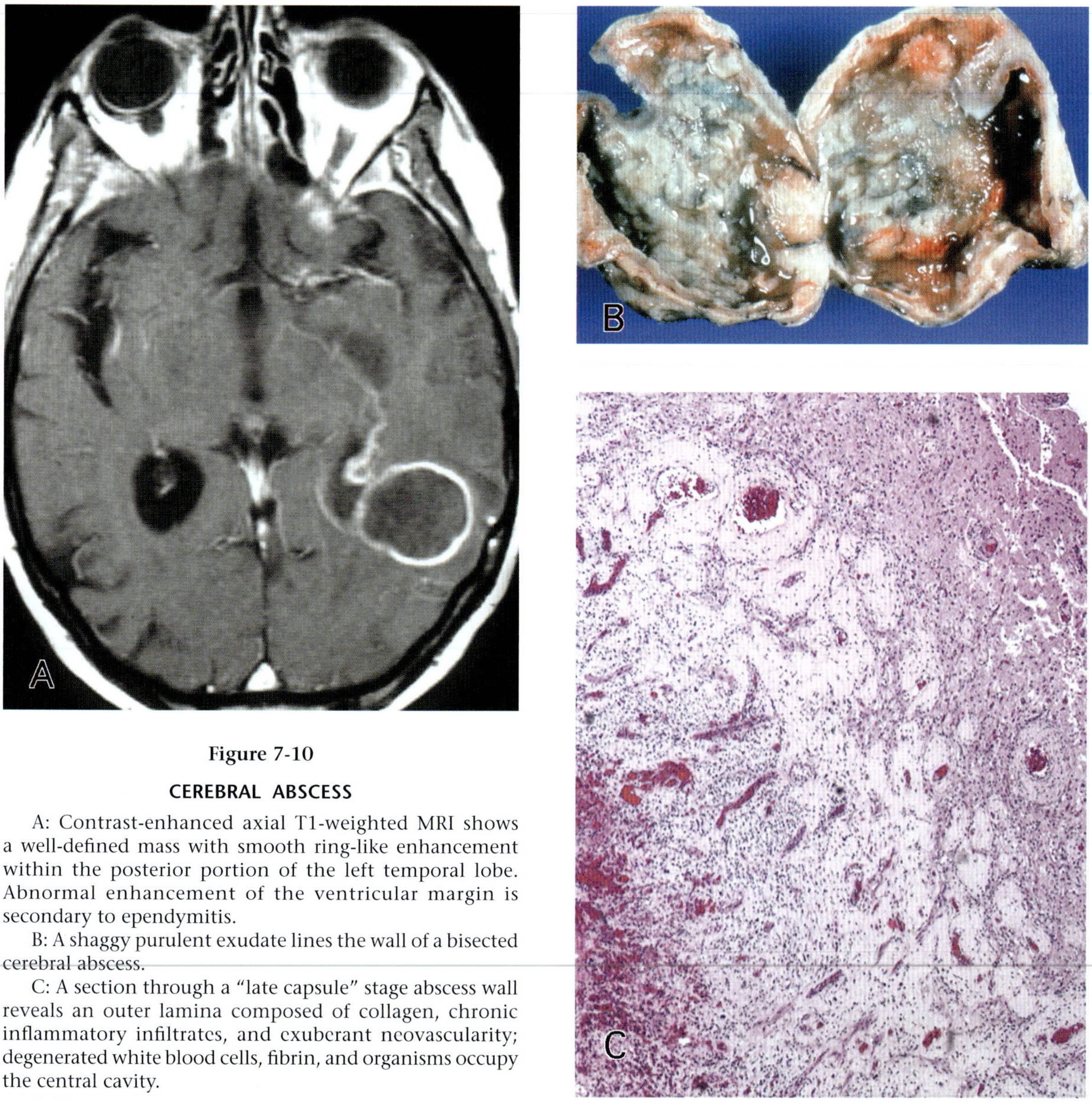

Figure 7-10

CEREBRAL ABSCESS

A: Contrast-enhanced axial T1-weighted MRI shows a well-defined mass with smooth ring-like enhancement within the posterior portion of the left temporal lobe. Abnormal enhancement of the ventricular margin is secondary to ependymitis.

B: A shaggy purulent exudate lines the wall of a bisected cerebral abscess.

C: A section through a "late capsule" stage abscess wall reveals an outer lamina composed of collagen, chronic inflammatory infiltrates, and exuberant neovascularity; degenerated white blood cells, fibrin, and organisms occupy the central cavity.

Gross Findings. Abscesses can be found anywhere but are more common in the cerebral hemispheres. They are usually solitary but may be multiple, particularly when the organism arrives by the hematogenous route. When abscesses arise as a complication of infections of the middle ear or paranasal sinuses, the temporal and frontal lobes, respectively, are common sites of involvement. Septic emboli that arise from hematogenous spread tend to localize in the perfusion territory of the middle cerebral artery, at the interface of the gray and white matter, and are often multiple. The lesion first appears as an irregular area of softening or hyperemia corresponding to the stage of early cerebritis, which gradually liquefies. The resultant cavitary lesion is discernable at 1 to 3 weeks and usually contains yellow-green pus surrounded by a capsule that gradually thickens (fig. 7-10B). The capsule tends to be thicker in superficial abscesses, especially the margin adjacent to the subcortical region. The surrounding brain parenchyma is edematous and congested. Complications include herniation and rupture of the abscess contents into the ventricular or subarachnoid spaces.

Microscopic Findings. Brain abscesses are typified by a sequence of histopathologic changes that vary over time. Four classic stages are recognized: 1) early cerebritis, 2) late cerebritis, 3) early capsule formation, and 4) late capsule formation. The initial stage of early cerebritis occurs from days 1 to 3 and is characterized by neutrophil accumulation, small foci of tissue necrosis, swelling of endothelial cells, and edema. Microthrombi, vascular congestion, and petechial hemorrhages may be identified within the involved area. A zone of microglial activation and astrogliosis around the inflammatory core is evident at this stage and generally persists throughout the maturation of the abscess.

The intermediate, or late cerebritis, stage occurs from days 4 to 7 and is associated with the arrival of abundant foamy macrophages and variable lymphoplasmacytic infiltrates. Pus is found inside a narrow rind of granulation tissue and is accompanied by variable numbers of neutrophils, lymphocytes, and macrophages.

The early capsule stage, recognized between days 10 and 13, consists of granulation tissue with lymphocytes, plasma cells, and macrophages. The portion of the abscess wall abutting deep white matter is less well organized and thinner than the subcortical wall. Circumferentially oriented reticulin deposition is evident as the wall of the abscess thickens.

The final, or late capsule, stage occurs from day 14 onward and is associated with the formation of a well-vascularized abscess wall with the proliferation of fibroblasts and collagen, in effect sequestering the lesion and protecting the surrounding normal brain parenchyma from additional damage (fig. 7-10C). The now firm capsule can be stripped from the surrounding edematous white matter. Microorganisms may be sparse and require special stains (e.g., Brown-Brenn, Brown-Hopps) for optimal visualization. Reactive astrocytes, neovascularization with plump endothelial cells, and variable numbers of perivascular inflammatory cells populate the surrounding brain tissue.

Although less contained, the morphologic features of subdural empyema are similar to those of parenchymal abscesses and consist of purulent material incompletely walled off by granulation tissue and a mixed inflammatory infiltrate. In some cases, there may be dystrophic calcification or even ossification. Most cases are supratentorial, although posterior fossa examples have been reported (16,45).

Actinomycosis

General Comments. Actinomycetes are bacteria that resemble fungi because of their filamentous, branching, hyphae-like appearance. *Actinomyces israelii* and *bovis* are the most common species that cause human disease.

Actinomycosis is a subacute or chronic bacterial infection that can affect immunocompetent or immunodeficient persons. Like other anaerobic infections, the organism thrives in the presence of necrosis or foreign bodies and is often involved in polymicrobial infections. Many diverse clinical forms have been recognized, but the majority are classified as cervicofacial. The mandible is most common site involved; other common sites are pulmonary and gastrointestinal. Specific risk factors include dental pathology, alcohol abuse, and Osler-Weber-Rendu disease. Involvement of the CNS is rare and the accompanying inflammatory response is often chronic, suppurative, or less commonly, granulomatous; abscesses tend to form (16,46).

Clinical Features. Patients present with mass lesions and neurologic findings. With prompt and vigorous antibiotic therapy the prognosis for patients with actinomycosis is good.

Microscopic Findings. Lesions consist of multilocular abscesses that show central necrosis and abundant neutrophils. The identification of sulfur granules distinguishes actinomycosis from nocardial infections. Sulfur granules can be identified grossly as small white to yellow particles and microscopically as masses of bacterial filaments arranged in ray-like projections within purulent material and surrounding granulation tissue (fig. 7-11). The organisms are Gram and Gomori methenamine silver (GMS) positive and acid-fast negative.

Nocardia

General Comments. *Nocardia* is a group of thin, gram-positive, variably acid-fast aerobic bacteria commonly found in the soil that form branching filaments that tend to fragment into coccobacilli. Cerebral *Nocardia abscesses*

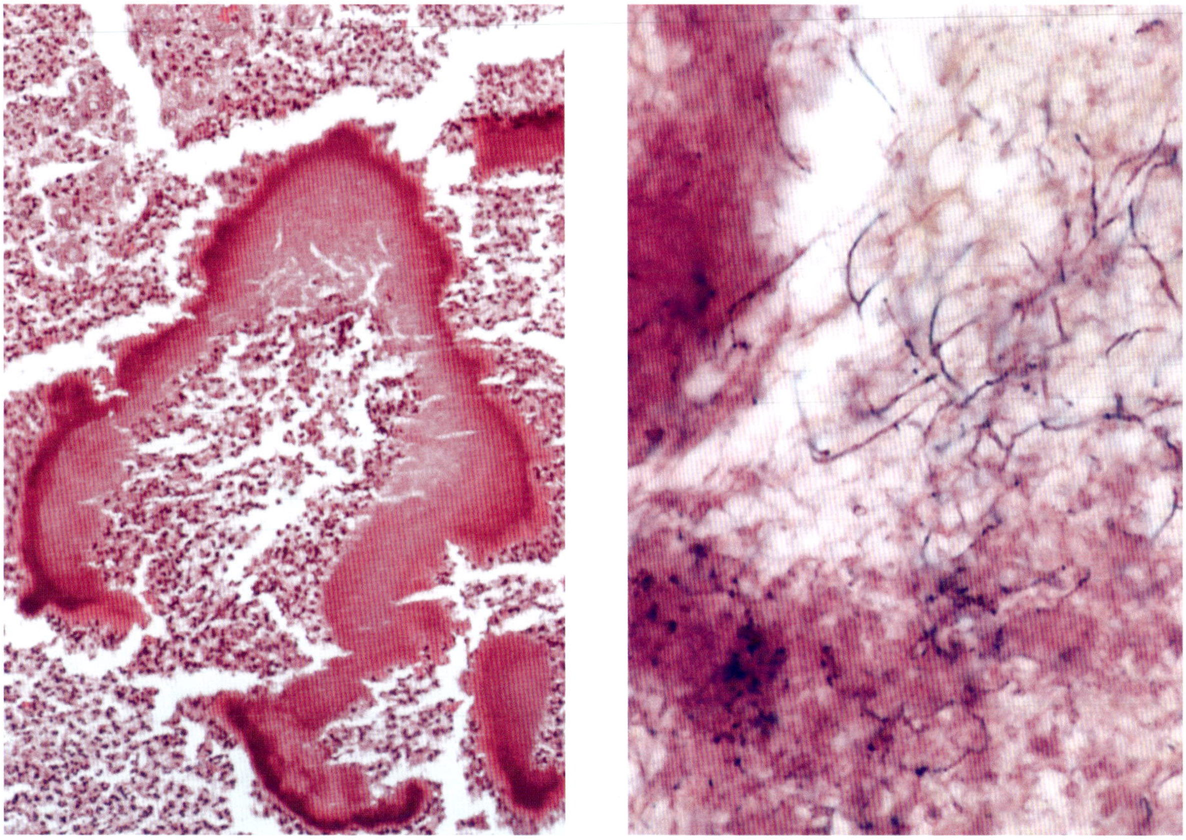

Figure 7-11

ACTINOMYCES ISRAELII INFECTION

The characteristic sulfur granule is a tangle of filamentous bacteria.

are secondary to hematogenous spread of systemic disease and are rare. The majority of CNS infections are due to *N. asteroids* complex. *N. brasiliensis* typically causes cutaneous and lymphocutaneous disease, but it may also cause systemic and, occasionally, CNS infection. HIV and organ transplantation are common predisposing conditions. *Nocardial meningitis* is a less common CNS manifestation and is often associated with brain abscess (16).

Clinical Features. Nocardial abscesses cause signs and symptoms of a typical mass lesion. Patients with meningeal involvement typically complain of stiff neck and headache. Appropriate treatment is often delayed, and mortality is high. Otherwise healthy persons who receive prompt antimicrobial therapy have a better prognosis.

Radiologic Findings. CT or MRI with contrast demonstrates ring-enhancing lesions, as observed with other causes of pyogenic brain abscess. In AIDS patients, brain abscess is often accompanied by an abnormal chest X ray, which suggests the diagnosis. With other patients, chest X-ray abnormalities are not always present. When detected, however, these combined findings are often mistaken for carcinoma with brain metastasis.

Microscopic Findings. Invasive procedures are generally required for diagnostic confirmation. As noted, CNS infection can cause either meningitis or abscesses. Histopathologic examination reveals acute inflammatory infiltrates with a predominance of neutrophils. Necrosis with minimal fibrosis results in the formation of multilocular abscesses with feeble attempts at capsule formation. In Gram- or Brown-Brenn–stained tissue sections, *Nocardia* organisms appear as beaded branching forms. GMS (fig. 7-12), modified Fite, and modified Gram demonstrate organisms well; culture is required for a definitive diagnosis.

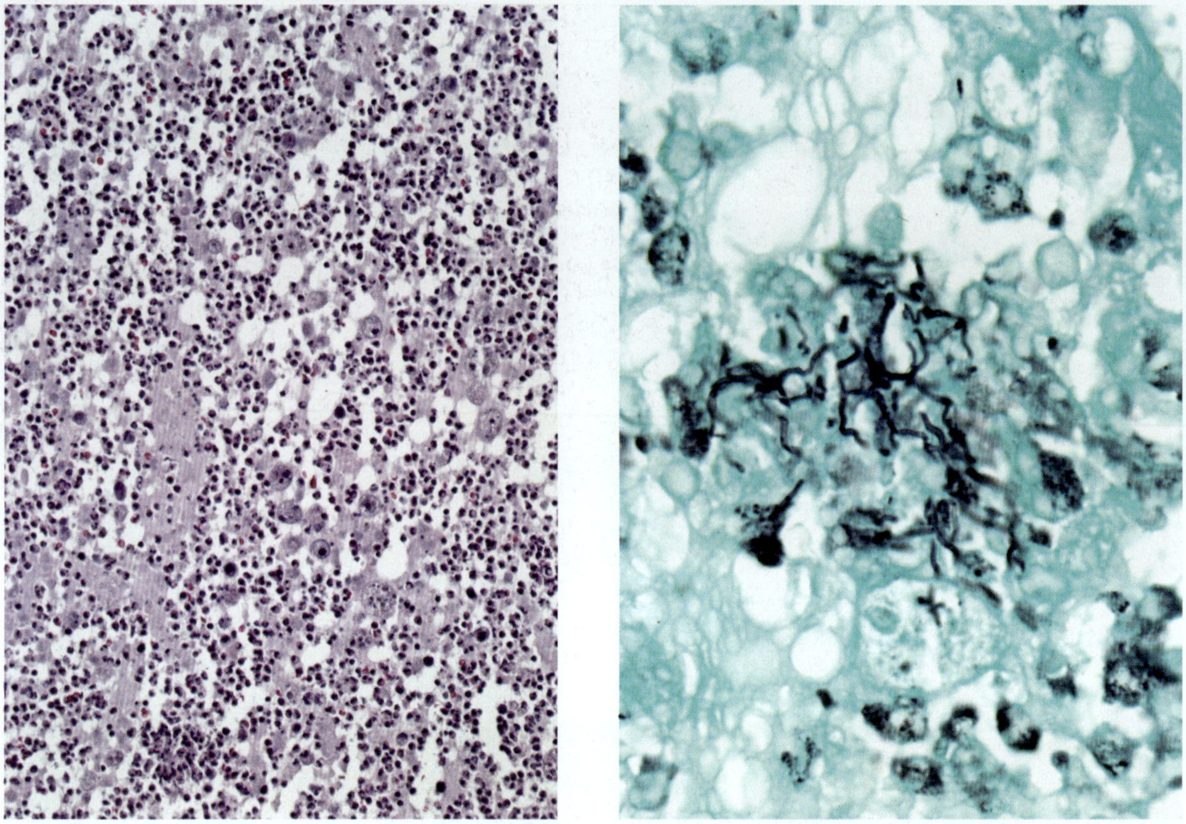

Figure 7-12

NOCARDIA INFECTION

Left: Microorganisms are inconspicuous within the abscess exudate from a renal transplant patient.
Right: Beaded filamentous bacteria are readily identified with methenamine silver impregnation.

Neurosyphilis

General Comments. Three genera of spirochetes cause CNS infections in humans: *Treponema*, which causes syphilis; *Borrelia*, which causes Lyme disease; and *Leptospira*, which causes leptospirosis. *Syphilis* is caused by the spirochete *Treponema pallidum*, a thin helical microorganism approximately 0.15 x 6 to 50 μm. Infection is usually acquired by sexual contact. Other modes of transmission include direct contact with an active lesion, passage through the placenta, and rarely, blood transfusion.

Clinical Features. The incidence and clinical spectrum of neurosyphilis have changed over time. Compared to the preantibiotic era, a lower frequency of late neurosyphilis has been observed. The most frequent clinical patterns are meningovascular (30.2 percent), meningeal (25.6 percent), and general paresis (25.6 percent).

The evolution of syphilitic infection proceeds in three stages. Primary syphilis presents as a painless ulcer (chancre) at the site of inoculation, which appears after about 3 weeks. Secondary syphilis occurs 3 to 6 weeks to 6 months after the resolution of primary syphilis and usually manifests as a diffuse maculopapular rash that affects the palms and soles. At this highly contagious stage, patients may also have syphilitic meningitis, optic neuritis, iritis, and uveitis. If left untreated, 10 percent of individuals get tertiary syphilis. Although symptomatic involvement of the nervous system is not restricted to any particular stage, it is more commonly encountered during the tertiary phase. Tertiary disease occurs 5 to 25 years after the initial infection and may manifest as parenchymatous neurosyphilis, meningovascular syphilis, and gummatous syphilis. Congenital neurosyphilis is acquired transplacentally, during the second and third trimesters, or through contact with an infectious lesion during delivery (47).

Classically, there are five recognized types of CNS disease: *acute syphilitic meningitis* and *meningovascular, parenchymatous, tabes dorsalis,* and *gummatous neurosyphilis*, which may occur alone or in combination with other variants. Most cases of syphilitic meningitis, noted in the primary and secondary stages, are associated with mild or no symptoms. Occasionally, patients develop symptoms of acute meningeal irritation, hydrocephalus, or cranial nerve palsies. Chronic meningovascular syphilis develops on average 7 years after the primary infection and may enter a phase of remission within weeks, even without treatment. Tabes dorsalis is the progressive degeneration of the dorsal roots and posterior columns of the spinal cord (myeloneuropathy). Affected individuals have disturbances of proprioception and periodic shooting or lancinating pain and/or paresthesias in the distribution of the involved nerve roots. Gummas are mass lesions that manifest as a hypersensitivity reaction to the presence of only scant treponemes (48,49).

Radiologic Findings. The neuroimaging features are nonspecific and depend largely on the clinical presentation. A wide range of imaging findings may be seen in neurosyphilis. Many cases of clinical neurosyphilis show no imaging abnormalities (49,50).

Meningovascular Neurosyphilis. The most common presentation of meningovascular neurosyphilis is a stroke syndrome in a relatively young adult, involving the middle cerebral artery or the branches of the basilar artery. Meningovascular syphilis refers to the combination of chronic meningitis and multifocal arteritis (Heubner endarteritis obliterans), which is prone to produce parenchymal infarctions (26,50).

Macroscopically, the leptomeninges are fibrotic and thickened, and sometimes accompanied by gummas. Accompanying brain fragments may be softened, suggesting possible infarcts.

The histologic response to the spirochete (*T. pallidum*) in this form of the disease is characterized by dense aggregates of lymphocytes and plasma cells rather than by histiocytes and epithelioid cells, which predominate in granulomatous reactions. The leptomeningeal fibrosis seen grossly may be evident. Arteries of different sizes may show marked concentric endothelial thickening (Heubner endarteritis obliterans) as well as thickening of the media and adventitia to the point of occlusion, with preservation of the elastic lamina (fig. 7-13, left). These vascular changes are responsible for infarcts within the subtended vascular territory. Detection of the organism requires the aid of special stains such as silver impregnation methods (fig. 7-13, right).

Parenchymatous Neurosyphilis. This disorder is more common in males and is characterized by progressive intellectual deterioration, seizures, and eventually death. Paretic dementia (of the insane) refers to the progressive intellectual deterioration. The surgical pathologist may encounter a specimen from a patient undergoing an evaluation for a treatable cause of dementia.

In parenchymatous neurosyphilis, brain fragments are shrunken and firm, and the overlying meninges are thickened and opacified. The atrophy observed grossly is due to the loss of cortical neurons accompanied by diffuse astrocytosis. This imparts "windblown" appearance to the sparsely populated cerebral cortex. In addition, there may be lymphocytic meningeal and perivascular inflammation and small infarcts. While not unique to this form of the disease, microglial proliferation with cytoplasmic iron deposits is characteristic.

Gummatous Neurosyphilis. A gumma is a well-circumscribed mass composed of a core of coagulative necrosis in which ghost-like outlines of the dead cells are still visible and are surrounded by a zone of lymphoplasmacytic inflammation that is encased in granulation tissue. Multinucleated giant cells and epithelioid cells are often identified. Gummas are usually confined to the dura, although the leptomeninges or cortex may be involved secondary to invasion and direct extension (50).

Congenital Neurosyphilis. Congenital syphilis affects the CNS in the majority of cases. The highest rate of transmission occurs during the primary and secondary stages of the disease. Clinical infection of the fetus occurs in months 4 to 7 of pregnancy. In the first 2 years of life, the most common lesion is acute or subacute meningitis, usually presenting at 4 to 5 months of age. The infection results in fetal or perinatal death in 40 percent of those infected. The

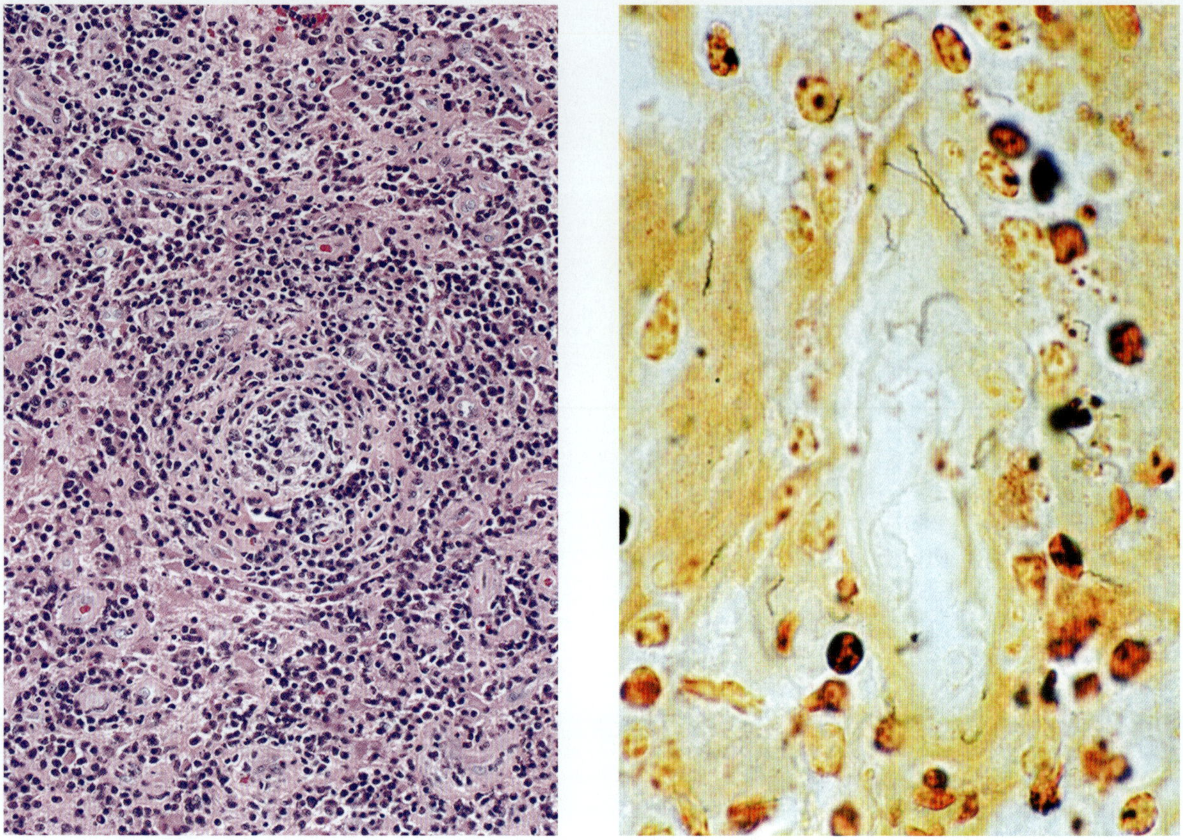

Figure 7-13

NEUROSYPHILIS

Left: The vasculopathy of meningovascular syphilis is marked by intimal thickening accompanied by perivascular and adventitial mononuclear inflammatory infiltrates.

Right: Spirochetes (Warthin-Starry stain).

characteristic features include interstitial keratitis, chorioretinitis, deafness, meningitis, and hydrocephalus (47).

Examination of the leptomeninges reveals mononuclear infiltrates that include lymphocytes, plasma cells, and macrophages. The infiltrates are the thickest at the base of the brain and extend along cranial nerve sheaths and the Virchow-Robin spaces. Parenchymal lesions are uncommon, although inflammatory infiltrates may be encountered in the superficial cortex. Chronic meningovascular syphilis generally develops after 2 years. The consequences are as follows: chronic arachnoiditis results in the development of hydrocephalus; obliterative vasculitis causes cerebral infarct, or rarely, aneurysm formation and cerebral hemorrhage; and the dense basilar infiltrates result in cranial nerve abnormalities, especially cranial nerve VII, but also III, IV, and VI. Late sequelae of congenital neurosyphilis include a form of juvenile "general paresis" and tabes dorsalis (48).

Leptospirosis

Leptospirosis is a zoonosis with a worldwide distribution that is caused by a species of the pathogenic bacteria belonging to the genus *Leptospira*, the family Leptospiraceae, and the order Spirochaetales. It is considered the most common zoonosis in the world. These spirochetes are finely coiled, thin, motile, obligate, slow-growing anaerobes.

Humans are accidental hosts that acquire the disease by direct contact with the body fluid of an acutely infected animal or by exposure to soil or fresh water contaminated with the urine of an animal that is a chronic carrier. During acute infection, bacteria are thought to multiply in the small blood vessel endothelium, resulting in damage and vasculitis. Leptospires also invade skeletal muscle, causing edema, vacuolization of myofibrils, and focal necrosis. The most common CNS manifestation is aseptic meningitis, which usually does not require the expertise of a surgical pathologist or radiologist for diagnosis.

Lyme Disease

General Comments. *Lyme disease* is a systemic infection caused by the tick-borne spirochete, *Borrelia burgdorferi*. The risk for infection is confined to regions that contain the deer (Ixodid) tick vector. This disease is currently the most commonly reported vector-borne illness in the United States. There are three major endemic areas: 1) southern New England, New York, and the middle Atlantic states; 2) Wisconsin, Minnesota, and Michigan; and 3) wooded areas of California and Oregon (51). The protean manifestations of this illness probably account for many unrecognized cases.

The inability to easily culture *B. burgdorferi* and the lack of a reliable assay for active infection have contributed to controversies in diagnosis and management. Because the vast majority of patients are seropositive, however, antibody testing is helpful to support the diagnosis of Lyme disease.

Clinical Features. Clinical disease involves characteristic skin, musculoskeletal, cardiac, ocular, and neurologic disorders that are associated with the local, early dissemination, and late stages of infection. The disease course proceeds through three stages: 1) days to weeks post-tick bite there is an evanescent skin lesion known as erythema migrans; 2) cardiac and neurologic effects present weeks to months post-tick bite; and 3) late manifestations occur months to years post-tick bite in the form of arthritis and CNS involvement.

The wide range of neurologic syndromes varies from mild to debilitating and can involve both the central and peripheral nervous systems. Meningitis and cranial and peripheral neuropathies are probably the most common syndromes ascribed to Lyme neuroborreliosis. Unilateral or bilateral facial palsy occurs in up to half of the patients. Peripheral neuritis has been reported, most frequently a motor or sensory radiculoneuritis that targets the extremities or trunk. Encephalitis may occur and present as emotional lability, depression, memory and concentration deficits, chorea in children, and cerebellar ataxia. Cerebral vasculitis and chronic encephalitis have also been attributed to Lyme disease. In Europe, lymphocytic meningoradiculitis (Bannwarth syndrome) is the most common manifestation.

Radiologic Findings. Although frequently abnormal, imaging features are nonspecific and rarely indicated in the workup of Lyme disease. MRI scans may demonstrate punctate white matter lesions on T2-weighted images, similar to those seen in demyelinating diseases or a variety of inflammatory disorders (51).

Laboratory Findings. Examination of the CSF shows lymphocytic pleocytosis with normal glucose and protein levels. *B. burgdorferi* DNA can be detected with PCR early in the infectious process (16,51).

Gross Findings. Grossly, specimens are remarkable for the dearth of morphologic changes.

Microscopic Findings. Lymphocytic infiltrates, microglial diffuse and nodular activation, spongiform changes, diffuse demyelination of the cerebral and cerebellar white matter, and diffuse astrocytosis are the characteristic microscopic features. Chronic inflammatory changes in the nuclei and roots of cranial nerves may also be present.

Whipple Disease

General Comments. *Whipple disease* is a rare multisystem disorder caused by infection with the gram-positive rod-shaped bacterium, *Tropheryma whippelii*. The disease is most frequently diagnosed in middle-aged to elderly men (52,53). Recent epidemiologic studies, including several familial cases, point to a genetic susceptibility related to certain human leukocyte antigen (HLA) loci. This finding suggests that host factors, such as defective T-helper cells, play a role in pathogenic events.

Clinical Features. The classic clinical presentation is dominated by profound weight loss, diarrhea, and low-grade fever. Transient episodes of arthralgias or nondeforming arthritis, uveitis, cutaneous hyperpigmentation, and lymphadenopathy are other clues to the diagnosis. Nervous system disease is a feature in 20 to 40 percent of patients. CNS manifestations are protean and usually develop in later stages of the illness, often with cranial nerve and cognitive manifestations, including dementia, supranuclear gaze palsy, movement disorders, hypothalamic dysfunction, and myorhythmia (53). On rare occasion, CNS Whipple disease presents as a mass lesion and thus mimics the presentation of a neoplasm (53,54).

Radiologic Findings. Cerebral Whipple disease has no characteristic imaging findings. The disease has a predilection for the temporal lobes. CT scans are frequently normal or show focal low-density areas that may enhance. MRI studies show various nonspecific lesions (53).

Laboratory Findings. The causative organism has been identified by RNA sequence analysis and can be cultured as a gram-positive actinomycete. The CNS infection is diagnosed by PCR of the CSF of 16S ribosomal RNA of *T. whippelii* (54).

Gross Findings. The diagnosis of Whipple disease can be made from a brain biopsy. Lesions have been reported in the basal ganglia, hypothalamus, periaqueductal gray matter, brain stem, dentate nucleus, and subpial regions. The gross features include cerebral atrophy and scattered small chalky nodules in the cortical and subependymal gray matter.

Microscopic Findings. At the histologic level, these nodules represent granulomas that contain PAS-positive foamy macrophages with coarsely granular cytoplasm; they harbor sickle-shaped PAS-positive diastase-resistant rods and reactive astrocytes (fig. 7-14A,B). Patchy perivascular inflammation and variable microglial proliferations are consistent features. Extensive areas of demyelination (resembling multiple sclerosis) and microinfarcts are sometimes identified in tissue specimens. A sensitive and specific immunohistochemical method for the diagnosis of Whipple disease in paraffin-embedded tissue has been recently described (55). Electron microscopic examination demonstrates the presence of rod-shaped structures (or bacilliform bodies), 0.3 x 1.5 to 2.5 μm, within the macrophages (fig. 7-14C).

FUNGAL INFECTIONS

Fungi are chlorophyll-deficient plants that occur in the soil worldwide and are responsible for a variety of diseases of the nervous system in both healthy and immunocompromised individuals. In simple terms, fungi are classified into yeasts and molds. The former are small, round or oval organisms and divide by budding, while the latter form tubular or filamentous structures called hyphae that grow by branching and longitudinal extension. There is some degree of overlap in the definition because certain fungi (e.g., *Histoplasma capsulatum, Coccidioides immitis, Blastomyces dermatitidis*) are dimorphic (i.e., grow as yeasts in tissues, but grow as molds under in vitro conditions).

Most fungi pathogenetic for humans cause infection when airborne spores are inhaled or when hyphae or spores are accidentally inoculated. Following the primary infection, most fungi spread to the CNS via the bloodstream. In immunocompetent hosts, CNS mycotic infections are most commonly caused by *Cryptococcus neoformans, Coccidioides immitis, Histoplasma capsulatum*, and *Blastomycetes dermatitidis*. The clinical presentation is usually as subacute or chronic basal meningitis, but intraparenchymal mycotic abscesses also occur and cause focal neurologic signs. Opportunistic fungal infections flourish in patients with AIDS (*Cryptococcus*), neutropenia, organ transplantation or diabetes (*Aspergillus*), or indwelling intravascular catheters (*Candida*) (55–57). The likelihood of CNS disease is also increased in the presence of systemic disease of kidney, lung, or skin.

To some extent, the type of CNS infection is related to the size of the organism. Because yeasts are smaller, they do not obstruct capillaries and more commonly cause leptomeningitis. Hyphal forms invade and obstruct medium-sized and large blood vessels, resulting in infarcts that develop into abscesses in the zone subtended by the affected blood vessel. CNS *Aspergillus* infections manifest either as mass lesions (e.g., brain abscess) or as cerebral infarcts, but rarely as meningitis (58).

The organisms may be elusive in H&E-stained specimens. Methods available for tissue identification of the organism include PAS and GMS stains as well as immunofluorescence and immunoperoxidase techniques (55–57).

Mucormycosis

General Comments. *Rhizopus* is the most common of three genera within the family Mucoraceae to cause human disease, followed by *Mucor* and

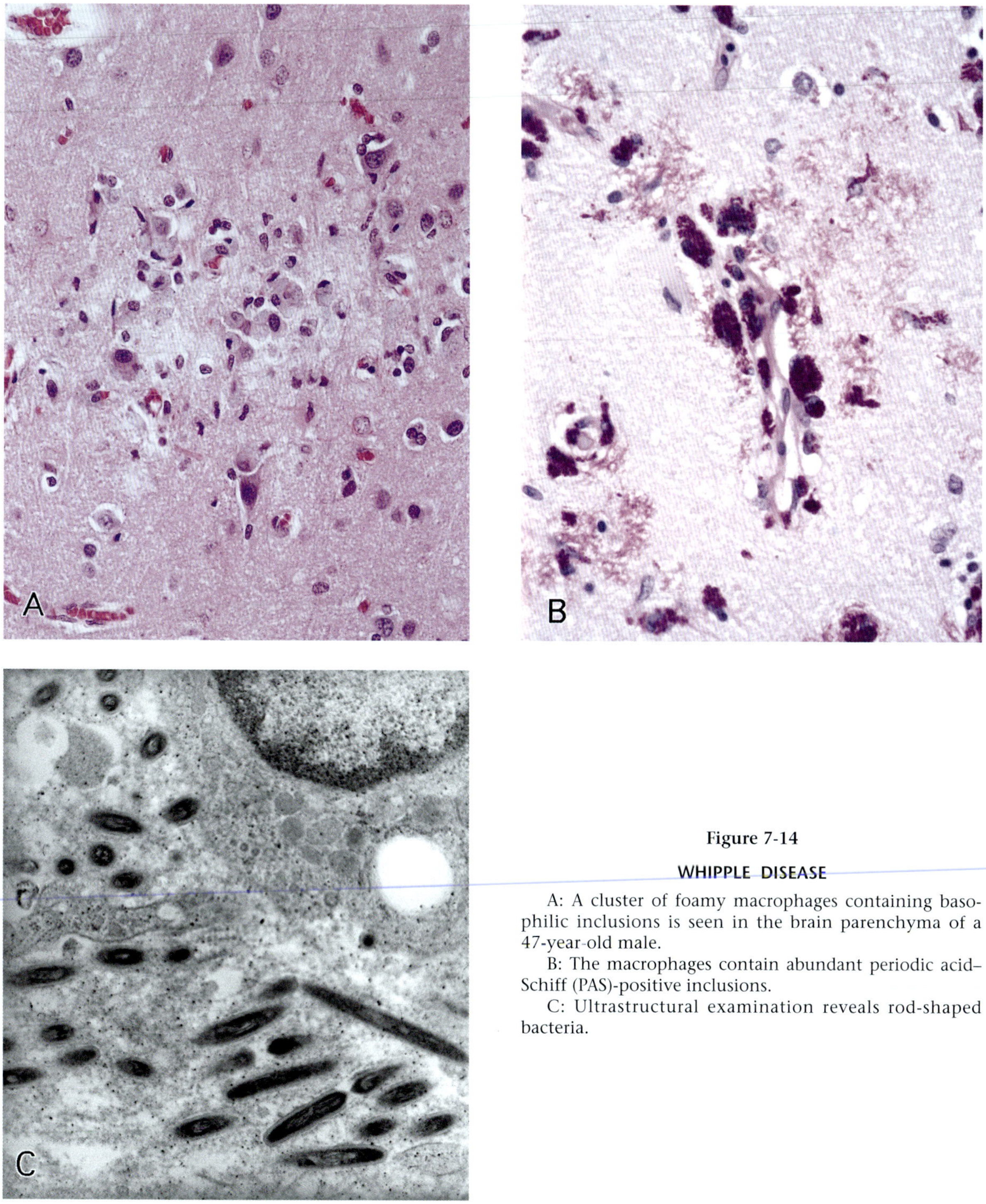

Figure 7-14

WHIPPLE DISEASE

A: A cluster of foamy macrophages containing basophilic inclusions is seen in the brain parenchyma of a 47-year-old male.

B: The macrophages contain abundant periodic acid–Schiff (PAS)-positive inclusions.

C: Ultrastructural examination reveals rod-shaped bacteria.

Absidia. *CNS mucormycosis* (also known as *phycomycosis* and *zygomycosis*) is an uncommon, aggressive infection usually limited to poorly controlled diabetics with ketoacidosis, intravenous drug abusers, and immunocompromised patients. Infection is acquired through the inhalation of this ubiquitous organism, found in soil, manure, and decaying vegetable matter. There are two recognized patterns of infection: *rhinocerebral mucormycosis*, which results from

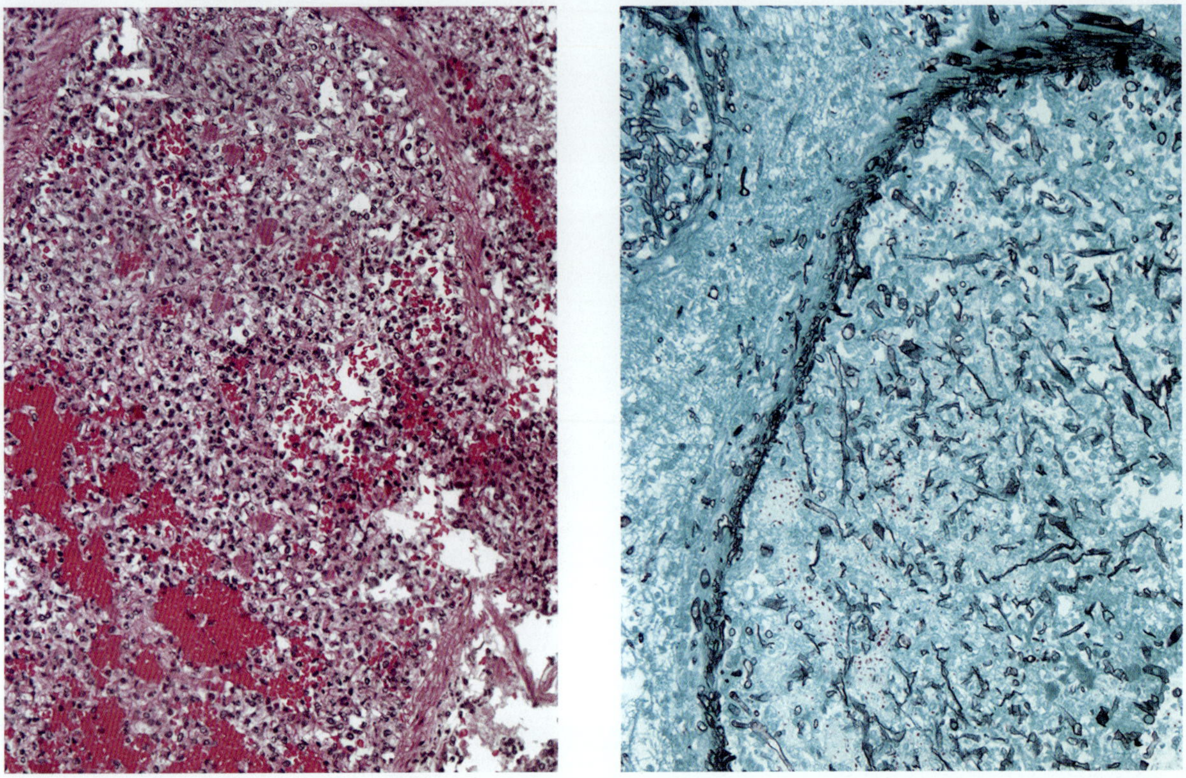

Figure 7-15

RHINOCEREBRAL MUCORMYCOSIS

Left: The wall of an artery shows florid chronic inflammation.
Right: Broad, septate hyphae of varying caliber are visualized by methenamine silver impregnation.

contiguous spread from sinus or skin infections, and hematogenous dissemination of mucormycosis. The rhinocerebral form with its characteristic spread is the most common. The infectious process progresses from the sinonasal cavity to the orbit, and later to the cavernous sinus.

Clinical Features. The most common clinical findings are headache, fever, orbitofacial cellulitis, cranial nerve palsy, altered mental status, and hemiparesis.

Gross Findings. Rhinocerebral mucormycosis generally gains access to the brain through the cavernous sinus, which may be thrombosed, or the orbital roof. Accordingly, foci of necrosis and hemorrhage are most prominent in tissue sampled from the orbitofrontal regions of the brain. Mycotic emboli from hematogenous dissemination have a predilection for the basal ganglia.

Microscopic Findings. Microscopic examination reveals numerous neutrophils and abundant, broad, nonseptate hyphae that branch at right angles around and within meningeal and parenchymal blood vessels (fig. 7-15).

Treatment. Although often fatal, aggressive surgical debridement, coupled with antifungal chemotherapy, ensures the best chance for a favorable outcome (59).

Aspergillosis

General Comments. *Aspergillus* is a ubiquitous mold. The species causing disease in humans are commonly *A. fumigatus, A. flavus,* and occasionally, *A. niger*. The modes of entry to the CNS are through hematogenous dissemination, through direct extension from the paranasal sinuses and middle ear or orbit, or through penetrating cranial trauma. *Aspergillus* species have a propensity for blood vessel invasion; CNS infection results from hematogenous dissemination usually following necrotizing pneumonia. This form of infectious cerebral vasculitis mainly involves thalamoperforating and lenticulostriate arteries, with a high frequency of thalamic or basal nuclei lesions (57,59).

Predisposing factors for invasive CNS infection include profound granulocytopenia, AIDS, prolonged corticosteroid or cytotoxic therapy, allogenic bone marrow transplantation, hematologic malignancy, diabetes mellitus, and liver failure. Complications include mycotic aneurysms, often seen within the basal ganglia and thalamus, subarachnoid hemorrhage, and vascular thrombosis (59).

Radiologic Findings. Typical imaging findings of intracranial aspergillosis include single or multifocal lesions involving the cerebral hemispheres, with hemorrhage in approximately 25 percent of lesions. On CT, the lesions generally have low attenuation. The lesions often appear hyperintense on T2-weighted or proton-density MRIs, and exhibit restricted diffusion on diffusion-weighted MRI, indicating infarction. Generally, the lesions exhibit no enhancement or only subtle peripheral enhancement. Lesional contrast enhancement tends to be stronger in immunocompetent hosts (57,59).

Gross Findings. Grossly, parenchymal lesions appear as necrotic zones, often in the domain of one or more blood vessels (fig. 7-16A).

Microscopic Findings. *Aspergillus* causes a distinctive, suppurative infection with a predilection for invading blood vessels walls and resulting in vascular thrombosis, necrosis, and infarction (fig. 7-16B). The nature of the inflammation varies over time. Initially, neutrophils predominate and are subsequently replaced by macrophages. Abscess formation, necrotizing nonsuppurative lesions, and granulomas may be seen, usually within the cerebral hemispheres. Granulomas consist of collections of lymphocytes, plasma cells, epithelioid cells, and Langhans type giant cells. The hyphae of *Aspergillus* organisms are septate and branch at acute angles. Fungal hyphae are associated with the destruction of the arterial elastic lamina.

Cryptococcosis

General Comments. *Cryptococcus neoformans* is a ubiquitous encapsulated, spherical, yeast-like fungus that has a worldwide distribution. It has been found in high concentrations in pigeon droppings and soil. Defects in cellular immunity or underlying disease are found in the majority of patients with *cryptococcosis*.

Predisposing factors to infection with *C. neoformans* include endogenous increases in corticosteroid production (Cushing syndrome), corticosteroid therapy (notably in transplantation immunosuppression), and hematological malignancies (particularly Hodgkin disease). Infection with *C. neoformans* may be seen as the AIDS-defining disease in patients with HIV infection and is associated with a high mortality rate (55,60–62).

Clinical Features. After the infection is acquired by inhalation of contaminated soil or bird droppings, the fungus reaches the CNS by hematogenous dissemination, usually from the lungs. CNS involvement can manifest either as meningitis, with or without parenchymal lesions, or as cryptococcal abscesses (*cryptococcomas*). Cryptococcomas are more common in individuals with a normal immune status.

Radiologic Findings. Contrast-enhanced MRI and CT scans may be normal or demonstrate hydrocephalus, atrophy, meningeal enhancement, or nonenhancing cryptococcomas. The areas of the brain most commonly affected are the meninges, basal ganglia, and dorsal cerebellum (62).

Laboratory Findings. The CSF profile varies with the immune status of the patient. In contrast to sporadic cryptococcal meningitis unrelated to AIDS, the CSF in patients with AIDS-related cryptococcal meningitis may have normal protein levels and no pleocytosis. Standardized diagnostic assays that detect cryptococcal capsular polysaccharide in samples of serum or CSF are highly specific and sensitive and should be performed on all HIV-seropositive patients with suspected meningitis (60–62).

Gross Findings. Mild or moderate leptomeningeal thickening and opacification frame tissue samples obtained from the basilar aspect of the brain (fig. 7-17, top). In some cases, small granulomas are seen. In the immunosuppressed population, surgical specimens are likely to contain basal ganglia or thalamus, and feature multiple, apparently intraparenchymal cysts that resemble soap bubbles (actually dilated Virchow-Robin spaces). The soap-bubble lesions are thought to represent organisms that grow in gelatinous masses within the meninges, often expanding the Virchow-Robin spaces. Cryptococcomas resemble bacterial abscesses but tend to be less purulent and may be found in the meninges, in the

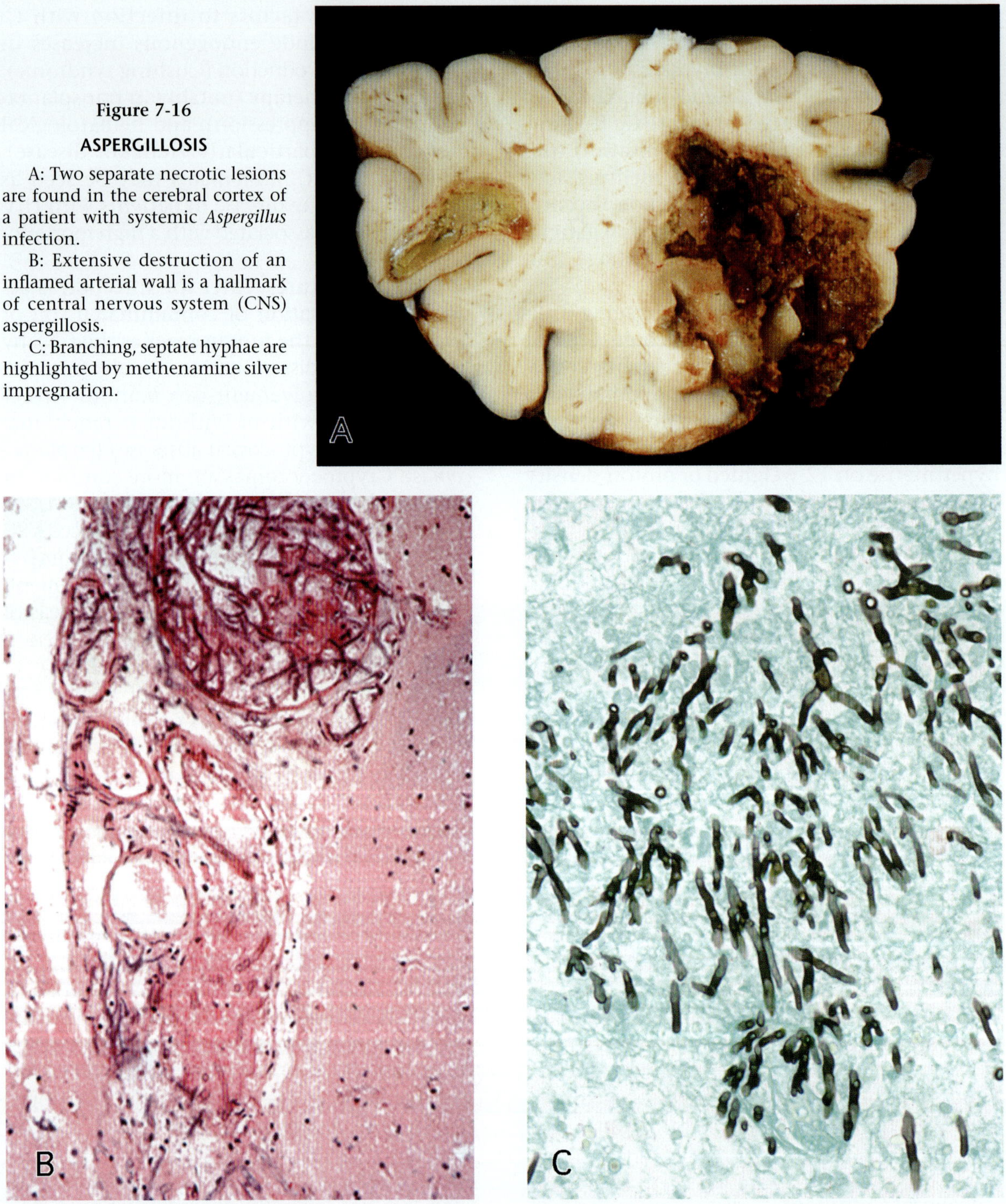

Figure 7-16

ASPERGILLOSIS

A: Two separate necrotic lesions are found in the cerebral cortex of a patient with systemic *Aspergillus* infection.

B: Extensive destruction of an inflamed arterial wall is a hallmark of central nervous system (CNS) aspergillosis.

C: Branching, septate hyphae are highlighted by methenamine silver impregnation.

choroid plexus, or within the brain parenchyma in individuals with normal immunity.

Microscopic Findings. Sites of involvement are marked by a variable cellular response, which ranges from a minimal or absent ("soap bubble" lesions) inflammatory cellular infiltrate to a brisk granulomatous reaction. The often sparse, mixed inflammatory infiltrate consists of lymphocytes, plasma cells, occasional eosinophils, and multinucleated giant cells (fig. 7-17, bottom). The organism is a 5- to 10-µm, round budding yeast that is surrounded by a

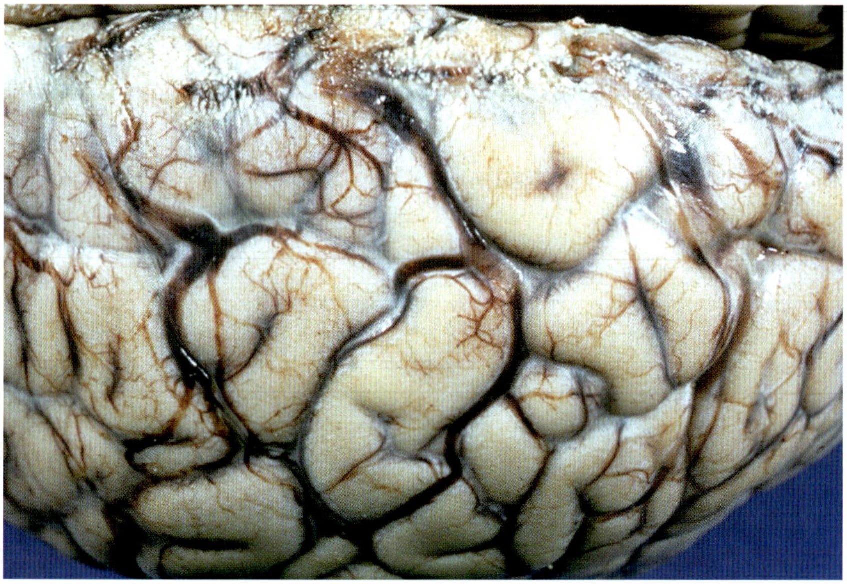

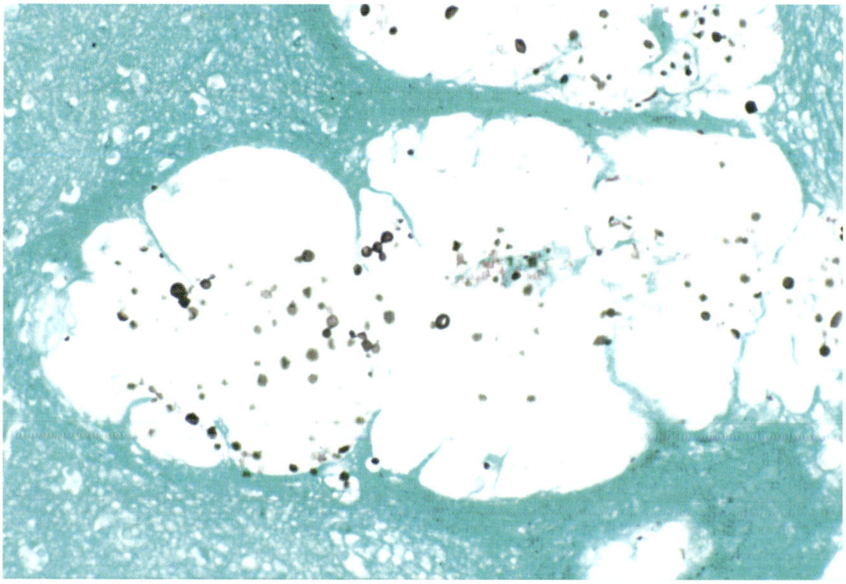

Figure 7-17

CRYPTOCOCCAL MENINGITIS

Top: Leptomeningeal opacification in a patient with cryptococcal meningitis.

Bottom: An enlarged perivascular space contains *Cryptococcus neoformans*. The surrounding brain tissue shows little reaction (Gomori methenamine silver [GMS] stain).

thick, gelatinous capsule. India ink, mucicarmine, Alcian blue, and PAS stains visualize the capsule. In patients with AIDS, the capsule is often deficient and difficult to identify with routine stains (63).

Coccidioidomycosis

General Comments. *Coccidioides immitis* flourishes in the soil in dry desert climates. The specific ecological areas are the semi-arid southwestern United States, certain areas of Central and South America, and Mexico. The mycelial form of the organism produces anthroconidia, which are highly infectious. Infection is acquired after inhalation of the arthroconidia into the alveoli. Immunosuppression due to a variety of causes sets the stage for developing disseminated infection and meningitis (64). Fewer than 100 patients in the United States die each year from infection; the majority are African-Americans. Higher but less dramatic risk for dissemination is noted in persons from the Philippines, Native Americans, and Hispanics. Complications include hydrocephalus, ventriculitis, subdural effusion or empyema, edema with or without herniation, cerebritis, abscess, and infarct because of either cortical vein thrombosis or arteritis (55,63,64).

Clinical Features. The disease syndrome most commonly associated with *C. immitis* infection is pneumonia. Meningitis is the most feared and most frequent presentation (one third to half of patients with disseminated coccidioidomycosis, although dissemination is a rare complication). CNS manifestations included headache, nuchal rigidity, mental status changes, and focal neurologic deficits. Of all the endemic mycoses, infection with *C. immitis* is the least responsive to currently available therapy (64). For patients with meningitis, cure is rare and therapy must be continued indefinitely.

Radiologic Findings. CT or MRI of the brain in patients with CNS involvement may demonstrate meningeal enhancement, predominantly in the basilar cisterns, granulomas, or abscesses. Patients also often have imaging signs of hydrocephalus (64).

Laboratory Findings. Patients with coccidioidal meningitis may have CSF pleocytosis with a mononuclear or, occasionally, eosinophilic predominance, decreased glucose levels, and elevated protein levels (64).

Gross Findings. The inflammatory exudates usually cover the base of the brain; the leptomeninges are thickened and opacified. In addition to meningitis, surgical specimens may reveal small caseating granulomas, abscesses, or vasculitis accompanied by ischemic lesions. Brain lesions may be superficial or deep and multiple or single. Involvement at any level of the spinal cord is common (55,65).

Microscopic Findings. On microscopic examination, *Coccidioides* organisms are usually numerous and form thick-walled, nonbudding spherules, 20 to 60 µm in diameter, often filled with endospores, which appear basophilic with the H&E stain (fig. 7-18, left). GMS and PAS stains highlight immature forms more effectively. Variable numbers of chronic inflammatory cells surround the spherules (fig. 7-18, right). A more acute inflammatory response may accompany spherule rupture.

Two patterns of vasculitis may complicate the infection. The first is a transmural inflammatory process of the intracranial blood vessels, which occurs early in the course of disease. Encroachment of the vessel lumen may result in thrombosis. The second process occurs with chronic disease and is associated with intimal thickening and luminal occlusion with minimal inflammation (55,65).

The definitive diagnostic test is growth of the organism. DNA probes can identify the organism once growth has occurred.

Blastomycosis

General Comments. *Blastomyces dermatitidis* is a dimorphic fungus that lives in moist soil in the southeastern United States and causes *North American blastomycosis*, which primarily affects agricultural workers. The major route of transmission to humans is via inhalation of airborne spores; the initial disease manifestations are usually pulmonary. Extrapulmonary blastomycosis of the skin may occur in conjunction with pulmonary infection and results from hematogenous dissemination. Primary cutaneous blastomycosis can also evolve after a dog bite, after inoculation in the laboratory, or during autopsy. Blastomycosis causes CNS disease on rare occasion, often in the setting of underlying chronic disease or immunosuppression. Living in endemic areas such as the Ohio or Mississippi River valley and exposure to dust from construction or excavation in these areas also augment the risk of infection (55,56).

Clinical and Radiologic Findings. Acute and chronic meningitis are the most common forms of CNS blastomycosis, but solitary mass lesions are a frequent presentation. In CNS blastomycosis, an intracranial dural-based granulomatous lesion is infrequent in comparison to chronic meningitis or encephalitis (56,67). A biopsy specimen of brain tissue is often necessary for the diagnosis. Survival is possible with timely therapeutic intervention.

MRI demonstrates progressive enhancement of the basal meninges and involvement of bilateral basal ganglia and thalami.

Gross Findings. Macroscopic features are dependent on the location and time course of the disease. Tissue specimens may be soft or firm, reflecting either acute suppurative disease or the fibrosis and gliosis associated with chronic infection. On cross section, isolated or multiple purulent mass lesions may involve the parenchyma.

Microscopic Findings. Lesions appear as abscesses or necrotizing granulomas. The

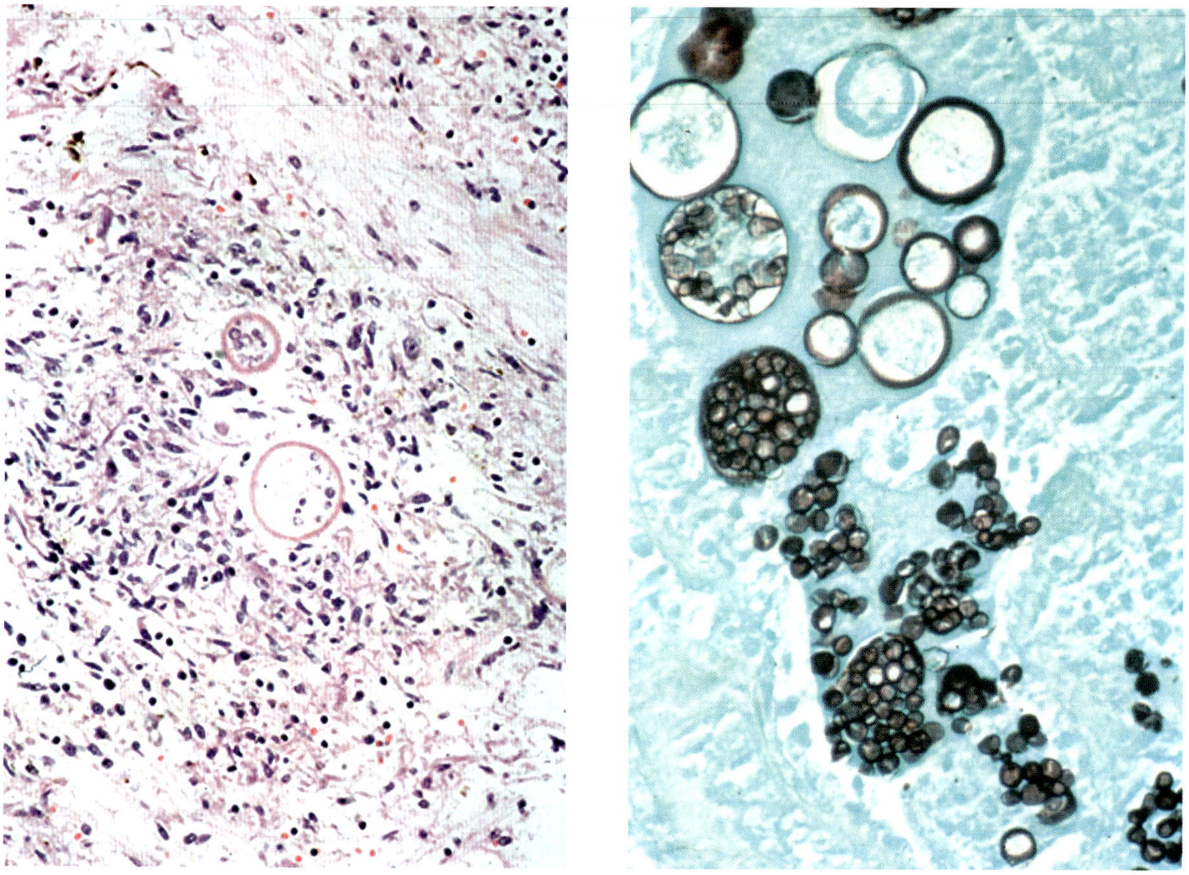

Figure 7-18

COCCIDIOIDOMYCOSIS

Left: Leptomeningitis with *Coccidioides* endospores.
Right: *Coccidioides* endospores are highlighted by methenamine silver impregnation.

organisms are round to oval, 5 to 25 µm in diameter, possess a double-contoured refractile wall, reproduce by characteristic broad-based budding, and elicit a mixed inflammatory reaction (fig. 7-19). The organisms are readily observed as basophilic bodies surrounded by a clear space with routine H&E staining, but PAS and GMS preparations highlight the thick-walled fungi. Central caseous necrosis and multinucleated giant cells are often identified (66,67).

Candidiasis

General Comments. Candidal species are ubiquitous in nature and are normal intestinal and skin commensals in humans. The organisms grow as single cells and reproduce by budding. The most common species is *Candida albicans*, but the incidence of non-*albicans* candidal infections (e.g., *C. tropicalis*) is increasing, including species with antifungal resistance (e.g., *C. krusei, C. glabrata*).

The disease is the most common nosocomial fungal infection, reflecting the dramatic change in prevalence during recent years. CNS involvement is a common manifestation and usually follows hematogenous dissemination. Important iatrogenic predisposing factors include the use of parenteral hyperalimentation, corticosteroids and other immunosuppressive therapies, broad-spectrum antibiotics, and indwelling devices such as neurosurgical shunts and urinary and vascular catheters. AIDS is another major risk factor (55,56).

Clinical and Radiologic Findings. CNS candidiasis is usually accompanied by fever, constitutional symptoms, and focal neurologic

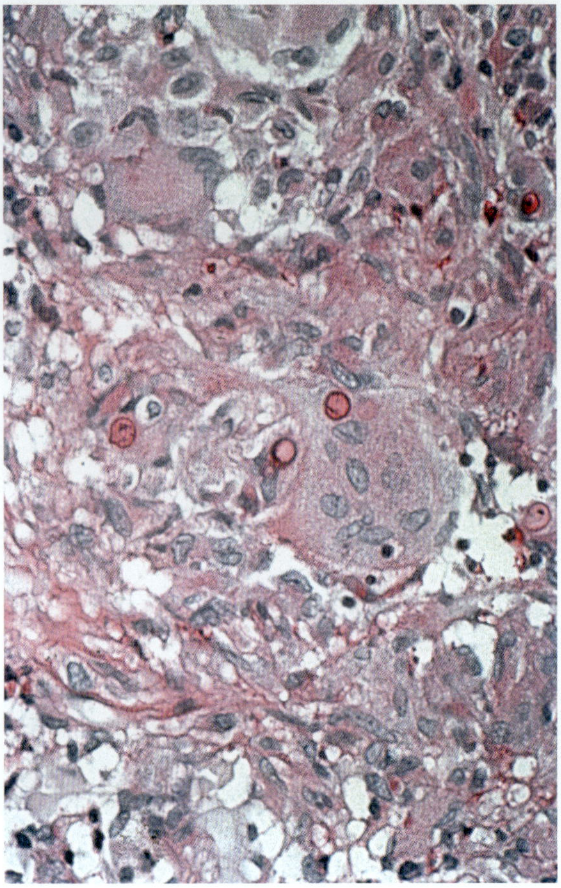

Figure 7-19

BLASTOMYCOSIS

Blastomyces yeast forms are surrounded by granulomatous inflammation, accompanied by multinucleated giant cells (PAS stain).

deficits. All parts of the CNS may be involved, with no apparent areas of predilection. Meningeal involvement is uncommon except in neonates. Candidal organisms tend to produce focal necrosis, resulting in microabscesses that are located mainly at the gray-white junction. Diagnosis requires blood cultures, radiographic imaging, and intraoperative culture. Management of candidal infection should include attempts to correct any predisposing factors. Aggressive systemic antifungal therapy is often necessary. Morbidity and mortality are usually high, due in part to the underlying conditions.

MRI is excellent for highlighting the microabscesses associated with vascular invasion and hemorrhage.

Laboratory Findings. Lumbar puncture is indicated for patients with suspected candidal meningitis. Findings include an elevated white blood cell count that is lymphocyte predominant and a low glucose level. Organisms are well seen with special stains (GMS or PAS). They can be identified in CSF cultures.

Gross and Microscopic Findings. The surgeon may sample tissue that harbors scattered hemorrhagic lesions resembling hemorrhagic infarcts, usually in the territory of the anterior and middle cerebral arteries. Histologic examination discloses the faintly basophilic *C. albicans,* which appears as tiny (2 to 5 μm) yeast-like forms, pseudohyphae, and true hyphae. Pseudohyphae are budding yeasts joined end to end at constrictions, thus simulating true hyphae. The organisms are visible with H&E stains, but a variety of special fungal stains (GMS, PAS) accentuate the pathogens (fig. 7-20). The organisms are more likely to be observed around blood vessels and adjacent to foci of hemorrhage and infarct (55,56).

Histoplasmosis

General Comments. *Histoplasma capsulatum* is one of the dimorphic fungi that exist in mycelial and yeast forms in the soil. *Histoplasmosis* has been reported from many areas of the world, with the Mississippi and Ohio River valleys being the major endemic regions in North America. Primary infection is usually asymptomatic and follows inhalation exposure. Dissemination occurs in individuals with underlying immune deficiency and at the extremes of age. Involvement of the CNS is rare but may occur as part of disseminated histoplasmosis and manifests most frequently as chronic meningitis. In some instances, the infection manifests as acute meningitis or as discrete, parenchymal mass lesions (55,56).

Clinical and Radiologic Findings. Symptoms are usually indolent and chronic, and include fever, headache, and mental status changes. Seizures and focal neurologic deficits occur. Imaging studies in CNS histoplasmosis consist of localized enhancing lesions (focal or multiple) (55,56).

Gross Findings. Mass lesions may be either soft and necrotic or firm and fibrotic, depending on the age of the process (fig. 7-21A).

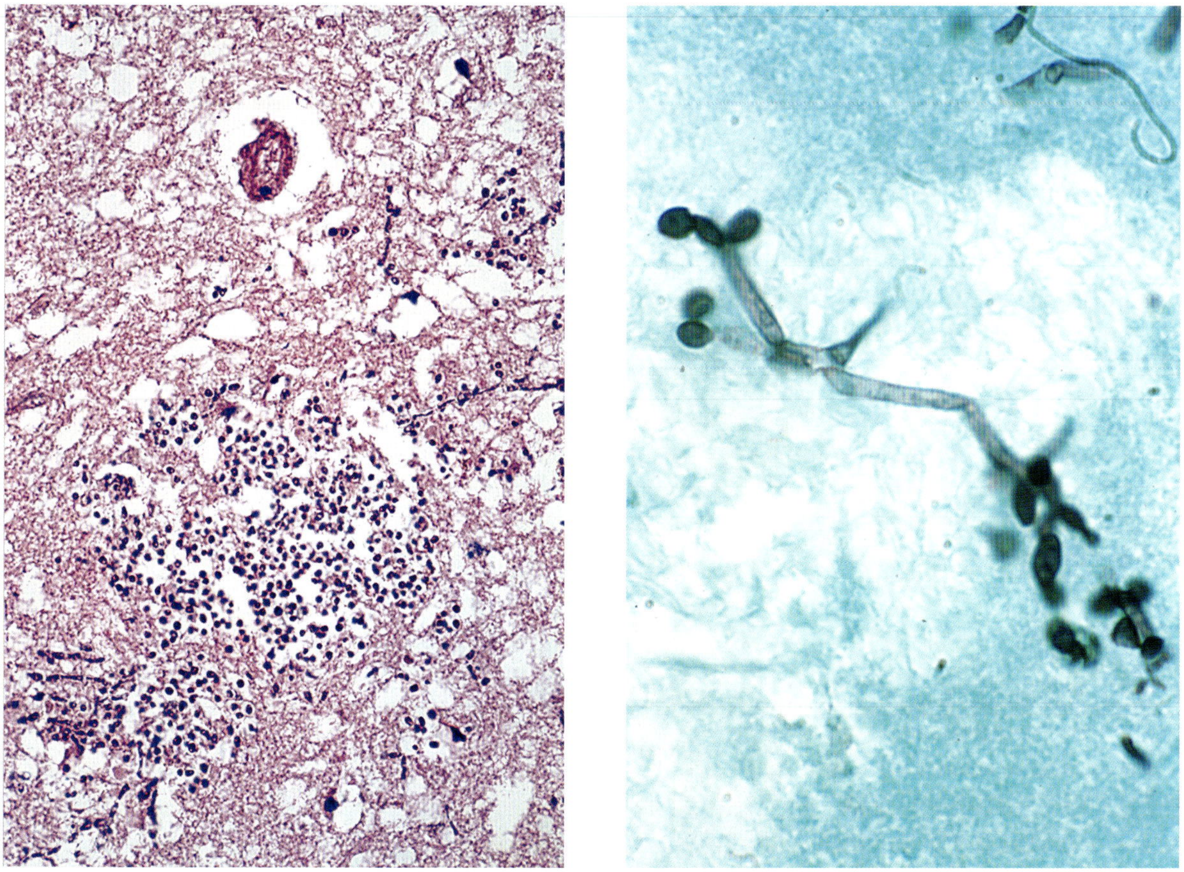

Figure 7-20

CANDIDIASIS

Left: Microabscesses are present. The inflammatory cells obscure fungal elements on routine H&E-stained sections. Right: Hyphal and pseudohyphal forms are optimally observed with methenamine silver impregnation.

Microscopic Findings. Microscopic examination of the involved leptomeninges or parenchyma reveals a dense collection of macrophages containing round to oval, intensely PAS- or GMS-positive *Histoplasma capsulatum*, small yeast forms that measure 2 to 5 μm in diameter (fig. 7-21B,C). Variable numbers of plasma cells, lymphocytes, and giant cells accompany the inflammatory reaction. Foci of necrosis and endothelial proliferation are common.

Chromoblastomycosis

General Comments. Although wordwide in distribution, *chromoblastomycosis* is primarily a disease of the tropics and subtropics. Most cases are caused by five genera of fungi: *Fonsecaea compactum, F. pedrosoi, Phialophora verrucosa, Cladosporium trichodes (bantianum),* and *Rhinocladiella aquaspersa*. CNS disease is most often caused by *C. trichodes* and usually occurs in healthy patients. The infection also manifests in the setting of debilitating disease or immunosuppression. The CNS portal of entry is hematogenous in the majority of cases (55,56).

Gross and Microscopic Findings. Brain involvement ranges from abscess formation, usually multifocal, to meningoencephalitis with extensive areas of hemorrhagic infarcts of the frontoparietal lobes. Abscesses are most frequent in the deep cerebral hemispheres or, less frequently, the thalamus, hypothalamus, brain stem, and cerebellum (fig. 7-22, top). Fungal elements are visible within the abscesses, which also contain a mixed inflammatory infiltrate consisting of neutrophils, lymphocytes, histiocytes, and giant cells surrounded by fibrosis and gliosis. Individual

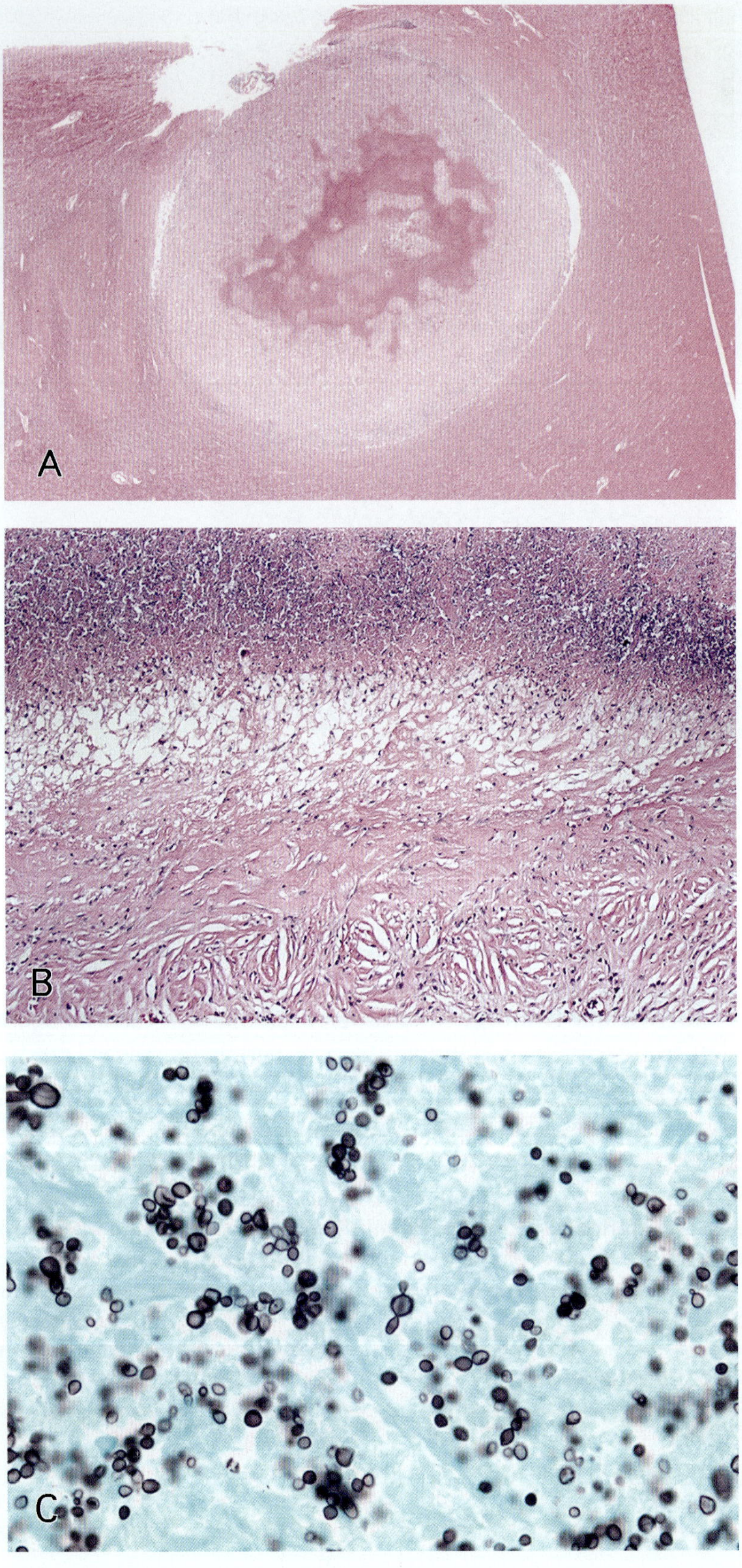

Figure 7-21

HISTOPLASMOSIS

A: Caseating granuloma (histoplasmoma) is a manifestation of histoplasmosis.

B: Macrophages at the edge of the granuloma aggregate contain numerous small, round *Histoplasma* yeasts.

C: The yeast forms are best visualized by methenamine silver impregnation.

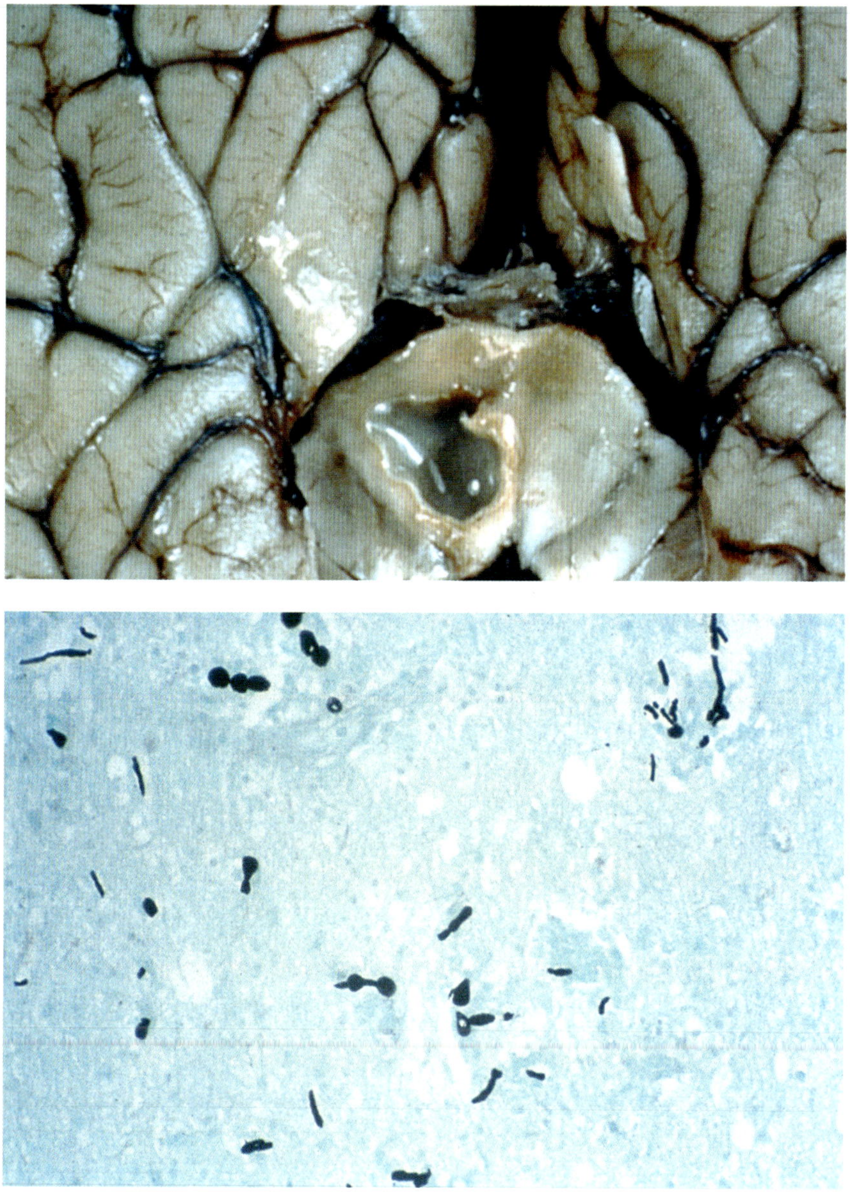

Figure 7-22

CHROMOBLASTOMYCOSIS

Top: A *Cladosporium* abscess is found within the midbrain.

Bottom: Hyphae show branching, 2- to 3-µm-thick septa with indentations at intervals of 5 to 15 µm on methenamine silver impregnation.

hypha, which may show branching, have 2- to 3-µm thick septa with indentations at 5- to 15-µm intervals (fig. 7-22, bottom) (55,56).

PARASITIC INFECTIONS

Toxoplasmosis

General Comments. *Toxoplasma gondii*, the cause of *toxoplasmosis*, is an obligate intracellular parasite that is worldwide in distribution. Cats and other feline species are the definitive hosts; human infection is acquired by eating undercooked meat or ingesting of cat feces. When the organism is ingested through lapses of hygiene, bradyzoites (the slowly growing form observed in cysts) are released from cysts or sporozoites are released from oocysts, and the organisms enter gastrointestinal cells. They multiply, rupture cells, and infect contiguous cells. The organisms are transported via the lymphatics and disseminated hematogenously throughout the body. Tachyzoites proliferate, producing necrotic foci surrounded by a mixed cellular reaction. With the development of a normal immune response, tachyzoites (the rapidly dividing form observed in the acute phase of infection) disappear from the tissues. Tissue cysts sometimes remain viable for decades without causing disease. In individuals with depressed cellular immunity, the acute infection progresses through reactivation of latent cysts and generation of many active tachyzoites (2,37,69).

Toxoplasmosis produces a wide range of clinical syndromes, the majority of which are asymptomatic in the immunocompetent. Those at risk for severe or life-threatening disease include fetuses, newborns, and immunologically impaired individuals. Among immunodeficient individuals, those with deficient T-cell–mediated immunity in the setting of hematologic malignancies, bone marrow and solid organ transplants, or AIDS are especially vulnerable. Toxoplasmosis ranks as the most common cause of focal brain lesions in AIDS patients and almost half of seropositive patients develop the disease. It is among the most common infectious diseases encountered by the surgical pathologist examining CNS tissues.

Clinical Features. The pattern of disease in fetuses and newborns is distinct from that in adults. *Congenital toxoplasmosis* arises only if maternal infection is acquired during pregnancy and is transmitted through the placenta. Susceptibility and severity vary during the course of the pregnancy. Transmission of the pathogen is more likely to occur after the third month and the resulting injury to the fetus is usually severe. As the pregnancy approaches term, the risk of infection remains high, but the fetus is seldom affected. Congenital toxoplasmosis can be diagnosed by serologic methods, PCR performed on amniotic fluid, or identification of the organism in the placenta or fetal tissues (2,37,69). The clinical manifestations in adults are protean and include headache, neuropsychiatric manifestations, and nonspecific features of increased intracranial pressure, seizures, movement disorders, and progressive focal neurologic deficits.

Radiologic Findings. The typical neuroimaging findings include single or multiple, rounded mass lesions; when a contrast agent is administered, most lesions display ring or nodular enhancement. MRI scans may reveal lesions not visualized by CT. Positron emission tomography (PET) may prove useful in distinguishing lesions of toxoplasmosis from lymphoma (69).

Gross and Microscopic Findings. *Adult Toxoplasmosis.* Cerebral toxoplasmosis may present as single, or more commonly, multiple lesions, which may be hemorrhagic, necrotic, or partially cavitated. The overlying leptomeninges are usually spared or show mild opacification. Lesions tend to favor the gray matter or localize along the corticomedullary junction, but often target the basal ganglia. In rare cases, brain involvement manifests as diffuse encephalitis without focal lesions.

The leptomeninges may harbor sparse mononuclear infiltrates. Microscopic examination of early (less than 2 weeks) untreated parenchymal lesions reveals necrotizing inflammation consisting of neutrophils, macrophages, and a few lymphocytes surrounded by reactive astrocytes and microglia (fig. 7-23, left). The surgical pathologist should give careful consideration to the possibility of cerebral toxoplasmosis in the setting of "dirty necrosis," in which there is extensive apparent karyorrhectic debris; some of the debris may reflect individual tachyzoites.

Intracellular and extracellular *Toxoplasma* pseudocysts or individual tachyzoites are usually readily found, and must be seen to confirm the diagnosis on tissue sections (7-23, right). On rare occasions, encysted *Toxoplasma* organisms are found in otherwise unremarkable brain samples and in the setting of other diseases (e.g., glioblastoma), perhaps representing dormant disease; for this reason, the demonstration of free tachyzoites is essential to implicating toxoplasmosis as the cause of active cerebral lesions. Giemsa stains have been the traditional method of visualizing the tachyzoites, but immunohistochemistry has now become the approach of choice, providing ready visualization of the free organisms. Tissue cysts containing bradyzoites are best visualized along the periphery of necrotic lesions.

After 4 weeks, the necrosis undergoes organization and organisms are rare. Chronic lesions consist of cystic spaces; organisms may be extremely difficult to demonstrate in previously treated cases. Another disease pattern is characterized by diffuse, non-necrotizing inflammation accompanied by microglial proliferation.

Congenital Toxoplasmosis. The histopathologic spectrum of findings ranges from extensive necrotizing lesions because of vascular thrombosis to limited, scattered necrotic foci. The

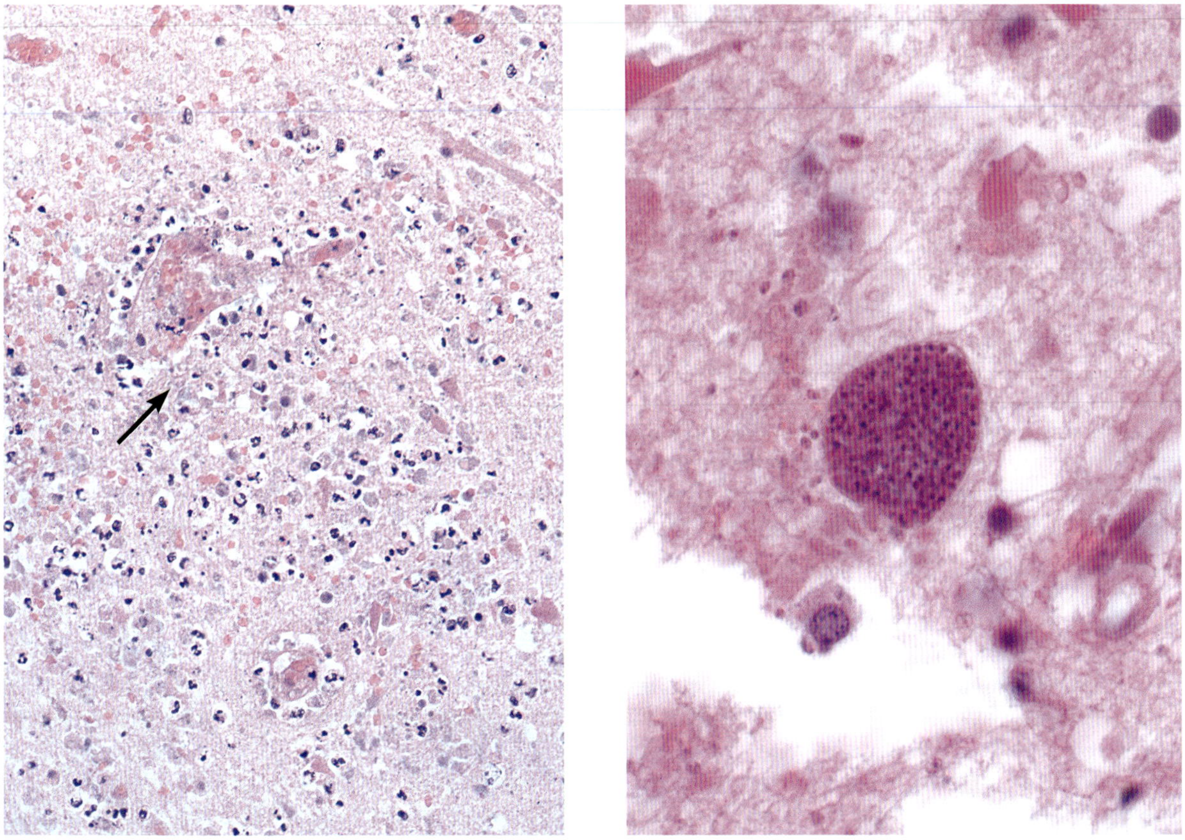

Figure 7-23

TOXOPLASMOSIS

Left: Necrotizing inflammation alerts the pathologist to search for *Toxoplasma* cysts or tachyzoites. Note the small collection of tachyzoites (arrow).

Right: A *Toxoplasma* cyst that contains numerous bradyzoites is readily visible with an H&E stain.

characteristic distribution of necrotic lesions is periventricular and periaqueductal, and often accompanied by calcification. The subarachnoid space contains mixed inflammatory infiltrates that cause obstructive hydrocephalus (69).

Cysticercosis

General Comments. *Neurocysticercosis* refers to the CNS infection caused by the larvae of the pork tapeworm *Taenia solium*. The disease has a worldwide distribution but is more common in Central and Latin America, Asia, Africa, and southern and eastern Europe. In the United States, states bordering Mexico have the highest incidence. Most infected patients in industrialized nations are immigrants from these endemic regions.

Humans are the only definitive hosts of *T. solium*. Human infection usually occurs by eating pork infected by viable larvae or cysticerci. Cysticerci are ovoid parasitic cysts containing an invaginated scolex, the larval head, surrounded by clear cystic fluid. The ingested cysticerci attach to the small intestine where they mature into adult tapeworms. The tapeworm sheds gravid proglottids into the stool. If contaminated food is ingested by the usual intermediate host, the pig, then the eggs hatch, burrow through the pig's gastrointestinal tract, enter the circulation, and encyst in systemic tissue, especially the brain, where they develop into the larval or cysticercus form. Humans, however, may become accidental intermediate hosts by ingesting food contaminated with *T. solium* eggs, shed either in the carrier's feces or in their own feces if they are infected by the adult tapeworm. If the resulting larvae encyst in the brain, neurocysticercosis develops. Skeletal muscle, skin, and eyes are other favored sites for the encysted larvae (56).

Clinical Features. The clinical presentation is highly variable and can mimic other CNS diseases, depending upon the number, size, and location of the cysts. In endemic regions, neurocysticercosis is a common cause of seizures and should be considered in the differential diagnosis of epilepsy. Other than epilepsy, presenting symptoms include focal neurologic deficits, increased intracranial pressure, and mental deterioration.

Subarachnoid lesions may cause meningitis, while intraventricular or aqueductal lesions may lead to hydrocephalus. Signs of increased intracranial pressure may be present. The manifestations of CNS cysticercosis are dependent upon the host immune response. Enlarging cysticerci may exert a mass effect, but as long as the larvae are viable, there are relative immune tolerance and minimal inflammatory response. Antigen exposure, however, occurs when the larvae degenerate. This unleashes an acute inflammatory response, with numerous eosinophils and edema. The inflammation gradually evolves into a granulomatous cellular response that eventually subsides, leaving a fibrous scar. The cysticerci undergo progressive involution during this process. By the stage of fibrous scarring, only rare entrapped and fragmented hooklets are seen or no identifiable structures are present within the cystic scar (56).

Radiologic Findings. The appearance of lesions on imaging studies varies with the stage of cyst formation and the corresponding host response. During the initial stages of development, the organism is still noncystic and often undetectable. Once the larvae have reached the vesicular stage, mature cysts are usually apparent on CT or MRI. CT may miss early lesions, which have the same density as brain, but hypodensity and contrast-enhancing ring lesions are seen with the development of inflammation around the lesion. CT images depict mature cysts as an enhancing nodule with surrounding edema, while MRI visualizes a thick enhancing ring or nodule, occasionally with edema surrounding it (fig. 7-24A). In the last stage, the nodule appears calcified on CT images and hypointense on MRI (68).

Laboratory Findings. CSF evaluation and enzyme-linked immunosorbent assays (ELISA) are used to confirm a diagnosis.

Gross Findings. Depending on the region sampled, gross examination reveals single or multiple, sometimes as many as several hundred, cysts localized to the superficial parenchyma, meninges, or ventricles. The so-called racemose form represents either an especially large cyst or grape-like coalescence of smaller ones, usually devoid of a scolex secondary to hydropic change. The lesions are located most frequently in the basal cisterns or inside the sylvian region, and can be as large as 100 mm in diameter. The organisms often protrude from the affected brain and appear as a glistening, translucent cyst with an opaque white scolex at one pole.

Microscopic Findings. Histologic sections often reveal the degenerating organism embedded in a necrotizing inflammatory infiltrate. The infiltrate consists of a central necrotic cavity surrounded by exuberant acute and chronic inflammation. Giant cells are an unusual feature. The exterior surface of the larval cyst is composed of a wavy, eosinophilic lamina whose inner surface rests on a cell layer containing infrequently spaced nuclei (fig. 7-24B). Internal to this layer, there may be loose connective tissue and portions of the larva armed with suckers and hooklets. In lesions that have undergone extensive degeneration, the remnants of the organisms appear as a calcified focus in which the organism is barely recognizable. The neighboring brain parenchyma is gliotic.

Treatment. Therapy may be medical or surgical. Surgical excision is reserved for viable cysts, although antihelminthic drugs are effective in some cases (56).

Amebiasis

General Comments. Free-living amebae are amphizoic protozoa that are widely distributed throughout the world in soil and water. They are linked to opportunistic and nonopportunistic infections in humans.

Amebae cause two distinct CNS infections: *primary amebic meningoencephalitis* (PAM) and *granulomatous amebic encephalitis* (GAE). *Naegleria fowleri* is the only recognized human pathogen associated with PAM. Victims are healthy young individuals with a history of recent water-related

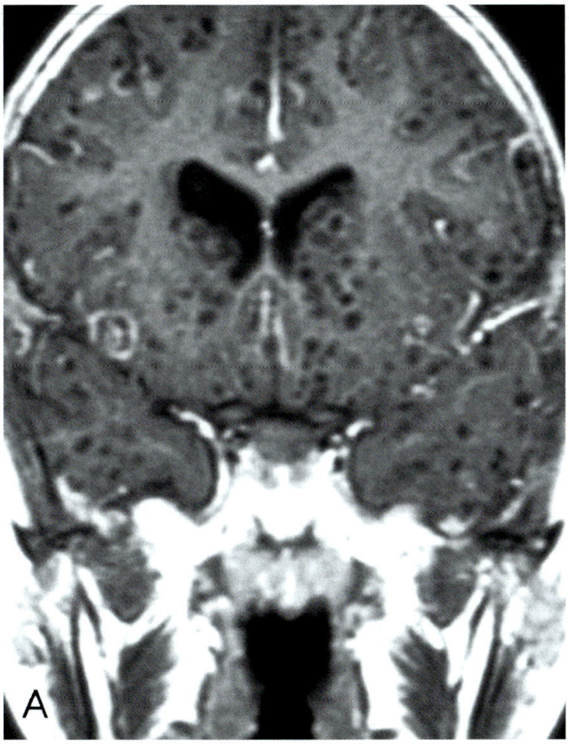

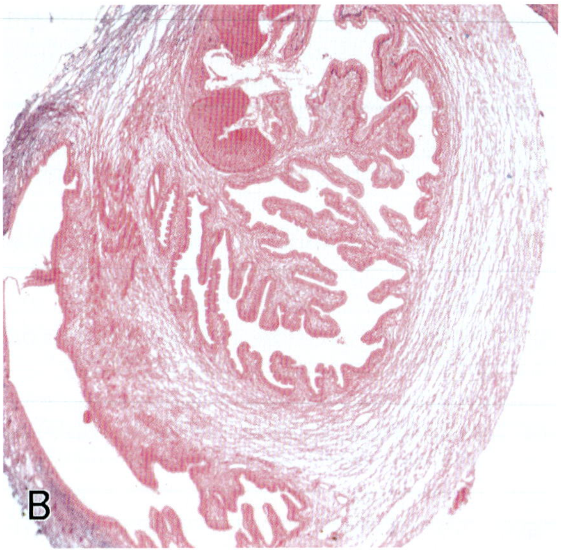

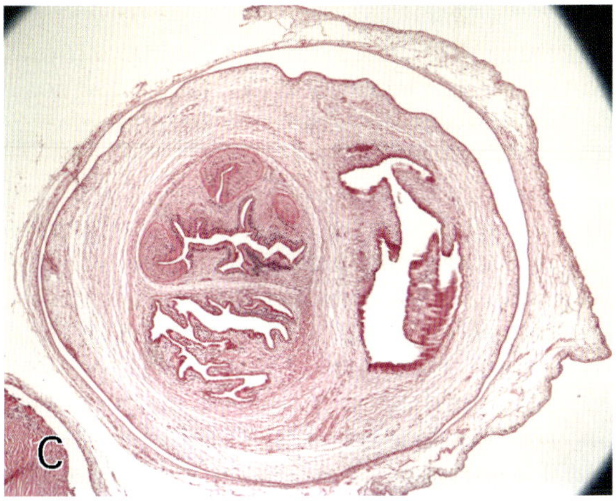

Figure 7-24

CYSTICERCOSIS

A: Contrast-enhanced coronal T1-weighted MRI demonstrates numerous small, well-defined focal areas of relative hypointensity consistent with the cystic change caused by neurocysticercosis.

B: The exterior surface of the larval cyst is composed of a wavy, eosinophilic lamina.

C: Three of four suckers are visible within the scolex.

sport activities. The pathogenetic amoebae invade the CNS through the nasal mucosa and cribriform plate. Dissemination occurs through the subarachnoid space and into the adjacent cerebral cortex, primarily at the base of the brain.

Infection with *Acanthamoeba* (*A. culbertsoni, A. castellanii*, and *A. polyphaga*) or *Balamuthia mandrillaris* often follows a more indolent course. These organisms cause GAE which targets debilitated, malnourished, chronically ill, or immunocompromised patients, e.g., those undergoing immunosuppressive therapy for organ transplants or having AIDS. Unlike the organisms responsible for PAM, the amebae causing GAE secondarily infect the CNS. There is no direct invasion through the nasal mucosa. In severely immunocompromised individuals, the granulomatous component may be negligible. On rare occasions, CNS infections due to *Entamoeba histolytica* are a life-threatening phenomenon that may be primary or secondary to amebiasis elsewhere in the body (70,71).

Clinical Features. After a short period of incubation, PAM rapidly progresses to seizures and coma, and most patients die within a week. Prompt diagnosis and early initiation of amebicidal therapy has been effective in isolated cases. Symptoms resulting from GAE resemble those of a single or multiple space-occupying CNS lesions and include hemiparesis, personality changes, seizures, and headaches. There is no proven effective therapy for this disease.

Secondary CNS amebiasis caused by *E. histolytica* usually presents in patients with a previous diagnosis of infection of the intestines, liver, or lung. This form of the disease tends to cause abscess formation and has a fulminant clinical course, culminating in the patient's death within 12 to 72 hours.

Radiologic Findings. In the majority of patients with GAE, imaging findings show multifocal CT abnormalities, although single lesions are frequent at initial presentation. The lesions are usually hypodense and show contrast enhancement. Mass effect is common, but hydrocephalus is not. Infarction is usually restricted to the territory of smaller vessels. The most common finding in PAM is cerebral edema (72,73).

Gross and Microscopic Findings. In PAM, the morphologic findings resemble those of fulminant bacterial meningoencephalitis: the acute hemorrhagic necrotizing infection produces modest purulent exudates, mainly in specimens taken from the base of the brain, brain stem, and cerebellum. Trophozoites are located within the CNS lesions, mainly around blood vessels. Definitive antemortem diagnosis depends on the detection of motile trophozoites in wet mount smears of CSF.

GAE is grossly characterized by multifocal necrotic lesions, hemorrhage, and sometimes abscess formation. The leptomeninges overlying these foci may be cloudy. GAE typically occurs in the cerebral hemispheres, basal ganglia, brain stem, and cerebellum. Microscopically, GAE lesions consist of lymphocytes, macrophages, and multinucleated giant cells accompanied by variable numbers of amebic trophozoites and cysts within necrotic CNS tissue. Vasculitis is invariably present due to amebic invasion of small blood vessels and the resulting thrombosis and fibrinoid necrosis.

The cysts of *Acanthamoeba* are rounded, are 10 to 15 µm in diameter, and have a thick, double-contoured, wrinkled wall. *Balamuthia* cysts are larger, 15 to 30 µm in diameter, and have a thicker wall and more globular refractile contents than the cysts of *Acanthamoeba*. The trophozoites of all the amebae have an irregular ameboid shape. *Acanthamoeba* trophozoites are 8 to 12 µm in greatest dimension. The cytoplasm is highly vacuolated and the nucleus has a large, round, dense karyosome with a halo around it (fig. 7-25A). *Balamuthia* trophozoites are larger, 15 to 35 µm in greatest dimension, with a less prominent nuclear karyosome (7-25B). Although sometimes mistaken for macrophages, amebae are readily identified in tissue sections stained with routine H&E, but are highlighted with GMS, PAS, and Masson trichrome stains (70–73).

Schistosomiasis

General Comments. *Schistosomiasis (bilharziasis)* is caused by one of several species of parasitic trematodes of the genus *Schistosoma*. After malaria, schistosomiasis is the second most prevalent tropical disease in the world. The clinical and pathologic sequelae of this helminthic infection are due to the immune response to the schistosome eggs. The clinical manifestations depend on the species of parasite, intensity of worm burden, and immunity of the host. Persons at risk include those who live or travel in areas where schistosomiasis occurs and who come into contact with fresh water where the appropriate type of snail (intermediate host) is present. Most cases of CNS schistosomiasis are observed with *S. japonicum* (brain lesions) and *S. mansoni* or *S. haematobium* (spinal cord disease). Although the presence of ova is an incidental finding in the majority of autopsied cases of schistosomiasis, only a minority of patients have CNS complications (56,74).

Clinical Features. The manifestations of CNS disease include headache, mental status changes, and focal and generalized seizures. Spinal schistosomiasis usually presents as a transverse myelitis or myeloradiculopathy. Patients typically present with progressive lower limb and back pain, bladder dysfunction, paresthesias, and lower limb weakness. Brain biopsy is the standard of reference for the diagnosis of CNS schistosomiasis (56,73,74).

Radiologic Findings. Although the findings are nonspecific, CT and MRI can be used to identify the granulomatous lesions induced by the host response to ova. Lesions appear hypointense on CT. They show low signal intensity on T1- and isointensity on T2-weighted MRIs (75).

Laboratory Findings. Laboratory evaluation can be difficult. Eosinophilia may not always be present. ELISA results are positive in the CSF (57).

Gross Findings. Lesions caused by *S. japonicum* are found throughout the CNS, although they are more abundant in the cerebral and cerebellar cortexes and deep gray matter. Miliary dissemination or solitary mass lesions are two

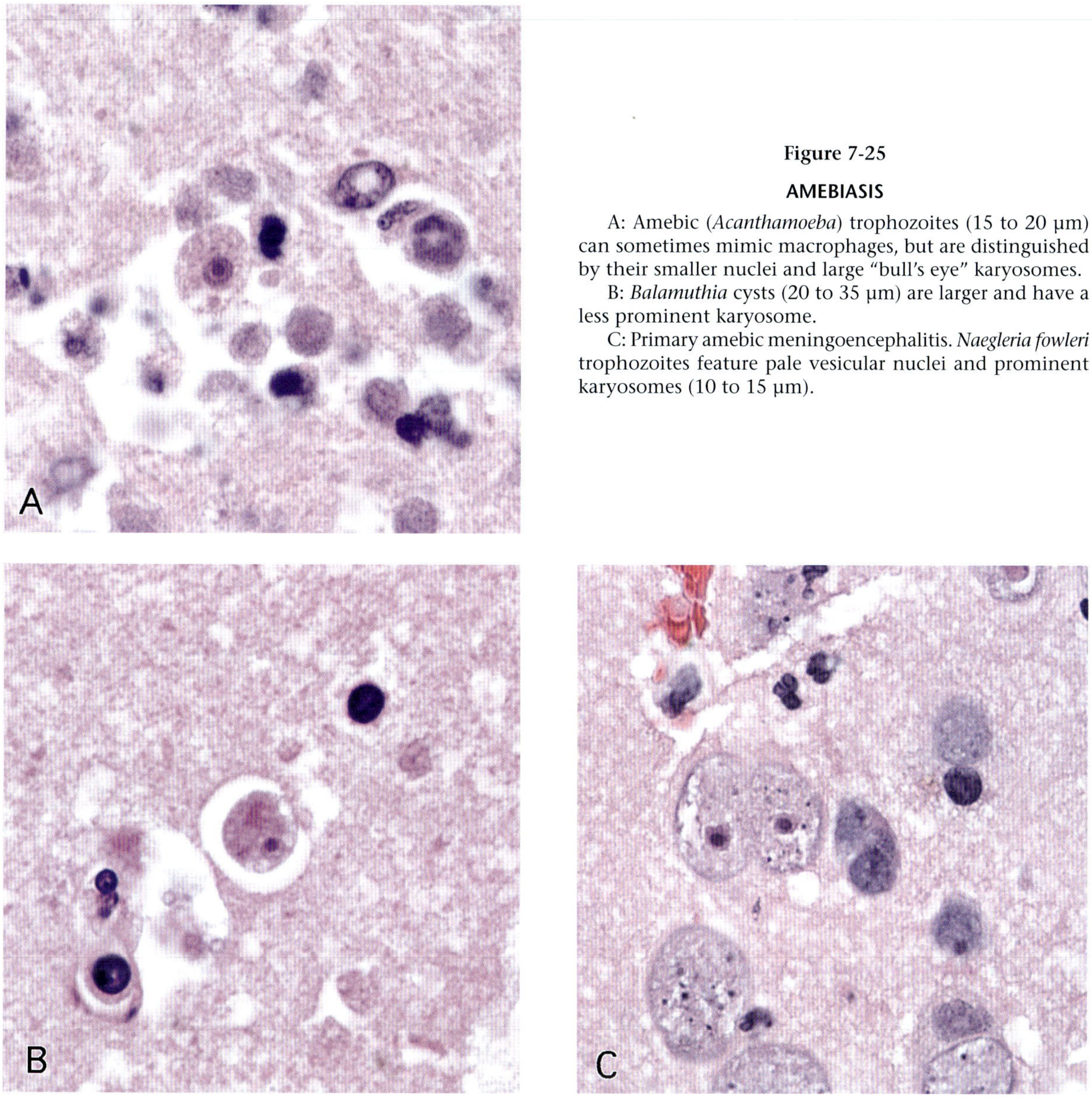

Figure 7-25

AMEBIASIS

A: Amebic (*Acanthamoeba*) trophozoites (15 to 20 µm) can sometimes mimic macrophages, but are distinguished by their smaller nuclei and large "bull's eye" karyosomes.

B: *Balamuthia* cysts (20 to 35 µm) are larger and have a less prominent karyosome.

C: Primary amebic meningoencephalitis. *Naegleria fowleri* trophozoites feature pale vesicular nuclei and prominent karyosomes (10 to 15 µm).

distinct patterns of CNS involvement. Grossly, miliary lesions appear as glistening yellow-orange nodules, ranging from 1 to 5 mm in diameter; solitary lesions can be up to 3 cm in diameter and mimic a neoplasm. Spinal cord lesions are seen in the thoracic and lumbar areas and appear as bulging, whitish masses.

Microscopic Findings. Histologically, the lesion is composed of a discrete area of granulomatous inflammation that involves the overlying meninges. Eosinophils, particularly prominent in the early stages of infection, and macrophages, populate the lymphoplasmacytic leptomeningeal infiltrate. Often enmeshed in fibroblasts or partially surrounded by multinucleated giant cells, the eggs of *S. japonicum* are oval, have a vestigial spine, and are typically smaller (68 to 100 x 45 to 80 µm) than those of the other species (fig. 7-26). Eosinophils are particularly prominent in the early stages of infection. The eggs of *S. mansoni* are large (length, 114 to 180 µm) and have a characteristic shape, with a prominent lateral spine near the posterior end (fig. 7-26). The anterior pole is tapered and slightly curved. *S. hematobium* eggs (55 to 65 x 170 µm) have an apical spine or knob (56,74).

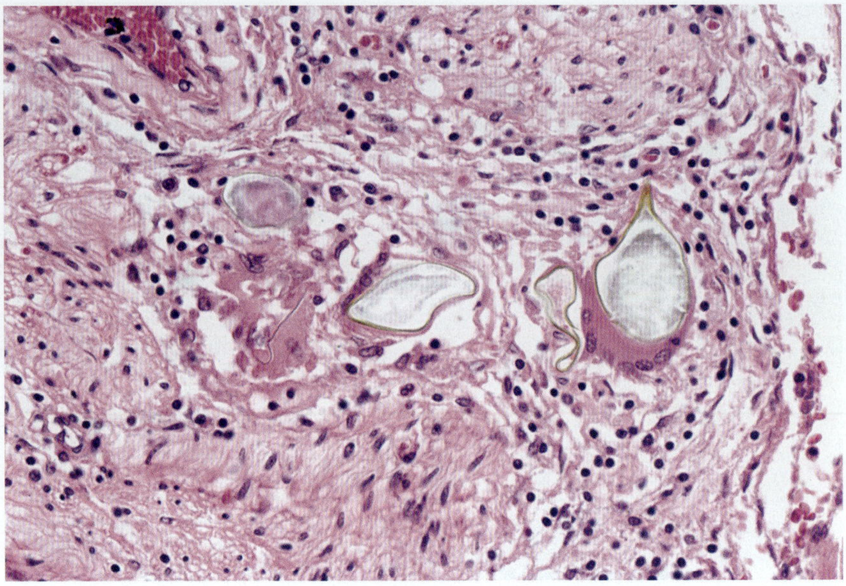

Figure 7-26

SCHISTOSOMIASIS

A chronic inflammatory infiltrate with *Schistosoma mansoni* ova (note lateral spine at 12 o'clock position).

Treatment. Antischistosomal drugs, corticosteroids, and surgery are the resources available for treating neuroschistosomiasis. The outcome is variable, but typically more favorable in cerebral disease.

Malaria

General Comments. It is estimated that more than 100 million people worldwide are infected by *malaria*, which causes 1 to 2 million deaths per year. When diagnosed in the United States, it is usually associated with travel to foreign countries or with recent immigration. Nonetheless, encountering cerebral malaria in the setting of surgical neuropathology is exceedingly rare.

Cerebral malaria is caused only by the obligate intracellular parasite, *Plasmodium falciparum*, which is transmitted to humans when bitten by an infected female *Anopheles* mosquito vector. Cases of congenital transmission or transmission secondary to transfusion of infected blood are extremely rare (76–78).

Knowledge of the parasite life cycle is important to understanding the pathogenesis of CNS infection. The *Plasmodium* parasite undergoes two cycles of replication: sporogony (the sexual cycle) and schizogony (the asexual cycle). After the mosquito bites the victim and ingests blood, the malarial sporozoites enter hepatocytes (liver phase) within minutes and reemerge into the bloodstream after a few weeks as a schizont containing myriad merozoites. These merozoites rapidly enter erythrocytes and develop into trophozoites and then schizonts over a period of days; this is the erythrocytic phase of the life cycle. Rupture of infected erythrocytes containing schizonts results in fever and merozoite release. Merozoites enter new red blood cells, and the process is repeated until immune clearance or sometimes, in the case of *P. falciparum* infection, death of the host occurs (76–78).

The virulence of *P. falciparum* is attributed to the high level of parasitemia that can occur and the property of "sequestration." Infection with *P. falciparum* alters the surface charge of red blood cells, which promotes adhesion to the endothelial surface. This property facilitates the attachment of trophozoite- and schizont-infected erythrocytes to endothelial cells of deep vascular beds within vital organs, especially the brain. Cytoadherence appears to be mediated by the electron-dense protuberances on the surface of the infected erythrocytes. These "knobs" are expressed during the trophozoite and schizont stages and are formed as a result of parasite proteins exported to the erythrocyte membrane. Electron microscopy demonstrates that these knobs are contact points between the infected erythrocyte and the endothelial cell (56,77).

Clinical and Radiologic Findings. After a 10- to 14-day incubation period, the fulminating onset of cerebral malaria is characterized by acute profound mental obtundation or psychosis. Prodromal symptoms may occur, including

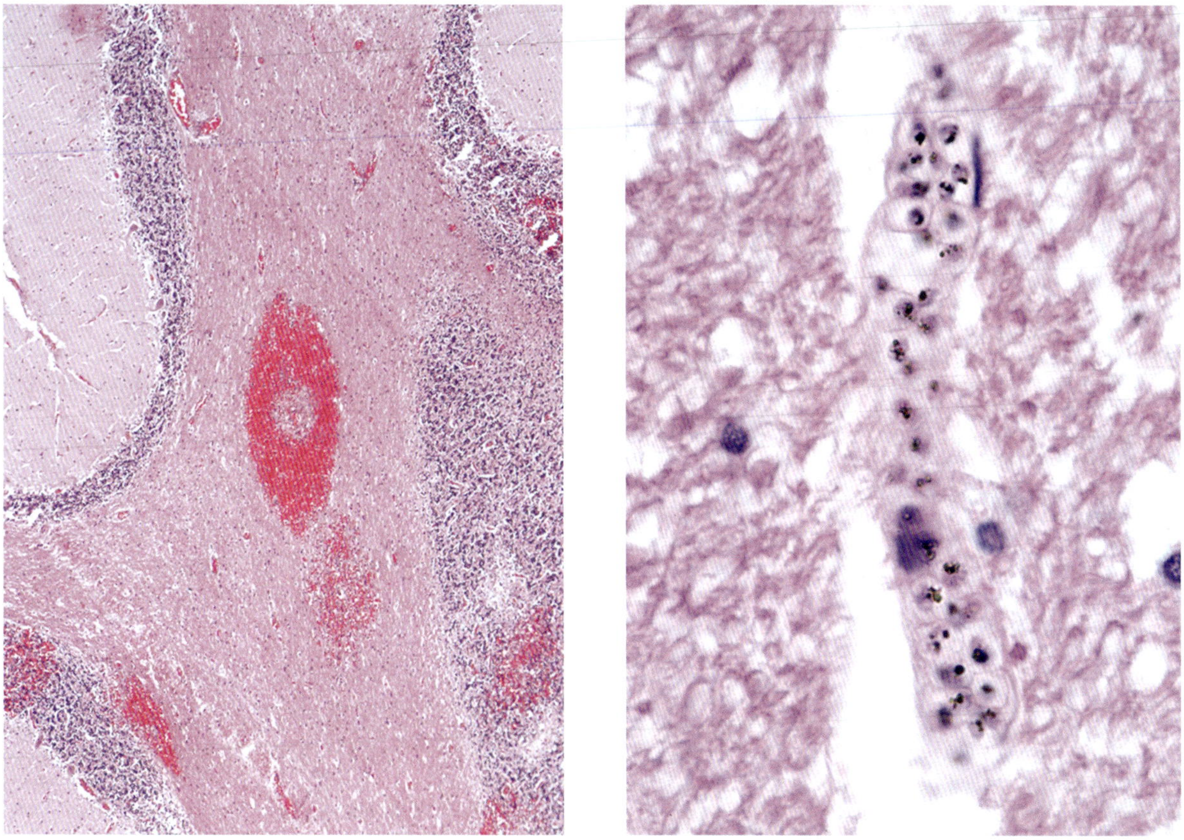

Figure 7-27

CEREBRAL *(PLASMODIUM FALCIPARUM)* MALARIA

Left: Perivascular ring hemorrhages are thought to be related to vascular stasis and inflammation of the parasitized vessel.

Right: A vessel engorged by ghost-like red blood cells contains malaria parasites and dark granules of malarial pigment (hematin).

intense headache and muscle pain. Seizures are common in the pediatric population.

MRI discloses either cortical infarcts or hyperintense areas of white matter on T2-weighted and FLAIR sequences (78).

Laboratory Findings. There is usually a mild elevation of protein levels in the CSF, but characteristically no pleocytosis.

Gross Findings. The involved brain is soft and shows opacification of the leptomeninges. There may be a slate gray discoloration from malarial pigmentation. Sectioning reveals dusky discoloration of the gray matter and widespread petechial hemorrhages. Hemorrhages are especially abundant in the periventricular white matter, and often surround necrotic arterioles and veins (fig. 7-27, left).

Microscopic Findings. Microscopic study discloses engorged cerebral vessels that are occluded by microthrombi, some of which are crowded with protozoa (fig. 7-27, right). Dark malarial pigment is found within the capillary lumens. Microglial proliferation may be generalized or focal, and surrounded by tightly packed reactive astrocytes, sometimes referred to as *Dürck granulomas*. These granulomas are usually found within cerebral white matter. Scattered mononuclear infiltrates and generalized hypoxic-ischemic changes are usually apparent. Ultrastructural studies show focal junctions between the knobs on infected red blood cells and endothelial cells (77).

REFERENCES

1. Morens DM, Folkers GK, Fauci AS. The challenge of emerging and re-emerging infectious diseases. Nature 2004;430:242-249.
2. Gray F, Chretien F, Vallat-Decouvelaere A, Scaravilli F. The changing pattern of HIV neuropathology in the HAART era. J Neuropathol Exp Neurol 2003;62:429-440.
3. Johnson RT. Emerging viral infections of the nervous system. J Neurovirol 2003;9:140-147.
4. Rutala WA, Weber DJ. Creutzfeldt-Jakob disease: recommendations for disinfection and sterilization. Clin Infect Dis 2001;32:1348-1356.
5. Fodor PA, Levin MJ, Weinberg A, Sandberg E, Sylman J, Tyler KL. Atypical herpes simplex virus encephalitis diagnosed by PCR amplification of viral DNA from CSF. Neurology 1998;51:554-559.
6. Lakeman FD, Whitley R. Diagnosis of herpes simplex encephalitis: application of polymerase chain reaction to cerebrospinal fluid from brain-biopsied patients and correlation with disease. National Institute of Allergy and Infectious Diseases Collaborative Antiviral Study Group. J Infect Dis 1995;171:857-863.
7. Richardson DC, Louie L, Louie M, Simor AE. Evaluation of a rapid PCR assay for diagnosis of meningococcal meningitis. J Clin Microbiol 2003;41:3851-3853.
8. Thomson RJ Jr, Bertram H. Laboratory diagnosis of central nervous system infections. Infect Dis Clin North Am 2001;15:1047-1071.
9. Weinberg A, Li S, Palmer M, Tyler K. Quantitative CSF PCR in Epstein-Barr virus infections of the central nervous system. Ann Neurol 2002;52:543-548.
10. Gold R. Epidemiology of bacterial meningitis. Infect Dis Clin North Am 1999;13:515-525.
11. Adams WG, Deaver KA, Cochi SL, et al. Decline of childhood Haemophilus influenzae type b (Hib) disease in the Hib vaccine era. JAMA 1993;269:221-226.
12. Gray BM, Converse GM 3rd, Dillon HC Jr. Epidemiologic studies of Streptococcus pneumoniae in infants. J Infect Dis 1980;142:923-933.
13. Roos K. Acute bacterial meningitis. Semin Neurol 2000;20:293-306.
14. Carpenter R, Petersdorf R. The clinical spectrum of bacterial infection. Am J Med 1962;33:262-275.
15. van de Beek D, de Gans J, Spanjaard L, Weisfelt M, Reitsma JB, Vermeulen M. Clinical features and prognostic factors in adults with bacterial meningitis. N Engl J Med 2004;351:1849-1859.
16. Gray F, Alonso JM. Bacterial infections of the central nervous system. In: Graham DI, Lantos PL, eds. Greenfield's neuropatholgy, Vol 2, 7th ed. New York: Arnold; 2002:151-189.
17. Bartt R. Listeria and atypical presentations of Listeria in the central nervous system. Semin Neurol 2000;20:361-373.
18. Mylonakis E, Hohmann EL, Calderwood SB. Central nervous system infection with Listeria monocytogenes: 33 years' experience at a general hospital and review of 776 episodes from the literature. Medicine (Baltimore) 1998;77:313-336.
19. Dunbar SA, Eason RA, Musher DM, Clarrridge JE 3rd. Microscopic examination and broth culture of cerebrospinal fluid in diagnosis of meningitis. J Clin Microbiol 1998;36:1617-1620.
20. Love S, Wiley C. Viral diseases. In: Graham DI, Lantos PL, eds. Greenfield's neuropatholgy, Vol 2, 7th ed. New York: Arnold; 2002:1-70.
21. Cheng TM, O'Neill BP, Scheithauer BW, Piepgras DG. Chronic meningitis: the role of meningeal or cortical biopsy. Neurosurgery 1994;34:590-595.
22. Leonard J, Des Prez R. Tuberculous meningitis. Infect Dis Clin North Am 1990;4:769-787.
23. Cassleman ES, Hasso AN, Ashwal S, Schneider S. Computed tomography of tuberculous meningitis in infants and children. J Comput Assist Tomogr 1980;4:211-216.
24. Offenbacher H, Fazekas F, Schmidt R, et al. MRI in tuberculous meningoencephalitis: report of four cases and review of the neuroimaging literature. J Neurol 1991;238:340-344.
25. Bernaerts A, Vanhoenacker FM, Parizel PM, et al. Tuberculosis of the central nervous system: overview of neuroradiological findings. Eur Radiol 2003;13:1876-1890.
26. Langford TD, Letendre SL, Larrea GJ, Masliah E. Changing patterns in the neuropathogenesis of HIV during the HAART era. Brain Pathol 2003;13:195-210.
27. Kennedy PG. Viral encephalitis: causes, differential diagnosis, and management. J Neurol Neurosurg Psychiatry 2004;75(Suppl 1):i10-15.
28. Schlitt MJ, Morawetz RB, Bonnin JM, Zeiger HE, Whitley RJ. Brain biopsy for encephalitis. Clin Neurosurg 1986;33:591-602.
29. Schiff D, Rosenblum M. Herpes simplex encephalitis (HSE) and the immunocompromised: a clinical and autopsy study of HSE in the settings of cancer and human immunodeficiency virus-type 1 infection. Hum Pathol 1998;29:215-222.
30. Morawetz RB, Whitley RJ, Murphy DM. Experience with brain biopsy for suspected herpes encephalitis: a review of forty consecutive cases. Neurosurgery 1983;12:654-657.
31. Martin JR, Mitchell WJ, Henken DB. Neurotropic herpesviruses, neural mechanisms and arteritis. Brain Pathol 1990;1:6-10.
32. Jemsek J, Greenberg SB, Taber L, Harvey D, Gershon A, Couch RB. Herpes zoster-associated encephalitis: clinicopathologic report of 12 cases and review of the literature. Medicine (Baltimore) 1983;62:81-97.

33. Schmidbauer M, Budka H, Pilz P, Kurata T, Hondo R. Presence, distribution and spread of productive varicella zoster virus infection in nervous tissues. Brain 1992;115:383-398.
34. Morgello S, Block GA, Price RW, Petito CK. Varicella-zoster virus leukoencephalitis and cerebral vasculopathy. Arch Pathol Lab Med 1988;112:173-177.
35. Gilden DH, Kleinschmidt-DeMasters BK, LaGuardia JJ, Mahalingam RJ, Cohrs R. Neurologic complications of the reactivation of varicella-zoster virus. N Engl J Med 2000;342:635-645.
36. Koralnik IJ. New insights into progressive multifocal leukoencephalopathy. Curr Opin Neurol 2004;17:365-370.
36a. Gray F, Bazille C, Adle-Biassette H, Mikol J, Moulignier A, Scaravilli F. Central nervous system immune reconstitution disease in acquired immunodeficiency syndrome patients receiving highly active antiretroviral treatment. J Neurovirol 2005;11(Suppl 3)16-22.
37. Lang W, Miklossy J, Deruaz JP, et al. Neuropathology of the acquired immune deficiency syndrome (AIDS): a report of 135 consecutive autopsy cases from Switzerland. Acta Neuropathol (Berl) 1989;77:379-390.
38. Schmidbauer M, Huemer M, Cristina S, Trabattoni GR, Budka H. Morphological spectrum, distribution and clinical correlation of white matter lesions in AIDS brains. Neuropathol Appl Neurobiol 1992;18:489-501.
39. Macedo de Oliveira A, Beecham BP, Montgomery SP, et al. West Nile virus blood transfusion-related infection despite nucleic acid testing. Transfusion 2004;44:1695-1699.
40. Guarner J, Shieh WJ, Hunter S, et al. Clinicopathologic study and laboratory diagnosis of 23 cases with West Nile virus encephalomyelitis. Hum Pathol 2004;35:983-990.
41. Sampson BA, Armbrustmacher V. West Nile encephalitis: the neuropathology of four fatalities. Ann N Y Acad Sci 2001;951:172-178.
42. Bouffard JP, Riudavets MA, Holman R, Rushing EJ. Neuropathology of the brain and spinal cord in human West Nile virus infection. Clin Neuropathol 2004;23:59-61.
43. Deresiewicz RL, Thaler SJ, Hsu L, Zamani AA. Clinical and neuroradiographic manifestations of eastern equine encephalitis. N Engl J Med 1997;336:1867-1874.
44. Morse RP, Bennish ML, Darras BT. Eastern equine encephalitis presenting with a focal brain lesion. Pediatr Neurol 1992;8:473-475.
45. Goodkin HP, Harper MB, Pomeroy SL. Intracerebral abscess in children: historical trends at Children's Hospital Boston. Pediatrics 2004;113:1765-1770.
46. Dailey AT, LeRoux PD, Grady MS. Resolution of an actinomycotic abscess with nonsurgical treatment: case report. Neurosurgery 1993;32:134-136.
47. Michelow IC, Wendel GJ Jr, Norgard MV, et al. Central nervous system infection in congenital syphilis. N Engl J Med 2002;346:1792-1798.
48. Conde-Sendin MA, Amela-Peris R, Aladro-Benito Y, Maroto AA. Current clinical spectrum of neurosyphilis in immunocompetent patients. Eur Neurol 2004;52:29-35.
49. Brightbill TC, Ihmeidan IH, Post MJ, Berger JH, Katz DA. Neurosyphilis in HIV-positive and HIV-negative patients: neuroimaging findings. AJNR Am J Neuroradiol 1995;16:703-711.
50. Holmes MD, Brant-Zawadzki MM, Simon RP. Clinical features of meningovascular syphilis. Neurology 1984;34:553-556.
51. Haass A. Lyme neuroborreliosis. Curr Opin Neurol 1998;11:253-258.
52. Adams M, Rhyner PA, Day J, DeArmond S, Smuckler EA. Whipple's disease confined to the central nervous system. Ann Neurol 1987;21:104-108.
53. De Coene B, Gilliard C, Indekeu P, Duprez T, Trigaux JP. Whipple's disease confined to the central nervous system. Neuroradiology 1996;38:325-327.
54. Baisden BL, Lepidi H, Raoult D, Argani P, Yardley JH, Dumler JS. Diagnosis of Whipple disease by immunohistochemical analysis: a sensitive and specific method for the detection of Tropheryma whipplei (the Whipple bacillus) in paraffin-embedded tissue. Am J Clin Pathol 2002;118:742-748.
55. Chimelli L, Mahler-Araujo MB. Fungal infections. Brain Pathol 1997;7:613-627.
56. Turner G, Scaravilli F. Parasitic and fungal diseases. In: Graham DI, Lantos PL, eds. Greenfield's neuropatholgy, Vol 2, 7th ed. New York: Arnold; 2002:107-141.
57. Boes B, Bashir R, Boes C, Hahn F, McConnell JR, McComb R. Central nervous system aspergillosis. Analysis of 26 patients. J Neuroimaging 1994;4:123-129.
58. Rumboldt Z, Castillo M. Indolent intracranial mucormycosis: case report. AJNR Am J Neuroradiol 2002;23:932-934.
59. Kim DG, Hong SC, Kim HJ, et al. Cerebral aspergillosis in immunologically competent patients. Surg Neurol 1993;40:326-331.
60. Chuck SL, Sande MA. Infections with Cryptococcus neoformans in the acquired immunodeficiency syndrome. N Engl J Med 1989;321:794-799.
61. Jones GA, Nathwani D. Cryptococcal meningitis. Br J Hosp Med 1995;54:439-445.
62. White MH, Armstrong D. Cryptococcosis. Infect Dis Clin North Am 1994;8:383-398.
63. Fish DG, Ampel NM, Galgiani JN, et al. Coccidioidomycosis during human immunodeficiency virus infection. A review of 77 patients. Medicine (Baltimore) 1990;69:384-391.
64. Banuelos AF, Williams PL, Johnson RH, et al. Central nervous system abscesses due to Coccidioides species. Clin Infect Dis 1996;22:240-250.
65. Mischel PS, Vinters HV. Coccidioidomycosis of the central nervous system: neuropathological and vasculopathic manifestations and clinical correlates. Clin Infect Dis 1995;20:400-405.

66. Friedman JA, Wijdicks EF, Fulgham JR, Wright AJ. Meningoencephalitis due to Blastomyces dermatidis: case report and literature review. Mayo Clin Proc 2000;75:403-408.
67. Tang TT, Marsik F,J Harb JM, Williams JE, Frommell GT, Dunn DK. Cerebral blastomycosis: an immunodiagnostic study. Am J Clin Pathol 1984;82:243-246.
68. Noujaim SE, Rossi MD, Rao SK, et al. CT and MR imaging of neurocysticercosis. AJR Am J Roentgenol 1999;173:1485-1490.
69. Martinez AJ, Visvesvara GS. Free-living, amphizoic and opportunistic amebas. Brain Pathol 1997;7:583-598.
70. Gardner HA, Martinez AJ, Visvesvara GS, Sotrel A. Granulomatous amebic encephalitis in an AIDS patient. Neurology 1991;41:1993-1995.
71. Seidel JS, Harmatz P, Visvesvara GS, Cohen A, Edwards J, Turner J. Successful treatment of primary amebic meningoencephalitis. N Engl J Med 1982;306:346-348.
72. Shirabe T, Monobe Y, Visvesvara GS. An autopsy case of amebic meningoencephalitis. The first Japanese case caused by Balamuthia mandrillaris. Neuropathology 2002;22:213-217.
73. Bassett R, Lowenberg K. Cerebral schistosomiasis. J Neuopathol Exp Neurol 1949;8:220-225.
74. Scrimgeour EM, Gajdusek DC. Involvement of the central nervous system in Schistosoma mansoni and S. haematobium infection. A review. Brain 1985;108(Pt 4):1023-1038.
75. Preidler KW, Riepl T, Szolar D, Ranner G. Cerebral schistosomiasis: MR and CT appearance. AJNR Am J Neuroradiol 1996;17:1598-1600.
76. Turner G. Cerebral malaria. Brain Pathol 1997;7: 569-582.
77. Oo MM, Aikawa M, Than T, et al. Human cerebral malaria: a pathologic study. J Neuropathol Exp Neurol 1987;47:223-231.
78. Millan JM, San Millan JM, Munoz M, Navas E, Lopez-Velez R. CNS complications in acute malaria: MR findings. AJNR Am J Neuroradiol 1993;14:493-494.

8 INFLAMMATORY DISEASES

The disease processes considered in this chapter share many clinical and pathologic features. In addition, their differential diagnoses nearly always include infectious processes and often neoplastic hematologic processes. These entities primarily present as mass lesions, and are separated on that basis from other inflammatory processes such as paraneoplastic processes (see chapter 10), Rasmussen encephalitis (see chapter 13), or other encephalitic diseases (see chapter 7).

Primary inflammatory diseases of the central nervous system (CNS) may involve the brain parenchyma (sometimes with a specific predilection for certain areas), the meninges (either leptomeninges or pachymeninges), the overlying skull, or a combination of these sites. The location of the lesion may guide the diagnosis, but cannot be relied upon to exclude most entities. Exceptions to this include, for example, the changes associated with intracranial hypotension, which are restricted to the dura mater. Many of these inflammatory processes are more commonly encountered at systemic sites; when CNS disease occurs in the setting of systemic involvement, the pattern may steer the clinician and pathologist toward a correct diagnosis.

The most critical decision to make regarding an apparent inflammatory lesion is to exclude an infectious or neoplastic process. Intraoperative consultation may be essential for the proper diagnosis of these disorders, enabling appropriate processing of tissues for additional studies both by the surgeon (sending tissue directly from the operating room to the microbiology laboratory) and by the pathologist. The final diagnostic decisions in the assessment of primary inflammatory diseases often combine diagnostic information from a mixture of microbiologic, light microscopic, including immunohistochemical, electron microscopic, and molecular diagnostic studies. Because the treatment of many of these entities involves a degree of immunosuppression, the exclusion of infectious processes is important in clinical decision making.

When the pathologic findings suggest an inflammatory process, preliminary information needs to be communicated in a timely manner to the relevant physicians involved in the patient's care. This is particularly true for dural-based lesions, which are often diagnosed preoperatively as meningioma. Since microbiology specimens are best submitted directly from the operative room, it is important to communicate the suggestion to prepare samples for culture during the ongoing surgical procedure. In the interval between intraoperative consultation and the final diagnosis, information must also be exchanged with physicians from other relevant clinical services as well as with pathologists with other expertise.

GENERAL DIAGNOSTIC APPROACH

The lesions considered here are those that present as a mass lesion or, in the case of some of skull lesions, a destructive process. The initial preoperative diagnosis usually includes more common mass lesions, such as meningioma or metastatic tumor. When an inflammatory process is unexpectedly diagnosed, optimally at the time of frozen section since surgical resection may not be fully indicated for some of these lesions, then the broader clinical exam, radiologic findings, and history are reexamined. In some settings, such as the solitary skull lesions of Langerhans cell histiocytosis, there may be a high degree of clinical suspicion of the correct diagnosis but surgery represents part of an appropriate therapeutic approach.

Clinical and Radiologic Findings

Knowledge of the clinical, laboratory, and imaging findings is particularly important for the accurate diagnostic evaluation of inflammatory lesions, and must be used as a complement to the histologic examination. The parameters that are informative and contributory toward a diagnosis, both in a positive and negative sense, include the peripheral markers of an inflammatory processes (e.g., sedimentation rate, C-reactive protein levels, angiotensin-converting enzyme [ACE] levels) as well as evidence of systemic involvement (e.g., pulmonary masses, lymphadenopathy, bony lesions).

Gross Findings

Although the gross appearance of a lesion does not provide major diagnostic information in the setting of brain biopsies, diagnostically useful findings may be gleaned from the appearance of dural lesions. Inflammatory lesions, although often containing a significant amount of reactive collagen deposition, are usually softer than many meningiomas or metastatic carcinomas. In addition, inflammatory cells, often with moderate to large numbers of histiocytes, may give the lesion a yellow hue.

Intraoperative Diagnosis

As is true for nearly all neuropathologic specimens, frozen section and touch/smear preparations are useful for the evaluation of inflammatory lesions. Smear preparations provide far greater cytologic detail than frozen section, which can be beneficial when assessing the cellular components of a lesion, particularly for the characterization of inflammatory cells (e.g., histiocytes). On the other hand, the architectural information that is gained from frozen section specimens provides equally important information (e.g., granuloma formation).

In addition to the routine hematoxylin and eosin (H&E) stain for frozen section specimens, water-based stains such as toluidine blue provide significant additional information. Water-based stains highlight macrophages because of the refractive appearance of the cytoplasmic lipid droplets in these cells, which exclude the stain, especially when histiocytes are few in number. Since there may be sampling differences between tissues used for frozen section and smear, the use of both smears and frozen sections, coupled with special stains on frozen section specimens, increases the likelihood of recognizing histiocytes.

Since the majority of inflammatory diseases require considerable workup, a firm diagnosis is usually not possible at the time of intraoperative consultation. Nonetheless, the "surprise diagnosis" of a possible inflammatory lesion mandates a conversation between the pathologist and the neurosurgeon for two main reasons: the neurosurgeon needs to be informed so that samples can be sent directly from the operating room for microbiologic studies, and the pathologist needs as much information as possible to determine appropriate processing of tissues.

Microscopic Findings

Although the various entities considered in this chapter have their own specific features, the presence of a mixture of inflammatory cells is their unifying aspect. To recognize and classify these diseases appropriately, it is essential to identify three major aspects of these lesions. The first is the specific cellular composition of the lesion. For instance, when histiocytic cells appear to be present, there is the possibility of Langerhans dendritic cells, which can be confirmed by immunohistochemistry and electron microscopy; alternatively, these cells may be true histiocytes in other lesions. The other cellular elements of the lesion can be nearly as informative about the general category of disease. The second essential element is the architecture. Well-formed granulomas must be contrasted with poorly formed granulomas; nongranulomatous patterns of inflammation are also commonly encountered. Finally, other specific histologic features, including the presence of necrosis and the relationship to blood vessels, should be evaluated.

Although the H&E stain remains the core of the diagnostic evaluation of inflammatory processes, particularly when combined with the immunohistochemical studies considered below, specific stains for organisms play an important role. The application of stains for bacteria (including tissue Gram stain equivalents, silver impregnations for spirochetes, stains for mycobacteria) and fungi is an essential step toward making a "diagnosis of exclusion," such as sarcoidosis. Stains for organisms, even when evaluated carefully in the context of appropriate positive controls, are only informative if positive; histologic staining for organisms has a lower level of sensitivity than culture or molecular diagnostic approaches. For this reason, failure to demonstrate the presence of a pathogen with appropriate staining is not overwhelming evidence of the absence of that particular agent as an underlying cause of the lesion.

Immunohistochemical Findings

Immunophenotyping has had a major influence on the classification of inflammatory diseases. Immunophenotyping is critical for distinguishing macrophages and other histiocytic-appearing cells, such as the Langerhans dendritic cell, although the exclusion of evidence of lymphoid malignancy as well as some forms of infection follows close behind. There may be significant benefit to retaining frozen tissue or to fixing tissue with methods other than buffered formalin, in keeping with local preferences for the relevant immunohistochemical studies. Among the key epitopes that are informative are S-100 protein, CD1a, and CD68; in addition, the full panoply of hematopathologic reagents often comes into use for the characterization of the components of the inflammatory infiltrate and for the exclusion of patterns associated with malignancy. Finally, because many of these lesions, when arising in the dura, are diagnosed preoperatively as meningioma, immunohistochemistry for markers such as epithelial membrane antigen (EMA) is used to evaluate the possibility of an underlying meningioma.

Ultrastructural Findings

Langerhans cell histiocytosis is one of the few diseases with a specific diagnostic abnormality that can be recognized only by electron microscopy. Ultrastructural identification of Birbeck granules had been a critical cornerstone of the diagnosis of this disease, but over the past two decades such studies have been supplanted by immunohistochemistry. Nonetheless, when adequate tissue is available, it is appropriate to consider fixation of small samples for potential electron microscopy. It is usual to refrain from processing such tissues, however, until light microscopic evaluation has been completed.

Laboratory and Molecular Findings. Microbiologic evaluation is often critical in the evaluation of inflammatory lesions, since some of these entities are diagnosed only after the exclusion of infection. This may require a wide range of cultures, as, for example, with sarcoidosis which may mimic mycobacterial and fungal granulomatous infections. With the increasing availability of molecular diagnostic approaches to infectious diseases, the long delay previously associated with difficult-to-culture and slow growing pathogens is now circumvented in some settings.

Flow cytometry may also play a role in the analysis of the inflammatory infiltrate, for example, to detect small populations of cells with combinations of epitopes that are usually interpreted as evidence of inappropriate marker expression. Similarly, searching for evidence of clonality of either B cells, through the examination of immunoglobulin gene rearrangements, or of T cells, with T-cell receptor (TCR) gene rearrangements, can be important for the evaluation of possible lymphoid malignancies. While clonality studies considered in this chapter have been pursued recently, such work remains investigational rather than of diagnostic importance.

Treatment and Prognosis. The absence of a clear understanding of the etiology of many of these lesions has not stood in the way of the development of relatively effective therapies. Since the disease coming to neuropathologic attention may be part of a multiorgan illness, therapies are often systemic. Various regimens of steroids and other immunosuppressive agents form the mainstay of treatment. Surgical approaches to therapy, such as curettage as in the case of solitary skull lesions of Langerhans cell histiocytosis, also contribute significantly to patient management. Similarly, there is often a role for the resection of discrete dural-based masses that have come to clinical attention because of symptoms referable to compression of underlying brain regions. Patients with the disorders considered in this chapter have a range of long-term prognoses, and even with specific entities, there may be significant variation in the clinical course and outcome.

PROCESSES WITH DISCRETE MASS LESIONS: GRANULOMATOUS LESIONS

Well-formed granulomas, either as discrete individual lesions or in the broader context of an inflammatory reaction, raise the possibility of several diagnostic entities when encountered in the brain and meninges. As is true in other sites in the body, exclusion of an infectious process remains the combined obligation of the pathologist and other physicians involved in the care of the patient. The standard battery of special stains and culture methods has been expanded over the recent past through the introduction both of immunohistochemical methods for some pathogens and the application of molecular methods. Polymerase chain reaction (PCR)-based pathogen detection from the cerebrospinal fluid (CSF) may occur prior to biopsy, and may preclude the need for tissue acquisition; alternatively, it may be performed on fresh or frozen tissue.

Apart from the infections that elicit a granulomatous response, the diseases that involve the brain and meninges considered here are sarcoidosis (often termed neurosarcoid), rheumatoid disease, and inflammatory pseudotumor (inflammatory myofibroblastic tumor). The granulomatous features of these diseases extend across the spectrum of this pattern of inflammation, with sarcoidosis demonstrating the classic well-formed noncaseating granulomas, rheumatoid disease showing necrobiosis with granulomatous inflammation around the edge, and pseudotumor featuring poorly formed granulomas. The histiocytoses may also show a granulomatous pattern, but these entities are distinguished by their specific cell types.

Sarcoidosis

Definition. Well known to pathologists because of its common presentation outside of the nervous system, *sarcoidosis* is an idiopathic disease recognized by the presence of noncaseating granulomas, often with widespread multiorgan involvement. Although CNS involvement (*neurosarcoidosis*) is an infrequent feature of the disease, it is usually a marker of aggressive disease.

General Comments. Often encountered by the general pathologist, sarcoidosis can involve the CNS in a variety of ways and in a variety of contexts. It is the combination of the setting and clinical findings that influences how likely lesions are to be biopsied as part of the evaluation; unfortunately for the pathologist, it is most commonly in those settings in which sarcoidosis is a less prominent entity in the differential diagnosis that it is encountered under the microscope (1). When sarcoidosis is known to involve other organs, presumptive neurosarcoid is often not biopsied. These lesions do, however, sometimes come to neurosurgical and pathologic attention if the clinical course does not follow the expected response to therapy. Pathologic examination in this setting may reveal neurosarcoid that was unresponsive to therapy or another entity from the clinical and imaging differential diagnosis.

Clinical Features. Sarcoidosis is a form of inappropriate immunologic response, dominated by a Th1 type constellation of immune cells and cytokines, resulting in the formation of granulomas in various organs. While a variety of inciting agents, including different potential pathogens and environmental exposures, has been assessed, there remains great uncertainty as to what serves as the trigger for this process. The varying incidences of the disease across ethnic groups as well as population- and family-based genetic studies suggest that there is a moderate heritable risk to developing the disease. These observations have been based on patient populations without a specific focus on neurosarcoidosis; there is little in the literature to suggest that patients with significant neurologic involvement differ from others with sarcoidosis.

With an overall average incidence rate estimated at 40 to 60/100,000 population, sarcoidosis is a relatively common illness; African-Americans and Scandinavians have an even higher incidence of the disease. There are several lines of evidence suggesting that there is a constellation of genetic risk factors that influence disease development, including studies linking distinct immunological loci in different populations and the well-documented increased risk of disease in first-degree relatives of affected individuals. Awareness of the appropriate high-risk populations can assist the pathologist in raising the possibility of a diagnosis of sarcoidosis, when the histologic findings are appropriate.

Well recognized for its pulmonary involvement, the frequency of neurologic involvement in sarcoidosis has been estimated in some clinical series as 5 to 15 percent of cases. This has been suggested to reflect an underrecognition of the disease burden, as a comparison between autopsy findings with the clinical diagnosis has suggested that only half of the cases of neurosarcoidosis are clinically evident (1).

In general, sarcoidosis presents in patients in the third to fifth decades, with some additional later spikes of incidence in specific ethnic groups. When the neurologic symptoms result in initial presentation, nearly all patients also have evidence of systemic disease. Conversely, 10 to 30 percent of individuals presenting with systemic sarcoidosis have neurologic involvement, if sought aggressively (2). The presence of isolated neurosarcoidosis, while extremely uncommon, represents the most problematic clinical situation and the one in which pathologic evaluation has the most to offer.

Cranial neuropathies are the most common manifestations of symptomatic neurosarcoidosis, although they rarely require biopsy for diagnosis. Involvement of cranial nerve VII, which may be bilateral, dominates the overall pattern of presentations. Multiple cranial nerves may be involved. There is little data available regarding the underlying pathologic mechanisms, but both direct involvement of the nerves as well as entrapment from involvement of the basal meninges and dura mater have been implicated. Other peripheral neuropathies can be observed in these patients, with small fiber neuropathies more common than large fiber ones. Involvement of these particular axons may result in pain or autonomic dysfunction; while the former may be disturbing to the patient, the latter can be associated with cardiac arrhythmias.

Although often grouped with the cranial neuropathies, optic nerve involvement has a closer relationship to the less common phenomenon of parenchymal involvement, as it is a discrete white matter tract of the CNS, with oligodendrocyte-derived myelin rather than Schwann cell myelin. Optic nerve involvement is less commonly bilateral than the other cranial neuropathies, and, particularly in young women, may suggest multiple sclerosis or Devic disease (neuromyelitis optica) when there is concurrent spinal cord involvement. While the response to immunosuppressive therapy may not distinguish between sarcoidosis and these demyelinating disorders, the presence of other systemic evidence of a granulomatous disease may be helpful.

The mass lesions of sarcoidosis may involve the dura and thus mimic meningioma, with symptoms referable to the site of involvement and associated compressive effects on adjacent brain or spinal cord or vascular elements. Dural-based lesions are sometimes multiple and do not show the same predilection for the basal skull region that is observed with parenchymal disease. Within the brain itself, the regions of the hypothalamus and pituitary gland are among the more common sites of symptomatic involvement, perhaps overrepresented because of the high likelihood of adequate symptoms to prompt neurologic and endocrinologic evaluation. There are also described cases of relatively rapid cognitive impairment or psychiatric symptoms in patients with widespread systemic sarcoidosis, which has been interpreted as reflecting widespread cortical involvement. Presentation of neurosarcoidosis is relatively uncommon among pediatric patients, but in this group there is an increase in presentation with mass lesions and seizures as compared to peripheral neuropathies (3).

Radiologic Findings. The advent of magnetic resonance imaging (MRI) increased the detection of neurosarcoidosis in patients with systemic involvement but without clear neurologic symptoms. The relatively characteristic patterns of signal intensity for sarcoidosis involving various brain structures have added to the preoperative diagnostic accuracy. Dural masses commonly show low signal intensity on T2-weighted images, which helps distinguish them from meningiomas, and they usually show homogeneous contrast enhancement on T1-weighted images. This same pattern of T1 enhancement can be seen with leptomeningeal and parenchymal disease as well.

Gross Findings. Surgical specimens from patients with neurosarcoidosis may be small, and are typically unremarkable grossly. When dural-based masses of neurosarcoid are resected because of a presumptive diagnosis of meningioma or other tumor, the lesions are yellow to white, depending on the degree of fibrosis present. The fibrosis also affects the relative firmness of the lesion. None of these features are predictable enough to discriminate between sarcoidosis and other lesions. Mass lesions can also be present in the leptomeninges and may be difficult to separate from the adjacent brain (fig. 8-1).

Intraoperative Diagnosis. When confronted with a dural mass of mildly fibrotic consistency, neurosurgeons are likely to assume that the lesion is a meningioma. When seen by the pathologist, the frozen section appearance of noncaseating granulomas should suggest the possibility of sarcoid involvement of the dura. With smear preparations, the typical meningothelial cells are absent, and instead, there is

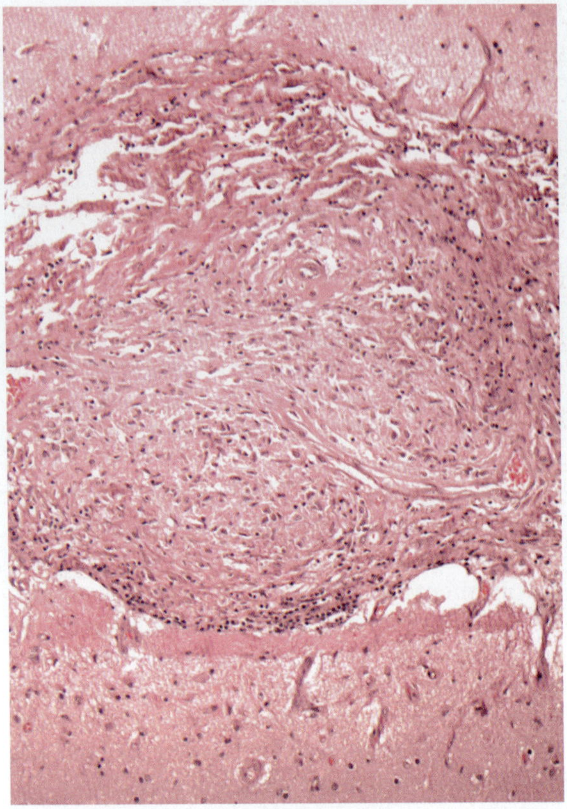

Figure 8-1

NEUROSARCOIDOSIS

Granulomas and nodules of fibrosis are in the leptomeninges.

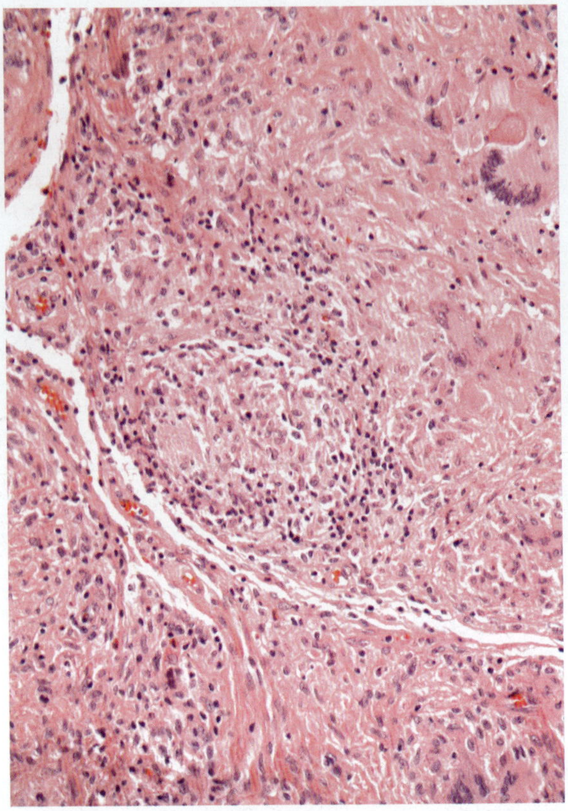

Figure 8-2

NEUROSARCOIDOSIS

Multiple noncaseating granulomas with a fibrous reaction characterize the lesion.

a mixed inflammatory background of disrupted granulomas—large histiocytic cells and small round lymphocytes. If there is significant fibrosis, it may be difficult to smear the specimen and this method may not yield a useful slide. An appropriately prepared smear from a meningioma, even a densely fibrotic meningioma, nearly always liberates some individual meningothelial cells. When present in this context, they are best found at the distal edge of the smear, sometimes right at the end of the slide.

Microscopic Findings. As elsewhere in the body, the defining pathologic lesion of sarcoidosis is the noncaseating granuloma (fig. 8-2). The central portion of the lesion contains a moderate number of epithelioid histiocytes, sometimes with the nonspecific cytoplasmic findings of asteroid bodies or stellate inclusions (fig. 8-3). These histiocytes are surrounded by a well-defined border of small round lymphocytes, sometimes with occasional plasma cells and macrophages (fig. 8-4). There can be a variable degree of fibrosis around the granuloma, with mass lesions often containing moderate amounts of paucicellular fibrous tissue. The overall architecture of the lesion sometimes is highlighted by a trichrome stain, which reveals the confluent nodular organization of the mass.

When present within the leptomeninges or the cerebral parenchyma, the granulomas often sit adjacent to the wall of a blood vessel, typically a small arteriole, but only rarely involve the full circumference of the vessel (figs. 8-5–8-7). It may be appropriate to consider these granulomas to be paravascular rather than perivascular (fig. 8-8). When the disease has been present for a prolonged period of time, there is often fibrosis as the cytokine profile evolves, and in some situations, nodules of fibrosis are the only remaining finding (fig. 8-9).

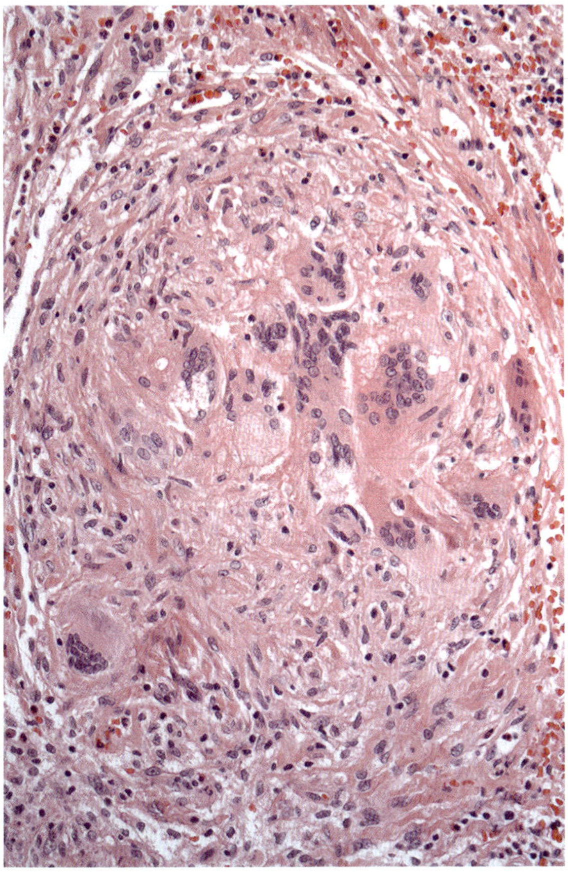

Figure 8-3

NEUROSARCOIDOSIS

Numerous multinucleated giant cells with nonspecific inclusion bodies are seen.

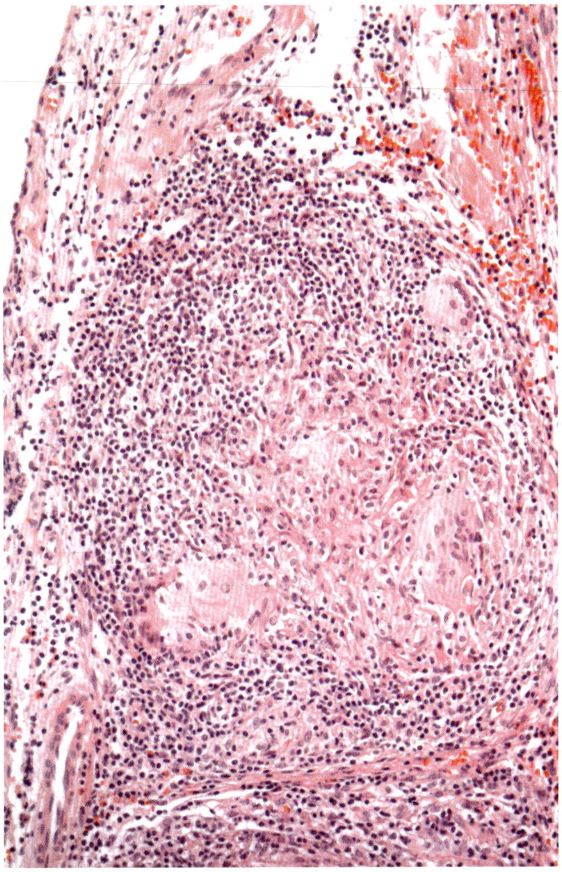

Figure 8-4

NEUROSARCOIDOSIS

A lymphocytic infiltrate is seen at the periphery of a well-formed granuloma.

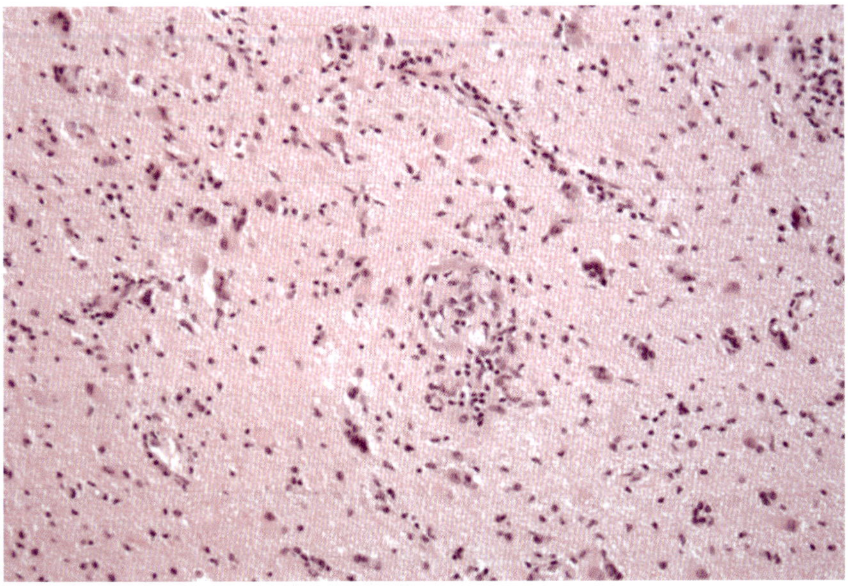

Figure 8-5

NEUROSARCOIDOSIS

A perivascular small granuloma is in the superficial cortex. Scattered perivascular inflammation is evident elsewhere. Reactive astrocytes are also present.

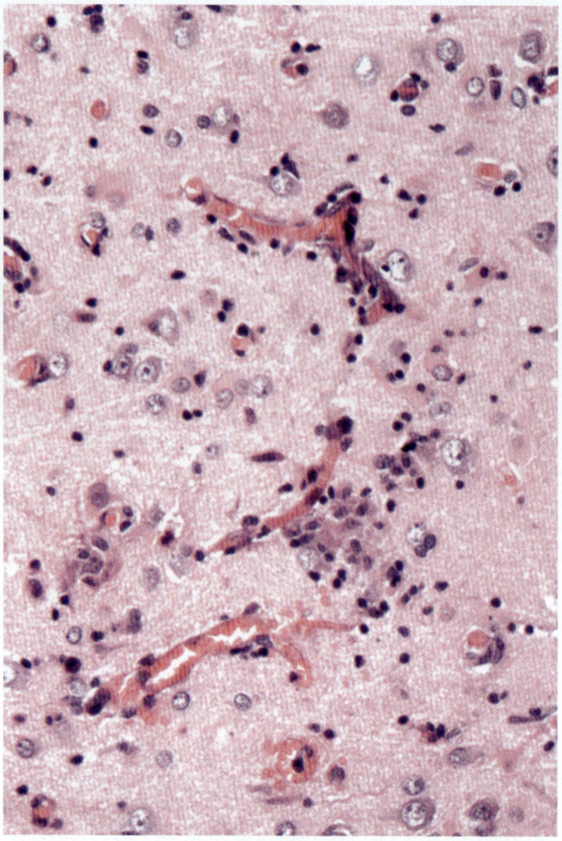

Figure 8-6

NEUROSARCOIDOSIS

Poorly organized collections of histiocytes, lymphocytes, and plasma cells are adjacent to intraparenchymal vessels.

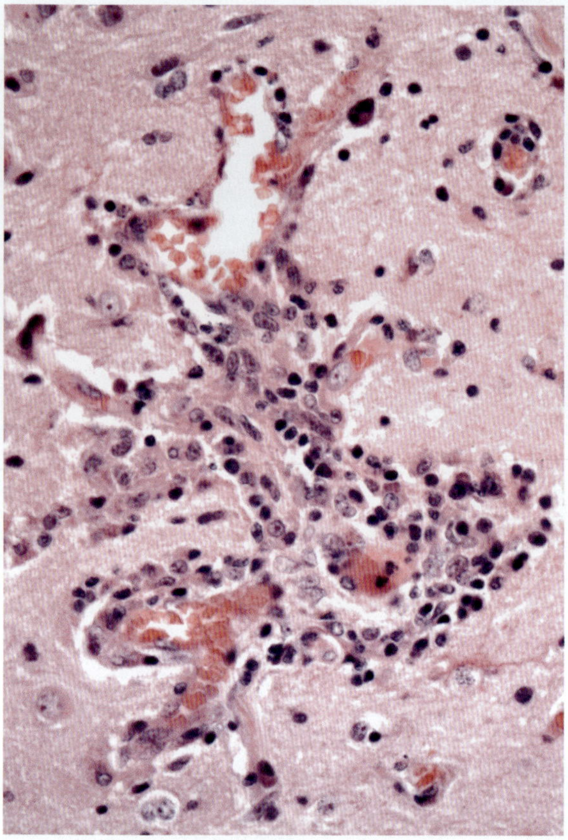

Figure 8-7

NEUROSARCOIDOSIS

Although the pattern suggests vasculitis, there is not necrosis of the vessel wall.

While necrosis at the center of a granuloma usually heralds the presence of an infectious agent, it may be found in sarcoidosis occasionally (figs. 8-10, 8-11). This is most commonly observed as a focal finding, in a sea of otherwise noncaseating granulomas. The presence of granulomatous inflammation, independent of the tissue integrity at the center of the lesion, should elicit a search for a pathogen by the pathologist. The most typical suspects are mycobacteria and fungi, and a combination of special staining, microbiology, and molecular diagnostics may be required to exclude them with confidence.

Immunohistochemical Findings. There are no specific markers that allow the identification of granulomas as being definitively associated with sarcoidosis. Instead, characterization of the cellular components of the distinctive lesions of the disease is important primarily for the exclusion of lesions that contain other histiocytic cells. The granulomas of sarcoidosis should be recognizable without the need to resort to immunohistochemical methods to demonstration the presence of CD68-positive histiocytes surrounded by predominantly CD4-positive T cells. The exclusion of infectious agents can be facilitated through the use of immunohistochemical methods, although the combination of standard special stains, culture, and molecular approaches dominates in this arena.

Laboratory Findings. Although elevated ACE levels in peripheral blood remain a hallmark of the diagnosis of sarcoidosis, attempts to make comparable use of ACE within the CSF as a marker for neurosarcoidosis have not been successful. The general consensus currently is that CSF ACE levels have overall low specificity and

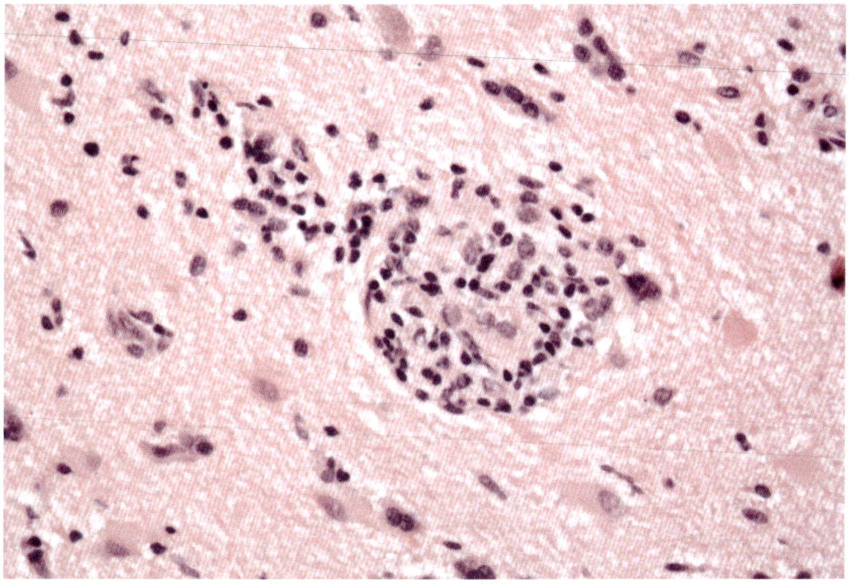

Figure 8-8

NEUROSARCOIDOSIS

Small granulomas extend into the parenchyma, away from blood vessels.

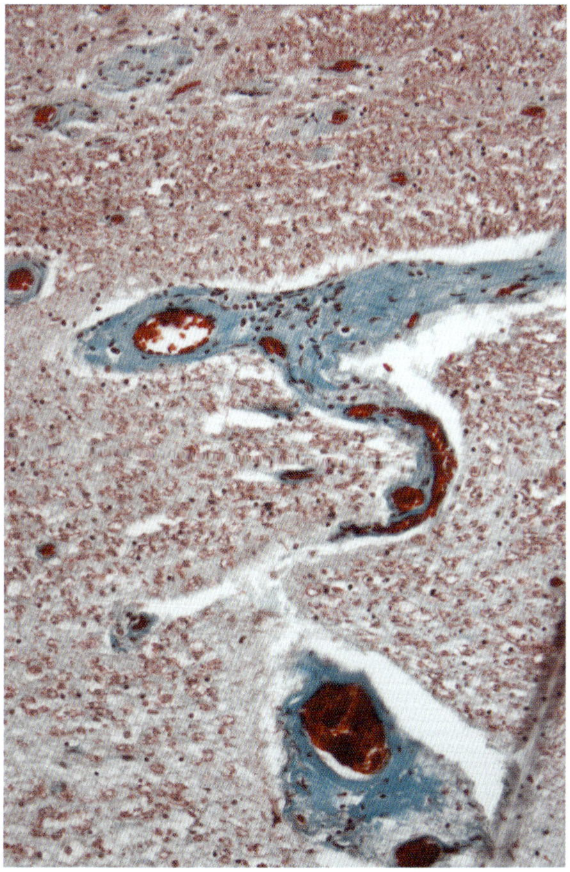

Figure 8-9

NEUROSARCOIDOSIS

As disease becomes inactive, the granulomas become sclerotic and hypocellular (trichrome stain).

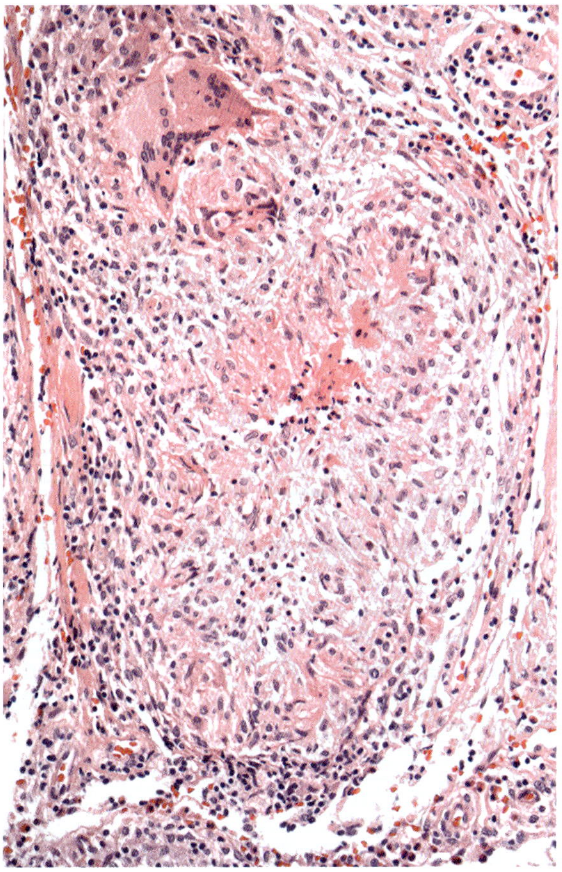

Figure 8-10

NEUROSARCOIDOSIS

Although uncommon, necrosis is found in granulomas on occasion.

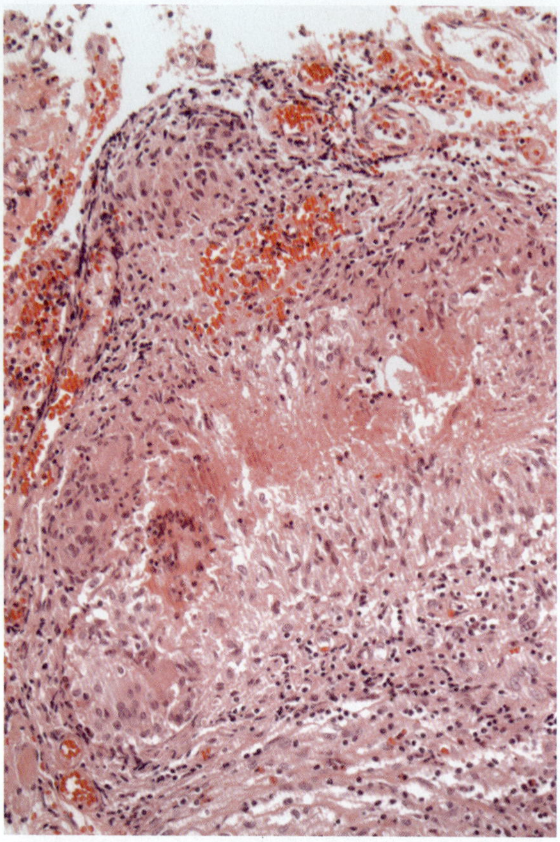

Figure 8-11

NEUROSARCOIDOSIS

The necrosis appears noncaseating.

sensitivity, with little role in the diagnosis of neurosarcoid (4,5). There may be a role for them in the assessment of disease progression once the diagnosis is established, although this needs to be balanced against the less invasive measures of skilled neurologic examination combined with appropriate serial imaging.

Differential Diagnosis. Determination of the differential diagnosis of the patient with neurosarcoid is influenced by whether there is evidence of sarcoidosis elsewhere in the body and by the presence of pathologic material from the CNS. When the diagnosis of systemic sarcoidosis is well established, the development of (or search for) neurologic symptoms may lead to studies that reveal the presence of a presumptive lesion of neurosarcoidosis. Such lesions have, in the absence of a tissue diagnosis of noncaseating granulomas, been suggested to meet criteria for probable neurosarcoidosis if there is exclusion of other likely causes for an otherwise typical lesion or presentation of neurosarcoid along with some evidence of inflammation within the CNS (1,6). Patients with sarcoidosis may also have other diseases, so if these presumptive lesions do not show the expected clinical features of neurosarcoid, subsequent efforts to obtain tissue for pathologic examination may be justified.

If a neurosurgical specimen demonstrates the typical findings of a noncaseating granuloma, then the differential diagnosis will depend on the site of involvement (2). If a dural mass lesion is sampled, then infectious agents need to be excluded; this remains true when there is systemic evidence of sarcoidosis, because of the potential for intercurrent infection, especially if there has been exogenous immunosuppressive therapy. With the parenchymal lesions of paravascular granulomas, the differential diagnosis includes granulomatous vasculitides such as Wegener granulomatosis, granulomatous angiitis of the nervous system (GANS), and cerebral amyloid angiopathy with granulomatous reaction. These can be distinguished from neurosarcoidosis, which lacks the vascular wall fibrinoid necrosis and the amyloid deposition of the last.

Treatment and Prognosis. Although systemic sarcoidosis often shows spontaneous remission, with as many as two thirds of patients having this desirable course within their first 2 years of disease (7), the increased morbidity and mortality associated with the presence of neurologic involvement, particularly in those patients with spinal cord involvement (6), typically prompts early and, often, more aggressive therapy. Recurrences are seen in many cases even after spontaneous remission.

In general, corticosteroids (at higher doses than used in cases without neurologic involvement) form the basis of initial therapy. Increasingly aggressive forms of immunosuppression may be needed. For lesions that are the most refractory to these approaches, data suggest a possible role for radiation therapy. Neurosurgery, apart from its role in assisting diagnosis, is most beneficial for altering the course of disease in cases of spinal cord compression from discrete masses or in the resection of treatment-resistant symptomatic masses elsewhere around the nervous system.

Rheumatoid Disease

Definition. Although most commonly considered a disease with symptoms referable to the joints, with inflammation and tissue injury, *rheumatoid arthritis* (RA) may affect the brain in any of several forms. Findings may be present in the pachymeninges (most commonly as dural nodules, with histologic features similar to the more common subcutaneous nodules of RA), leptomeninges (most commonly as a lymphocytic infiltrate presenting as aseptic meningitis), parenchyma (as vasculitis), or a combination of these.

General Comments. RA is a common disease, affecting roughly 1 percent of the population, yet direct involvement of the CNS is a rare complication. The presentations, pathologies, and diagnostic issues considered here exclude those in which the effects of RA on the nervous system are manifest through the inflammation, tissue proliferation, and eventual destruction of synovial surfaces. Involvement of the spine represents the most critical pattern of impact of RA on the CNS, and those processes that involve the upper cervical spine (in particular, at the atlantoaxial joint) have the potential for catastrophic impingement on the spinal cord (8).

Clinical Features. Involvement of the brain and its coverings may occur early in the course of RA, but is more commonly observed in patients with a longstanding disease, often for more than a decade. Although there is a strong overall female predominance among cases of RA, there is much less of a gender difference when it comes to CNS involvement. At the time of presentation with neurologic signs and symptoms referable to rheumatoid disease, not all patients have active disease elsewhere: in one series, only roughly half showed active synovitis at the time of CNS presentation, with a larger fraction having subcutaneous nodules (9).

When RA gives rise to disease within the brain and its coverings, multiple forms of pathology are observed. There is usually some combination of rheumatoid nodules (which are histologically similar to those that are found in traumatized subcutaneous areas), mild chronic leptomeningitis, and vasculitis. As would be expected, the nodules, which are typically located in the dura, mimic meningioma in many respects (10). They give rise to symptoms based primarily on the mass effect related to compression of underlying regions of the brain. Similar lesions have been described within the choroid plexus (11,12) and even within meningiomas (13).

When the presentation is dominated by the more diffuse processes of inflammation in the meninges and is associated with vessels, there are the expected diffuse symptoms of headache and altered mental status. It has been suggested that, even in the absence of complaints, there may be cognitive impairments in patients with RA which can be elicited with formal testing and may be associated with parenchymal changes (14). From a series that included several cases in which the diagnosis of RA involvement of the nervous system was made only at autopsy in asymptomatic individuals, it was observed that vasculitis did not appear to be present without causing symptoms; this suggests that vasculitis is an important pathologic mechanism of CNS injury rather than a nonspecific accompaniment to the underlying illness (9). It is also important to recognize that methotrexate, one of the more common agents used in the treatment of patients with RA (15), can itself result in a set of diffuse symptoms that resemble those of direct involvement of the CNS (16). As the effects of methotrexate on cognitive function are typically reversible, it should be possible to exclude this effect without needing to proceed to a neurosurgical procedure.

Radiologic Findings. As would be expected, rheumatoid nodules of the dura fall into a broad differential diagnosis centered on meningioma and its mimics. Dural involvement by RA typically shows contrast enhancement with imaging studies; it is hypointense compared to brain with T1-weighted sequences and hyperintense with T2-weighted sequences. In general, there are commonly white matter abnormalities and cortical atrophy in patients who come to neurologic attention because of cognitive or other diffuse symptoms, but the existence of such findings of similar frequency and severity in controls as well as RA patients raises some questions about the specificity of such findings (17).

Gross Findings. As would be expected from the imaging findings and the histologic changes, the involved dura is typically thickened. The necrobiotic zone at the center of a rheumatoid nodule may not be easily appreciated on gross examination.

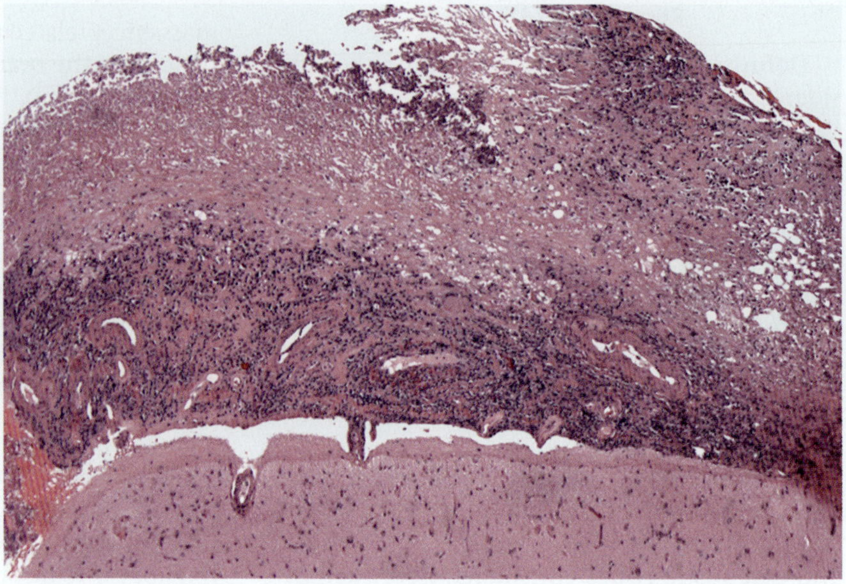

Figure 8-12

RHEUMATOID DISEASE

The combination of areas of abundant inflammatory cells and zones of necrosis characterizes these lesions.

Intraoperative Diagnosis. Specimens that represent CNS involvement by RA are most likely to be dural masses that have mimicked meningioma or other tumors. The central areas of necrosis and the organized layers of surrounding inflammatory elements should allow the adequately prepared mind to recognize the lesion as likely to be a rheumatoid nodule. When this does not occur, the pathologist is most likely to focus on the presence of the necrotic material and the histiocytic response, with the subsequent alarms suggesting potential mycobacterial infection demanding attention. The helpful features of the lesion that can reassure the pathologist and neurosurgeon are often the overall size of the area of necrosis (larger in rheumatoid nodules than in many caseating granulomas) and the usual absence of nuclear debris within the necrosis.

Patients with RA often have an intrinsic degree of immunocompromise, with the superimposed effects of therapy. This increases the risk for reactivation of tuberculosis; thus, the existence of a known diagnosis of RA should not be taken as evidence of the absence of mycobacterial infection.

Microscopic Findings. The most characteristic and specific finding of RA is the rheumatoid nodule, typically occurring in the dura. As in other sites, these nodules are characterized by a central area of necrosis with surrounding layers of inflammatory cells (figs. 8-12, 8-13). The area of necrosis is typically large, with an irregular contour, and is characterized by the presence of degenerating material, without cell ghosts. This latter feature is helpful in distinguishing these nodules from areas of tumor necrosis. The surrounding cells are usually a layer of macrophages arranged in a loose palisade at the edge of the necrobiotic zone, surrounded by a second rim of lymphocytes and polyclonal plasma cells (figs. 8-14, 8-15).

In contrast to the rheumatoid nodules, which have a distinctive appearance that may be diagnostic once unusual infectious processes are excluded, the other manifestations of RA in the CNS are nonspecific. There can be an inflammatory leptomeningeal infiltrate, which is usually composed of lymphocytes and plasma cells (fig. 8-16), but may even contain neutrophils; a similar mixed infiltrate has been described in cases of parenchymal vasculitis (9).

Immunohistochemical Findings. There are no specific markers that identify these lesions as being a direct manifestation of rheumatoid disease. Instead, the role of immunohistochemical studies is predominantly for the exclusion of other diseases in the differential diagnosis, either unusual infectious agents or lymphoproliferative diseases.

Differential Diagnosis. When typical rheumatoid nodules are identified, and there is systemic evidence of RA, there are few entities in the differential diagnosis. Because of a predilection for the basal meninges, the other inflammatory

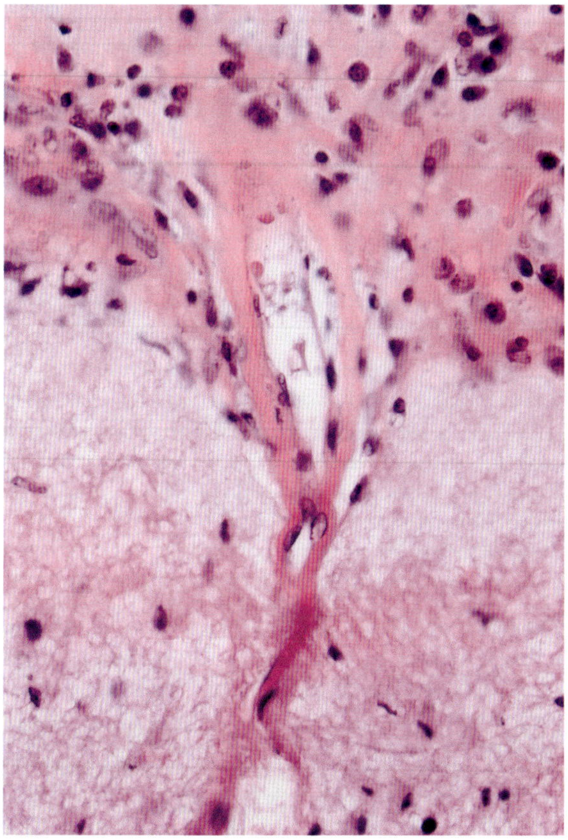

Figure 8-13

RHEUMATOID DISEASE

The inflammatory cell infiltrate involves leptomeninges and may extend into the parenchyma.

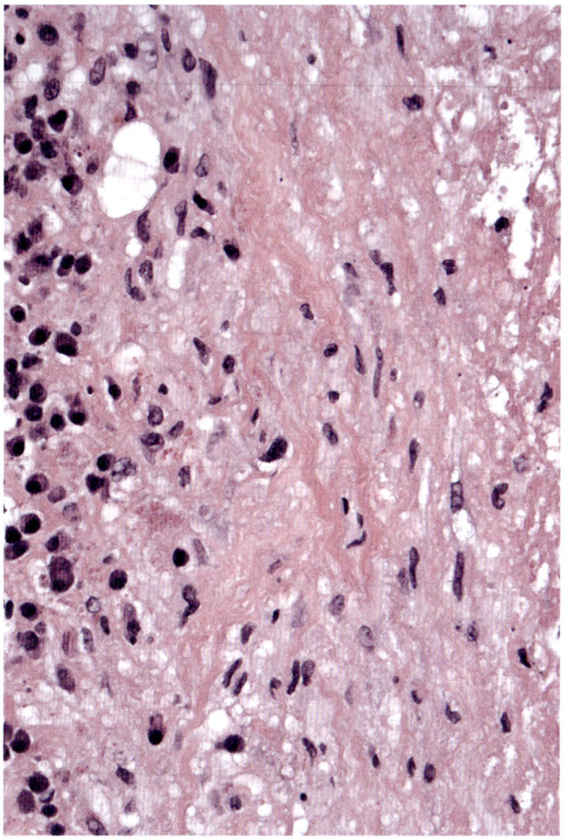

Figure 8-14

RHEUMATOID DISEASE

The transition between inflammation and necrosis is typically devoid of cellular debris, in contrast to an infectious process.

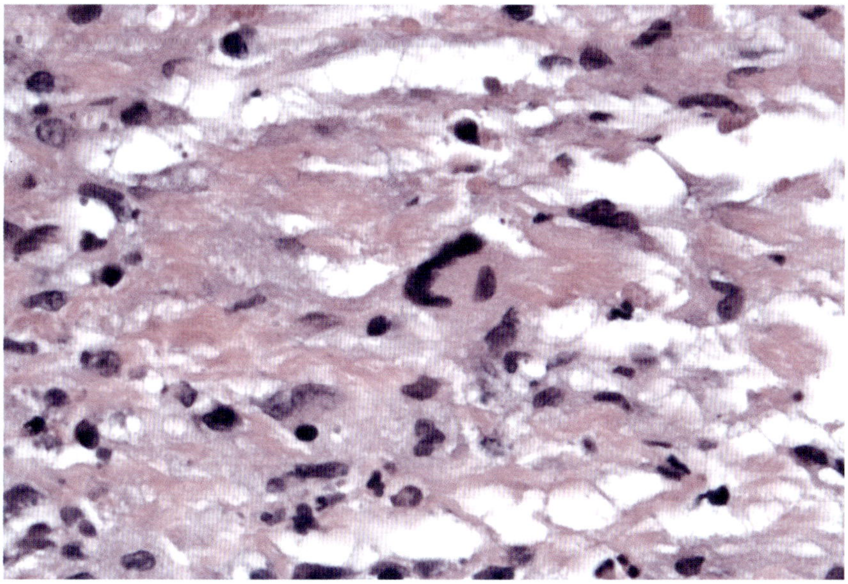

Figure 8-15

RHEUMATOID DISEASE

Occasional giant cells are present.

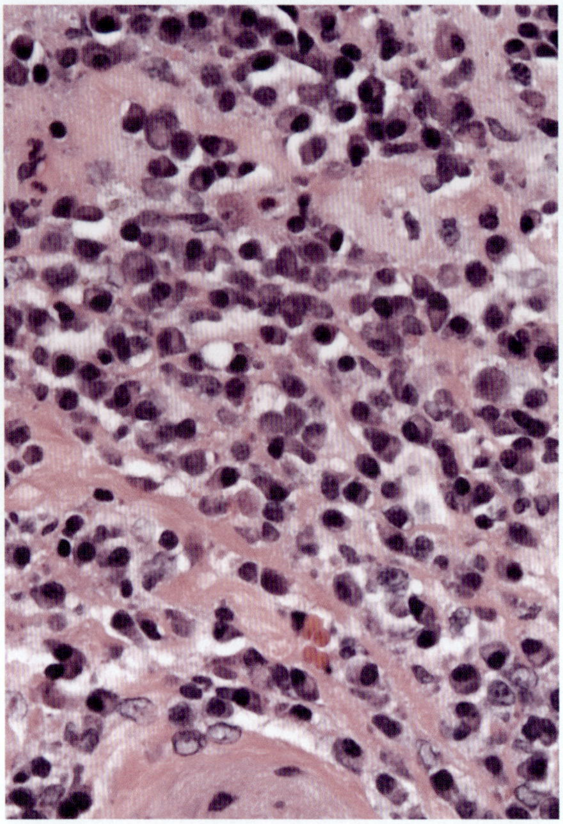

Figure 8-16

RHEUMATOID DISEASE

Plasma cell-rich areas of inflammation are common.

processes that tend to involve this region, such as sarcoidosis, tuberculosis, and some other infectious processes, need to be excluded. The pattern of the rheumatoid nodule is sufficiently characteristic that, in the proper clinical context, it is diagnosable. The need to exclude infectious processes derives from the therapeutic approaches; prior to significant immunosuppressive therapy, rigorous efforts should be made to eliminate the possibility of a missed diagnosis of an infectious process.

The problem is significantly more complex when the pathologist is confronted with the nonspecific meningitis or vasculitis that may be present. While a preexisting or newly recognized diagnosis of RA may reassure the pathologist that these histologic findings are a component of the rheumatoid disease, the absence of specificity requires that efforts be made to exclude other similar-appearing disease processes. In addition to a search for potential pathogens, as in the evaluation of any meningitis, the evaluation of vasculitis should include the assessment for the presence of amyloid in the affected vessel walls. This problem may be simplified when the different components of the rheumatoid pathology are present together; in particular, once a rheumatoid nodule is recognized, there can be a readier acceptance of the presence of either the meningitis or the vasculitis.

Treatment and Prognosis. When symptoms are referable to a nodule that is creating a mass effect, surgical resection may be a successful intervention. For more diffuse processes, the same therapies that are appropriate for RA in general can be applied.

Much of the published literature on the outcome of patients with documented RA involvement of the CNS is more than a decade old, and does not necessarily represent the overall prognosis with current therapeutics. From one review of the literature (9), there was a high overall mortality rate, of which only a portion was directly attributed to the neurologic component of the RA.

HISTIOCYTIC LESIONS

There are several disease processes that tend to cause discrete space-occupying lesions, either attached to the dura or within the brain parenchyma, in which the diagnostic and sometimes dominant cellular component is the histiocyte. These include the relatively well-known Langerhans cell histiocytoses, as well as two diseases, Rosai-Dorfman disease and Chester-Erdheim disease, which are better recognized for their non-neurologic manifestations. These three processes are considered as a group here since they arise in the same differential diagnostic considerations. There are both specific features that assist in their diagnosis, as well as distinct immunophenotypes of the histiocytes.

Langerhans Cell Histiocytosis

Definition. *Langerhans cell histiocytosis* (LCH) is a lesion characterized by the presence of inflammatory cell infiltrates with recognizable Langerhans type dendritic cells.

General Comments. Among the histiocytoses, LCH is the most common and well recognized by pathologists and other clinicians. This familiarity can be attributed to the existence of several stereotypic patterns of presentation, which in the past have been graced with eponymous designations and linked with differing clinical courses. Although they are now recognized to share critical histologic and immunologic phenotypes, resulting in the current unity of nomenclature, there is a long history of separating eosinophilic granuloma (the solitary lesion, typically in bone or soft tissue), Hand-Schüller-Christian disease (with skull lesions as well as exophthalmos and diabetes insipidus), and the most aggressive, Letterer-Siwe disease (with infantile onset and widespread systemic involvement). All are considered manifestations of the same overall disease process, although to treat them as a continuum is probably not ideal since there is often no transition from one form to another. Much of the recent investigative literature has been built around the childhood forms of these diseases, which are the most common, and has focused on defining high- and low-risk forms of LCH and on the appropriate treatments for them.

An additional aspect of LCH that has recently come under study is the clonal nature of the Langerhans cells. These cells may show loss of heterozygosity, even though standard cytogenetic abnormalities are extremely rare (18,19); whether this is enough evidence to redefine this disease as a neoplasm remains uncertain.

Clinical Features. The current categorization of LCH recognizes localized and multifocal forms of the disease, with or without organ dysfunction (20). As mentioned above, the localized form is the well-recognized painful destructive lesion of bone, often with involvement of the skull. This tends to occur in children and young adults and is often a readily manageable disease. On occasion, it recurs locally after incomplete curettage or reappears at a different site. When the disease involves multiple organs, it typically arises in a younger age group and may have a more aggressive course. The nature of the clinical course of the disease is mostly related to the distribution of the organs involved, with lungs and gastrointestinal tract associated with the worst outcome.

In addition to involvement of the calvarium, LCH can involve the CNS in a variety of ways. The most common clinical manifestation, typically occurring in the setting of multifocal disease, is diabetes insipidus. It is observed in roughly 10 percent of patients with LCH, and is either found at the time of clinical manifestation or develops over the course of the illness (21). It has also been suggested that LCH represents the most common cause of central diabetes insipidus (22). Exophthalmos, when present, typically marks the existence of a mass lesion of LCH in the orbital cavity. CNS involvement by LCH may occur in isolation or as part of multifocal disease. CNS involvement is more common in older patients, with many cases occurring in the fourth decade or later (23–26).

Radiologic Findings. Imaging studies reveal several patterns of LCH involving the brain and its coverings (27). These include the well-recognized involvement of the skull or hypothalamic/infundibular abnormalities in more than half of the cases. Lesions in the meninges, including the stroma of the choroid plexus, are found in about a third of cases and distinct parenchymal mass lesions are seen in less than 10 percent. The discrete mass lesions, mostly found in the dura, are typically isointense or hypointense relatively to brain on T1-weighted images and consistently hypointense on T2-weighted images.

There may also be changes that represent a distinct pattern of neurodegeneration, in that they are not characterized by space-occupying lesions (23). Lesions of white matter, most commonly in the pons, with a high T2 signal, are present in about a quarter of patients, almost always in association with lesions with similar characteristics in the cerebellar dentate. The latter lesions are more common, and are seen even in the absence of changes in the pons. Sometimes accompanying the cerebellar signal abnormalities are comparable changes in the putamen and globus pallidus. While these degenerative changes have sometimes been noted in patients who received therapy, including chemotherapy and radiation, they have also been observed in untreated subjects. The majority of those patients with diffuse white or gray matter lesions have neurologic symptoms.

Gross Findings. Specimens of LCH are most commonly encountered after curettage of skull lesions, where the pathology specimen shows a friable, often hemorrhagic collection of soft tissue. When meningeal or cerebral masses are resected, they are typically soft and friable, and do not have distinguishing characteristics.

Intraoperative Diagnosis. When examining either frozen section or smear preparations from the typical lytic lesion of the skull or the less commonly encountered masses from within the cranial vault, it is reasonable to suggest the diagnosis when confronted with the mixed inflammatory infiltrate, often with abundant eosinophils and neutrophils, in addition to the characteristic Langerhans type cell. These cells have a reniform, sometimes deeply cleaved, nucleus. Immunophenotyping (CD68 negative, S-100 protein positive, CD1a positive), which forms the backbone of the current formal diagnostic criteria, does not play a role in intraoperative diagnosis.

Diagnosing LCH may be more problematic when examining a biopsy specimen from a lesion that has come to surgery as a possible metastatic tumor from an unknown primary, based on the presence of multiple rounded lesions near the gray-white junction. While the inflammatory cell background can suggest an infectious etiology, the displacement of brain elements, in a manner similar to that seen in metastatic lesions, may be enough to suggest an alternative. Once that pattern has been recognized, it is sometimes possible to identify the characteristic nuclei of the Langerhans cells.

There is a suggestion that, over time, there may be a natural regression of the Langerhans cell component of these lesions, resulting in a comparable lesion with a distinct but related cellularity of T cells and CD68-positive macrophages and the near absence the CD1a-positive cells (23). These lesions are nearly impossible to diagnose at the time of frozen section unless an extensive clinical history is provided; even then, it is appropriate only to treat them as "not inconsistent with" a late-stage lesion of LCH.

Microscopic Findings. The diagnostic feature of LCH is, not surprisingly, the Langerhans cell, with its specific ultrastructural finding of the Birkbeck granule and its immunophenotype. These cells are single nucleated, large histiocytes without overly vacuolated cytoplasm. The characteristic feature of the Langerhans cell, as accessible to the pathologist with H&E staining, is the reniform (bean-shaped) nuclei, often with a crisp groove at the midpoint. Langerhans cells may be abundant in the lesions, or they may be a relatively minor component, being swamped by the presence of macrophages (CD68 positive, S-100 protein negative, CD1a negative), lymphocytes, eosinophils, and occasionally, neutrophils (figs. 8-17, 8-18). The chemokine secretion profile of the Langerhans cell may be responsible for the mixed infiltrate that accompanies the lesion.

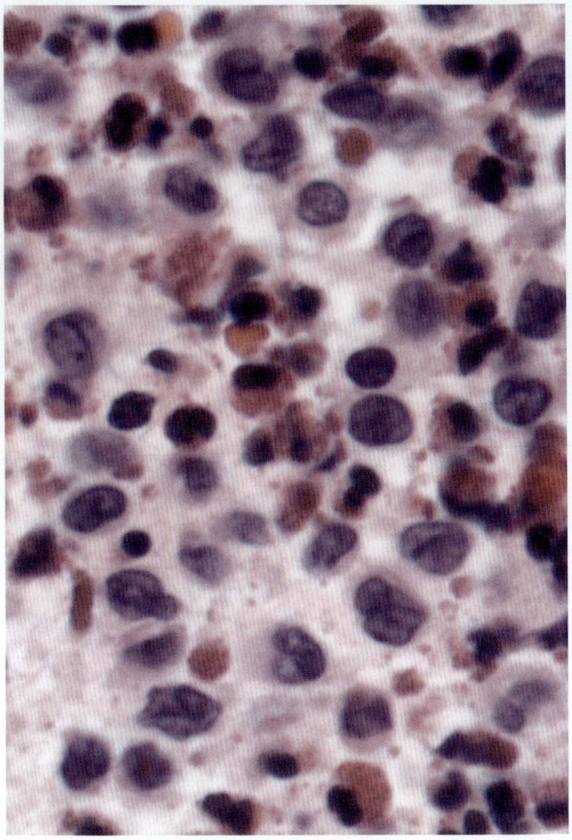

Figure 8-17

LANGERHANS CELL HISTIOCYTOSIS

Along with the characteristic Langerhans cells are lymphocytes, eosinophils, and neutrophils.

In addition to the well-recognized mass lesions of LCH, a form of neurodegenerative disease that is characterized by tissue damage with gliosis, neuronal loss, axonal loss, and injury in the form of spheroids, all putatively associated with a CD8-positive T-cell infiltrate in some cases, is often centered on the cerebellar dentate nucleus and the basal ganglia (23,27,28). While only limited neuropathologic findings of these lesions have been reported, there appears to be a striking absence of the CD1a-positive, S-100 protein-positive cells that characterize the more

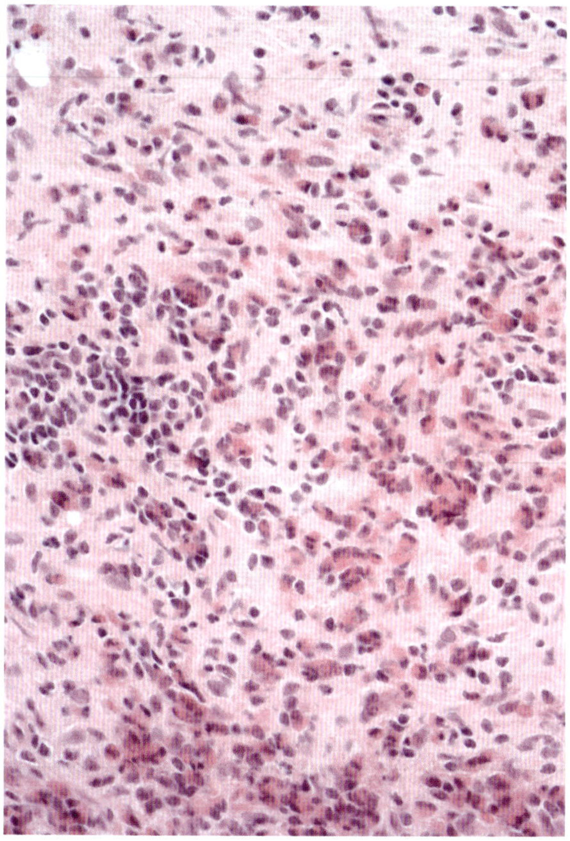

Figure 8-18

LANGERHANS CELL HISTIOCYTOSIS

Occasionally, eosinophils are abundant, in part accounting for the term eosinophilic granuloma.

standard LCH lesions. Whether these cases represent the local effects of cytokines or the elicited immune cells on the brain parenchyma, or whether they represent a localized response to a systemic abnormality of immune regulation, cannot be determined currently.

Immunohistochemical Findings. The Langerhans cell is CD68 negative, S-100 protein positive, and CD1a positive. In addition, these cells are positive for CD207/langerin, a surface marker that is also related to the formation of Birbeck granules (29,30). The inflammatory cell infiltrate, in addition to eosinophils and neutrophils, often contains CD8-positive T cells (23). With involvement of the brain parenchyma, there is often marked surrounding gliosis that can be highlighted by staining for glial fibrillary acidic protein (GFAP), although this is purely a reactive and nonspecific change.

Ultrastructural Findings. LCH is one of the few diseases with a specific ultrastructural finding: the Birbeck granule. This is often described as a tennis racket–shaped cytoplasmic organelle, although sometimes only the handle of the racket is visible. Within the elongated portion of the granule, a trilaminar appearance is often visible. Although there remains some uncertainty as to the function of the Birkbeck granule, it appears to be a cycling endosomal compartment associated with the internalization of CD207/langerin. Despite these uncertainties, this rare structure remains specific enough to support the diagnosis of LCH.

Differential Diagnosis. With the identification of the Langerhans cells in a lesion, there is scarcely a differential diagnosis. Until the specific cells are recognized with routine staining such as H&E or identified by immunohistochemistry, however, the differential diagnosis includes other histiocytic processes that can involve the brain and its coverings, such as Rosai-Dorfman disease and Chester-Erdheim disease. In the suprasellar region, consideration should also be given to the possibility that the inflammation represents a component of a germ cell tumor. In addition, limited samples that contain mostly reactive inflammatory cells and CD68-positive macrophages may suggest either infection or infarction. As mentioned previously, it is the space-occupying nature of the lesion that can assist the pathologist in shifting away from infarct, while the clinical setting usually helps to exclude infection.

Treatment and Prognosis. Even though the relatively distinct subtypes of this disorder contain similar cellular components, there is little progression from the more limited forms of the disease to the most widespread. Many of the bony lesions can be treated with curettage, and sometimes with extremely low-dose radiation. Similarly, discrete meningeal masses without cerebral involvement can be treated with local surgical approaches, holding other therapies for subsequent use for recurrences. Treatment options for more widespread disease tend to involve chemotherapeutic options, some of which have been found to reduce recurrence rates as well as to limit the appearance of new symptoms such as diabetes insipidus (20).

Rosai-Dorfman Disease

Definition. *Rosai-Dorfman disease* (RDD) is characterized by the presence of a histiocytic cell with a specific immunophenotype (CD68 positive, S-100 protein positive, CD1a negative) and emperipolesis of lymphocytes.

General Comments. The original description of this disorder by Rosai and Dorfman in 1969 (31) identified the characteristic cellular composition and morphologic features within lymph nodes, which came to clinical attention because of enlargement. The histiocytes that comprised much of the cellularity of the lesion were localized to the sinuses, hence, the alternative name *sinus histiocytosis with massive lymphadenopathy* (SHML). Extranodal disease is relatively common, both in combination with nodal involvement or in isolation. Given that the term SHML makes little sense when discussing disease that involves non-nodal sites (such as the dura mater), the eponymous designation of Rosai-Dorfman disease is used here.

Clinical Features. RDD is a rare disorder, and there are few large series that help define the natural history of the disease. A registry of cases has been established, and various publications have drawn from these data (32). From what has been reported in the literature, RDD is a disease of older children and young adults, without a gender bias (33). Although nearly all patients have painless nodal involvement, which typically includes the cervical nodes and may involve other nodes as well, multisystem involvement with extranodal disease occurs in nearly half of the patients (32). Among the extranodal sites, skin is the most common, including a form of RDD limited to cutaneous involvement. Intracranial involvement has been reported in fewer than 10 percent of patients; recent publications suggest that fewer than 50 reported cases are in the literature, although the significance of this number may be limited by the biases that influence such reports (34).

Intracranial involvement by RDD, either in combination with nodal disease, other extranodal diseases, or in isolation, typically involves the dura. Presentation is as an extraaxial mass lesion that most commonly mimics a meningioma (34–42). The age of onset appears to be slightly older for patients with isolated intracranial RDD than for those with nodal presentations (43). Intracranial RDD has a relatively low rate of associated nodal disease (only about 30 percent) and in about half of the cases there is no other site of disease (39). A few lesions directly involve the parenchyma (36,43–45), although some of these were felt to be extraaxial masses with possible brain invasion.

Radiologic Findings. The lesions of RDD have imaging characteristics similar to those of meningiomas, often enhancing on both computerized tomography (CT) and MRI. The lesions may be multiple and involve the dural sinuses on rare occasions (46).

Gross Findings. RDD is often a mildly polypoid, dural-based lesion that may be difficult to distinguish from meningioma. A yellowish color is commonly described, in keeping with the presence of histiocytes in the lesion.

Intraoperative Diagnosis. Since intracranial forms of RDD are most commonly brought to neurosurgical attention under the belief that they are meningiomas, frozen sections yield an unexpected diagnosis. As is common with lesions containing large numbers of histiocytes, a diverse set of processes, including infections, hematologic neoplasia, and nonspecific inflammation enter the differential diagnosis. Although the morphologic features of RDD usually declare themselves (47), with the presence of emperipolesis as the most dramatic feature, allocation of tissue for microbiologic studies may be indicated. If adequate tissue is available, then direction of some tissue for flow cytometry studies for surface markers may be appropriate, both to characterize the cells of RDD and to exclude other immunophenotypes that would suggest a hematologic malignancy.

Microscopic Findings. Unlike in the lymph nodes, RDD involving the dura elicits a fibroblastic response to the cellular infiltrate. Within the fibrotic reaction there is typically a mixed inflammatory cell infiltrate, which has been variously observed to include plasma cells, lymphocytes, and the large histiocytic cells that are the diagnostic feature (figs. 8-19–8-21) (33). These large histiocytes usually have single nuclei and abundant cytoplasm, often with mild vacuolation; they may be only a minor component of the infiltrate.

Emperipolesis involving these histiocytes is the hallmark of RDD, and is defined by the presence

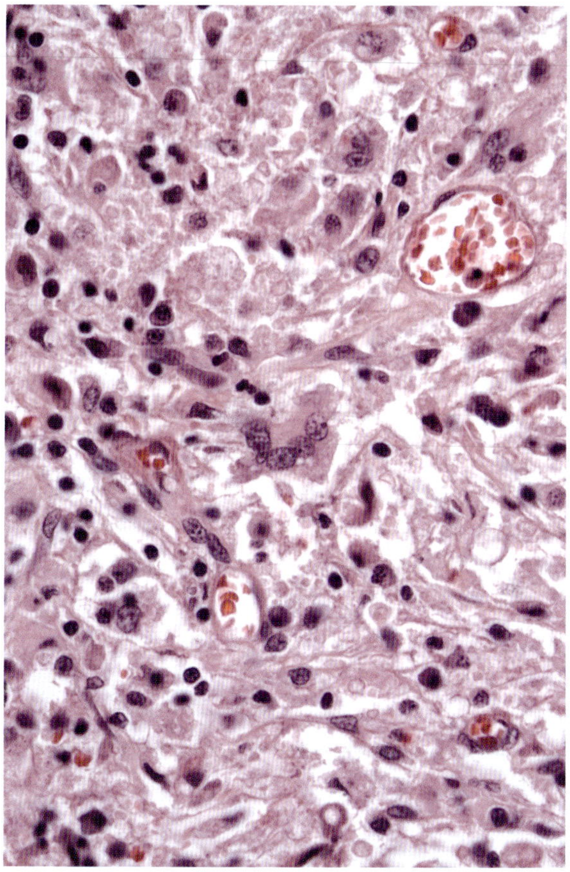

Figure 8-19

ROSAI-DORFMAN DISEASE

The infiltrate has a predominant macrophage component, with scattered lymphocytes and plasma cells.

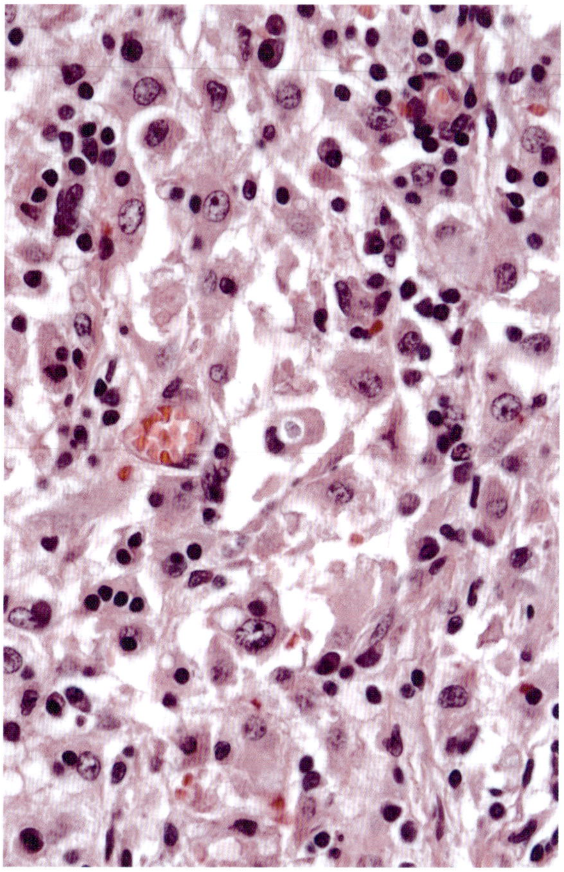

Figure 8-20

ROSAI-DORFMAN DISEASE

In some areas, plasma cells are more abundant.

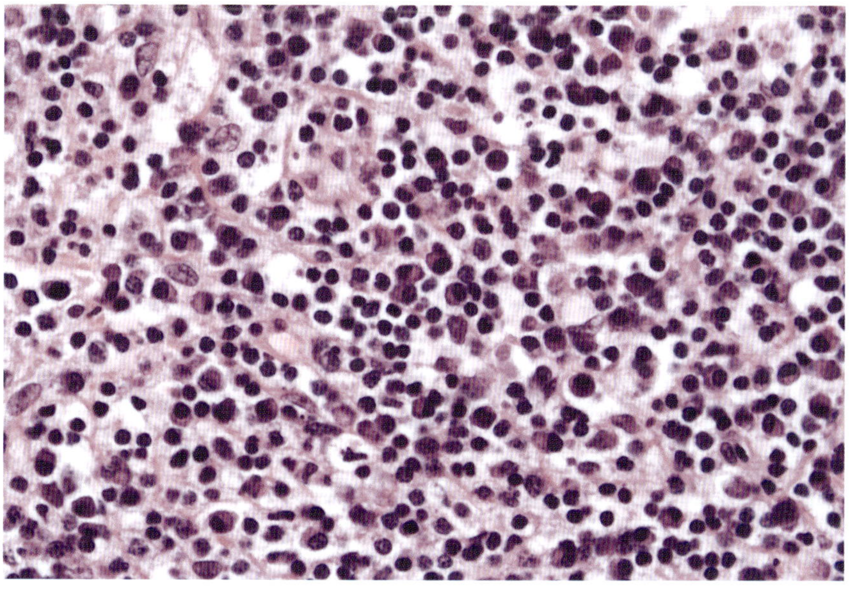

Figure 8-21

ROSAI-DORFMAN DISEASE

A rich lymphoplasmacytic infiltrate occurs in some lesions.

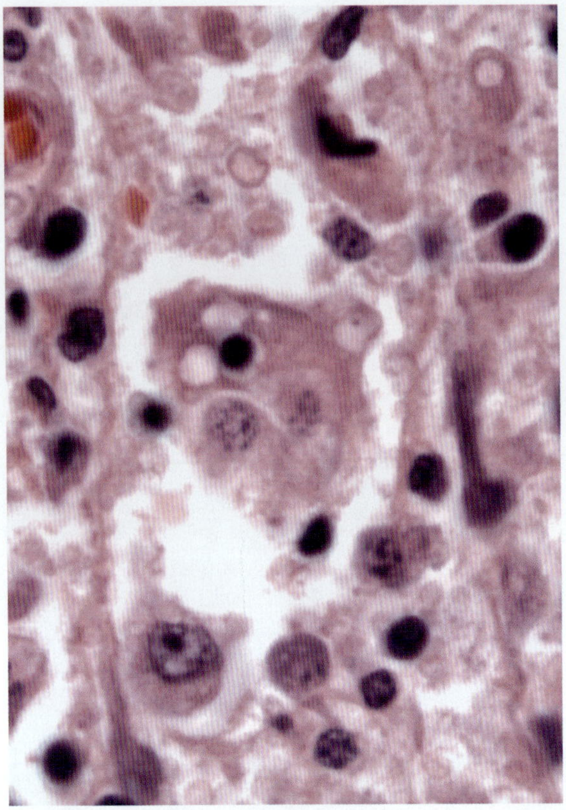

Figure 8-22

ROSAI-DORFMAN DISEASE

Emperipolesis is the hallmark of this disorder.

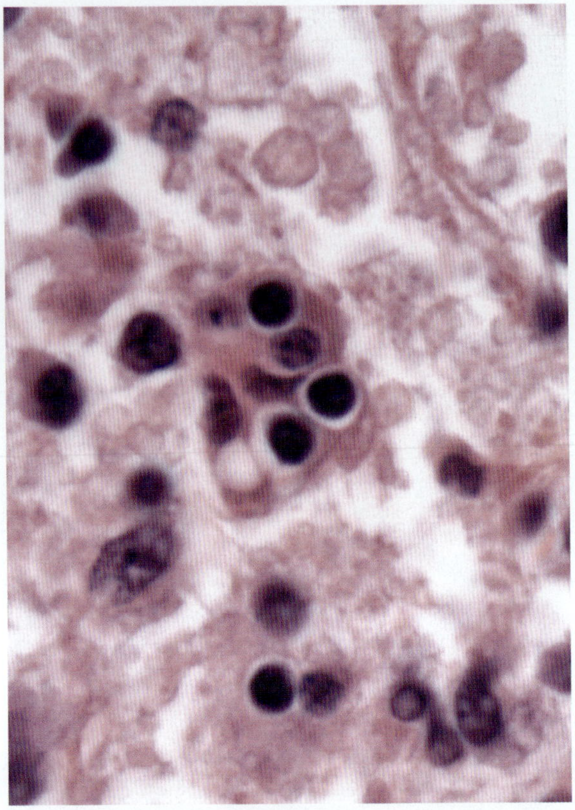

Figure 8-23

ROSAI-DORFMAN DISEASE

Some of the large histiocytic cells contain multiple internalized lymphocytes.

of viable-appearing lymphocytes within the cytoplasm of the large histiocytes (figs. 8-22, 8-23). The phenomenon is also termed lymphophagocytosis, again highlighting the importance of identification of lymphocytes within the histiocyte cytoplasm as part of the diagnosis (as opposed to erythrophagocytosis, in which intact red blood cells are found in the cytoplasm of phagocytic cells) (48). Other components of the inflammatory cell infiltrate may also be found within the cytoplasm of the histiocyte; in addition to plasma cells and neutrophils, there may also be some intact red blood cells.

Immunohistochemical Findings. The pattern of markers expressed by the histiocytes of RDD is usually a strong complement to the morphologic features of the lesion and is critical in establishing a firm diagnosis. Because these cells are part of the true histiocytic/macrophage lineage, they express CD68. The coexpression of this marker with S-100 protein sets the histiocytes of RDD apart from those of other lesions (fig. 8-24) (33,49). Given the presence of S-100 protein-positive cells in these lesions, it is important to exclude LCH by demonstrating that the RDD histiocytes do not express CD1a.

While other markers can be observed on the histiocytic cells of RDD, including other macrophage lineage molecules such as CD14, CD15, CD64, lysozyme, and alpha-1-antitrypsin, these do not play a prominent role in the diagnostic evaluation (50,51).

Ultrastructural Findings. Although there are no specific positive findings that support a diagnosis of RDD, the absence of Birbeck granules is important when attempting to make the distinction between RDD and LCH. Nonetheless, the morphologic features and immunophenotype are sufficiently distinct that electron microscopy has little role in the diagnosis of RDD.

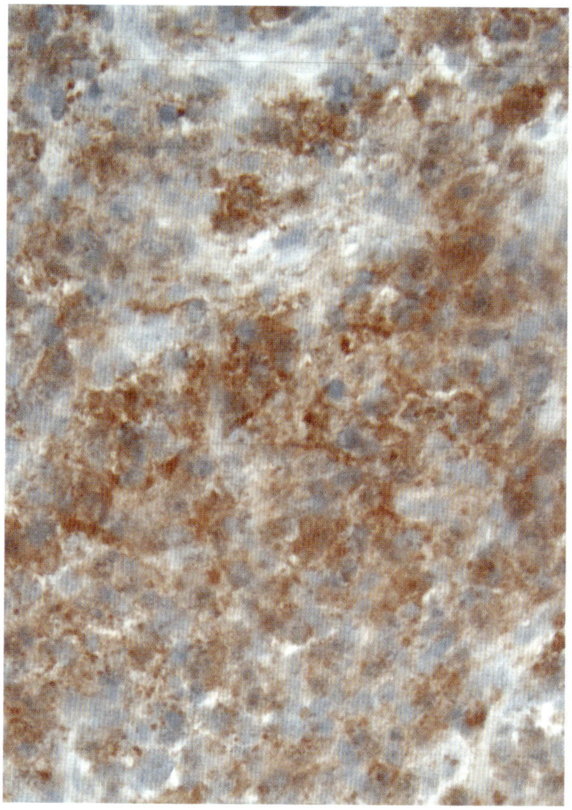

Figure 8-24

ROSAI-DORFMAN DISEASE

The histiocytic elements of this lesion express S-100 protein in addition to CD68 (S-100 immunohistochemistry).

Laboratory Findings. Fever can be both a presenting symptom and a cause of significant morbidity but is more commonly seen in the setting of nodal disease. An elevated sedimentation rate is typically observed, but this is a nonspecific finding. Hypergammaglobulinemia is found in nearly all patients (33).

Differential Diagnosis. While the differential diagnosis of RDD in the lymph node can be complicated, the issues relating to neurosurgical specimens are typically more straightforward. Although the preoperative diagnosis usually suggests meningioma, the morphologic evaluation can rapidly exclude that possibility and shift attention to the histiocytic group of lesions. Within this set of disorders, the combination of the immunophenotype and the presence of emperipolesis usually allows the pathologist to distinguish RDD from LCH or other histiocyte-rich lesions. While emperipolesis may be focal or difficult to find, the CD68-positive, S-100 protein-positive cells should allow for the diagnosis.

In the absence of these two specific findings, additional disorders in the differential diagnosis include various macrophage-rich storage diseases (although the presence of the mixed inflammatory cell infiltrate argues against this), reactive inflammatory processes (such as may be associated with trauma and foreign bodies), and the usual array of infectious processes.

Treatment and Prognosis. No firm data from randomized clinical trials exist to guide the treatment of patients with RDD. In general, resection plays an important role in the care of patients with intracranial RDD. The literature, as it exists, suggests that most of these patients do not have symptomatic recurrence of their disease (39). This may reflect, in part, the usual absence of other extranodal diseases in these patients, as it has been suggested that some forms of visceral involvement are associated with greater morbidity and mortality (33).

Chester-Erdheim Disease

Definition. *Chester-Erdheim disease* (CED) is a systemic disorder characterized by vaguely granulomatous histiocytic and mixed inflammatory aggregates, typically affecting the long bones, resulting in symmetric sclerosis.

General Comments. Another of the relatively rare lesions that may affect the CNS and its covering with aggregates of histiocytes as part of a mixed inflammatory process, CED has predominantly nonspecific findings. The diagnosis rests on the presence of other systemic abnormalities as much as on the exclusion of other disease processes. Because the original description of this disorder was published by Chester, there has been a recent shift in the eponymous designation of the disorder; however, much of the relevant literature refers to Erdheim-Chester disease. Although there are conflicting reports as to whether CED is a clonal disorder, little convincing data suggest that the lesions are clonal (52,53).

Clinical Features. CED is a sporadic disease that typically presents as osteosclerotic lesions of long bones, with epiphyseal sparing, usually in a symmetric distribution and associated with a xanthogranulomatous inflammatory cell infiltrate of the bone marrow space. The lesions are often painful, which prompts clinical evaluation and diagnosis, but the bony lesions may be clinically silent until discovered during evaluation because of systemic involvement (54). Patients with CED (mean age of 56 years; range, 7 to 84) are usually adults, and are typically older than patients with LCH.

Nervous system involvement is most commonly evident as a secondary effect of retro-orbital disease, presenting as exophthalmos, or as lesions in the region of the pituitary stalk/hypothalamus, presenting as diabetes insipidus. Lesions may be multiple, occurring throughout the brain parenchyma (54–62); the literature suggests a relatively high frequency of posterior fossa involvement, but this may reflect a bias of case reports. When lesions are present in the dura, the fibrosis and xanthogranulomatous foci may result in mass effect that can mimic a meningioma. This is associated with signs and symptoms appropriate to the site of involvement. Rare cases of isolated parenchymal involvement by CED have been reported, although this remains a diagnosis of exclusion in the absence of the other hallmarks of systemic involvement (61). Lesions of the CNS have also been described in patients with no neurologic symptoms but with other organ involvement, seen both by imaging studies and at autopsy (57,62).

Radiologic Findings. The lesions of CED can usually be visualized by both CT and MRI. They are often best demonstrated by their strong enhancement with gadolinium and hyperintensity on T2-weighted imaging (54,57,59,62,63).

Gross Findings. While large resection specimens are rarely encountered, information from autopsy studies suggests that the lesions of CED may be yellow, consistent with the xanthogranulomas that are present, or whiter and firmer, if the fibrosing component is more extensive (57).

Intraoperative Diagnosis. At the time of surgery, it is difficult to establish a diagnosis of CED unless there is clear evidence from other aspects of the clinical history and exam that the patient has other evidence of the disease. If that is the case, then it is possible to suggest that a histiocyte-rich lesion represents another manifestation of the disease. In addition to the other histiocytic lesions that may affect the CNS, the differential diagnosis at the time of frozen section includes xanthomatous change/degeneration in a meningioma, collections of macrophages associated with infarct or demyelination in brain parenchyma, and macrophage-rich infectious processes. As with most of the inflammatory disorders, the collection of tissue for microbiologic studies and for potential electron microscopy (for demonstration of Birbeck granules in support of a diagnosis of LCH) may be appropriate. The histiocytic elements of CED on smear preparations (foamy macrophages, moderate nuclear pleomorphism, and Touton-like giant cells admixed with round benign-appearing lymphocytes) may aid in the recognition of the disease (64).

Microscopic Findings. The characteristic cell of CED is the foamy histiocyte, typically present in a mildly fibrotic background, with small numbers of plasma cells and lymphocytes (figs. 8-25, 8-26). The histiocyte is the dominant cellular element of the infiltrate and may form discrete tumor-like masses within the meninges or brain parenchyma. Touton-like giant cells may also be part of the infiltrate.

A perivascular distribution of the histiocytes is often found when the brain is directly involved (fig. 8-27). Exclusion of parenchymal elements by the space-occupying lesion is typical, and there are reactive changes observed around the lesions. In some cases, the reactive changes include the presence of Rosenthal fibers, as is typically associated with longstanding mass lesions. In some lesions, there may be a predominantly microglial appearance to the histiocytic cells, with elongated cells diffusely involving the parenchyma (fig. 8-28).

In addition to the discrete masses of CED within the brain, there are changes observed in the parenchyma at autopsy (57). Clusters of the histiocytic elements that characterize these lesions are found in grossly unremarkable, and radiographically unremarkable, regions of the brain. In this setting, these cells are present as a diffuse infiltrate, with a moderate perivascular predisposition.

Immunohistochemical Findings. In addition to the characteristic systemic findings of CED, the immunoprofile of the histiocytes of the lesion is an important aspect of establishing the diagnosis. In this sense, the entity is a diagnosis by exclusion, as the critical aspect is to demonstrate that these cells are CD68 positive, CD1a negative, and S-100 protein negative.

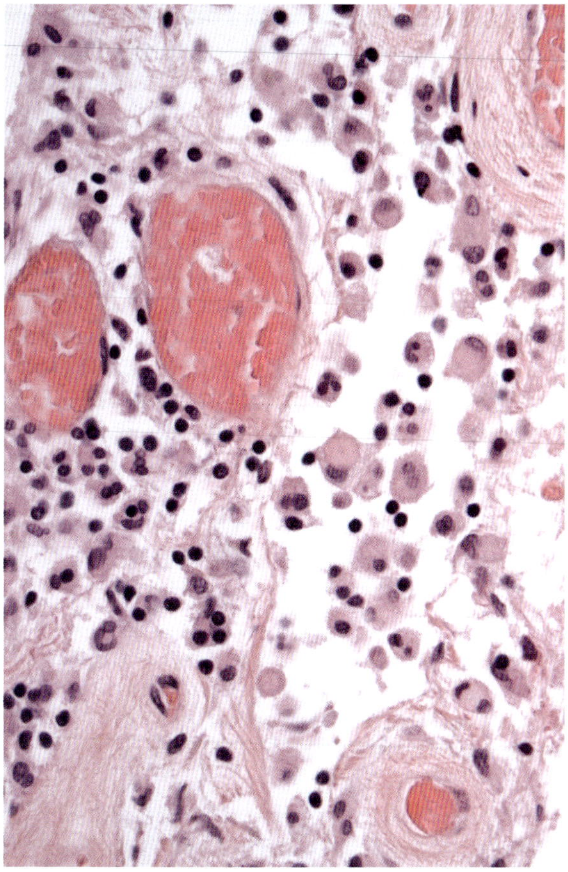

Figure 8-25

CHESTER-ERDHEIM DISEASE

Scattered histiocytes, lymphocytes, and plasma cells in the leptomeninges are associated with a mild fibrotic reaction.

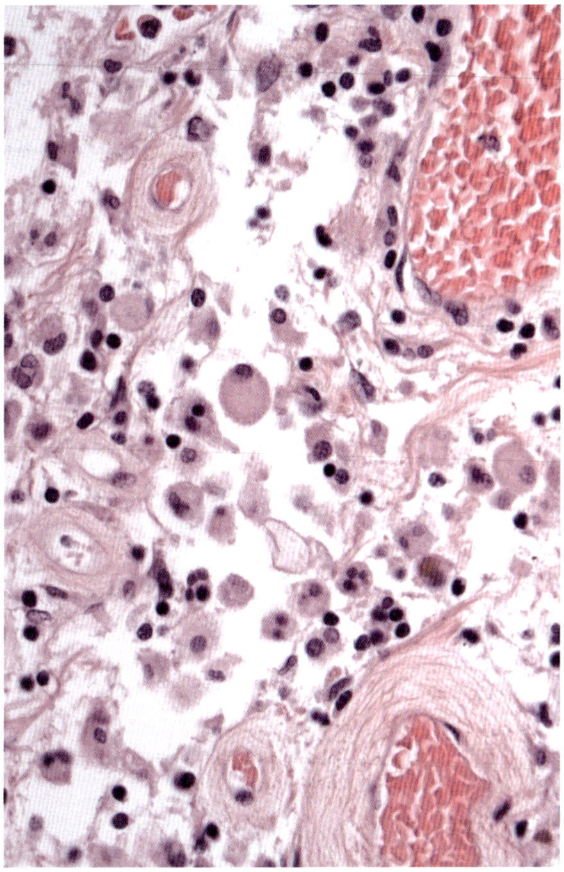

Figure 8-26

CHESTER-ERDHEIM DISEASE

The infiltrate in the meninges is diffuse and poorly cohesive.

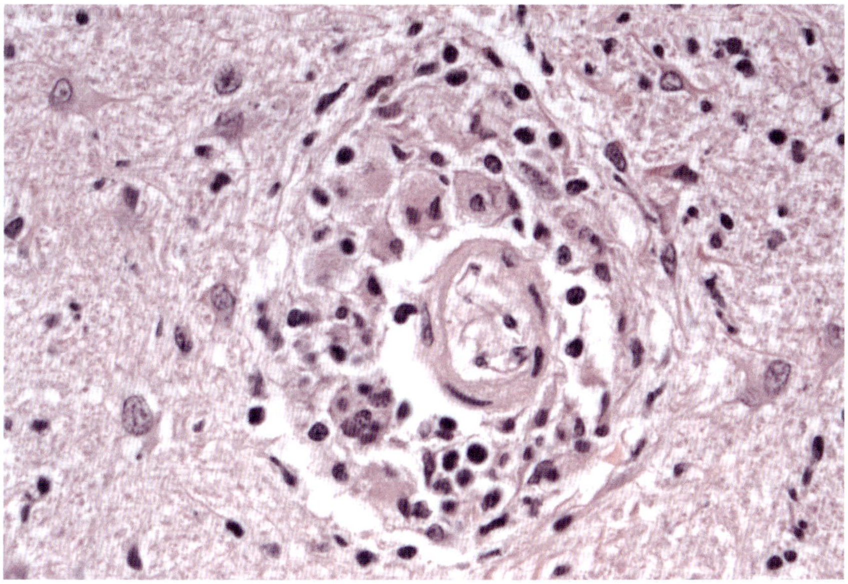

Figure 8-27

CHESTER-ERDHEIM DISEASE

Extension of the lesion into the brain parenchyma often occurs around penetrating vessels. Cells are present in the Virchow-Robin space, with surrounding reactive astrocytosis.

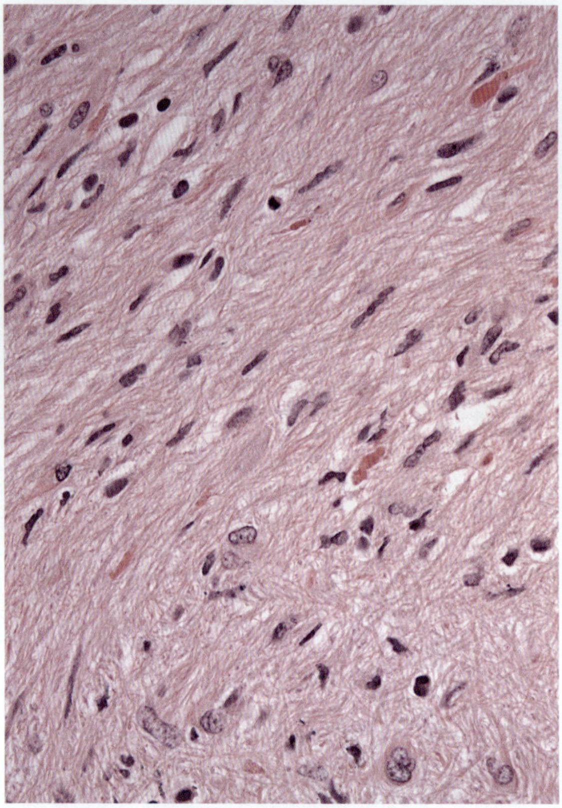

Figure 8-28

CHESTER-ERDHEIM DISEASE

When direct brain infiltration occurs, the histiocytic cells acquire a microglial appearance. Reactive changes with Rosenthal fibers are common.

Mixed lesions have been reported, with scattered LCH type cells present (57,65,66), suggesting that there may be situations in which the distinction cannot be made with certainty.

Ultrastructural Findings. Although no electron microscopic findings are present that support a diagnosis of CED, the presence of Birbeck granules within the cytoplasm of the histiocytic cells should be taken as strong evidence that the disease process is more likely LCH than CED.

Differential Diagnosis. Depending on the site of the lesion, various entities fall into the differential diagnosis of CED. The distinction between CED and the other histiocytic lesions of the brain and its coverings (LCH and RDD) can be made through the application of immunohistochemistry and the systemic findings. For parenchymal lesions associated with diabetes insipidus associated with hypothalamic or infundibular dysfunction, the differential diagnosis includes granulomatous hypophysitis and germinoma. CED can be separated from these, respectively, by its presence primarily as a mass-occupying lesion rather than as an infiltrative process and by the absence of the large tumor cells and appropriate markers of germinoma.

Treatment and Prognosis. No adequate studies have assessed objectively the efficacy of various forms of therapy for intracranial CED. There have been reports of the use of corticosteroids, as well as reports of varying success with radiotherapy. The course of progression of CED is that of a slow but relentless disease, with many patients succumbing to its complications (54).

Juvenile Xanthogranuloma

Definition. Primarily a pediatric self-limited cutaneous disease of dermal dendrocytes (67), *juvenile xanthogranuloma* (JXG) is characterized by accumulations of histiocyte-rich inflammatory masses. When it occurs within the CNS, it may have a less benign natural history, although the scarcity of the disease makes this difficult to assess with confidence.

Clinical Features. Two distinct patterns of presentation of JXG are recognized: isolated brain involvement or in combination with disease at other sites, most typically skin (68). Both are extremely unusual, with only a handful of case reports in the literature. JXG remains a disease found in the pediatric age group. It has been suggested that CNS involvement occurs as solitary lesions when cutaneous lesions are absent and as multiple foci when there is systemic disease (68), although exceptions have been reported (69). As with the majority of mass lesions that involve the CNS, the clinical manifestations are governed more by location than by pathology, although the pace of growth may influence this rule.

Radiologic Findings. With imaging studies, the masses of JXG are typically circumscribed and discrete, often with rounded contours. They enhance homogeneously with contrast on CT scans and similarly with gadolinium.

Gross Findings. Because of the xanthomatous nature of the lesion, the gross appearance of tissue samples is typically described as yellow. The lesion is usually well encapsulated and can be separated from the adjacent structures without significant difficulty.

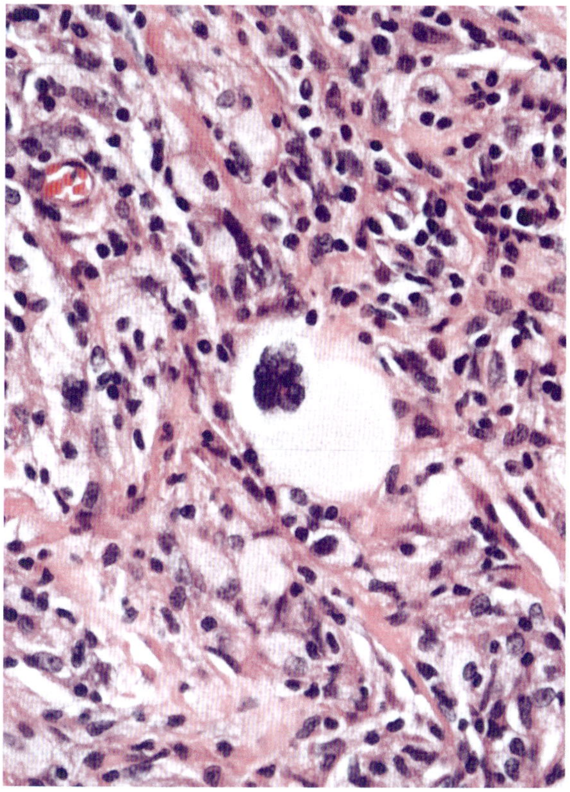

Figure 8-29

JUVENILE XANTHOGRANULOMA

Numerous lipid-laden macrophages admixed with a polymorphous inflammatory cell infiltrate characterize the lesion.

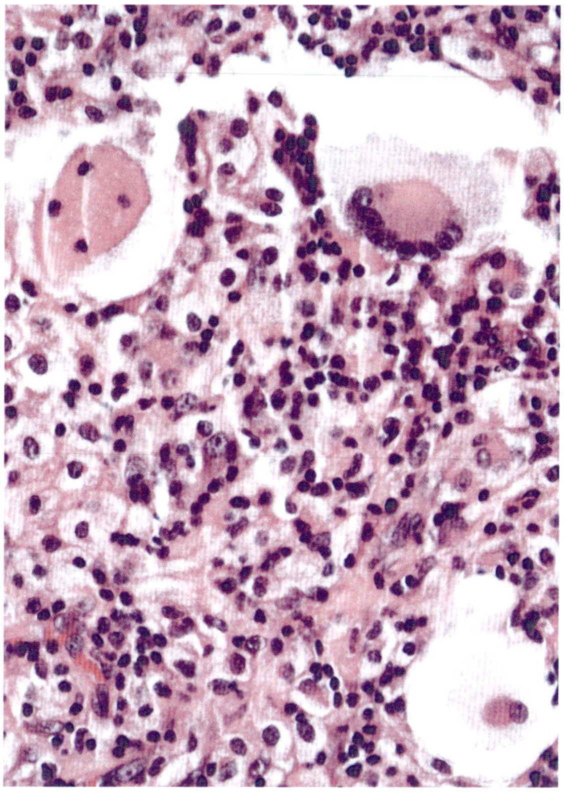

Figure 8-30

JUVENILE XANTHOGRANULOMA

Touton giant cells are present, sometimes as part of the xanthomatous component.

Intraoperative Diagnosis. When confronted on smear preparation and frozen section with the sheets of histiocytes that comprise this lesion, the pathologist is likely to have a difficult time reaching a specific diagnosis. The differential diagnosis includes infection, other histiocytoses, and, in the case of intraparenchymal lesions, demyelination and infarction. The presence of other inflammatory cells, in addition to the macrophages and the absence of the expected architectural features of other parenchymal disorders, helps argue against these last two entities.

Microscopic Findings. It is the abundance of xanthomatous cells, foamy macrophages filled with lipid, that gives rise to the name of the lesion and constitutes the dominant feature of the histology of these lesions (fig. 8-29). Unlike the cutaneous form of the disease, in which there is often a moderate amount of fibrosis associated with a spindle cell component, only scattered elongated cells are present in these lesions. There is a minor population of other inflammatory cells, which may accompany the sheets of macrophages, and these are primarily lymphocytes but may also include a few eosinophils. Touton type giant cells may be present as well (figs. 8-30, 8-31). As expected, stains for organisms are negative.

Immunohistochemical Findings. The cells of JXG share the pattern of markers with traditional macrophages, rather than with any of the specialized histiocytic cells that mark some of the other diseases considered here. As such, they are immunoreactive for CD45 and CD68 and negative for CD1a and S-100 protein.

Ultrastructural Findings. As the cells of JXG are not Langerhans cells, they do not contain Birbeck granules. Given this, electron microscopy only has a role in the attempt to exclude a form of

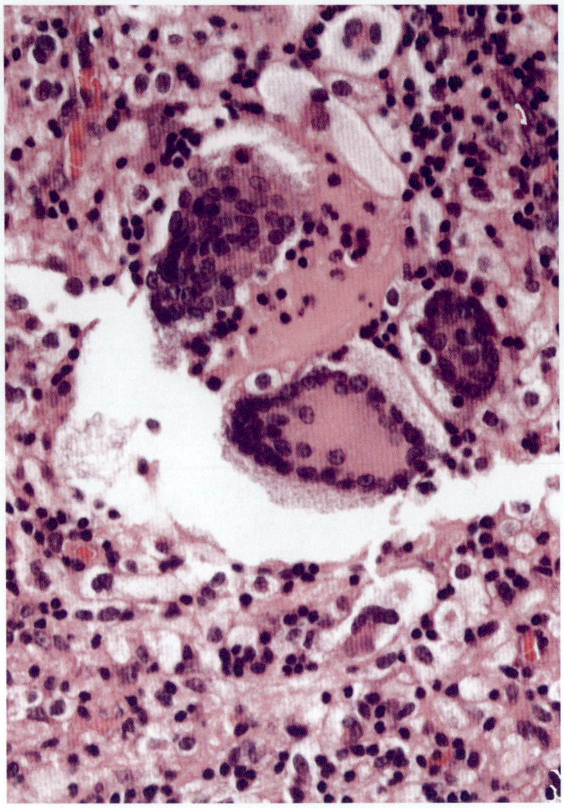

Figure 8-31

JUVENILE XANTHOGRANULOMA

The giant cells contain numerous nuclei.

LCH. With the advances in immunohistochemical characterization of Langerhans cells, the role for ultrastructural analysis has diminished.

Differential Diagnosis. JXG must be distinguished from LCH. This is achieved by the distinct immunophenotype of the histiocytic elements of these two processes. When JXG occurs within the parenchyma of the brain, the accumulation of lipid-rich macrophages needs to be distinguished from demyelination, and is done through the demonstration of the absence of axons within the lesion (see chapter 4). Cerebral infarction also results in large areas of macrophages, but this is usually associated with evidence of tissue loss.

Treatment and Prognosis. While the cutaneous lesions of JXG are expected to regress over the first few years of life (70,71), the natural history of lesions affecting the CNS is less clear (68). Whether this is associated with the consequences of location in regions that preclude resection or with the subsequent effects of aggressive therapies in a developing brain remains uncertain.

Choroid Plexus Xanthogranuloma

Definition. *Choroid plexus xanthogranuloma* (CPX) is an often incidental lesion of the choroid plexus that is typically identified at autopsy in older individuals. CPX is characterized by the presence of abundant cholesterol clefts, hemosiderin, and reactive changes.

General Comments. Typically incidental and asymptomatic, CPX is found in 1 to 7 percent of patients at autopsy (72). The lesion is benign, but in rare instances grows large enough to come to clinical attention. The etiology is uncertain. It is possible that these lesions begin as areas of focal hemorrhage within the choroid plexus (73). Xanthogranulomatous lesions also occur within the third ventricle where they cause obstructive hydrocephalus and likely come more rapidly to clinical attention (72,74).

Clinical Features. Most are incidental lesions discovered at autopsy or on neuroimaging performed for other reasons. In rare instances, the lesion may grow large enough to cause clinical symptoms. Alternatively, if the mass occurs in regions of the ventricular system and blocks the flow of CSF, particularly the region of the foramina of Munro, patients may become symptomatic (75).

CPXs typically are seen in adults, but childhood cases have been reported (76). The lesions may be unilateral or bilateral. In the rare instances where these lesions have become symptomatic, headache is the most common presenting symptom (73). Other reported manifestations include seizures, syncope, ataxia, memory problems, parageusia, and parosmia, and may have a significant duration before the lesions are identified. CPX has been associated with death in at least one case (72).

Radiologic Findings. By MRI, the lesions seen as incidental findings at autopsy appear as tiny plaques within the choroid plexus (77). More extensive symptomatic lesions are characterized by high signal intensity on T1-weighted images and low signal intensity on T2-weighted images (72,77). CPX is typically an enhancing lesion located in the trigone of the lateral ventricle (72). A lesion in the anterior third ventricle can

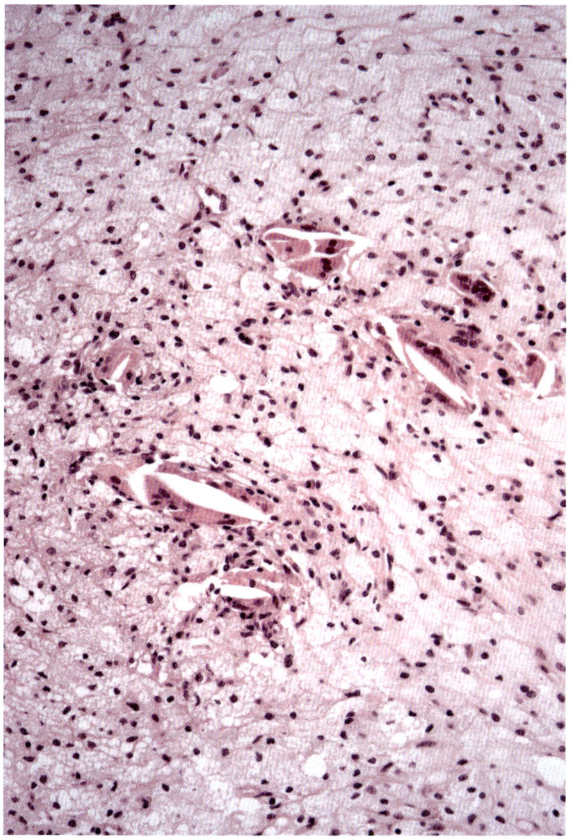

Figure 8-32

CHOROID PLEXUS XANTHOGRANULOMA

Lesions contain macrophages and giant cells.

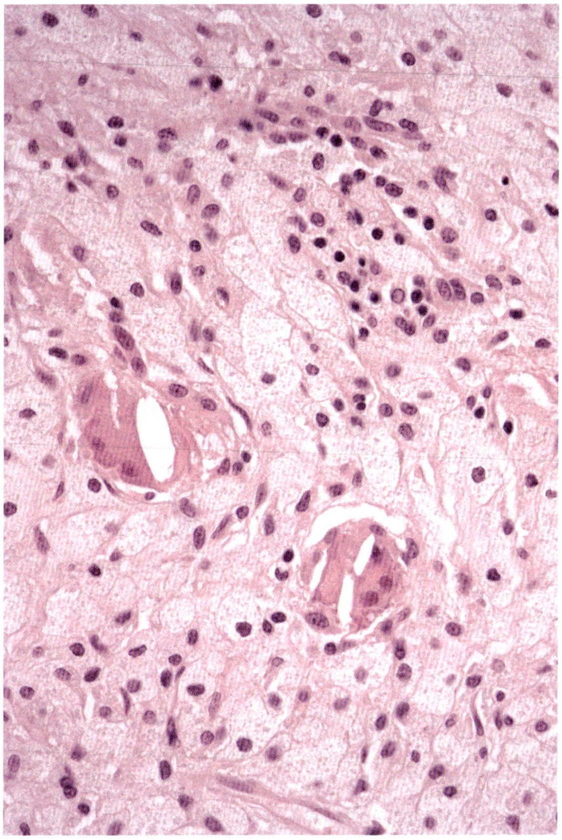

Figure 8-33

CHOROID PLEXUS XANTHOGRANULOMA

Giant cells contain often multiple cholesterol clefts.

mimic a colloid cyst (75). CPX is typically well circumscribed and does not involve the adjacent brain parenchyma in most cases (73).

Gross Findings. CPX is generally a small (2 to 3 cm), well-circumscribed nodular lesion. It is typically firm or rubbery and may have adherent fragments of choroid plexus. The presence of blood breakdown products often imparts a yellow-orange color to the specimens. The center of these specimens may contain grumous debris.

Intraoperative Findings. There is relatively little demand for routine intraoperative evaluation of CPX. Frozen sections of these lesions, however, should readily demonstrate the characteristic histologic features described below.

Microscopic Findings. Smaller lesions seen at the time of autopsy are characterized primarily by the presence of xanthoma cells. This distinguishes them from the larger lesions that are surgically resected where xanthoma cells are, at best, a variably prominent feature. CPX is characterized by the presence of cholesterol clefts, a foreign body giant cell reaction, hemosiderin and other blood breakdown products, dense fibrosis, lymphocytic infiltrates, and calcifications including psammoma bodies (figs. 8-32, 8-33) (72). Based on these histologic observations, it has been suggested that CPX might better be considered a cholesterol granuloma of the lateral ventricle (73). Lesions in the third ventricle show a slightly different histology. In addition to the xanthogranulomatous changes, these lesions are typically cystic and are often associated with the presence of a single or multilayered ciliated or cuboidal epithelium. Incidental xanthomas are not encountered in this location. As a result, many of these lesions are described as combined colloid cysts and xanthogranulomas, in which the later changes are presumed to arise within or are secondary to the cystic lesion.

Differential Diagnosis. While CPX is encountered, although rarely, in surgical neuropathology, there are several pathologic processes that occur with greater frequency in the lateral ventricle. These include meningioma, choroid plexus tumors, ependymoma, and vascular malformations. The imaging characteristics of CPX typically allow for ready distinction between these entities (77). In addition, there is little overlap at the microscopic level between choroid plexus tumor, meningioma, and CPX. While arteriovenous malformations may be associated with reactive changes, fibrosis, and hemosiderin deposits, CPX is not characterized by abnormal blood vessels.

When these lesions arise in the third ventricle, the major differential diagnosis is colloid cyst. Specimens should be carefully examined for minute collections of colloid material or the characteristic epithelial lining of colloid cyst. As noted above, the distinction between these lesions may be imprecise.

Treatment and Prognosis. The treatment for CPX is surgical. These are benign lesions that are not reported to recur after resection. Resolution of symptoms is reported in some, but not all, patients following surgery (73).

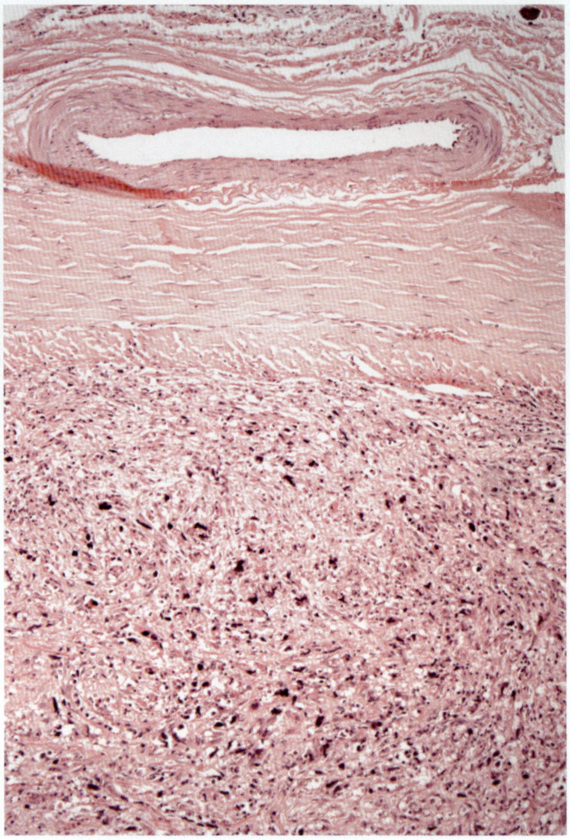

Figure 8-34

DURAL EXTRAMEDULLARY HEMATOPOIESIS

The mass is identified on the subdural side of the dural connective tissue, based on the location of the large muscular artery.

EXTRAMEDULLARY HEMATOPOIESIS OF THE DURA MATER

Definition. *Extramedullary hematopoiesis* (EMH) is a focus of developing hematopoietic cells located in a site other than the bone marrow.

General Comments. EMH develops as a compensatory mechanism to generate blood cells when the normal hematopoietic bone marrow space is replaced. The most common diseases to produce EMH are the myeloproliferative disorders, but thalassemia is a predominant cause in regions of the world in which thalassemia is common (78). Involvement of the CNS typically occurs late in the disease process, when there is EMH affecting other organs, most notably the spleen, liver, and lymph nodes. EMH in the CNS is nearly always dural based, affecting the intracranial and paraspinal dura mater. In many cases, the involvement is incidental and only discovered at autopsy (79). EMH is also occasionally found as microscopic foci within intracranial tumors, particularly hemangioblastomas.

Clinical Features. Most cases are discovered incidentally at autopsy as small subdural nodules scattered over the cerebral convexities. When symptomatic, signs and symptoms relate to the location of the mass or masses. Patients with intracranial subdural deposits often present with seizures and those with spinal tumors have manifestations of cord compression (78). The subdural masses, if confluent, can resemble a subdural hematoma (fig. 8-34) (80). Rare cases have diffusely involved the subarachnoid space, including the Virchow-Robin spaces (81). The most common spinal location is the lower or mid-thoracic region (78), and spinal disease may be either subdural or epidural.

Radiologic Findings. The lesions are strongly enhancing on MRI. They are isointense on T1- and hyperintense on T2-weighted images.

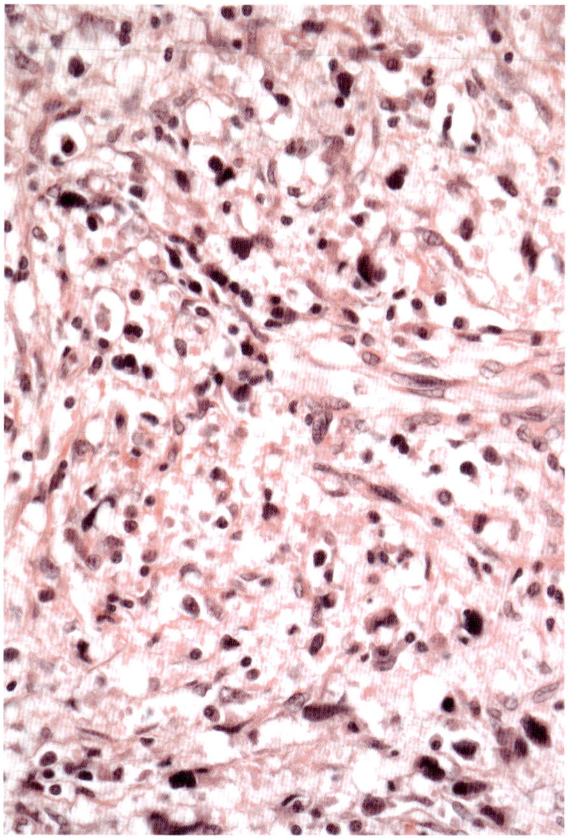

Figure 8-35

DURAL EXTRAMEDULLARY HEMATOPOIESIS

All lineages of developing bone marrow elements should be present.

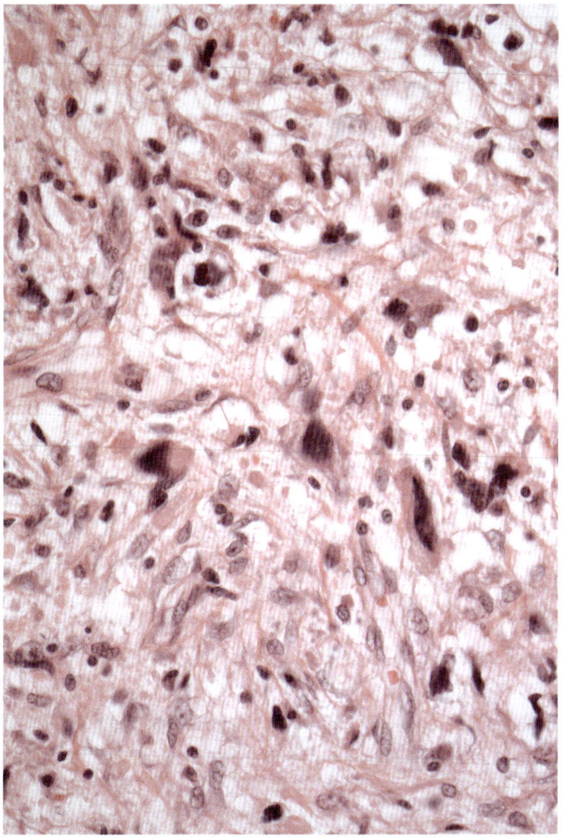

Figure 8-36

DURAL EXTRAMEDULLARY HEMATOPOIESIS

In some areas, one hematopoietic lineage is predominant (megakaryocytes are often easiest to recognize).

Gross Findings. Cases seen by the surgical pathologist are dural-based, rounded, white-tan or reddish brown, often firm masses, although those affecting the spinal cord may be sausage shaped. The variability in the gross appearance relates to the amount of fibrosis present. At autopsy, multiple dural-based nodules are typically less than 1 cm and relatively firm.

Intraoperative Diagnosis. The preoperative diagnosis is usually meningioma or nerve sheath tumor. Cells from EMH, if the lesion is not fibrotic, smear in a more even manner than either meningioma or schwannoma, and the marked pleomorphism of the megakaryocytes is readily apparent. In addition, the granular and varied cytoplasm of myeloid precursors, in combination with the large megakaryocytes, suggests EMH. Cases in which fibrosis is prominent will not smear well. In these cases, frozen section demonstrates the large megakaryocytes, but this may suggest a poorly differentiated malignancy.

Microscopic Findings. The lesions feature sheets of hematopoietic cells, including the broad range of myeloid, megakaryocytic, and erythroid precursors (figs. 8-35, 8-36). The most striking are the megakaryocytes because of their size and multiple nuclei. These cells, coupled with the small hyperchromatic nuclei of the red blood cell precursors and the granular cytoplasm of the developing myeloid cells, should direct the pathologist to the correct interpretation. Some lesions are extensively fibrotic and the hematopoietic cells are scattered singly and in small groups in a dense collagenous background.

Immunohistochemical and Ultrastructural Findings. Immunohistochemistry for factor VIII-related antigen helps identify the megakaryocytic nature of the large cells. If needed, immunohistochemistry for keratins and other markers can exclude desmoplastic carcinomas as well as sarcomas from the differential diagnosis. Ultrastructural analysis should not be needed to arrive at the correct diagnosis, but will demonstrate the hematopoietic nature of the cells and can exclude the possibility of epithelial or mesenchymal differentiation in a malignancy.

Laboratory Findings. The laboratory diagnosis is linked to the underlying cause of the bone marrow dysfunction, in most cases either a myeloproliferative syndrome or thalassemia. The results of such a workup, including bone marrow biopsy, are usually present at the time of neurosurgical intervention.

Differential Diagnosis. In a patient with known bone marrow dysfunction and hepatosplenomegaly, the diagnosis of EMH is straightforward. The initial intraoperative diagnosis should call into question the preoperative possibilities of meningioma or schwannoma. Recognition of the unusual elements as hematopoietic precursors seals the diagnosis, and immunohistochemistry for factor VIII is helpful in this regard. Failure to recognize these elements correctly may raise the possibility of a desmoplastic metastasis from a carcinoma if the lesion is fibrotic, or a poorly differentiated sarcoma. Obtaining a full clinical history and performing immunohistochemical workup should exclude these entities.

Treatment and Prognosis. Surgical removal of symptomatic masses is the primary therapy, particularly for spinal tumors causing cord compression, but radiation is also used. Other therapy is directed toward the underlying condition that fostered the EMH. The prognosis is related to the underlying disease.

CASTLEMAN DISEASE

Definition. *Castleman disease* (CD) is a lymphoproliferative disorder, most commonly thought of as a disorder of mediastinal lymph nodes, with a rich component of plasma cells in the inflammatory cell infiltrate. Although rare, it has been reported as a mass lesion affecting the CNS.

General Comments. Originally described on the basis of clinicopathologic correlations as a unique disease process often resulting in lymphadenopathy and systemic symptoms, there have been significant recent advances in the classification of histologic patterns of CD (separation of the hyaline vascular and plasma cell variants) and the patterns of involvement (unifocal and multifocal). The recognition of a strong association of the plasma cell variant with human immunodeficiency virus (HIV) infection and, beyond that, human herpesvirus (HHV)-8 infection, has also clarified some of the mechanisms of the development of the disease as well as guiding therapies (33,82,83). In addition, the term *Castleman syndrome* has entered the literature to describe some of the systemic findings that were traditionally associated with CD (microcytic hypochromic anemia and polyclonal hypergammaglobulinemia). These may be directly attributable to altered levels of cytokines, particularly interleukin (IL)-6. These clinical findings are most commonly associated with chordoid meningiomas, often when there is a robust lymphoplasmacytic infiltrate associated with the tumor (84). The association of CD with HHV-8 has been linked to a viral-derived form of IL-6 (vIL-6) (85).

Clinical Features. There are several distinct presentations of CD that may be encountered clinically, which are best separated as unifocal and multifocal disease. Superimposed on this division, CD is also usually classified by the primary pathologic pattern: *hyaline vascular* (matching the original cases of Castleman) and *plasma cell rich*. As is true for many forms of disease classification based on histology, cases with intermediate features are also seen. The hyaline vascular pattern is found in the setting of unifocal disease, and is only rarely associated with the systemic manifestations (86). This combination of distribution and morphology constitutes the most common form of this disease, accounting for roughly 70 percent of cases (82). These cases, which include some of the reported cases of CNS involvement, are typically found in adults in their fourth decade.

Of the remaining roughly 30 percent of cases of CD, which have the plasma cell-rich morphologic findings, roughly twice as many are unifocal as are multifocal. There is a slight shift toward younger patients with the unifocal form of the disease and a shift in the other direction when multifocal (82). Anemia, often in association with an elevated sedimentation rate, often accompanies unifocal plasma cell-rich CD. More severe systemic signs and symptoms are found with the multifocal pattern of disease, and these are often the reason the patient comes to clinical attention. The most problematic of these, in addition to fever, is the POEMS (polyneuropathy, organomegaly, endocrinopathy, monoclonal gammopathy, and skin changes) syndrome.

CD that occurs in HIV-infected individuals tends to be multicentric, and therefore has a plasma cell-rich histology (87). There is little evidence to suggest that antiviral therapy for HIV, with the consequent benefit for immune function and CD4 cell counts, has comparable consequences for CD. In the HIV-infected population, CD is strongly associated with HHV-8 infection (88). Studies that have attempted to demonstrate clonality in CD lesions have had conflicting results, suggesting that if it does occur, it is not an essential step in the pathogenesis of the disease (82).

When CD involves the CNS, most commonly as a dural-based or spinal extradural mass, the local mass effect of the lesion is the typical reason for coming to medical attention. Neurologic manifestations are related to the relevant area of the CNS, such as the spinal cord (89–91), orbit (92), or cerebral cortex, as with other dural masses (93–97).

Radiologic Findings. CD of the pachymeninges radiologically presents as a discrete mass lesion with the features of a meningioma. The lesion often shows enhancement and there may be evidence of infiltration of the lesion into the surface of the brain, which is not typically seen with lower-grade meningiomas. CD may be hypointense on T2-weighted MRI.

Gross Findings. Although little information exists, resected lesions of CD from the dura are usually described as moderately firm, often polypoid masses with color ranging from tan to yellow to gray. As such, the appearance of these lesions does not have any specific characteristics that assist in the diagnosis.

Intraoperative Diagnosis. Diagnostic interpretation during surgery is assisted by the exclusion of meningioma through frozen section and smear preparations. Since there are lymphocyte and plasma cell-rich meningiomas, it is important to consider the possibility of inadequate sampling on frozen section. With appreciation of the follicular organization of the lesion and the abundance of plasma cells, the suggestion of a reactive lesion can be made. Because of the presence of the prominent component of plasma cells in the lesion, a hematologic malignancy, such as multiple myeloma, may be considered. Appropriate tissue handling for immunophenotyping, either frozen or fixed, sometimes with fixatives other than formalin, which may differ according to institutional preferences, is appropriate, along with retention of frozen tissue for potential molecular studies for clonality.

Microscopic Findings. CD lesions are inflammatory cell lesions, with focal or extensive development of the follicular architecture (figs. 8-37–8-39). When this occurs in an enlarged lymph node, evaluation of the underlying disease can pose a significant challenge; when it occurs in the coverings of the nervous system, the challenge is to remember to consider CD as a diagnostic possibility.

The hyaline vascular form of CD tends to have an abnormal follicular architecture with a moderately depleted lymphoid population, but with vascular proliferation and hyalinization (figs. 8-40, 8-41). This increased vascularity is thought to be associated with increased levels of vascular endothelial growth factor (VEGF) in the lesions. The common prominence of a single dominant vessel penetrating to the center of a depleted follicle has been likened in appearance to a lollipop. The mantle zone around these follicles is usually larger than expected, corresponding to the expansion that is seen in lymph nodes. In contrast, the plasma cell-rich form of CD is marked by the presence of larger, hypercellular follicles with sheets of plasma cells.

Immunohistochemical Findings. As expected, the abundant plasma cells can easily be marked with the appropriate surface markers, with polyclonal expression of both kappa- and lambda-expressing cells. There is often a background of predominantly B-cell lymphocytes (CD20 positive) and a minor population of CD3-positive T cells.

Laboratory Findings. When systemic symptoms are present, particularly with the plasma cell variant of CD, the most common findings are microcytic hypochromic anemia and polyclonal hypergammaglobulinemia. While these are not specific markers of the disease, the abnormalities typically normalize after

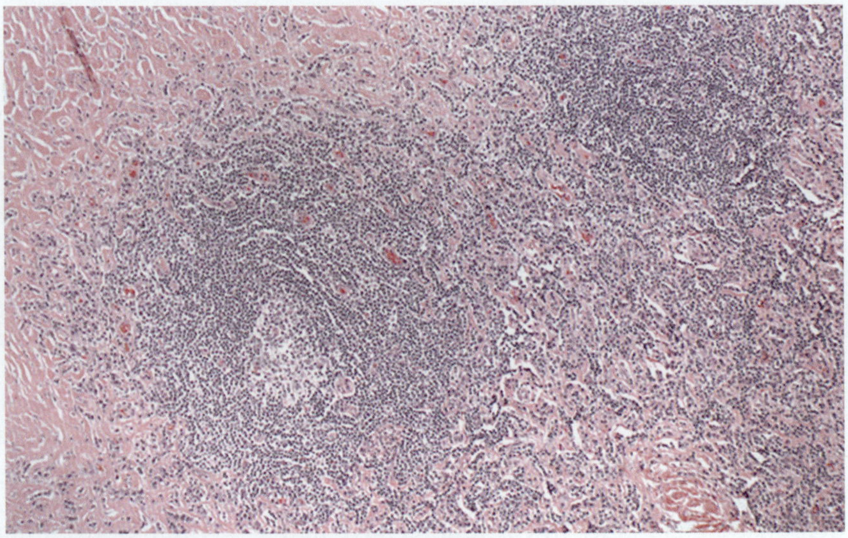

Figure 8-37

CASTLEMAN DISEASE

Nodules of organized inflammatory cells in a moderately fibrotic, thickened dura.

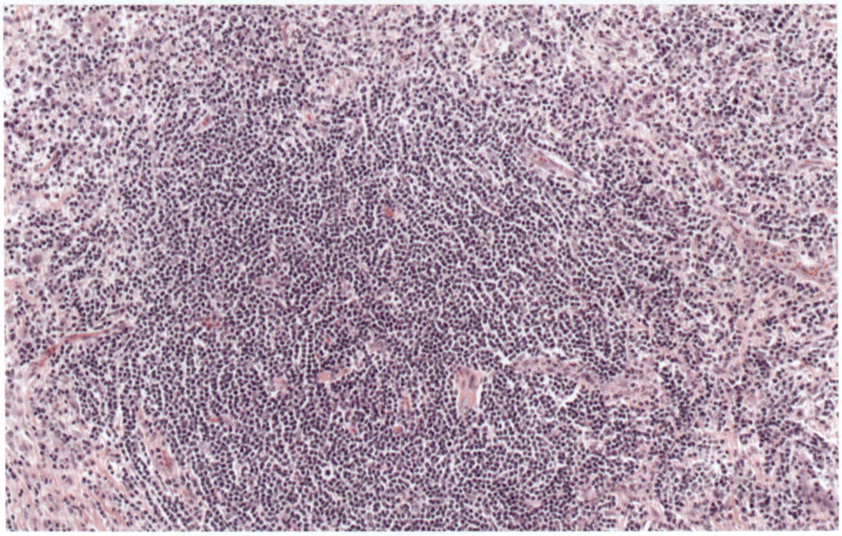

Figure 8-38

CASTLEMAN DISEASE

Some nodules are not well organized into lymphoid follicles but show vascular sclerosis.

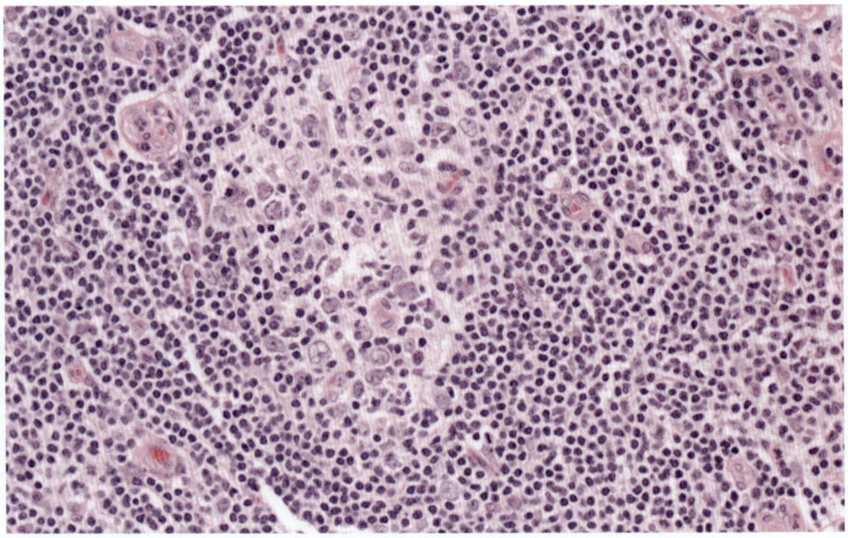

Figure 8-39

CASTLEMAN DISEASE

Lymphoid follicles can be well developed.

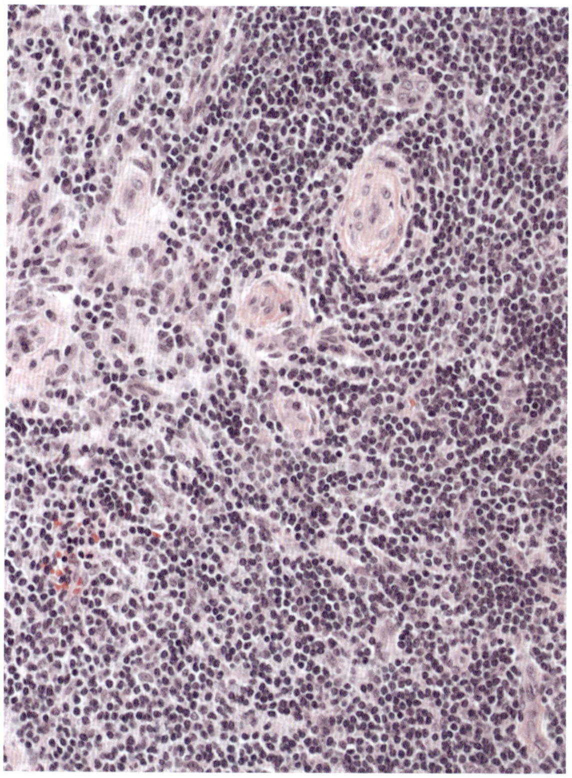

Figure 8-40

CASTLEMAN DISEASE

Abnormal follicular architecture is seen in the hyaline vascular form.

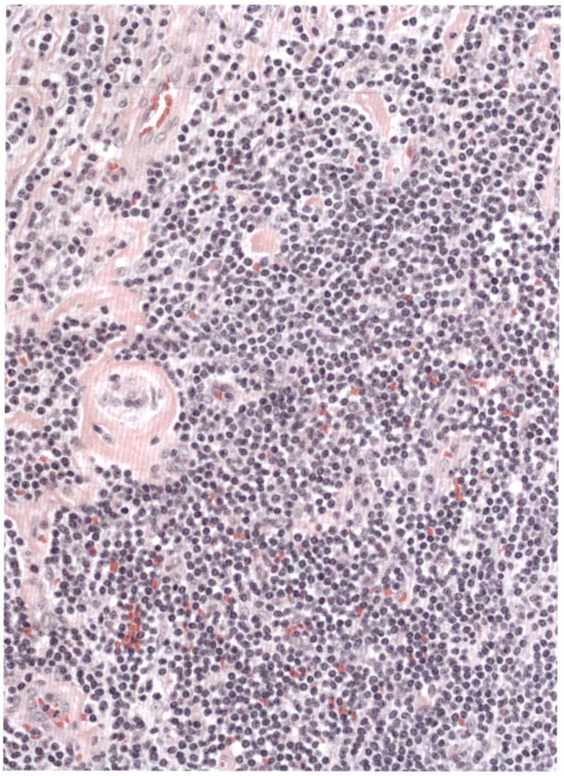

Figure 8-41

CASTLEMAN DISEASE

Marked vascular hyalinization is found in the follicles.

treatment of CD, either by surgical resection, radiation, or systemic therapy.

CD is associated with the POEMS syndrome. The increased size of the spleen and lymph nodes associated with CD pathology and this syndrome appears to also be associated with elevations of IL-6 as well as other circulating mediators (98). There are insufficient data to determine whether CD involving the CNS is associated with POEMS.

Differential Diagnosis. Given the typical presentation of CD as a discrete mass, the preoperative diagnosis usually centers on meningioma, with possible consideration of dural metastases. Recognition of the inflammatory nature of the lesion should begin to shift the pathologist away from meningioma and toward the general category of reactive inflammatory lesions. It is important, however, particularly in light of the association of some of the systemic symptoms associated with CD with some subtypes of meningioma, to evaluate lesions fully to exclude the presence of such a tumor. Since this pattern of symptoms is most often associated with chordoid meningioma, which is a World Health Organization (WHO) grade II/IV lesion, this has particular importance (119).

Once meningeal tumors have been excluded, it is necessary to consider dural involvement by a plasma cell dyscrasia or multiple myeloma. The architectural features of CD, the relative absence of atypical plasma cells, and the lack of clonality support a diagnosis of CD over the malignant alternative lesion of plasma cells. Similarly, it is the architectural features that distinguish these lesions from other plasma cell-rich processes, such as plasma cell granuloma.

Treatment and Prognosis. When the CNS is the only site involved by CD, then surgical resection may provide adequate therapy, if the location of the lesion makes this feasible (90). When surgery is not possible, localized radiation therapy may be used with success (99). With systemic disease, a variety of therapies may be indicated, ranging from corticosteroids through the use of agents directed against circulating IL-6 (82). Although the literature for CNS involvement by CD is solely based on case reports, owing to its rarity, the implications of these reports is that these lesions are typically successfully treated through one of these approaches, and do not usually result in increasing symptoms or morbidity once a diagnosis is established.

INFLAMMATORY MYOFIBROBLASTIC TUMOR/ INFLAMMATORY PSEUDOTUMOR/ PLASMA CELL GRANULOMA

Definition. *Inflammatory myofibroblastic tumor* (IMT), known by many names, is a lesion that has been found in the CNS as well as elsewhere in the body. It is characterized by a combination of a collagenous stroma with a mixed population of myofibroblastic cells and inflammatory cells, often with a prominent plasma cell component.

General Comments. The nomenclature for this lesion has been multiple and continues to evolve, often with the neuropathology literature trailing behind the contributions of pathologists more experienced with lower organs. This is a poorly understood proliferative lesion that may occur nearly anywhere in the body, as well as affecting the brain, spinal cord, and meninges. Even as the terminology becomes more homogeneous across different disciplines within pathology, there is emerging evidence of likely molecular heterogeneity within this group of lesions. Given that there are few positive diagnostic findings for these tumors, it can be expected that their classification will continue to evolve.

Clinical Features. IMT has a wide variety of clinical presentations, which depend in large part on the portion of the neuroaxis involved. While many of these lesions are dural-based tumors that mimic meningiomas in terms of clinical and radiographic signs, IMTs can involve various structures. From the largest review of cases in the literature, it was determined that meningeal involvement was the most common, accounting for roughly 60 percent of CNS cases, although more than a third of these also superficially infiltrated the parenchyma (100). Isolated intraparenchymal tumors were described less frequently, as were intraventricular lesions. The latter were assumed to be associated primarily with the choroid plexus. There were also several cases described in which the tumor extended from the intracranial compartment to other regions of the skull and associated structures (sphenoid sinus, nasal cavity, temporalis muscle). In a separate description of cases involving the spinal cord, lesions have been described in all three anatomic sites: extradural, intradural/extramedullary, and intramedullary (101). Given this wide range of sites, it is to be expected that there is a comparable wide range of presentations.

The age range for reported patients is wide, extending from 3 years to greater than 70 years, although pediatric cases are rare. The median age at presentation is 32 years, and there is a slight male predominance (100,102,103). A single lesion at presentation is the rule, with only 6 of 38 patients in one series having disease at two sites; of these, involvement of two regions of the CNS is less common than the pairing of a CNS and extraneural site (102).

Radiologic Findings. When growing in the dura, an IMT may extend as a discrete mass or mimic the en plaque pattern of meningioma. Contrast enhancement has been described in many of these tumors, ranging from homogeneous to patchy.

Gross Findings. Descriptions of the lesion often emphasize the fibrous nature, in keeping with the histologic presence of significant amounts of spindle cells and collagen deposition. Unlike most meningiomas and many other inflammatory lesions that arise in the dura, IMTs are more often associated with superficial infiltration of the adjacent brain, resulting in a more complicated neurosurgical dissection.

Intraoperative Diagnosis. Specimens from IMT can be perplexing. The mixture of spindle cells and inflammatory cells may suggest a range of lesions, extending from tumors with a spindle cell component (such as meningioma, solitary fibrous tumor, or metastasis) to infectious lesions if the inflammatory cell component dominants. While the combination of the different cell types in the lesion may suggest the diagnosis, it is not likely that this diagnosis will be rendered by the pathologist facing an IMT at frozen section. The combination of the need to exclude other entities through the application

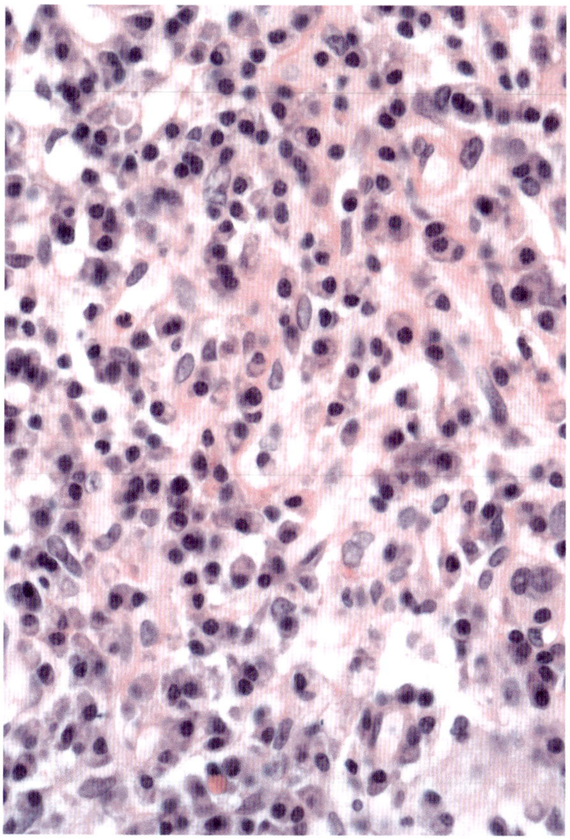

Figure 8-42

INFLAMMATORY MYOFIBROBLASTIC TUMOR

Lesions contain easily recognized, abundant plasma cells.

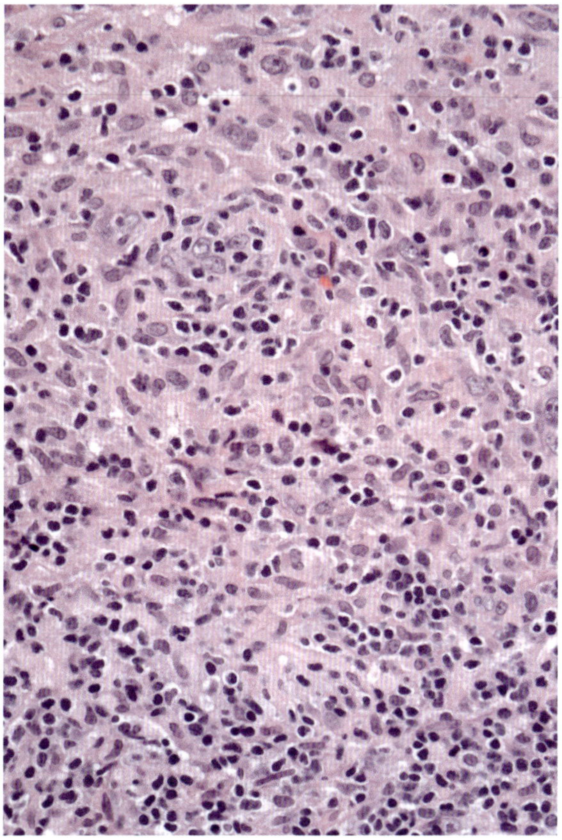

Figure 8-43

INFLAMMATORY MYOFIBROBLASTIC TUMOR

Fibroblastic, elongated cells are the predominant component.

of immunohistochemistry and the overall rarity of the lesion preclude establishing a diagnosis at the time of intraoperative consultation.

Depending on the pattern of histology, it is often considered appropriate to sample these lesions for electron microscopy (when the differential diagnosis focuses on spindle cell neoplasms), for immunohistochemistry and molecular studies (when the differential is directed by a prominent plasma cell component), or for microbiologic studies (when a mixed inflammatory cell infiltrate dominates). Appropriate negative results from these studies aid the pathologist in reaching the diagnosis, which is often a surprise to all involved in the patient's care.

Microscopic Findings. As to be expected from the panoply of names that have been applied to this group of lesions, there is considerable variability in the histologic appearance, with either the plasma cell component (fig. 8-42) or the spindle cell component (fig. 8-43) dominating (at least in the eye of the classifying pathologist). The spindle cell component, which is properly considered myofibroblastic based on the immunophenotype of these cells, is typically bland with minimal nuclear pleomorphism. Mitotic figures are usually rare or absent, and reported proliferation indices are low (1 to 3 percent), even in recurrent tumors (100). The collagenous stroma varies in amount. Necrosis has been described in rare cases (104), but is unusual. The plasma cell component, which is often accompanied by other inflammatory cells including lymphocytes and macrophages, may include Russell bodies and some binucleated cells (fig. 8-44). While both cell types are present in most lesions (fig. 8-45), tumors are typically skewed in one direction or the other (103).

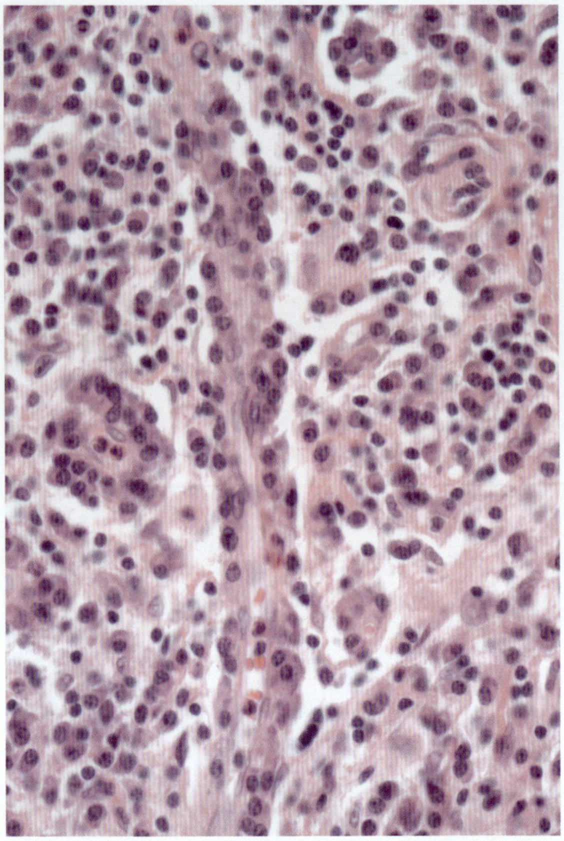

Figure 8-44

INFLAMMATORY MYOFIBROBLASTIC TUMOR

Binucleated plasma cells as well as Russell bodies are present.

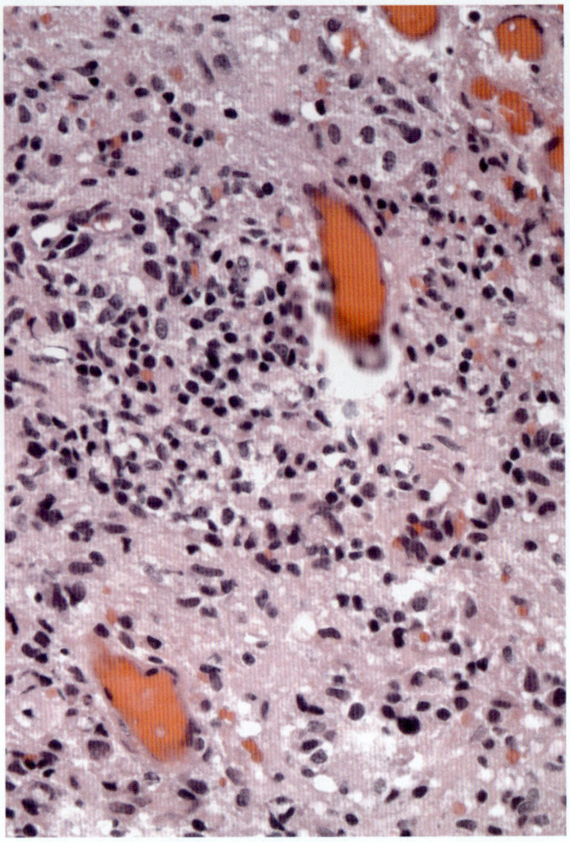

Figure 8-45

INFLAMMATORY MYOFIBROBLASTIC TUMOR

Some lesions show myofibroblastic elements and plasma cells.

Parenchymal infiltration from primarily dural-based lesions is a more common finding in an IMT than in other lesions (fig. 8-46). The tight relationship between the dural-based mass and the surface of the brain, which the neurosurgeon may find so troubling, has its origin in the extension of the inflammatory cell component of the lesion along the Virchow-Robin spaces into the parenchyma (fig. 8-47). This is sometimes accompanied by myofibroblasts, with the development of apparent fibrovascular septa within the brain (fig. 8-48).

Immunohistochemical Findings. There are several ways that immunohistochemical staining plays a useful role in distinguishing IMT from other entities in the differential diagnosis. First, in order to assess the potential presence of a meningioma with extensive lymphoplasmacytic infiltration, EMA is used since it is absent in IMT while usually positive to some extent in the more meningothelial areas of a meningioma. The spindle cells of IMTs affecting the CNS and from other regions of the body are nearly always immunoreactive for smooth muscle actin (SMA) and vimentin (100,103). In contrast to non-CNS tumors where the rate of cytoplasmic immunoreactivity for alkaline lymphoma kinase (ALK)1 antibody is present in the majority of cases (105,106), it was not present in any CNS cases in one series of 10 tumors (103) and was present in one of two lesions from another study (100). Given this uncertainty, the role of ALK1 in confirming a diagnosis of IMT is uncertain.

In addition to the spindle cell population, there is a role for immunophenotyping the inflammatory cell infiltrates in these lesions, mostly in order to exclude the presence of a

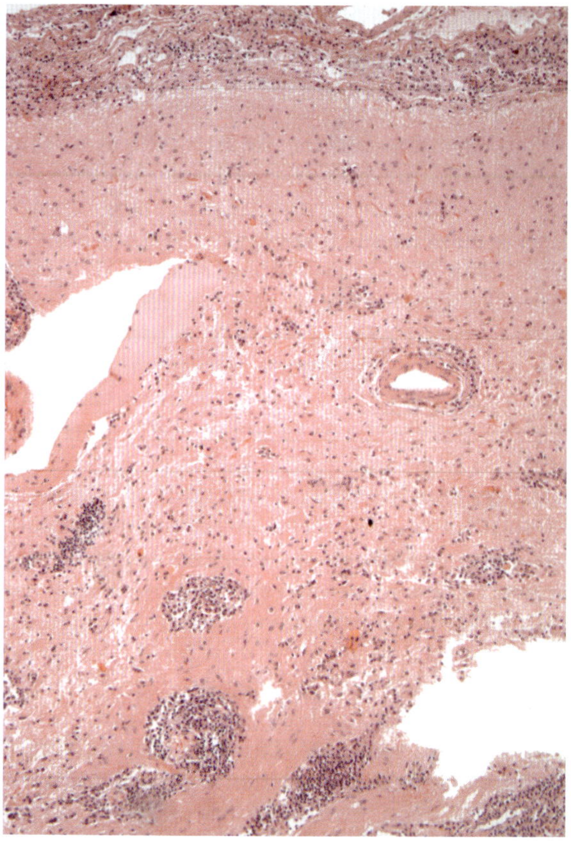

Figure 8-46

INFLAMMATORY MYOFIBROBLASTIC TUMOR

The lesion can bind the dura to the surface of the brain, as the inflammatory process extends into the parenchyma.

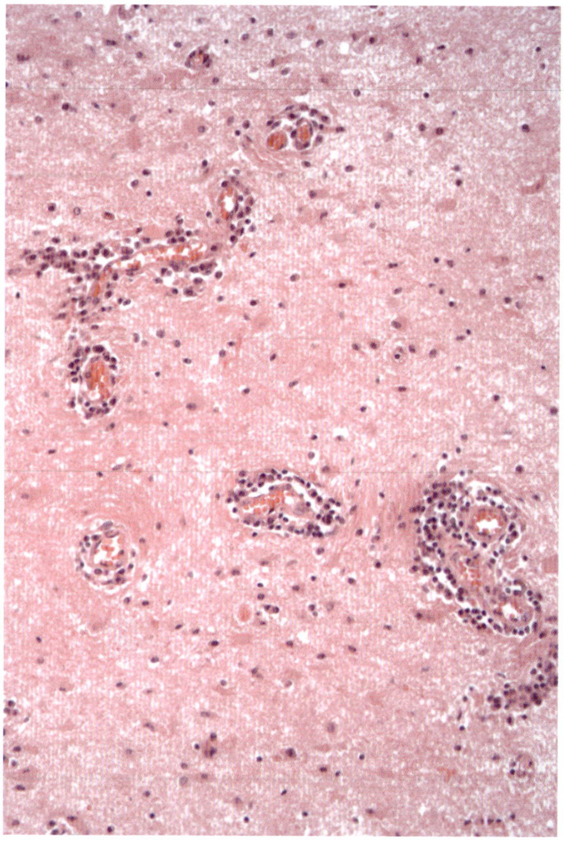

Figure 8-47

INFLAMMATORY MYOFIBROBLASTIC TUMOR

Spread into the brain along the Virchow-Robin spaces.

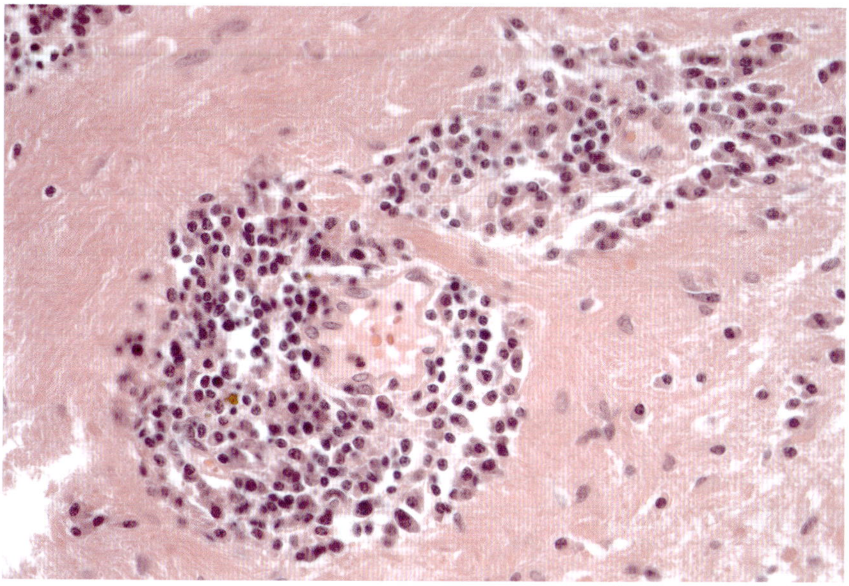

Figure 8-48

INFLAMMATORY MYOFIBROBLASTIC TUMOR

Fibrous septa may develop in brain parenchyma in association with an inflammatory myofibroblastic tumor (IMT).

clonal lymphoid population. IMTs are characterized by the presence of plasma cells (CD79a positive) expressing both kappa and gamma light chains. In addition, there is a mixture of B cells (CD20 positive), T cells (CD3 positive), and macrophages (CD68 positive).

Laboratory Findings. Given the finding of ALK1 expression and associated translocations involving the corresponding gene on chromosome 2p23 for anaplastic large cell lymphoma (107) and the similar findings for IMTs of other sites in the body (105,108,109), it might be expected that similar results would be detected for the *ALK1* gene in IMTs of the CNS. There is little data to support this, however, and the low frequency of reported IMTs of the CNS showing ALK1 expression (103) suggests that this may not be the pathway of histogenesis of this subset of tumors. As it has been suggested that, even at those anatomic sites in which the translocations are relatively common, there is no histologic difference between tumors with and without this specific genetic alteration, the absence of the chromosomal alteration does not require a reclassification of these tumors. As additional cases are studied, and as more molecular and cytogenetic studies are performed, there remains the potential for the development of new markers for IMT.

Differential Diagnosis. When these lesions have a dominant inflammatory cell component, with a particularly plasma cell-rich infiltrate, then plasmacytoma is considered as part of the differential diagnosis. Assessment of the presence or absence of clonality of the plasma cell component aids in this distinction. There are also two other plasma cell-rich lesions in the differential diagnosis: various forms of meningioma in which this pattern of inflammatory cell infiltrates is common (chordoid and lymphoplasmacyte-rich meningiomas) as well as the plasma cell-rich form of CD. The latter is excluded by the absence of a follicular architecture in IMTs, while a diligent search for meningothelial differentiation within the spindle cell component of the lesion is required. As mentioned above, there can be an important role here for the combination of EMA and SMA immunohistochemistry.

Many of the IMTs associated with the CNS have a dominant spindle cell population, which raises a slightly different differential diagnosis. Here there is a need to distinguish IMTs from other spindle cell neoplasms, including fibroblastic meningiomas, solitary fibrous tumors, gliomas with prominent spindle cell morphology, and primary meningeal or metastatic sarcomas. When a focus of parenchymal extension around Virchow-Robin spaces is examined, the differential diagnosis may include meningioangiomatosis. For all of these distinctions, the combination of positive staining of vimentin and SMA, with the absence of other markers, is helpful.

Treatment and Prognosis. Although there are no reports from single institutions on IMTs involving the CNS, an analysis of 43 cases (allowing for the basis of small series and case reports) suggested that roughly 40 percent of patients experience a recurrence within 2 years after surgery (100). The effect of incomplete resection was strong, a factor that suggests that some of these recurrences should be considered residual lesions with regrowth (101). Recurrence was not restricted to the prior site of the lesion, however, with both intracranial and distant locations being involved in rare cases.

There are no clear data on which to base therapeutic decisions. Patients are often treated with a combination of resection followed by radiation therapy and/or steroids.

OTHER ENTITIES

Inflammatory lesions of the brain and its coverings are not restricted to the lesions already considered. In addition to infectious processes, which may be confused with many of these entities, there are two patterns of inflammatory disease that have unique presentations and fall into distinct categories of pathology.

Paraneoplastic syndromes, which may cause cognitive impairment ("limbic encephalitis"), cerebellar dysfunction, seizures, sensory neuronopathy, and opsoclonus-myoclonus syndrome among others, are characterized by the presence of parenchymal inflammation. This is mostly manifest as an anatomically localized combination of perivascular inflammation with benign T cells and parenchymal activation of microglia, sometimes associated with microglial nodules and neuronophagia. These syndromes are most commonly encountered when biopsies are performed for the diagnosis of neurologic problems without specific anatomic lesions, such as in the evaluation of patients with suspected meningoencephalitis, vasculitis, or other causes of diffuse dysfunction. The specific pathologic changes of paraneoplastic syndromes are discussed in chapter 10.

Inflammation, with some combination of perivascular lymphocytic cuffing and microglial activation, in association with extensive neuronal loss and gliosis, can be found in *Rasmussen encephalitis*. This is a relatively unusual form of pathologic change, associated with unilateral hemispheric devastation and a relentlessly progressive seizure disorder. This disease is discussed in the context of the neuropathology of epilepsy in chapter 13.

PROCESSES WITH DIFFUSE DURAL ABNORMALITIES

The presence of widespread dural abnormalities on imaging studies (most commonly MRI and usually evident as contrast enhancement) in patients with persistent headaches may result in biopsy. Under these circumstances, the most common entities in the differential diagnosis are infection and involvement of the dura by metastatic tumor, usually carcinoma. The next two entities present similarly, but require different therapeutic approaches and carry significantly different prognoses.

Intracranial Hypotension

Definition. Low CSF pressure, either as a spontaneously arising disorder *(spontaneous intracranial hypotension)* or as a secondary event, is associated with relatively stereotypic orthostatic headaches as well as other neurologic signs and symptoms (110). The imaging characteristics are consistent and the combination of these clinical studies nearly always allows for a diagnosis without the need for a biopsy, although not always (111).

General Comments. While the disease process is clearly not new, the recognition of it as a specific entity was facilitated by the widespread use of MRI approximately two decades ago. Given the nonspecific findings reported in meningeal biopsies from patients with intracranial hypotension, surgical pathology makes its contribution by excluding conditions that can clinically and radiologically mimic intracranial hypotension. This is most likely when a patient has other diseases that might cause the clinical symptoms and radiologic findings.

Clinical Features. The most common presenting feature of intracranial hypotension is orthostatic headache, with relief elicited by lying down. This may be associated with nausea and vomiting, which is often relieved in the same manner. Among other neurologic findings, abducens nerve palsies with horizontal diplopia as well as alterations in hearing are moderately common (110). The most common underlying cause of spontaneous intracranial hypotension is the development of a CSF leak, most of which occur around the spinal cord.

Radiologic Findings. The combination of the above symptoms with the MRI findings constitutes the diagnostic criteria for this disorder. MRI shows consistent gadolinium enhancement of the pachymeninges, which is usually continuous, diffuse, and smooth. It may vary in thickness but is only occasionally nodular. It should be easily distinguished from a process involving the leptomeninges through its relationship with the dural contours and the absence of a gyral or folial pattern. Associated with this enhancement is downward displacement of the brain parenchyma, which may be so significant as to displace the cerebellar tonsils into the foramen magnum and resemble a Chiari type 1 malformation. Another typical finding is enlargement of the pituitary gland, which in turn may mimic an adenoma.

Accumulation of fluid in the subdural space is a relatively common abnormality which may be seen on imaging studies, and which may motivate a neurosurgical procedure. These are nearly always hygromas, collections of fluid, without evidence of prior hemorrhage and associated with altered CSF and vascular hydrodynamics, rather than hematomas.

Gross Findings. Gross alterations in the dura or leptomeninges are usually not evident (112–114). There may be leptomeningeal fibrosis that develops over the course of the disease, although there is uncertainty as to how long it takes to develop.

Intraoperative Diagnosis. Specimens from patients with intracranial hypotension are most likely to come for intraoperative consultation because of the concern about an infectious process. Given that the histologic features of the lesion, as described below, are minimal and nonspecific, it is mostly the absence of a strong

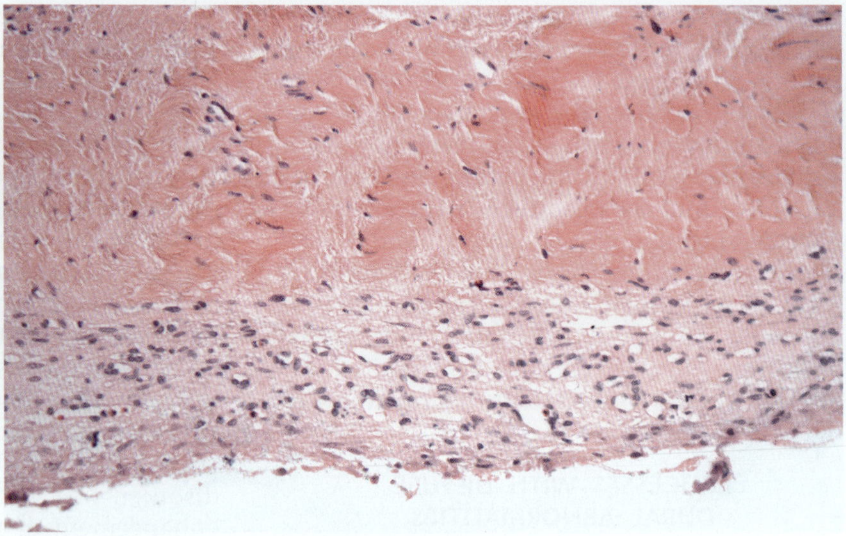

Figure 8-49

INTRACRANIAL HYPOTENSION

The thin subdural fibrous tissue layer resembles an organized subdural hematoma but lacks hemosiderin.

inflammatory process that should catch the pathologist's eye.

Microscopic Findings. Abnormalities have been described in both the pachymeninges and leptomeninges, although the latter appear to be associated with more longstanding disease (112–114). Within the dura, the abnormality is localized to the face of the dura adjacent to the leptomeninges, with no changes in the periosteal side of the dura mater. The changes seen in the dura tend to resemble those of an organizing subdural hematoma, with a discrete region of fibroblast proliferation associated with loose matrix and thin-walled blood vessels (fig. 8-49). It is the absence of evidence of prior hemorrhage, as revealed by the failure to identify hemosiderin, that distinguishes these changes from those of the more commonly encountered subdural membranes.

When leptomeningeal abnormalities are encountered, they resemble those in the dura, with fibrosis in the absence of evidence of prior hemorrhage. As leptomeningeal bland fibrosis is a common concomitant of normal aging, and is found without evidence either of related symptoms or inciting events, it can be difficult to interpret such changes.

Laboratory Findings. As expected from the descriptive name of the disorder, the opening CSF pressure with lumbar puncture is typically low (often less than 60 mm of water), although it may only be at the lower end of the normal range in some cases. The CSF may show a mild elevation in protein, with a normal glucose level. Mild lymphocytic pleocytosis can be seen, and there may be evidence of hemorrhage with either red blood cells (indicative of a recent event) or xanthochromia (for a more remote event).

When performed, evidence of the underlying CSF leak can be observed with radioisotope cisternography. With the increasing recognition of the features of the disorder, this is less often required to make the diagnosis.

Differential Diagnosis. When the clinical context and imaging results match the characteristics described for the syndrome, there is little uncertainty as to the diagnosis. Diagnostic neurosurgical procedures are most likely to be performed when there is a history or evidence of either an underlying malignancy (raising the possibility of meningeal carcinomatosis) or infection (such as tuberculosis). Distinguishing the bland pathology of this disorder from these entities is straightforward for the pathologist.

Another setting in which the pathologist may need to distinguish this disease from others occurs when a patient with headaches, in the absence of the typical orthostatic alterations, is found to have subdural fluid accumulations. When the pathologist finds the typical features of intracranial hypotension without evidence of prior hemorrhage, then it is possible to suggest that the underlying etiology of the headaches is not the presence of the putative subdural hematoma but may be associated with an otherwise unsuspected CSF leak.

Treatment and Prognosis. Given the underlying etiology of CSF leak, several approaches have been employed to treat these patients. Patients may respond to conservative management, treatment through obliteration of the leak (as with an epidural blood patch), or surgical repair of a dural breech.

Idiopathic Hypertrophic Pachymeningitis

Definition. *Idiopathic hypertrophic pachymeningitis* (IHP) is a disease in which there is thickening of the dura and enhancement on appropriate imaging studies. While this pattern may be observed in a variety of infectious diseases (including mycobacterial infection, fungal infection, and syphilis) or other inflammatory diseases (such as rheumatoid arthritis), it is considered idiopathic when there is neither clinical nor pathologic evidence of these other potential etiologies.

General Comments. Although the descriptions of these pathologic findings has a long history in neuropathology and clinical neurology, extending back as far as Charcot, the need to exclude underlying causes of the pathologic changes has resulted in an ever-narrowing set of cases that are considered truly idiopathic. The diagnosis of IHP is most commonly considered by the pathologist when, after a biopsy is performed with the intent of establishing a diagnosis of metastatic dural disease, inflammatory changes are present without evidence of an underlying pathogen.

Clinical Features. Headache is a common presenting complaint of patients with IHP, with cranial nerve dysfunction, as a consequence of entrapment, the most common accompanying sign (115). Optic nerves can be involved along with true cranial nerves. Involvement is also prominent along the tentorium or falx (116). When spinal dura mater is involved, the distribution tends to center on the cervical or upper thoracic cord (117).

Because the clinical differential diagnosis includes infection and malignancy, CSF sampling is part of the presurgical evaluation. Opening pressure is typically normal or slightly elevated, in contrast to intracranial hypotension. There may be a slight pleocytosis and an elevated protein level. Culture and molecular studies for the detection of pathogens are negative.

Systemic markers of inflammatory disease, such as sedimentation rate and C-reactive protein, may be elevated (115,116). Various autoantibodies typically associated with collagen vascular disease syndromes have also been reported in some patients; whether this suggests that the dural abnormality is part of this systemic illness remains a question.

Radiologic Findings. Radiographic studies show dural thickening, which may be diffuse or nodular. There is a predilection for the regions of the dura away from the cerebral convexities, with common regions of involvement including the falx, tentorium, parasellar region, cavernous sinus, and orbital fissures. Dural thickening can be seen on T2-weighted images and shows striking enhancement with the administration of gadolinium. Unlike the changes in intracranial hypotension, the brain is properly positioned. The radiologic differential diagnosis remains wide; only rarely does IHP present with a single localized mass suggesting meningioma.

Gross Findings. The few clinical reports that comment on the gross appearance of the dura describe it as thickened and discolored (118). The normal tan-white, glistening appearance is altered, showing a more yellow color. Unlike most neoplastic masses involving the dura, the changes observed in IHP do not typically appear as a discrete mass.

Intraoperative Diagnosis. The inflammatory nature of the process often suggests an infectious etiology. For this reason, neurosurgical colleagues must be advised to submit tissue directly from the operating room for appropriate cultures. Given the need to exclude both infectious and collagen vascular disorders prior to making a diagnosis of IHP, the diagnosis is not possible based on frozen section or smear preparations alone.

Microscopic Findings. Biopsies of the affected regions of the dura demonstrate a mixed inflammatory infiltrate, often including a combination of plasma cells and small round lymphocytes (fig. 8-50). Neutrophils have been reported in some cases, but appear to be a less common component of the infiltrate. There are also often scattered histiocytes present, but typically not granulomas. The thickening of the dura is associated with increased fibrosis and collagen deposition in a rough proportion to the

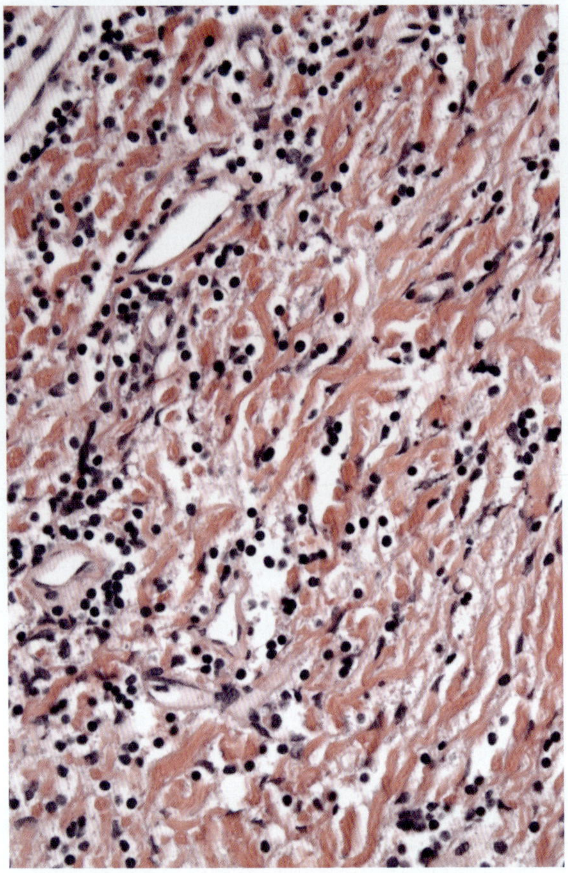

Figure 8-50

IDIOPATHIC HYPERTROPHIC PACHYMENINGITIS

Inflammatory infiltrates are in the dura, without evidence of organization.

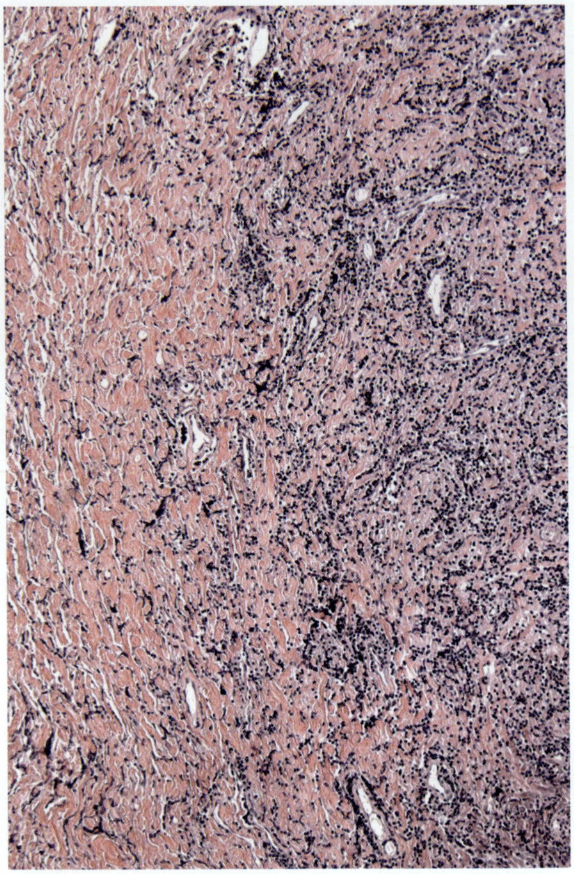

Figure 8-51

IDIOPATHIC HYPERTROPHIC PACHYMENINGITIS

Dural fibrosis accompanies more severe areas of inflammation.

volume of the inflammatory infiltrate (fig. 8-51). Special stains for organisms are negative, but must be performed to establish the diagnosis.

Differential Diagnosis. This idiopathic process brings with it a wide differential diagnosis, which can be grouped into three categories: infectious, other inflammatory diseases, and tumors. While most tumors that involve the dura are readily distinguished from IHP on radiologic appearance, en plaque meningioma may occasionally be part of the preoperative diagnosis. The exclusion of meningioma is usually straightforward, but foci of meningioma must be searched for carefully since some meningiomas are rich in inflammatory infiltrates. Rarely, metastatic carcinoma (such as lobular carcinoma of the breast) may present with a diffusely thickened dura; histologically, scant tumor cells infiltrate the dura in narrow strands or small nests, accompanied by marked fibrosis and an inflammatory infiltrate. While this may be difficult to distinguish at the time of intraoperative consultation, paraffin sections and wider sampling usually reveal recognizable nests of carcinoma. Immunohistochemical staining for keratin often helps to resolve challenging cases.

Infection, most prominently mycobacterial or fungal but also including other agents, is the most prominent entity in the differential diagnosis, and requires special attention because of the use of immunosuppression as therapy for IHP. Some combination of special stains, cultures, and serologic and molecular studies, all of which may draw on tissue collected at surgery as well as serum and CSF, is often required to provide reassurance that the inflammation and dural thickening are not attributable to a pathogen.

The other inflammatory processes that can result in comparable clinical and radiologic presentations, and may have overlapping pathologic features, include vasculitides (such as Wegener granulomatosis, chapter 6), other inflammatory diseases in which granulomatous inflammation may be present (such as sarcoidosis and rheumatoid disease), and other entities such as Behcet disease (chapter 6). In general, these processes have either systemic findings (such as sinopulmonary involvement in Wegener granulomatosis or hilar adenopathy in sarcoidosis) or serologic abnormalities. Although the therapeutic approach to IHP may well overlap with the nonspecific immunosuppressive treatment of these other diseases, it is probably most appropriate to retain the diagnosis of IHP for those cases in which no other disease process is identifiable. Given this, there may eventually be a decrease in the number of cases considered as IHP, as other diagnostic entities subsume cases previously considered as such.

Treatment and Prognosis. Leaving aside those cases that have been reported as IHP responsive to antimycobacterial agents (which most likely represent cases of infection in which culture and morphologic methods were inadequate to identify organisms), the use of immunosuppressive agents is the most appropriate form of therapy (115). Because of the contraindication to such treatment in the face of an infectious process, there is a significant burden on the pathologist, working with infectious disease and microbiology colleagues, to exclude an infectious process prior to therapy. In the absence of treatment, the typical course of the illness is that of progressive symptoms and clinical deficits. While steroids are typically the first form of therapy, the natural history of the disease may require more aggressive immunosuppresion.

REFERENCES

1. Hoitsma E, Faber CG, Drent M, Sharma OP. Neurosarcoidosis: a clinical dilemma. Lancet Neurol 2004;3:397-407.
2. Nowak DA, Widenka DC. Neurosarcoidosis: a review of its intracranial manifestation. J Neurol 2001;248:363-372.
3. Baumann RJ, Robertson WC Jr. Neurosarcoid presents differently in children than in adults. Pediatrics 2003;112:e480-486.
4. Schweisfurth H, Schioberg-Schiegnitz S, Kuhn W, Parusel B. Angiotensin I converting enzyme in cerebrospinal fluid of patients with neurological diseases. Klin Wochenschr 1987;65:955-958.
5. Dale JC, O'Brien JF. Determination of angiotensin-converting enzyme levels in cerebrospinal fluid is not a useful test for the diagnosis of neurosarcoidosis. Mayo Clin Proc 1999;74:535.
6. Zajicek JP, Scolding NJ, Foster OR, et al. Central nervous system sarcoidosis—diagnosis and management. QJM 1999;92:103-117.
7. Gullapalli D, Phillips LH 2nd. Neurologic manifestations of sarcoidosis. Neurol Clin 2002;20:59-83, vi.
8. Nadeau SE. Neurologic manifestations of connective tissue disease. Neurol Clin 2002;20:151-178, vi.
9. Bathon JM, Moreland LW, DiBartolomeo AG. Inflammatory central nervous system involvement in rheumatoid arthritis. Semin Arthritis Rheum 1989;18:258-266.
10. Guermazi A, Lafitte F, Miaux Y, Adem C, Bonneville JF, Chiras J. The dural tail sign—beyond meningioma. Clin Radiol 2005;60:171-188.
11. Kim RC, Collins GH, Parisi JE. Rheumatoid nodule formation within the choroid plexus. Report of a second case. Arch Pathol Lab Med 1982;106:83-84.
12. Guermazi A, De Kerviler E, Zagdanski AM, Frija J. Diagnostic imaging of choroid plexus disease. Clin Radiol 2000;55:503-516.
13. Kepes JJ, Dunlap MD, O'Boynick P, Terreros D. Meningioma with multiple rheumatoid nodules. A case report. Acta Neuropathol (Berl) 1986;70:314-319.
14. Bartolini M, Candela M, Brugni M, et al. Are behaviour and motor performances of rheumatoid arthritis patients influenced by subclinical cognitive impairments? A clinical and neuroimaging study. Clin Exp Rheumatol 2002;20:491-497.
15. Doan T, Massarotti E. Rheumatoid arthritis: an overview of new and emerging therapies. J Clin Pharmacol 2005;45:751-762.
16. Wernick R, Smith DL. Central nervous system toxicity associated with weekly low-dose methotrexate treatment. Arthritis Rheum 1989;32:770-775.

17. Bekkelund SI, Pierre-Jerome C, Husby G, Mellgren SI. Quantitative cerebral MR in rheumatoid arthritis. AJNR Am J Neuroradiol 1995;16:767-772.
18. Dacic S, Trusky C, Bakker A, Finkelstein SD, Yousem SA. Genotypic analysis of pulmonary Langerhans cell histiocytosis. Hum Pathol 2003;34:1345-1349.
19. Willman CL, Busque L, Griffith BB, et al. Langerhans'-cell histiocytosis (histiocytosis X)—a clonal proliferative disease. N Engl J Med 1994;331:154-160.
20. Arceci RJ, Longley BJ, Emanuel PD. Atypical cellular disorders. Hematology (Am Soc Hematol Educ Program) 2002:297-314.
21. Grois N, Flucher-Wolfram B, Heitger A, Mostbeck GH, Hofmann J, Gadner H. Diabetes insipidus in Langerhans cell histiocytosis: results from the DAL-HX 83 study. Med Pediatr Oncol 1995;24:248-256.
22. Prosch H, Grois N, Prayer D, et al. Central diabetes insipidus as presenting symptom of Langerhans cell histiocytosis. Pediatr Blood Cancer 2004;43:594-599.
23. Grois N, Prayer D, Prosch H, Lassmann H, CNS LCH Cooperative Group. Neuropathology of CNS disease in Langerhans cell histiocytosis. Brain 2005;128:829-838.
24. Grois N, Tsunematsu Y, Barkovich AJ, Favara BE. Central nervous system disease in Langerhans cell histiocytosis. Br J Cancer Suppl 1994;23:S24-28.
25. Vital A, Loiseau H, Kantor G, Vital C, Cohadon F. Primary Langerhans' cell histiocytosis of the central nervous system with fatal outcome. Case report. J Neurosurg 1996;85:1156-1160.
26. Hund E, Steiner H, Jansen O, Sieverts H, Sohl G, Essig M. Treatment of cerebral Langerhans cell histiocytosis. J Neurol Sci 1999;171:145-152.
27. Prayer D, Grois N, Prosch H, Gadner H, Barkovich AJ. MR imaging presentation of intracranial disease associated with Langerhans cell histiocytosis. AJNR Am J Neuroradiol 2004;25:880-891.
28. Steiner M, Prayer D, Asenbaum S, et al. Modern imaging methods for the assessment of Langerhans' cell histiocytosis-associated neurodegenerative syndrome: case report. J Child Neurol 2005;20:253-257.
29. Chikwava K, Jaffe R. Langerin (CD207) staining in normal pediatric tissues, reactive lymph nodes, and childhood histiocytic disorders. Pediatr Dev Pathol 2004;7:607-614.
30. Romani N, Holzmann S, Tripp CH, Koch F, Stoitzner P. Langerhans cells—dendritic cells of the epidermis. APMIS 2003;111:725-740.
31. Rosai J, Dorfman RF. Sinus histiocytosis with massive lymphadenopathy. A newly recognized benign clinicopathological entity. Arch Pathol 1969;87:63-70.
32. Foucar E, Rosai J, Dorfman R. Sinus histiocytosis with massive lymphadenopathy (Rosai-Dorfman disease): review of the entity. Semin Diagn Pathol 1990;7:19-73.
33. McClain KL, Natkunam Y, Swerdlow SH. Atypical cellular disorders. Hematology (Am Soc Hematol Educ Program) 2004:283-296.
34. Kayali H, Onguru O, Erdogan E, Sirin S, Timurkaynak E. Isolated intracranial Rosai-Dorfman disease mimicking meningioma. Clin Neuropathol 2004;23:204-208.
35. Deodhare SS, Ang LC, Bilbao JM. Isolated intracranial involvement in Rosai-Dorfman disease: a report of two cases and review of the literature. Arch Pathol Lab Med 1998;122:161-165.
36. Gaetani P, Tancioni F, Di Rocco M, Rodriguez y Baena R. Isolated cerebellar involvement in Rosai-Dorfman disease: case report. Neurosurgery 2000;46:479-481.
37. Griffiths SJ, Tang W, Parameswaran R, Kelsey A, West CG. Isolated intracranial Rosai-Dorfman disease mimicking meningioma in a child. Br J Neurosurg 2004;18:293-297.
38. Huang HY, Huang CC, Lui CC, Chen HJ, Chen WJ. Isolated intracranial Rosai-Dorfman disease: case report and literature review. Pathol Int 1998;48:396-402.
39. Kattner KA, Stroink AR, Roth TC, Lee JM. Rosai-Dorfman disease mimicking parasagittal meningioma: case presentation and review of literature. Surg Neurol 2000;53:452-457.
40. Kim M, Provias J, Bernstein M. Rosai-Dorfman disease mimicking multiple meningioma: case report. Neurosurgery 1995;36:1185-1187.
41. Panicker NK, Sabhikhi AK, Rai R. Rosai-Dorfman disease presenting as a meningioma. Indian J Cancer 1996;33:192-194.
42. Resnick DK, Johnson BL, Lovely TJ. Rosai-Dorfman disease presenting with multiple orbital and intracranial masses. Acta Neuropathol (Berl) 1996;91:554-557.
43. Andriko JA, Morrison A, Colegial CH, Davis BJ, Jones RV. Rosai-Dorfman disease isolated to the central nervous system: a report of 11 cases. Mod Pathol 2001;14:172-178.
44. Natarajan S, Post KD, Strauchen J, Morgello S. Primary intracerebral Rosai-Dorfman disease: a case report. J Neurooncol 2000;47:73-77.
45. Juric G, Jakic-Razumovic J, Rotim K, Zarkovic K. Extranodal sinus histiocytosis (Rosai-Dorfman disease) of the brain parenchyma. Acta Neurochir (Wien) 2003;145:145-149; discussion 149.
46. Toh CH, Chen YL, Wong HF, Wei KC, Ng SH, Wan YL. Rosai-Dorfman disease with dural sinus invasion. Report of two cases. J Neurosurg 2005;102:550-554.

47. Chen KT. Crush cytology of Rosai-Dorfman disease of the central nervous system. A report of 2 cases. Acta Cytol 2003;47:1111-1115.
48. Larroche C, Mouthon L. Pathogenesis of hemophagocytic syndrome (HPS). Autoimmun Rev 2004;3:69-75.
49. Bonetti F, Chilosi M, Menestrina F, et al. Immunohistological analysis of Rosai-Dorfman histiocytosis. A disease of S-100+ CD1-histiocytes. Virchows Arch A Pathol Anat Histopathol 1987;411:129-135.
50. Eisen RN, Buckley PJ, Rosai J. Immunophenotypic characterization of sinus histiocytosis with massive lymphadenopathy (Rosai-Dorfman disease). Semin Diagn Pathol 1990;7:74-82.
51. Paulli M, Rosso R, Kindl S, et al. Immunophenotypic characterization of the cell infiltrate in five cases of sinus histiocytosis with massive lymphadenopathy (Rosai-Dorfman disease). Hum Pathol 1992;23:647-654.
52. Al-Quran S, Reith J, Bradley J, Rimsza L. Erdheim-Chester disease: case report, PCR-based analysis of clonality, and review of literature. Mod Pathol 2002;15:666-672.
53. Chetritt J, Paradis V, Dargere D, et al. Chester-Erdheim disease: a neoplastic disorder. Hum Pathol 1999;30:1093-1096.
54. Veyssier-Belot C, Cacoub P, Caparros-Lefebvre D, et al. Erdheim-Chester disease. Clinical and radiologic characteristics of 59 cases. Medicine (Baltimore) 1996;75:157-169.
55. Evidente VG, Adler CH, Giannini C, Conley CR, Parisi JE, Fletcher GP. Erdheim-Chester disease with extensive intraaxial brain stem lesions presenting as a progressive cerebellar syndrome. Mov Disord 1998;13:576-581.
56. Tashjian V, Doppenberg EM, Lyders E, et al. Diagnosis of Erdheim-Chester disease by using computerized tomography-guided stereotactic biopsy of a caudate lesion. Case report. J Neurosurg 2004;101:521-527.
57. Adle-Biassette H, Chetritt J, Bergemer-Fouquet AM, Wechsler J, Mussini JM, Gray F. Pathology of the central nervous system in Chester-Erdheim disease: report of three cases. J Neuropathol Exp Neurol 1997;56:1207-1216.
58. Bohlega S, Alwatban J, Tulbah A, Bakheet SM, Powe J. Cerebral manifestation of Erdheim-Chester disease: clinical and radiologic findings. Neurology 1997;49:1702-1705.
59. Martinez R. Erdheim-Chester disease: MR of intraaxial and extraaxial brain stem lesions. AJNR Am J Neuroradiol 1995;16:1787-1790.
60. Pautas E, Cherin P, Pelletier S, Vidailhet M, Herson S. Cerebral Erdheim-Chester disease: report of two cases with progressive cerebellar syndrome with dentate abnormalities on magnetic resonance imaging. J Neurol Neurosurg Psychiatry 1998;65:597-599.
61. Rushing EJ, Bouffard JP, Neal CJ, et al. Erdheim-Chester disease mimicking a primary brain tumor. Case report. J Neurosurg 2004;100:1115-1118.
62. Wright RA, Hermann RC, Parisi JE. Neurological manifestations of Erdheim-Chester disease. J Neurol Neurosurg Psychiatry 1999;66:72-75.
63. Caparros-Lefebvre D, Pruvo JP, Remy M, Wallaert B, Petit H. Neuroradiologic aspects of Chester-Erdheim disease. AJNR Am J Neuroradiol 1995;16:735-740.
64. Rushing EJ, Kaplan KJ, Mena H, Sandberg GD, Koeller K, Bouffard JP. Erdheim-Chester disease of the brain: cytological features and differential diagnosis of a challenging case. Diagn Cytopathol 2004;31:420-422.
65. Vital C, Bioulac-Sage P, Tison F, et al. Brain stem infiltration by mixed Langerhans cell histiocytosis and Chester-Erdheim disease: more than just an isolated case? Clin Exp Pathol 1999;47:71-76.
66. Waite RJ, Doherty PW, Liepman M, Woda B. Langerhans cell histiocytosis with the radiographic findings of Erdheim-Chester disease. AJR Am J Roentgenol 1988;150:869-871.
67. Favara BE, Feller AC, Pauli M, et al. Contemporary classification of histiocytic disorders. The WHO Committee On Histiocytic/Reticulum Cell Proliferations. Reclassification Working Group of the Histiocyte Society. Med Pediatr Oncol 1997;29:157-166.
68. Freyer DR, Kennedy R, Bostrom BC, Kohut G, Dehner LP. Juvenile xanthogranuloma: forms of systemic disease and their clinical implications. J Pediatr 1996;129:227-237.
69. Bostrom J, Janssen G, Messing-Junger M, et al. Multiple intracranial juvenile xanthogranulomas. Case report. J Neurosurg 2000;93:335-341.
70. Gianotti F, Caputo R. Histiocytic syndromes: a review. J Am Acad Dermatol 1985;13:383-404.
71. Tahan SR, Pastel-Levy C, Bhan AK, Mihm MC Jr. Juvenile xanthogranuloma. Clinical and pathologic characterization. Arch Pathol Lab Med 1989;113:1057-1061.
72. Bruck W, Sander U, Blanckenberg P, Friede RL. Symptomatic xanthogranuloma of choroid plexus with unilateral hydrocephalus. Case report. J Neurosurg 1991;75:324-327.
73. Hicks MJ, Albrecht S, Trask T, Byrne ME, Narayan RK, Goodman JC. Symptomatic choroid plexus xanthogranuloma of the lateral ventricle. Case report and brief critical review of xanthogranulomatous lesions of the brain. Clin Neuropathol 1993;12:92-96.

74. Tomita H, Tamaki N, Korosue K, Kokunai T. Xanthogranuloma with massive hematoma in the third ventricle: case report. Neurosurgery 1996;39:591-594.
75. Tatter SB, Ogilvy CS, Golden JA, Ojemann RG, Louis DN. Third ventricular xanthogranulomas clinically and radiologically mimicking colloid cysts. Report of two cases. J Neurosurg 1994;81:605-609.
76. Mendez-Martinez OE, Luzardo-Small GD, Cardozo-Duran JJ. Symptomatic bilateral xanthogranulomas of choroid plexus in a child. Br J Neurosurg 2000;14:62-64.
77. Kadota T, Mihara N, Tsuji N, Ishiguro S, Nakagawa H, Kuroda C. MR of xanthogranuloma of the choroid plexus. AJNR Am J Neuroradiol 1996;17:1595-1597.
78. Rutherfoord GS, Lamprecht D, Hewlett RH. October 2001: 40-year-old Xhosa male with back pain and leg weakness. Brain Pathol 2002;12:263-264, 269.
79. Ligumski M, Polliack A, Benbassat J. Myeloid metaplasia of the central nervous system in patients with myelofibrosis and agnogenic myeloid metaplasia. Report of 3 cases and review of the literature. Am J Med Sci 1978;275:99-103.
80. Brown JA, Gomez-Leon G. Subdural hemorrhage secondary to extramedullary hematopoiesis in postpolycythemic myeloid metaplasia. Neurosurgery 1984;14:588-591.
81. Brouland JP, Megarbane B, Kafe H, Brouet JC, Mikol J. Cerebro-meningeal localization of extramedullary haematopoiesis (EMH), a rare complication of chronic idiopathic myelofibrosis (CIM). Neuropathol Appl Neurobiol 2004;30:396-401.
82. Casper C. The aetiology and management of Castleman disease at 50 years: translating pathophysiology to patient care. Br J Haematol 2005;129:3-17.
83. Greiner T, Armitage JO, Gross TG. Atypical lymphoproliferative diseases. Hematology (Am Soc Hematol Educ Program) 2000:133-146.
84. Kepes JJ, Chen WY, Connors MH, Vogel FS. "Chordoid" meningeal tumors in young individuals with peritumoral lymphoplasmacellular infiltrates causing systemic manifestations of the Castleman syndrome. A report of seven cases. Cancer 1988;62:391-406.
85. Nicholas J, Ruvolo VR, Burns WH, et al. Kaposi's sarcoma-associated human herpesvirus-8 encodes homologues of macrophage inflammatory protein-1 and interleukin-6. Nat Med 1997;3:287-292.
86. Waterston A, Bower M. Fifty years of multicentric Castleman's disease. Acta Oncol 2004;43:698-704.
87. Oksenhendler E, Duarte M, Soulier J, et al. Multicentric Castleman's disease in HIV infection: a clinical and pathological study of 20 patients. AIDS 1996;10:61-67.
88. Oksenhendler E, Boulanger E, Galicier L, et al. High incidence of Kaposi sarcoma-associated herpesvirus-related non-Hodgkin lymphoma in patients with HIV infection and multicentric Castleman disease. Blood 2002;99:2331-2336.
89. Alper G, Crumrine PK, Hamilton RL, Albright AL, Wald ER. Unusual case of inflammatory spinal epidural mass (Castleman syndrome). Pediatr Neurol 1996;15:60-62.
90. Kachur E, Ang LC, Megyesi JF. Castleman's disease and spinal cord compression: case report. Neurosurgery 2002;50:399-402; discussion 402-403.
91. Lee HY, Lee SH, Kim SN. Castleman's disease: unusual case of inflammatory spinal dorsal epidural mass: case report. Neurosurgery 2002;50:396-398.
92. Rivas DM, Saint Blancat P, Marjou F, Van Effenterre R, Poirier J. Intra-orbital Castleman's disease. Clin Neuropathol 2004;23:91-94.
93. Delmont E, Lonjon M, Michiels JF, et al. [Castleman's disease located in the central nervous system]. Rev Neurol (Paris) 2003;159:581-585. [French]
94. Gianaris PG, Leestma JE, Cerullo LJ, Butler A. Castleman's disease manifesting in the central nervous system: case report with immunological studies. Neurosurgery 1989;24:608-613.
95. Lacombe MJ, Poirier J, Caron JP. Intracranial lesion resembling giant lymph node hyperplasia. Am J Clin Pathol 1983;80:721-723.
96. Matsumura K, Nakasu S, Tanaka T, Nioka H, Matsuda M. Intracranial localized Castleman's disease. Case report. Neurol Med Chir (Tokyo) 2005;45:59-65.
97. Sotrel A, Castellano-Sanchez AA, Prusmack C, Birchansky S, Brathwaite C, Ragheb J. Castleman's disease in a child presenting with a partly mineralized solitary meningeal mass. Pediatr Neurosurg 2003;38:232-237.
98. Gherardi RK, Belec L, Soubrier M, et al. Overproduction of proinflammatory cytokines imbalanced by their antagonists in POEMS syndrome. Blood 1996;87:1458-1465.
99. Gulati P, Sun NC, Herman BK, Said JW, Cornford ME. Isolated leptomeningeal Castleman's disease with viral particles in the follicular dendritic cells. Arch Pathol Lab Med 1998;122:1026-1029.
100. Hausler M, Schaade L, Ramaekers VT, Doenges M, Heimann G, Sellhaus B. Inflammatory pseudotumors of the central nervous system: report of 3 cases and a literature review. Hum Pathol 2003;34:253-262.

101. Despeyroux-Ewers M, Catalaa I, Collin L, Cognard C, Loubes-Lacroix F, Manelfe C. Inflammatory myofibroblastic tumour of the spinal cord: case report and review of the literature. Neuroradiology 2003;45:812-817.
102. Buccoliero AM, Caldarella A, Santucci M, et al. Plasma cell granuloma—an enigmatic lesion: description of an extensive intracranial case and review of the literature. Arch Pathol Lab Med 2003;127:e220-223.
103. Jeon YK, Chang KH, Suh YL, Jung HW, Park SH. Inflammatory myofibroblastic tumor of the central nervous system: clinicopathologic analysis of 10 cases. J Neuropathol Exp Neurol 2005;64:254-259.
104. al-Sarraj S, Wasserberg J, Bartlett R, Bridges LR. Inflammatory pseudotumour of the central nervous system: clinicopathological study of one case and review of the literature. Br J Neurosurg 1995;9:57-66.
105. Cook JR, Dehner LP, Collins MH, et al. Anaplastic lymphoma kinase (ALK) expression in the inflammatory myofibroblastic tumor: a comparative immunohistochemical study. Am J Surg Pathol 2001;25:1364-1371.
106. Tsuzuki T, Magi-Galluzzi C, Epstein JI. ALK-1 expression in inflammatory myofibroblastic tumor of the urinary bladder. Am J Surg Pathol 2004;28:1609-1614.
107. Duyster J, Bai RY, Morris SW. Translocations involving anaplastic lymphoma kinase (ALK). Oncogene 2001;20:5623-5637.
108. Cessna MH, Zhou H, Sanger WG, et al. Expression of ALK1 and p80 in inflammatory myofibroblastic tumor and its mesenchymal mimics: a study of 135 cases. Mod Pathol 2002;15:931-938.
109. Coffin CM, Patel A, Perkins S, Elenitoba-Johnson KS, Perlman E, Griffin CA. ALK1 and p80 expression and chromosomal rearrangements involving 2p23 in inflammatory myofibroblastic tumor. Mod Pathol 2001;14:569-576.
110. Mokri B. Low cerebrospinal fluid pressure syndromes. Neurol Clin 2004;22:55-74, vi.
111. Schievink WI. Misdiagnosis of spontaneous intracranial hypotension. Arch Neurol 2003;60:1713-1718.
112. Good DC, Ghobrial M. Pathologic changes associated with intracranial hypotension and meningeal enhancement on MRI. Neurology 1993;43:2698-2700.
113. Mokri B, Parisi JE, Scheithauer BW, Piepgras DG, Miller GM. Meningeal biopsy in intracranial hypotension: meningeal enhancement on MRI. Neurology 1995;45:1801-1807.
114. Mokri B, Piepgras DG, Miller GM. Syndrome of orthostatic headaches and diffuse pachymeningeal gadolinium enhancement. Mayo Clin Proc 1997;72:400-413.
115. Kupersmith MJ, Martin V, Heller G, Shah A, Mitnick HJ. Idiopathic hypertrophic pachymeningitis. Neurology 2004;62:686-694.
116. Riku S, Kato S. Idiopathic hypertrophic pachymeningitis. Neuropathology 2003;23:335-344.
117. Ashkenazi E, Constantini S, Pappo O, Gomori M, Averbuch-Heller L, Umansky F. Hypertrophic spinal pachymeningitis: report of two cases and review of the literature. Neurosurgery 1991;28:730-732.
118. D'Andrea G, Trillo G, Celli P, Roperto R, Crispo F, Ferrante L. Idiopathic intracranial hypertrophic pachymeningitis: two case reports and review of the literature. Neurosurg Rev 2004;27:199-204.
119. Kepes JJ, Chen WY, Connors MH, Vogel FS. "Chordoid" meningial tumors in young individuals with peritumoral lymphoplasmacellular infiltrates causing systemic manifestations of the Castleman syndrome. A report of seven cases. Cancer 1988;62:391-406.

9 DEMYELINATING DISEASES

ACUTE DEMYELINATING DISEASES

Demyelinating diseases are common diseases of the central nervous system (CNS), and are among the most commonly encountered non-neoplastic diseases in surgical neuropathology. In our consultation practices, demyelinating diseases constitute the single largest group of diseases mistakenly biopsied with the suspicion of malignant glioma, and the largest group of diseases histologically mistaken for malignant glioma. For these reasons, it is essential for the pathologist to have a working knowledge of the cardinal histologic features of demyelinating diseases.

Demyelinating diseases, as the name denotes, are primary diseases in which the myelin is preferentially destroyed, with relative sparing of the underlying axons. The preservation of the axons is relative, that is, there may be some axonal destruction concomitant with myelin loss. The pathologic hallmark of these diseases is, therefore, not apparent on standard hematoxylin and eosin (H&E)-stained sections, but requires special stains for visualization. A number of myelin stains are available, the most popular and easily applied being based on Luxol fast blue, either as Luxol fast blue combined with H&E (LHE) or as a Kluver-Barrerra stain, which combines Luxol fast blue with cresyl violet. For intraoperative diagnosis, the rapid toluidine blue stain allows visualization of myelin as light brownish purple material, and may suggest myelin loss if the transition zone at the edge of the lesion is sampled.

Axons are not seen with myelin stains and require either silver impregnation stains or immunohistochemical detection of axonal proteins. Different silver preparations have varying affinities for different components of the CNS, with some more robustly depositing silver on axons. The most popular silver impregnation used over the past few decades to highlight axons in surgical biopsy specimens is the Bodian preparation, with others, such as the Bielschowsky, less commonly used. These techniques are not straightforward, varying with the expertise of the individual technician, and obviously rely on the use of silver, which is expensive and can be difficult to dispose. For these reasons, many hospitals (and most hospitals lacking a neuropathology service) do not perform Bodian silver impregnations. With the advent of immunohistochemistry, Bodian impregnations have further waned in popularity. Now, in many centers, immunostaining for axonal components, predominantly neurofilaments, is the most practical, first-line approach to visualizing axons. Neurofilaments are the intermediate filaments associated with neurons, and are abundant in most axonal processes. Most diagnostic assays use a "neurofilament cocktail," a combination of antibodies directed against the high, medium, and low molecular weight neurofilaments, easily highlighting axonal processes in a more reproducible and less fickle manner than the silver-based approaches.

The diagnostic approach to samples suspected of harboring a demyelinating disease involves combined staining for both myelin and axons. In most conditions (see below for details of individual conditions), myelin loss is nearly complete in affected areas, although the extent of the affected regions varies widely between the different conditions. For example, the lesions of multiple sclerosis often take up sizeable portions of neurosurgical biopsy specimens, whereas the lesions of acute disseminated encephalomyelitis are typically localized to perivascular locations. In addition, the interface between the demyelinated and normal brain tissue varies considerably in its nature between the different diseases. For instance, in acute multiple sclerosis, the border is usually sharp, with an abrupt transition to myelinated brain. In progressive multifocal leukoencephalopathy, the border is irregular and there is often a transition zone of less affected brain between the overt lesion and the normal-appearing parenchyma. Nonetheless, as mentioned above, within these areas, the myelin loss tends to be nearly complete, with a few wisps of remaining myelin along axonal structures.

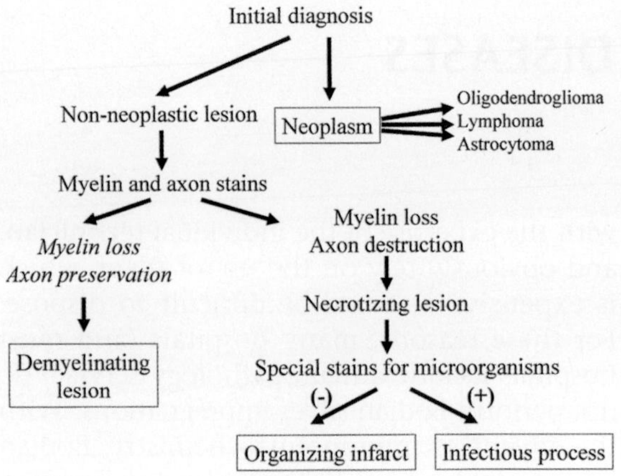

Figure 9-1

DEMYELINATING DISEASES

The flow chart shows the differential diagnosis of demyelinating diseases. The hallmarks of demyelinating diseases are myelin loss and axon preservation.

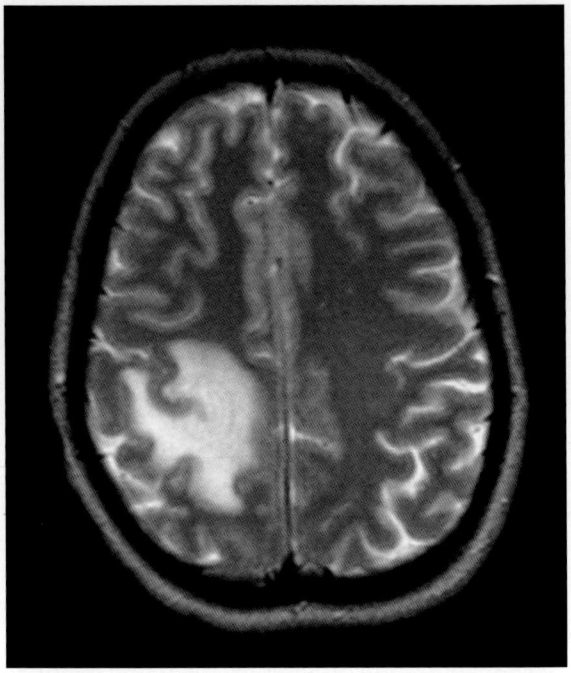

Figure 9-2

ACUTE DEMYELINATION/MULTIPLE SCLEROSIS

A large area of increased T2 signal associated with mass effect in the right frontal parietal white matter surrounds the right central sulcus and extends into cortex. Subtle concentric rings of low T2 signal may indicate rings of demyelination.

Certain histologic features raise "red flags" when the pathologist is considering a diagnosis of malignant glioma (see chapter 2), and such red flags are often found in primary demyelinating diseases. These include reactive astrocytes and macrophages in general as well as more specific features such as Creutzfeldt cells (see below) and viral inclusions. The histologic characteristics of reactive astrocytes and macrophages are covered in chapter 2. There are, however, distinctive features of the reactive astrocytes and macrophages in demyelinating diseases that might steer the pathologist toward this diagnostic possibility. For macrophages, myelin stains often reveal myelin debris (i.e., Luxol fast blue-positive material) within the foamy macrophages—not a specific, but certainly a suggestive, finding. For the astrocytes, in addition to the uniformly distributed reactive astrocytes with their prominent nucleolus and copious eosinophilic cytoplasm with processes, there are the so-called Creutzfeldt cells. These striking cells are astrocytic in nature and are characterized by glassy eosinophilic cytoplasm and an "exploded" nucleus that sometimes looks like an atypical mitosis and sometimes like a cell with numerous, minute nuclei. Again, these are highly suggestive, but not absolutely diagnostic, features of acute demyelinating disease. A flow chart for the differential diagnosis of demyelinating diseases is given in figure 9-1.

Acute Demyelinating Disease and Multiple Sclerosis

Definition. *Multiple sclerosis* (MS) is a demyelinating disease in which the lesions, known as plaques, are separated in both space and time: the demyelinating lesions are multiple and present at different times. Based on the timing and progression of the lesions, there are different clinical subtypes of MS, the most common and characteristic of which is the relapsing-remitting form. In this form, each episode is followed by only partial recovery, thus leading to progressive neurological worsening during the course of the disease.

The clinically and radiologically typical forms of MS are almost never biopsied. Thus, the most common variant to be biopsied is an acute demyelinating disease presenting as a single mass lesion (fig. 9-2). Because such cases do not suffice for a formal diagnosis of MS and because such cases do not necessarily progress to classic

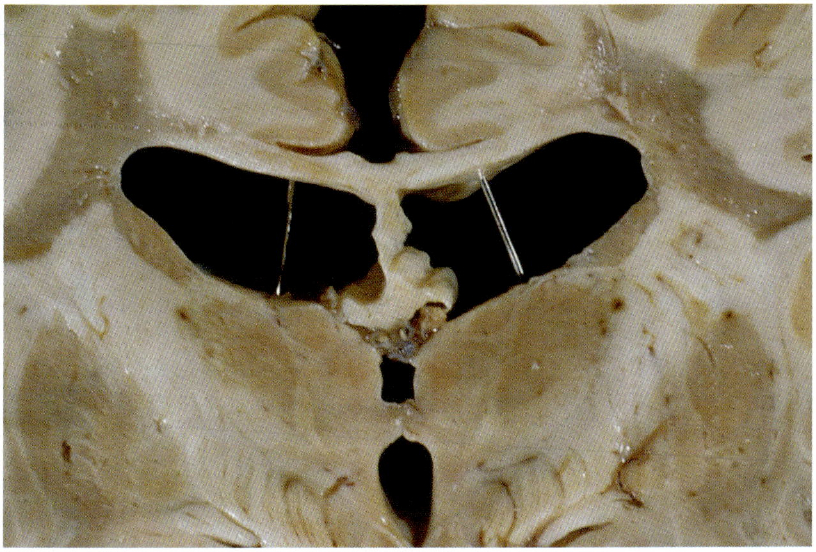

Figure 9-3

ACUTE DEMYELINATION/ MULTIPLE SCLEROSIS

Bilateral periventricular areas of demyelination are firm, tan, slightly depressed plaques at the corners of the ventricles. The ventricles are kept open with thin metal clips.

MS, some prefer the less committal term *acute demyelinating disease* to describe these cases. Given the implications of assigning a diagnosis of MS to a patient, we prefer the term acute demyelinating disease if the patient does not already have a diagnosis of MS.

General Comments. In our experience, acute demyelinating diseases, including acute variants of MS, are the most common conditions misdiagnosed by pathologists as gliomas. In general, only those demyelinating conditions that radiologically resemble gliomas are biopsied; as a result, the submitting diagnosis is usually malignant glioma. These lesions are often contrast-enhancing, single, large lesions that occur in the absence of either a clinical history of MS or radiologic findings suggesting MS. In other words, only those cases that are diagnostically challenging from a clinical and radiologic point of view make it to biopsy. This chapter focuses on those cases that are biopsied and therefore come to the attention of the surgical pathologist.

Clinical Features. MS usually presents in young adults, but both children and older adults are affected; there is a female predominance. Because MS plaques affect a wide variety of white matter sites, the clinical signs and symptoms vary widely. The most characteristically affected sites are the periventricular regions, particularly the corners of the lateral ventricles (Wetterwinkel, or storm center of Steiner) (figs. 9-3, 9-4); but these lesions do not necessarily cause clinical problems. Commonly affected sites that lead to clinical presentation include the optic nerve, the spinal cord, the brain stem, and the cerebellum, with signs and symptoms depending

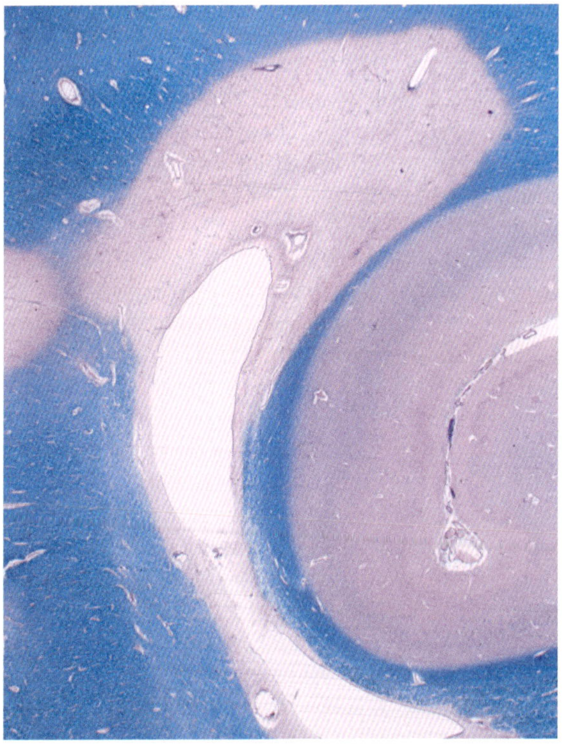

Figure 9-4

ACUTE DEMYELINATION/MULTIPLE SCLEROSIS

Periventricular demyelination appears as an eosinophilic area adjacent to the occipital horn of the lateral ventricle (Luxol fast blue-hematoxylin and eosin [H&E] stain).

on the site affected. The onset of symptoms is usually subacute or acute, sometimes worsening over a period of days. In many instances, there is slow, partial recovery of function, but the partial nature of the recovery brings about gradual worsening of overall neurological function with repeated episodes over time.

MS has been separated into different clinicopathologic variants (1–3). Chronic forms include the *relapsing-remitting type* as well as more gradually progressive forms. Acute forms include the *Marburg type* (acute MS with a typical distribution of plaques), *Balo concentric sclerosis* (in which plaques and regions of preserved myelin have a roughly concentric appearance), *Devic neuromyelitis optica* (with acute onset of optic nerve and spinal cord disease), *Schilder type* (acute MS consisting of giant plaques that may involve much of both hemispheres), and the single, often large lesions that lead to biopsy. Significantly, the Schilder type may also be biopsied and the histologic features are identical to those of the single, large acute plaques. Only clinical and radiologic differences allow distinction of these entities, and they may represent parts of a spectrum.

For the nonclassic cases that most often come to biopsy, the signs and symptoms are usually those of a mass lesion affecting either the cerebral hemisphere or spinal cord, and less often, the brain stem or cerebellum. The clinical presentation can be identical to that of any other mass lesion of subacute onset in these regions, thus closely mimicking a neoplasm.

Radiologic Findings. Neuroimaging is helpful in establishing a diagnosis in classic cases (4), but may be misleading in those cases coming to biopsy. T2-weighted magnetic resonance images (MRIs) are sensitive to detecting plaques, and finding plaques in the characteristic, periventricular locations is virtually pathognomonic of MS. Contrast enhancement may be found in active plaques. The single, acute lesions that are biopsied, however, usually occur in the absence of classic MS, and appear rather as large, enhancing masses that mimic malignant glioma (fig. 9-2). There may be ring enhancement and mass effect with surrounding edema.

Gross Findings. The macroscopic features of classic, chronic MS are most readily appreciated at autopsy. The plaques have a firm, tan, sharply demarcated appearance, with the tissue assuming a concave depression on the cut surface of fixed brain tissue (fig. 9-3). The lesions have a characteristic distribution, most commonly affecting periventricular regions such as the corners of the lateral ventricles as well as the superficial white matter tracts of the brain stem and spinal cord. Subacute lesions may have less well-demarcated borders, sometimes with a pinkish hue, reflecting ongoing myelin loss and inflammation. Rare plaques have reduced myelin "shadowing" the main plaque, which may represent remyelination. In some larger plaques, it is possible to discern fingers of demyelinated tissue extending outward from the main plaques, around large blood vessels (Dawson fingers) (fig. 9-5).

On gross examination of surgical specimens, a border between intact white matter and a plaque is often appreciated, with the plaque sometimes mistaken for normal gray matter (fig. 9-3). Plaques are often somewhat darker and more rubbery, however, than normal gray matter.

Intraoperative Diagnosis. Smear preparations demonstrate foamy macrophages, often in large numbers (fig. 9-6). The macrophages vary in size from small, round cells with cytoplasm only twice the size of the nucleus, to larger, irregularly rounded cells, sometimes having more than one nucleus. The cytoplasm is characteristically foamy, consisting of numerous, minute vacuoles. Prominent reactive astrocytes are often noted in the center of small smeared pieces of cerebral parenchymal tissue ("tissuelets"), with the central astrocyte appearing to hold the tissue fragment together. If inflammation is present, small, bland-appearing lymphocytes may be plentiful on the smears.

Frozen sections also demonstrate the macrophages, often arranged in broad sheets as a so-called "sea of macrophages." In some cases, particularly when an edge is sampled, the macrophages are clustered around blood vessels. Toluidine blue–stained sections may show refractile myelin debris within the macrophages, and oil red O stains highlight the lipid from ingested myelin occupying the foamy cytoplasm. Oil red O stains are particularly helpful in cases in which the cytologic features of the macrophages are less characteristic, assuring the pathologist that the numerous cells are lipid laden and therefore more likely to be macrophages

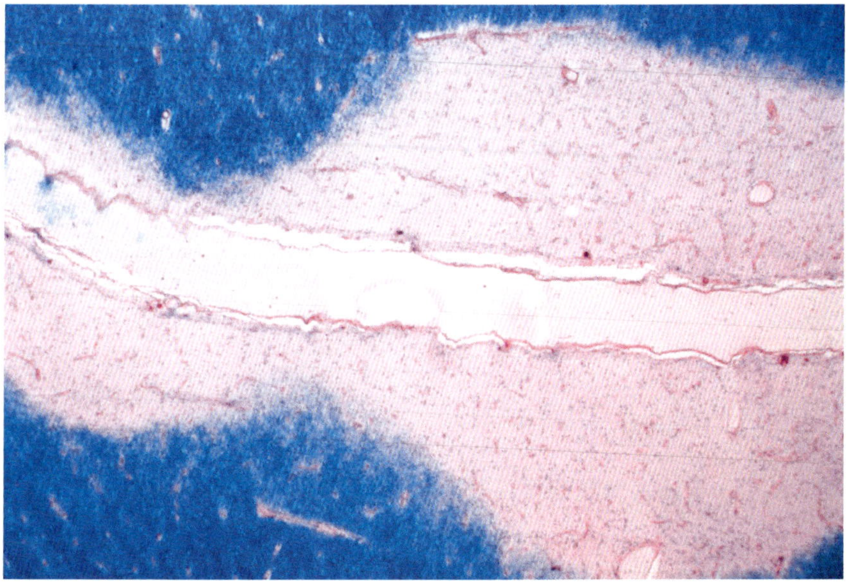

Figure 9-5

ACUTE DEMYELINATION/ MULTIPLE SCLEROSIS

Demyelination often occurs in a perivascular distribution at the edge of larger plaques, as a so-called Dawson finger (Luxol fast blue-H&E stain).

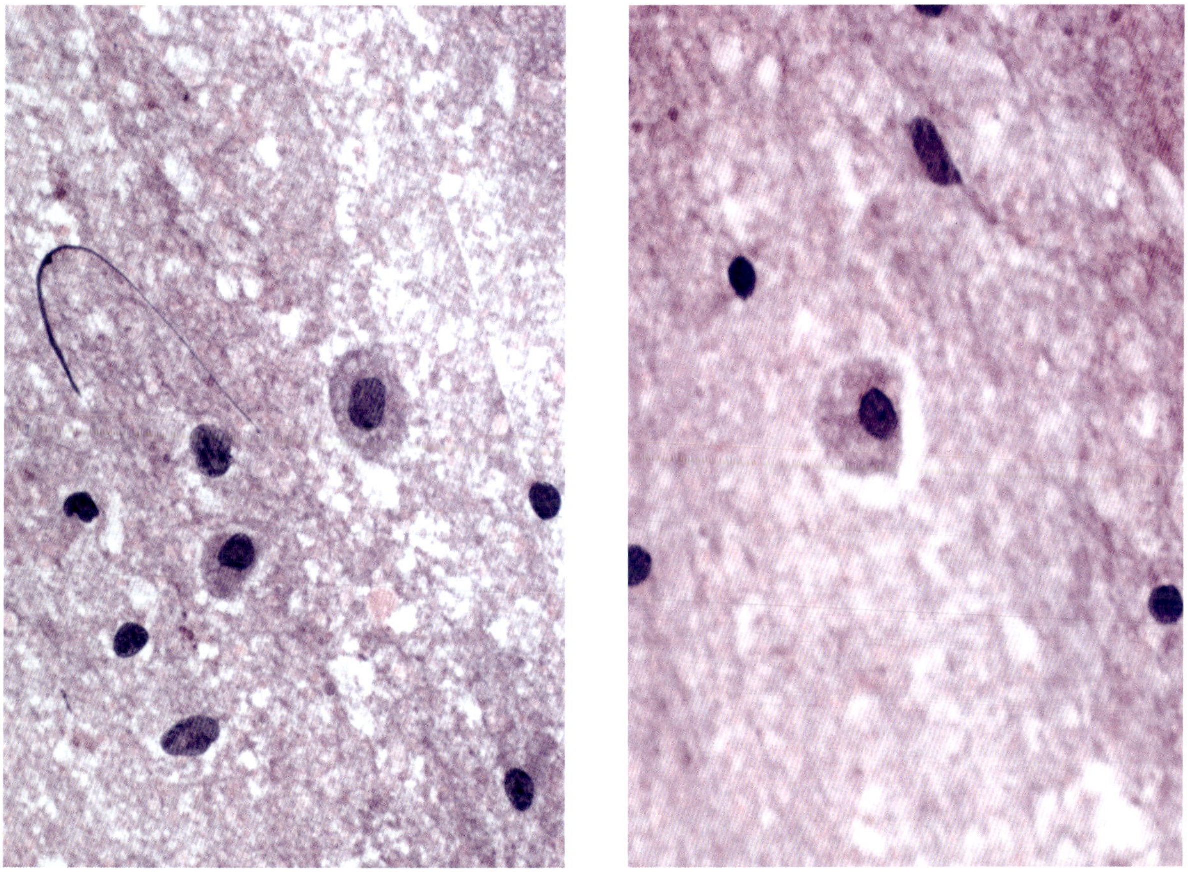

Figure 9-6

ACUTE DEMYELINATION/MULTIPLE SCLEROSIS

Smear preparations demonstrate macrophages, with their distinct rounded contours and granular cytoplasm.

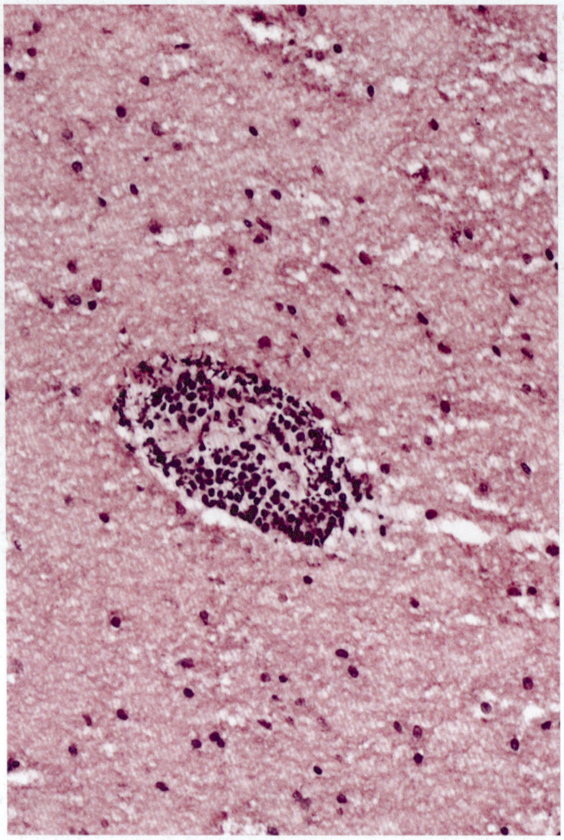

Figure 9-7

ACUTE DEMYELINATION/MULTIPLE SCLEROSIS

The frozen section specimen illustrates a conspicuous perivascular lymphocytic cuff.

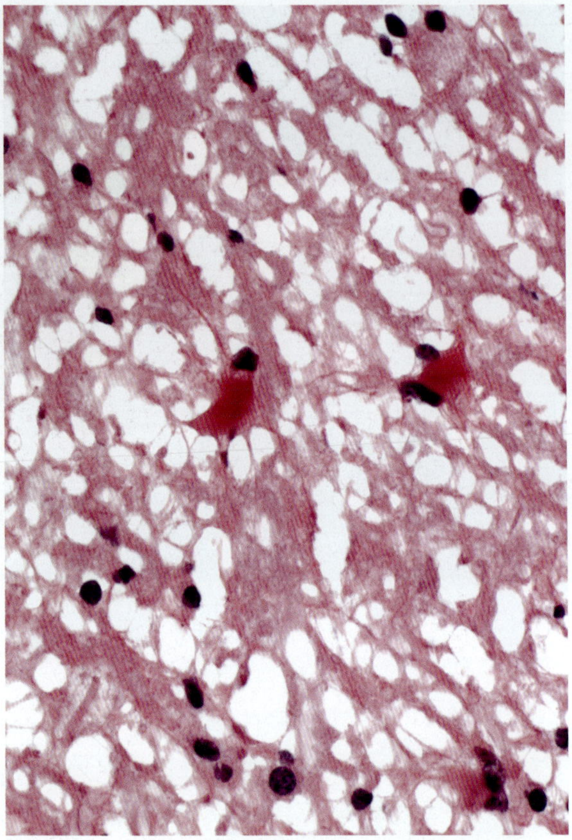

Figure 9-8

ACUTE DEMYELINATION/MULTIPLE SCLEROSIS

The presence of reactive astrocytosis on a frozen section smear is a feature of demyelinating disease.

than tumor cells. The toluidine blue–stained sections also demonstrate the change from intact myelin to digested myelin if the edge of the lesion is sampled, with the myelin appearing as light refractile purple-brown material along axons surrounding the lesion. Standard H&E-stained frozen sections further demonstrate the macrophages, reactive astrocytes, and perivascular lymphocytes, strongly suggesting that the lesion represents a reactive, possibly demyelinating process (figs. 9-7–9-9). Sometimes, Creutzfeldt cells are seen in frozen sections.

Microscopic Findings. The general microscopic findings of the acute demyelinating diseases have been detailed above. In classic MS, different plaques may have different appearances, reflecting the spectrum from acute to chronic lesions. The histologic findings in those cases that come to biopsy, however, are remarkably uniform. The hallmark features include extensive collections of foamy macrophages, which can be shown to have myelin in their cytoplasm by oil red O staining of frozen section specimens and Luxol fast blue staining of paraffin-embedded specimens (figs. 9-10, 9-11). Periodic acid–Schiff (PAS) staining is also a sensitive stain for demonstrating the granular macrophage contents. Indeed, the presence of numerous macrophages on any biopsy suspected to represent a malignant glioma should raise the strong suspicion that the lesion may instead be a demyelinating disease. Reactive astrocytes may be prominent (fig. 9-11), often with Creutzfeldt cells (fig. 9-12). In some lesions, perivascular lymphocytic cuffs are present; these range from rare lymphocytes to dense aggregates (fig. 9-13), and are composed of bland-appearing T cells. There is often a sharp margin between the macrophage-dense

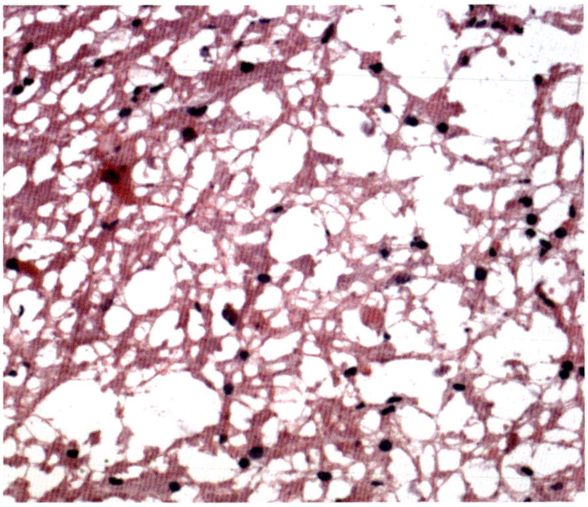

Figure 9-9

ACUTE DEMYELINATION/MULTIPLE SCLEROSIS

The edges of frozen section specimens are particularly informative, with reactive astrocytes of brain (upper left) adjacent to the spongy appearing lesion.

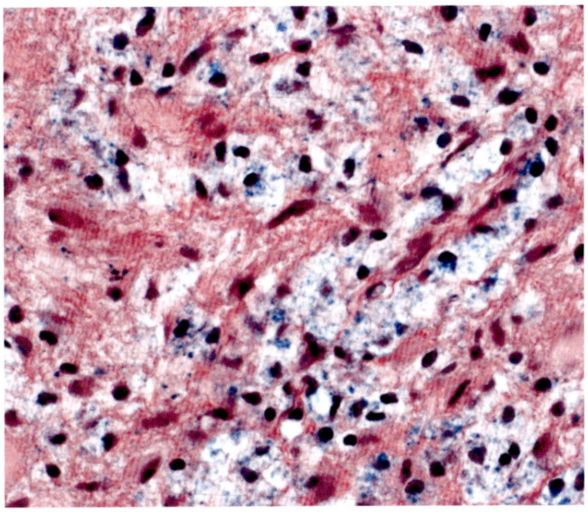

Figure 9-10

ACUTE DEMYELINATION/MULTIPLE SCLEROSIS

Foamy macrophages filled with myelin debris, sometimes around blood vessels (right), and reactive astrocytes are keys to diagnosis (Luxol fast blue-H&E stain).

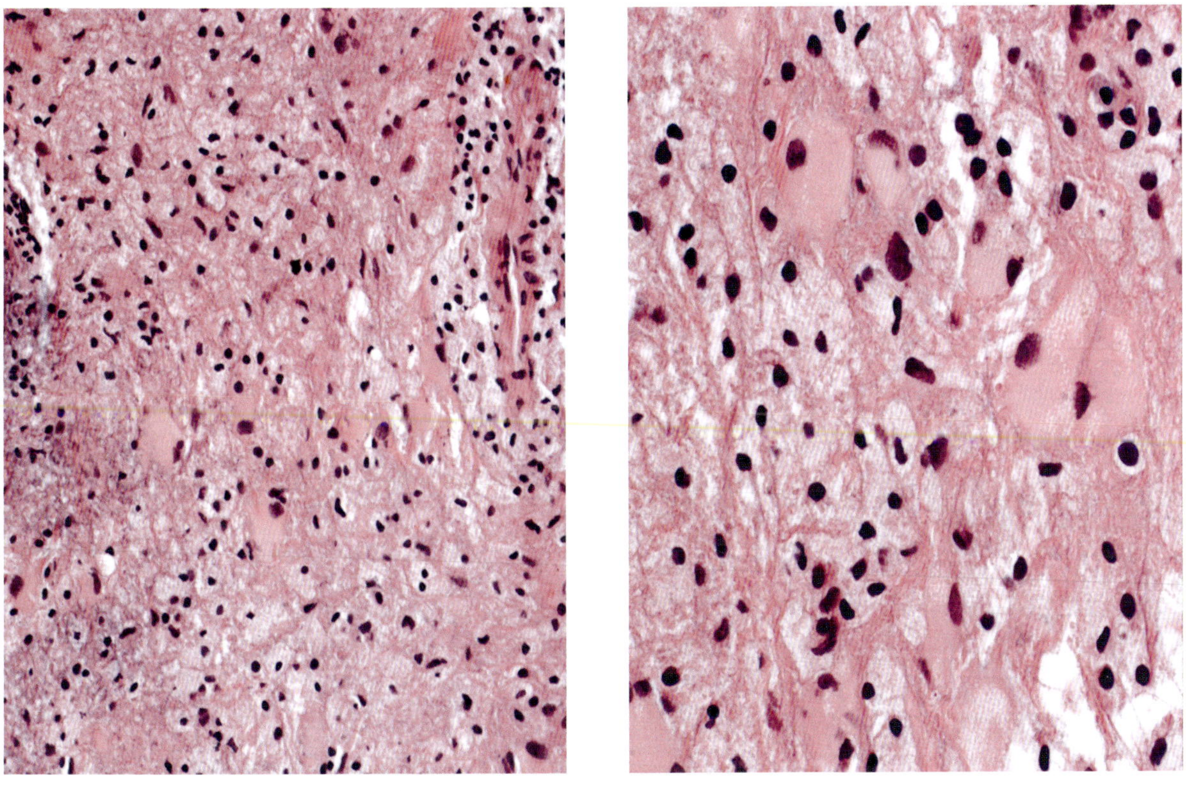

Figure 9-11

ACUTE DEMYELINATION/MULTIPLE SCLEROSIS

Left: Reactive astrocytes and macrophages in the parenchyma, and a perivascular accumulation of macrophages (top right).

Right: Reactive astrocytes are seen along with parenchymal macrophages.

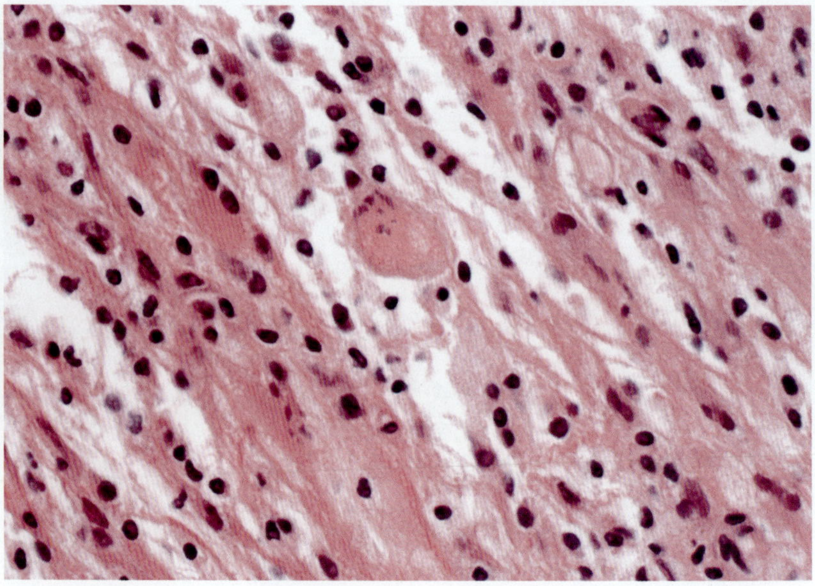

Figure 9-12

ACUTE DEMYELINATION/ MULTIPLE SCLEROSIS

A Creutzfeldt cell has eosinophilic cytoplasm and an "exploded" nucleus. (Also see fig. 2-20.)

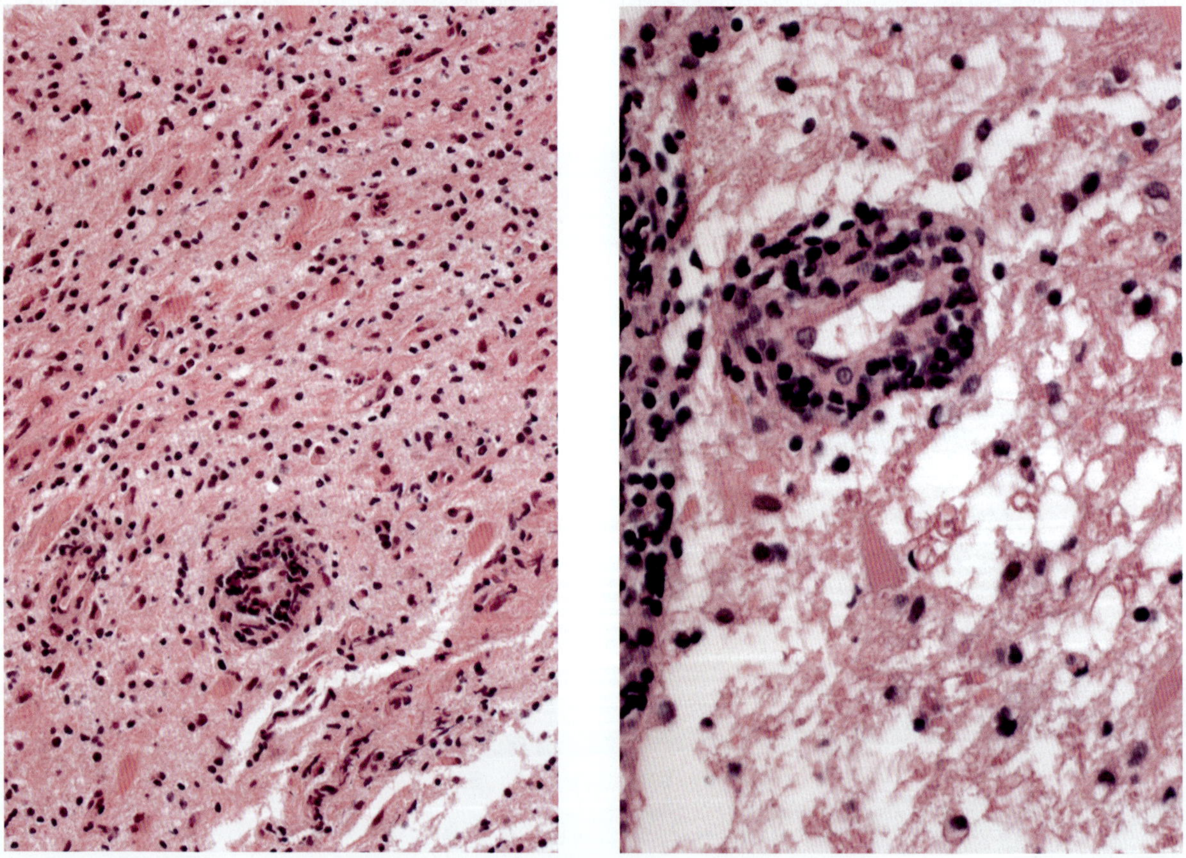

Figure 9-13

ACUTE DEMYELINATION/MULTIPLE SCLEROSIS

Left: Inflammatory cuffs, macrophages, and reactive astrocytes are seen.
Right: High-power microscopy of an inflammatory cuff shows small, bland lymphocytes.

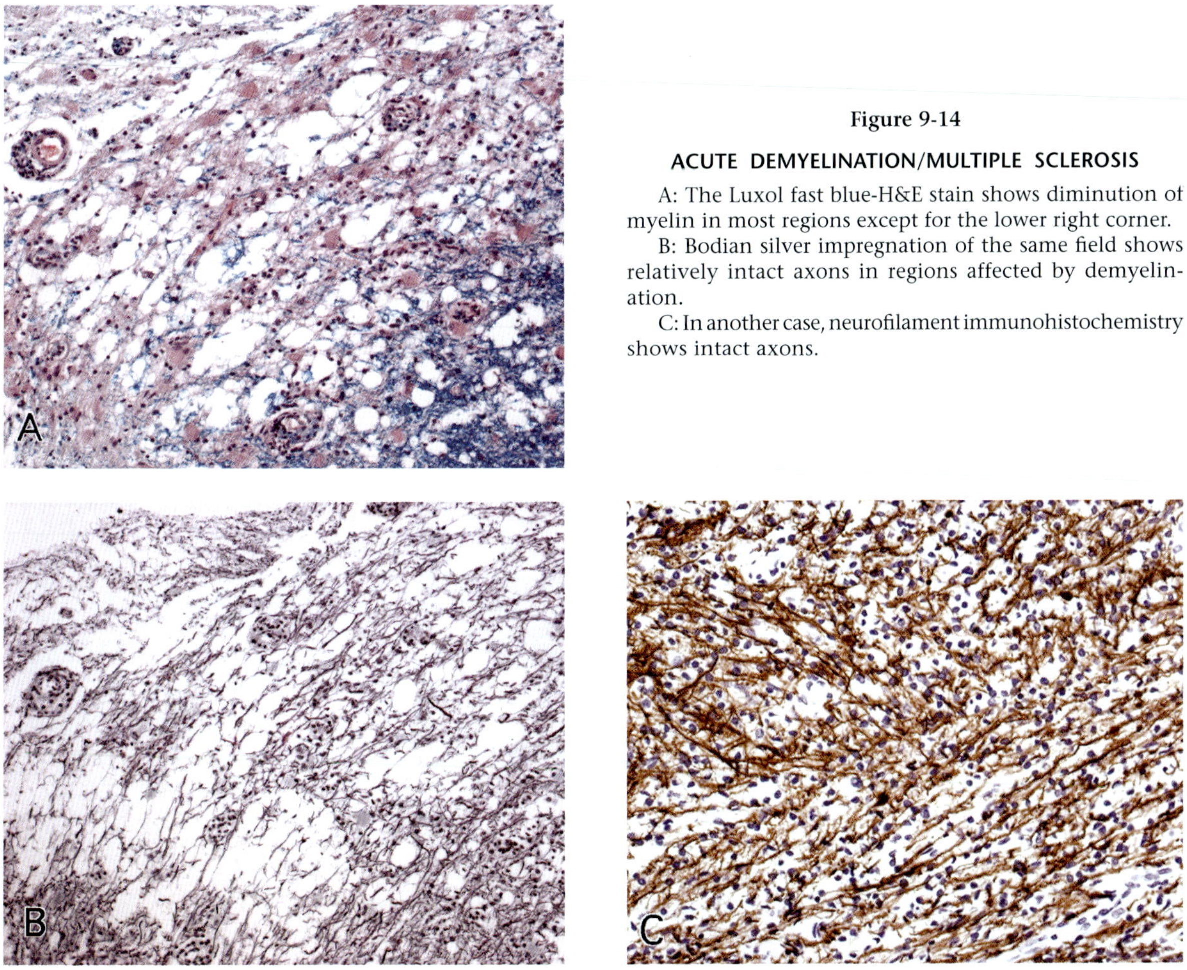

Figure 9-14

ACUTE DEMYELINATION/MULTIPLE SCLEROSIS

A: The Luxol fast blue-H&E stain shows diminution of myelin in most regions except for the lower right corner.

B: Bodian silver impregnation of the same field shows relatively intact axons in regions affected by demyelination.

C: In another case, neurofilament immunohistochemistry shows intact axons.

plaque and the surrounding brain, although the immediately adjacent brain often harbors reactive astrocytes and T-cell infiltrates.

The diagnosis is secured by comparing myelin and axon stains to document loss of myelin and relative preservation of axons (figs. 9-14, 9-15). In general, myelin loss is nearly complete in plaques that consist of dense, back-to-back macrophages, sometimes with only scattered myelinated fibers remaining, with the myelin resuming an essentially normal appearance at the plaque margin. Although there may be axonal loss, it does not often approach the severity of the myelin loss. Notably, however, some particularly acute plaques may undergo necrosis and nearly complete axonal loss, but such destructive changes are usually focal, with other areas displaying more characteristic relative axonal preservation. Oligodendroglial loss is often extensive in chronic plaques; in surgically biopsied cases, however, possible oligodendroglial loss is overshadowed by the other histologic alterations.

Some have postulated that active plaques occur in four patterns: those that are well demarcated and centered around blood vessels, with (pattern I) or without (pattern II) immunoglobulin and complement deposition; and those that are less well demarcated and are not vasculocentric (pattern III, with widespread apoptosis and pattern IV, with central apoptosis only). Myelin protein loss and the degree of remyelination vary between these types. It seems likely, however, that each person only develops one general type of pattern (I/II or III/IV) (5,6).

Immunohistochemical Findings. Immunohistochemistry for neurofilaments may be helpful in diagnosing acute demyelinating diseases since, as mentioned above, it is an easy and reproducible means for demonstrating axons (fig. 9-14C). Macrophages are readily highlighted

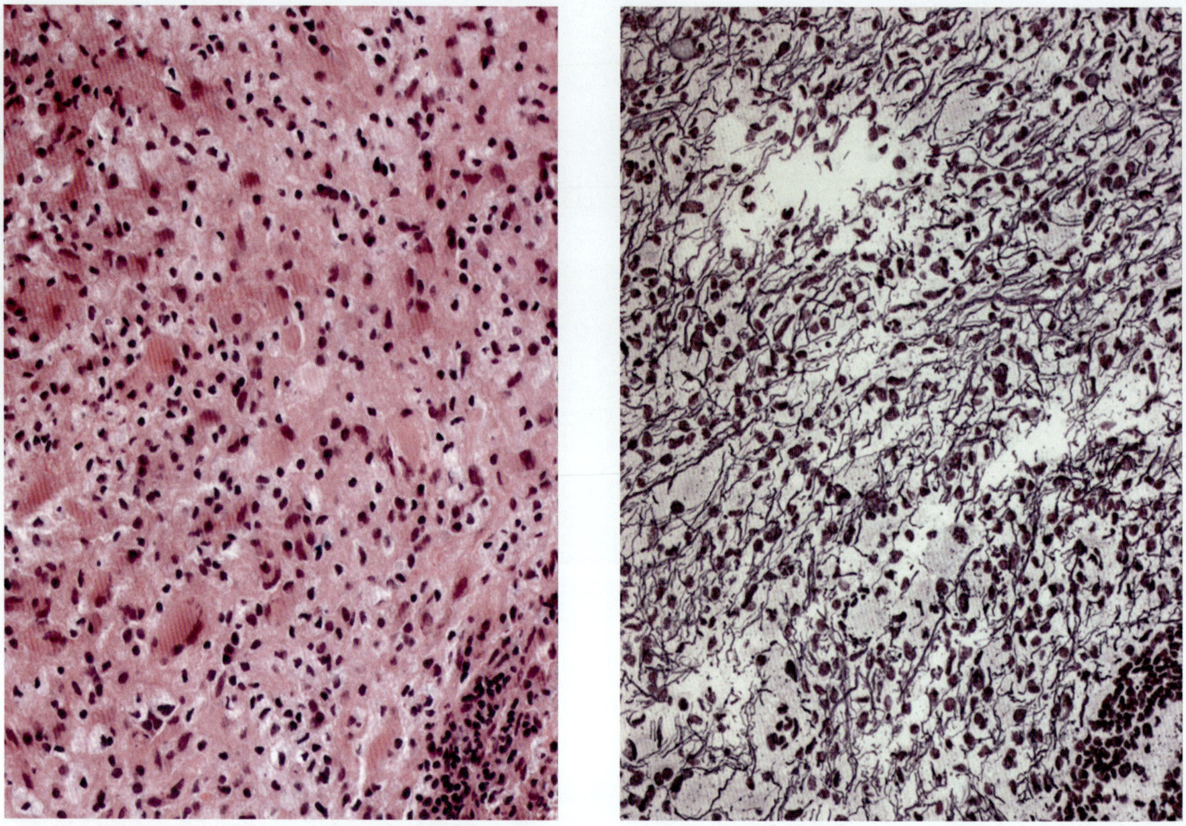

Figure 9-15

ACUTE DEMYELINATION/MULTIPLE SCLEROSIS

Left: The Luxol fast blue-H&E stain shows complete loss of myelin except in occasional macrophages (note inflamed vessel in lower right).

Right: Bodian silver impregnation shows intact axons from the same field (note inflamed vessel in lower right).

using CD68 (KP1) staining (fig. 9-16A,B) and lymphocytes using leukocyte common antigen (LCA). Since most of the small lymphocytes are T cells, T-cell markers may be of use in accenting the lymphocytes (fig. 9-16C). Although not necessary in most instances, glial fibrillary acidic protein (GFAP) demonstrates the usual even spacing and long processes of the reactive astrocytes.

Ultrastructural Findings. Ultrastructural examination is not needed for the diagnosis of acute demyelinating conditions. If undertaken, the hallmark finding is macrophages containing myelin debris intercalated amid intact axons. In particularly acute cases that include axonal destruction, some dilated axons containing whorled filaments and microtubules (axonal spheroids) are seen.

Laboratory Findings. Cerebrospinal fluid (CSF) examination for the presence of oligoclonal bands is a sensitive diagnostic test for MS. Oligoclonal bands are present in approximately 95 percent of patients with MS (7). Visual evoked potentials are also abnormal in many patients, and may provide indirect evidence of deep-seated lesions.

Differential Diagnosis. The differential diagnosis includes neoplasms, other demyelinating conditions, and other inflammatory, nondemyelinating conditions. Of initial importance is the distinction of primary demyelinating disease from neoplasms. As indicated above, this is one of the most commonly encountered difficulties leading to misdiagnosis by pathologists not familiar with neuropathology (8–11). Neoplasms that are mimicked by acute

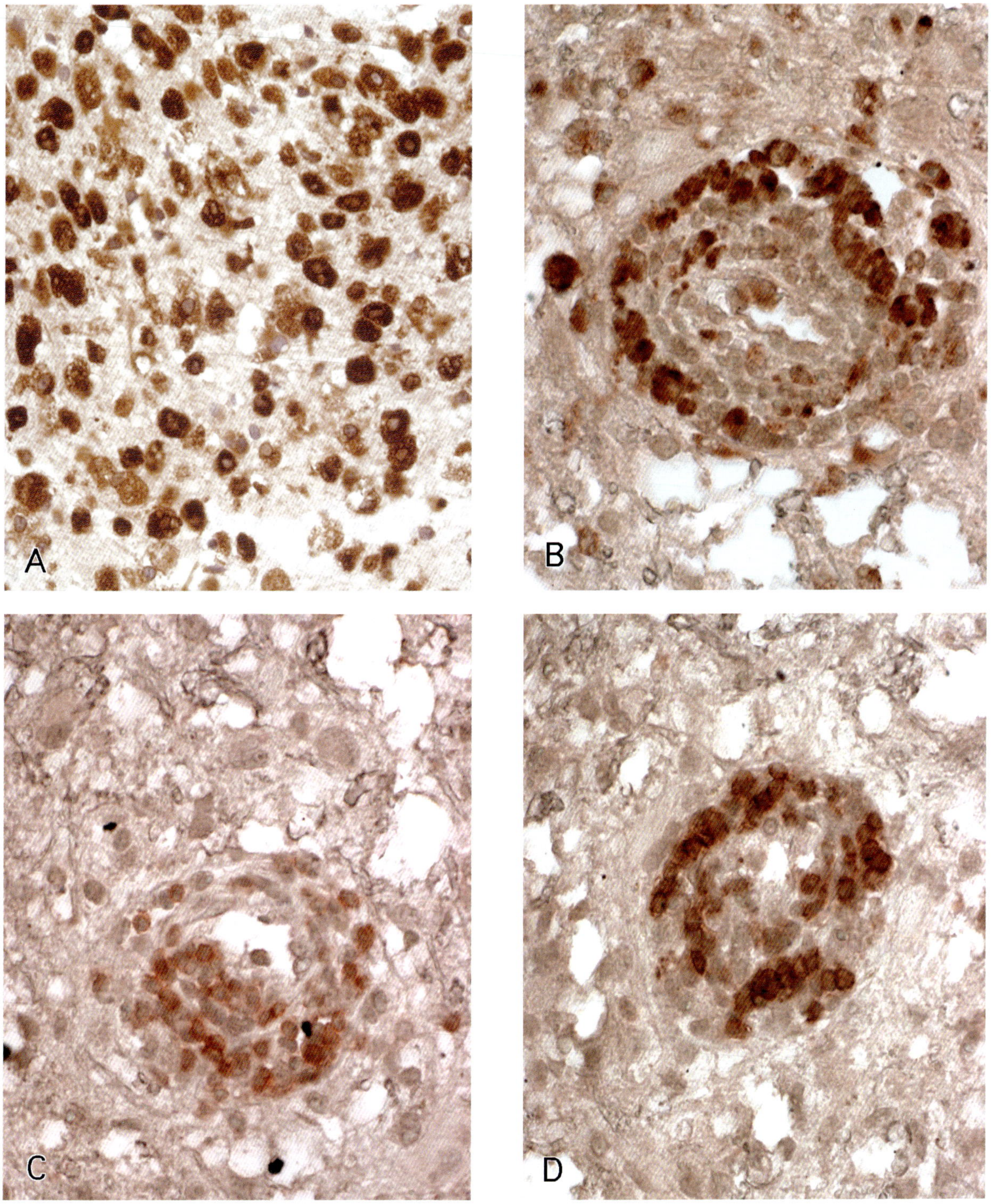

Figure 9-16

ACUTE DEMYELINATION/MULTIPLE SCLEROSIS

A: CD68 immunohistochemistry highlights parenchymal macrophages.
B: Perivascular macrophages seen with CD68 immunohistochemistry (same case as C and D).
C: Many perivascular cells are T lymphocytes (CD3 immunohistochemistry).
D: B cells may also be present (CD20 immunohistochemistry).

demyelinating disease include gliomas as well as hematopoietic lesions.

Macrophages can be mistaken, particularly at low-power microscopic examination, for the sheets of "fried egg" cells characteristic of oligodendroglioma. This distinction can usually be made in a variety of ways, most commonly and easily by observing the typical cytologic features of macrophages (copious, granular or bubbly cytoplasm and distinct cell borders) on smear preparations or on standard sections of well-fixed, nonfrozen tissue and by using immunohistochemistry for macrophage markers such as CD68. Although uncommon, untreated oligodendroglial tumors may have perivascular collections of typical macrophages. Malignant astrocytic tumors sometimes feature granular tumor cells or macrophage infiltrates, even prior to therapy, and may thus be histologically reminiscent of demyelinating disease. Finally, although exceedingly uncommon, glial tumors such as oligodendrogliomas may coexistent with demyelinating lesions, sometimes abutting one another (12).

The other demyelinating conditions are most readily distinguished on the basis of clinical and radiologic differences; the histologic features may be indistinguishable. Nonetheless, the smaller lesions of acute disseminated encephalomyelitis (see below) may be preferentially perivascular in location and acute hemorrhagic leukoencephalitis (see below) features vasculocentric collections of proteinaceous fluid and polymorphonuclear leukocytes, and sometimes, vascular damage. Infectious demyelinating conditions, in particular progressive multifocal leukoencephalopathy, should display evidence of viral infection, such as viral inclusions, immunohistochemical positivity for viral antigens, or ultrastructural presence of viral particles. Hereditary demyelinating conditions usually have clinical courses that do not lead to biopsy, have specific genetic or biochemical diagnostic features, and sometimes have specific histologic findings (see chapter 12). Secondary demyelination as a sequela of therapy for primary CNS lymphoma may be indistinguishable from primary demyelinating disease, and only rebiopsy of recurrent lesions months later may yield the correct diagnosis (13,14).

Other rare conditions that may lead to myelin loss with relative axonal preservation, and which are essentially never biopsied, include subacute sclerosing panencephalitis, human immunodeficiency virus (HIV) encephalopathy, phenylketonuria, Marchiava-Bignami disease, vitamin B12 deficiency, central pontine myelinolysis, toxic encephalopathies (hexachlorophene, chemotherapy, radiation, solvent vapors), prolonged cerebral edema, and hypoxic-ischemic encephalopathy (2).

Reactive conditions that feature prominent macrophage infiltrates must also be considered in the differential diagnosis of acute demyelinating diseases. The most common condition encountered in surgical neuropathology is subacute cerebral infarction (see chapter 5). Infarcts are usually only biopsied when subacute, not of sudden onset, and not radiologically typical. Given the subacute nature of these infarcts, it is common to find numerous macrophages, particularly if the lesion is more than 1 week of duration. Careful examination for infarcted tissue, including hypoxic-ischemic "red" neurons, and for equal destruction of axons and myelin, usually points to a correct diagnosis. In addition, as opposed to the central regions of demyelinated plaques, reactive astrocytes are not found within the center of liquefactive infarcts. Other reactive conditions include infectious diseases featuring numerous macrophages, such as Whipple disease.

Treatment and Prognosis. Treatment of classic MS involves attempts to modulate the immune system as well as supportive care. The classes of compounds used to some benefit have included antiinflammatory, immunomodulatory, and immunosuppressive drugs (15).

About 50 percent of patients die of complications of MS, with estimates suggesting that the disease reduces life expectancy by 7 to 14 years. Patients may have a worse prognosis in a number of settings: older age, frequent or closely spaced attacks during the early years, incomplete remissions, and rapid progression (15).

There has been some controversy concerning the prognosis of those patients who present with acute demyelinating disease, i.e., whether those patients have less likelihood of going on to develop classic MS. Some authors have suggested that patients with single, large lesions that result in biopsy often have a single episode, without necessarily progressing to chronic MS (2,14).

Postinfectious/Inflammatory Demyelinating Diseases: Acute Disseminated Encephalomyelitis and Acute Hemorrhagic Leukoencephalitis (Weston Hurst Syndrome)

Definition. *Acute disseminated encephalomyelitis* (ADEM) is an acute, monophasic, inflammatory demyelinating disease that typically affects the brain in a diffuse manner, and often follows a viral infection or immunization. *Acute hemorrhagic leukoencephalitis* (AHL), or *Weston Hurst syndrome,* is an acute, monophasic, inflammatory and hemorrhagic demyelinating condition that may be related to ADEM, often with a preceding viral illness, but which features microscopic evidence of vascular damage (necrotic venules, polymorphonuclear infiltrates, fibrin, and small hemorrhages) and which usually follows an aggressive clinical course.

General Comments. The etiologies of ADEM and AHL are not known, but multiple lines of evidence point to an acute (ADEM) or hyperacute (AHL) immunologic reaction: the frequent history of viral infection or immunization; the monophasic course; animal models that recapitulate the histologic findings after the triggering of an immune response; and the inflammatory infiltrates and myelin loss. Many studies have attempted to find evidence of infectious agents, but results have not conclusively implicated any specific ones.

Given the often characteristic combination of clinical and radiologic findings, these entities are only rarely biopsied. In nearly all situations, a biopsy is undertaken to rule in another condition, for which treatment options might depend on the biopsy results; the perivascular demyelination then raises the alternative diagnosis of ADEM or AHL. The other conditions in the clinical and radiologic differential diagnosis are primary diffuse gliomas, CNS lymphoma, vasculitis, and infectious encephalitides. The most tricky situations are those in which a low-grade glioma is entertained in the differential diagnosis prior to biopsy, and the unwary pathologist is drawn by the history into considering the hypercellularity as neoplastic.

Clinical Features. ADEM presents, usually in children or young adults, with rapid onset of neurologic difficulties (16). The diffuse involvement of the CNS usually causes nonlocalizing neurologic problems, similar to those seen with infectious encephalomyelitis. Occasionally, prominent disease in the optic nerve or spinal cord causes more focal neurologic symptoms and signs. Other patient have a more meningitic picture, including prominent headaches. Fever can be present as well. There is usually a history of recent viral illness or immunization between 2 days and 2 weeks prior to neurologic onset. ADEM is typically monophasic, but rare patients suffer multiple bouts over a few months, which has been termed *multiphasic ADEM*. The relationship of multiphasic ADEM to MS remains controversial. AHL also typically presents in children or young adults, with a rapid course of acute onset of fever, seizures, neurologic impairment, and subsequent coma.

Radiologic Findings. In both conditions, diffuse involvement of the white matter is noted by patchy high-signal intensity on T2-weighted images and fluid-attenuated inverse recovery (FLAIR) sequences (figs. 9-17, 9-18) (17). Lesions are found throughout the CNS, with an emphasis on posterior fossa structures in children. Thalamic involvement, as well as lesions in other gray matter areas, has been noted in many patients with ADEM.

Gross Findings. Postmortem examination of fatal cases has demonstrated edematous brains, often with evidence of cerebral herniation. Macroscopic lesions are not visible in ADEM, but the small hemorrhages of AHL may be visible, and AHL may feature more confluent hemorrhages and regions of necrosis (figs. 9-19, 9-20). Surgical biopsies usually appear grossly within normal limits.

Intraoperative Diagnosis. As with other acute demyelinating diseases, smear preparations show foamy macrophages, reactive astrocytes occasionally forming the cores of parenchymal "tissuelets" (see chapter 2), and perivascular lymphocytes (more in ADEM than AHL). Frozen sections demonstrate similar features but, importantly, show that the macrophage collections are more restricted to perivascular regions than in other acute demyelinating diseases. The relative restriction of demyelinated foci to the perivascular region necessarily means fewer macrophages and possibly fewer reactive astrocytes, making these diagnoses more challenging than that of acute MS. The examination of routine toluidine blue–stained, rapid frozen sections allows the rough assessment of myelin content in the

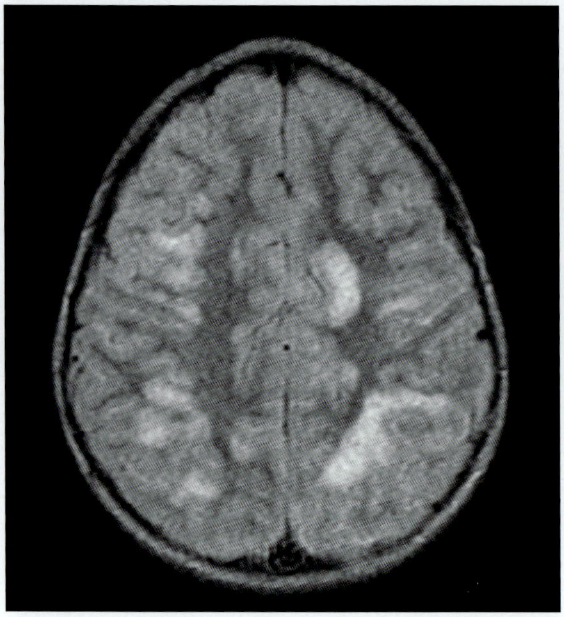

Figure 9-17

ACUTE DISSEMINATED ENCEPHALOMYELITIS

In this fluid-attenuated inverse recovery (FLAIR) image, multiple regions of white matter disease are noted, particularly affecting the subcortical white matter.

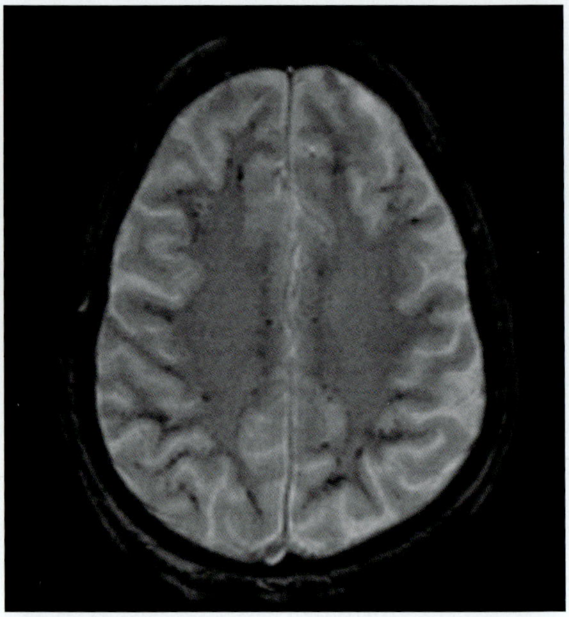

Figure 9-18

ACUTE HEMORRHAGIC LEUKOENCEPHALITIS

Small subcortical hemorrhages are evident as dark spots in this gradient echo T2-weighted magnetic resonance image (MRI).

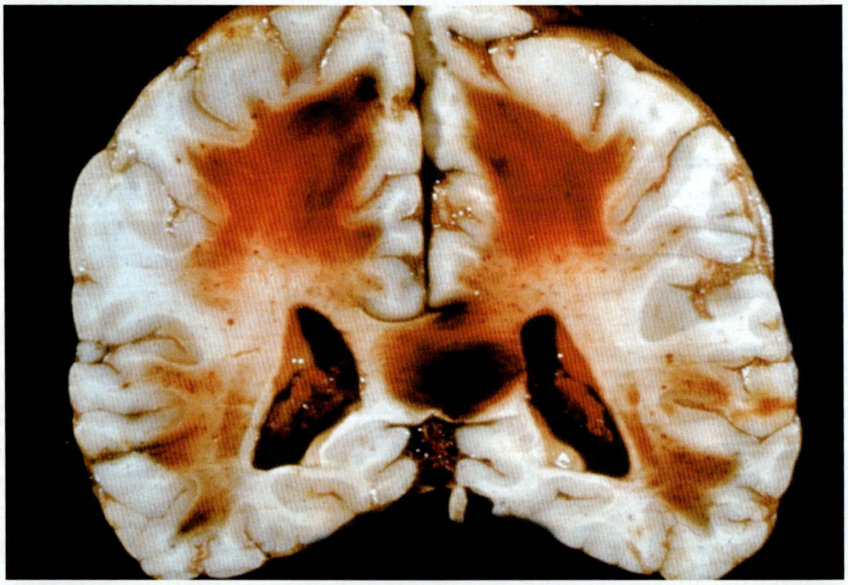

Figure 9-19

ACUTE HEMORRHAGIC LEUKOENCEPHALITIS

The cerebral white matter has both diffuse minute petechial hemorrhages as well as focal larger hemorrhages.

frozen section laboratory, but the subtlety of the myelin loss typical of these conditions makes it difficult to use such stains in a diagnostic sense during intraoperative consultation.

Microscopic Findings. Both ADEM and AHL are lesions that appear similarly acute, consistent with the monophasic clinical course. Biopsies of both conditions demonstrate demyelination that is primarily perivascular, with small perivascular cuffs of myelin loss and relative axonal preservation (figs. 9-21–9-23). The cuffs tend to have more irregular, less

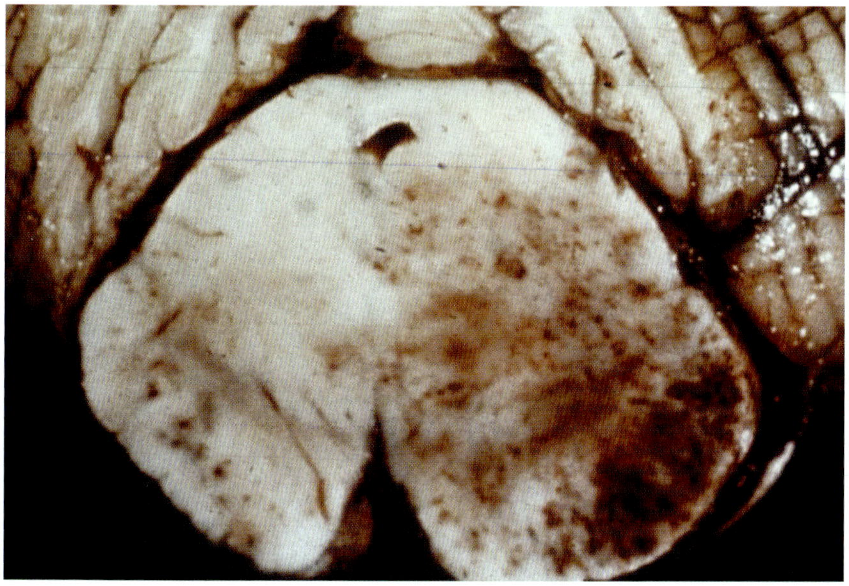

Figure 9-20

ACUTE HEMORRHAGIC LEUKOENCEPHALITIS

The midbrain has numerous petechial hemorrhages.

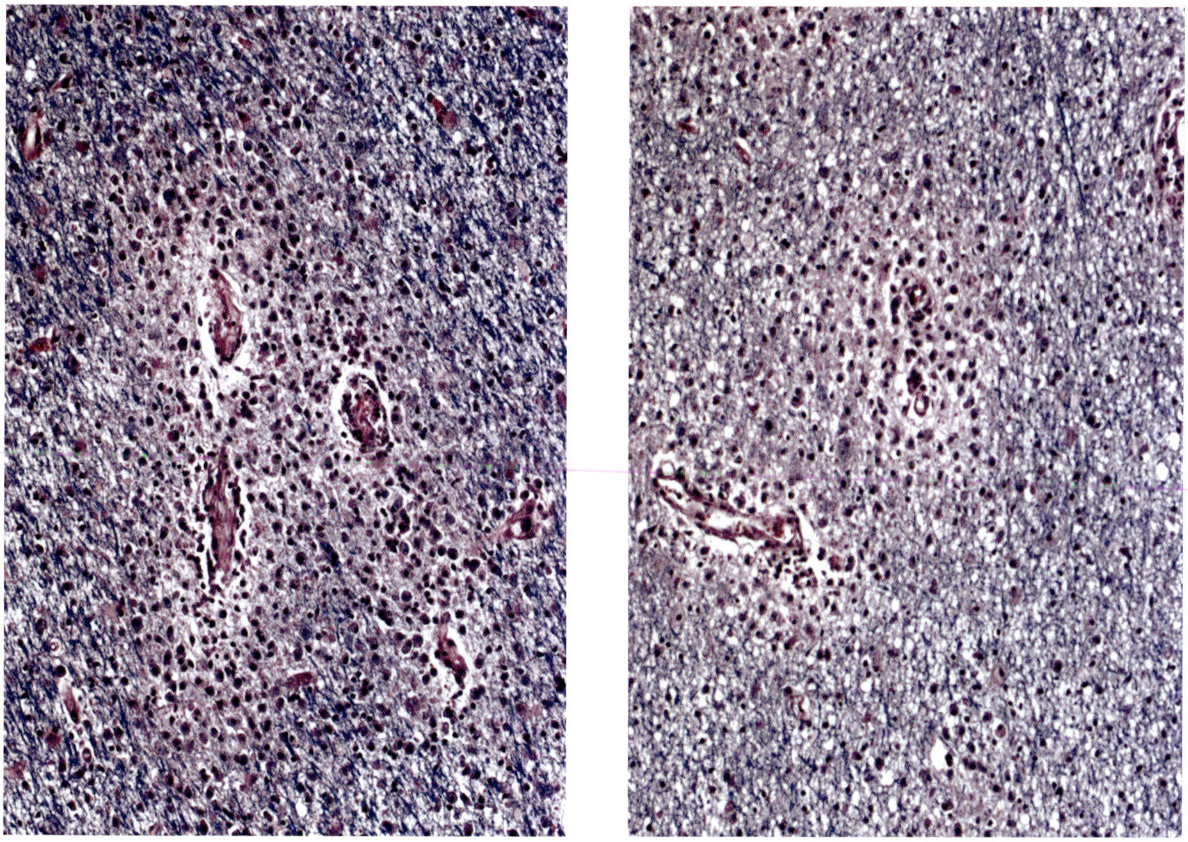

Figure 9-21

ACUTE DISSEMINATED ENCEPHALOMYELITIS

Perivascular demyelination can be subtle and lack sharp borders. Parenchymal macrophages are evident (Luxol fast blue-H&E stain).

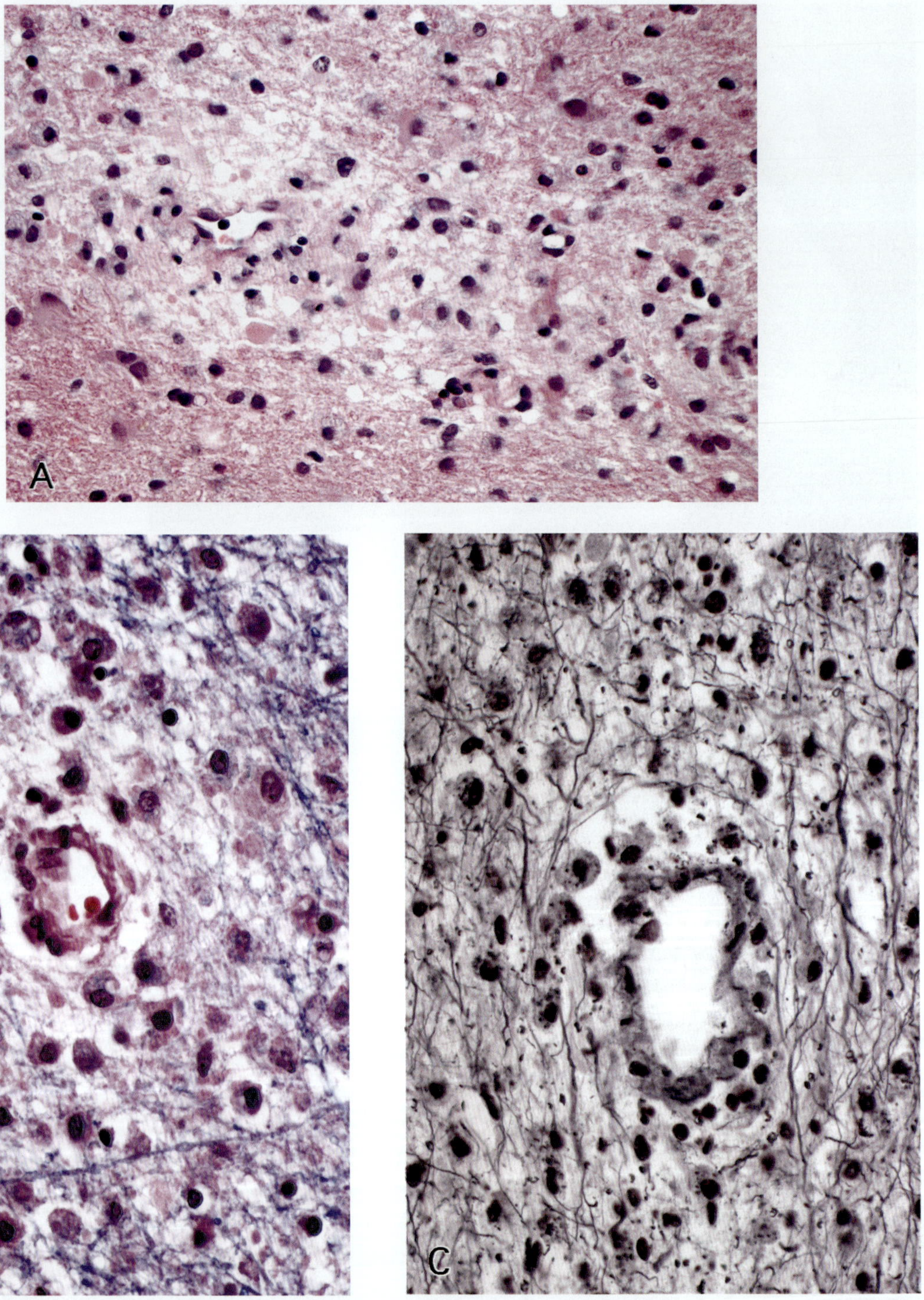

Figure 9-22

ACUTE DISSEMINATED ENCEPHALOMYELITIS

A: With H&E stains, perivascular demyelination gives a spongy appearance to the tissue, with accompanying macrophages and occasional axonal spheroids.

B: Luxol fast blue-H&E stain highlights the irregular, patchy perivascular myelin loss and myelin debris in the macrophages.

C: Axons are relatively intact on Bodian silver impregnation.

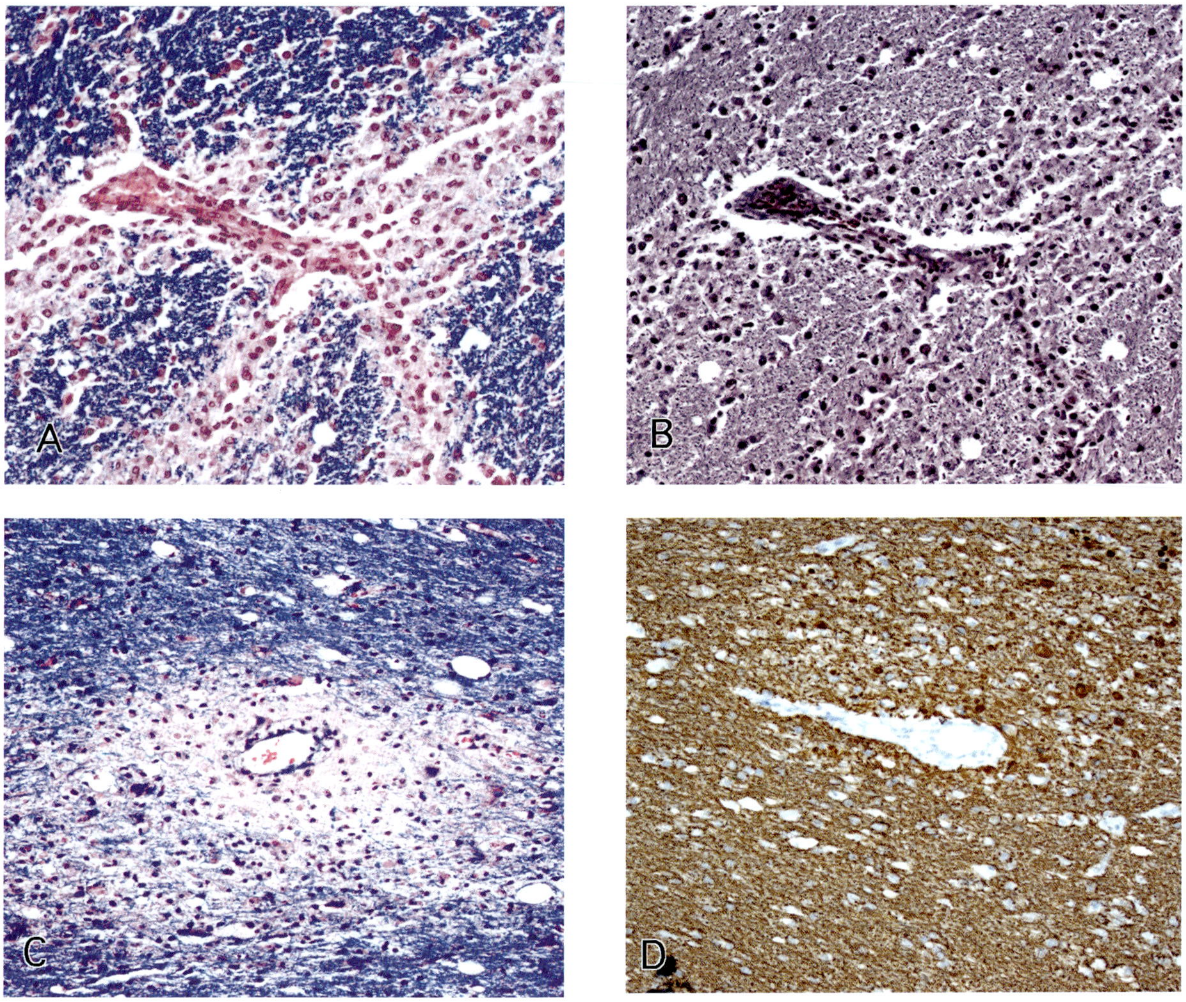

Figure 9-23

ACUTE DISSEMINATED ENCEPHALOMYELITIS

A: The demyelination radiates along small vessels, away from the larger vessel (Luxol fast blue-H&E stain).

B: Surrounding the same vessel seen in A, axons appear intact (Bodian silver impregnation).

C: In another case, a Luxol fast blue-H&E stain shows perivascular demyelination.

D: In the same case as C, the axonal architecture appears entirely intact surrounding an affected vessel (neurofilament immunohistochemistry).

defined borders than are found in MS. In more destructive lesions, axonal spheroids may be present, and may be highlighted on silver impregnation preparations or by neurofilament immunohistochemistry. The macrophages are similar to those noted in MS, and may be visualized in similar ways (fig. 9-24). Sometimes, perivascular lesions become confluent, creating larger, plaque-like areas. Demyelination may not be apparent in patients dying after only a few days. Perivascular inflammation is nearly always present; T cells and microglia may be prominent in the adjacent brain. Reactive astrocytes are found at the edges of lesions biopsied after a few days, but gliosis is usually not as prominent as in MS or other less acute demyelinating conditions. Creutzfeldt cells are not characteristic, but mitotic figures may be observed in astrocytes or macrophages. Occasionally, subpial demyelination is seen in the spinal cord and brain stem, and lymphocytic meningitis is usually present.

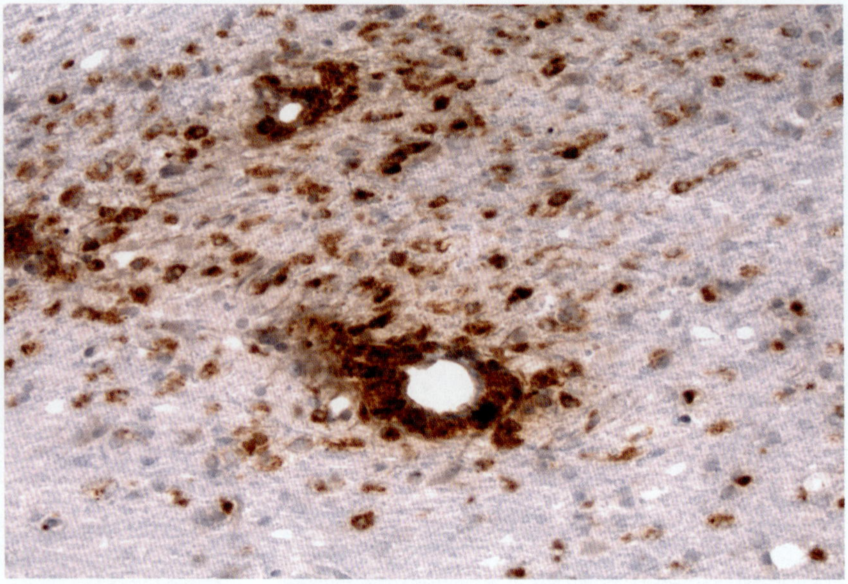

Figure 9-24

ACUTE DISSEMINATED ENCEPHALOMYELITIS

CD68 immunohistochemistry highlights perivascular macrophages.

AHL features more destructive histologic changes in which small venules are necrotic and surrounded by cuffs of polymorphonuclear leukocytes and fibrin pools, as well as small ring or ball hemorrhages (figs. 9-25, 9-26). The fibrin can be highlighted with phosphotungstic acid-hematoxylin (PTAH) stains (fig. 9-27). Demyelination is perivascular but may not be apparent in patients whose disease follows an aggressive short course. In addition, the demyelination may be overshadowed by the prominent perivascular acute inflammation and hemorrhage. Edema also may be noted in biopsies that include perilesional brain. Biopsies that sample the superficial CNS may show neutrophilic meningitis.

Laboratory Findings. CSF examination in both ADEM and AHL may reveal high opening pressures, pleocytosis, high protein levels, and occasional oligoclonal bands. In AHL, the pleocytosis typically includes many polymorphonuclear leukocytes (although these may be seen in ADEM as well) and red blood cells.

Differential Diagnosis. The primary histologic differential diagnosis for ADEM is MS. The histologic features may be identical. Although restriction of demyelination to perivascular foci favors a diagnosis of ADEM, MS plaques often have perivascular demyelination at their periphery and, therefore, sampling issues must be considered. In most cases, clinical (e.g., age of patient and antecedent viral illness) and radiologic differences aid in the distinction of ADEM from MS, but some cases of ADEM may represent the first episode of subsequent MS.

Given that demyelination may be difficult to document in some cases of AHL, an important differential diagnostic feature of AHL is the absence of gray matter involvement, which may be common in other entities in the differential diagnosis. The differential diagnosis of AHL includes entities that produce small vessel destruction, including vasculitis. Primary vasculitis should not produce demyelination, and is more likely to lead to cerebral infarction. Infectious diseases include those that affect small cerebral vessels and result in microhemorrhages, such as malaria and rickettsia; clinical correlations and special stains typically aid in making such distinctions. Fat emboli can also produce multiple small cerebral hemorrhages, preferentially in the white matter, but neutrophils and demyelination should not be present; furthermore, a clinical history of trauma and oil red O–positive fat particles support this diagnosis. Drug hypersensitivity reactions with histologic findings similar to those of AHL have been reported, and may represent a similar hyperacute immunologic reaction.

Treatment and Prognosis. Treatment is aimed at suppressing the immune response that is presumably causative. The majority of patients with ADEM respond well to intravenous steroids, but some require additional therapy, such as plasmapheresis. The prognosis of most

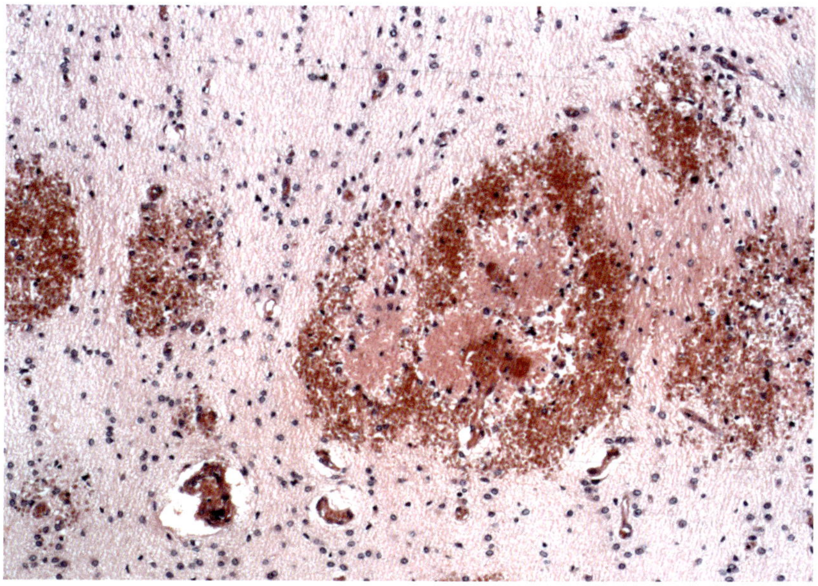

Figure 9-25

ACUTE HEMORRHAGIC LEUKOENCEPHALITIS

Ring hemorrhages with perivascular fibrin deposits.

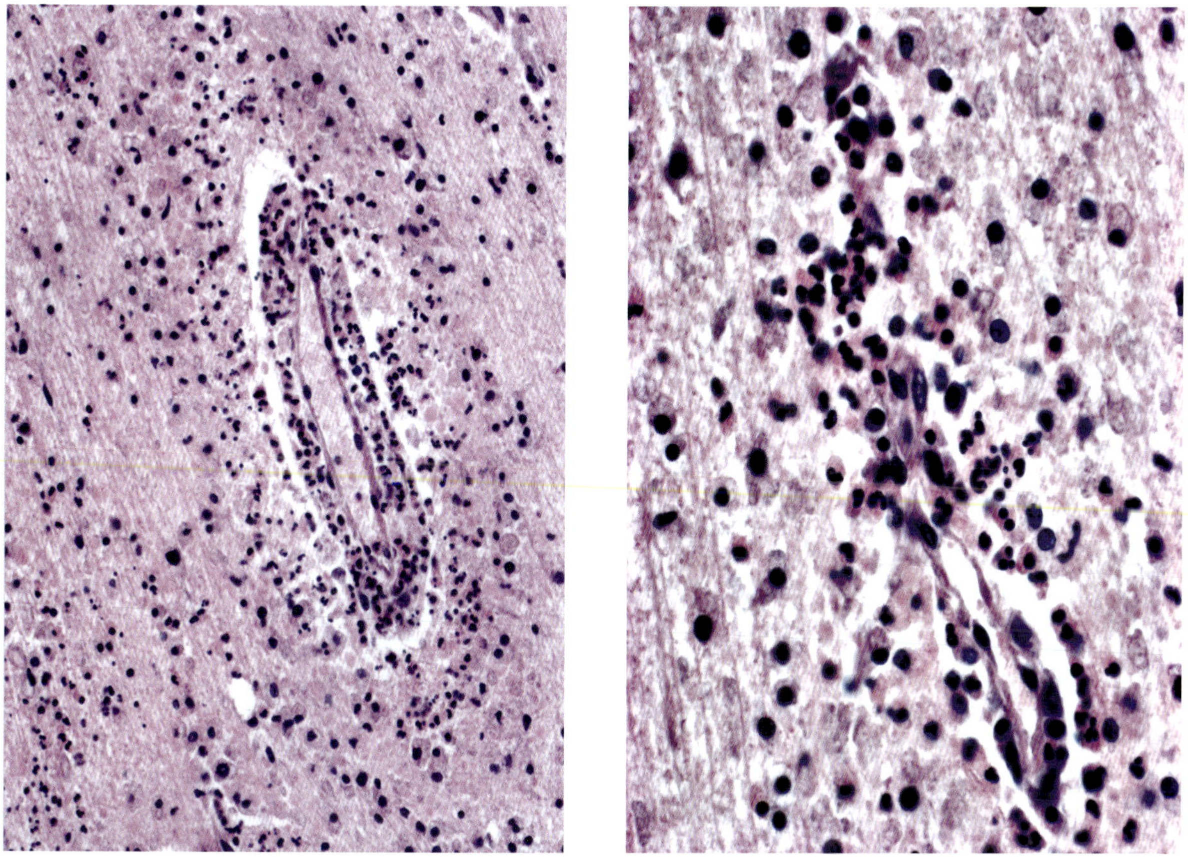

Figure 9-26

ACUTE HEMORRHAGIC LEUKOENCEPHALITIS

Left: At medium power, a vessel is surrounded by numerous polymorphonuclear leukocytes and some macrophages. Right: At high power, both polymorphonuclear leukocytes and macrophages are apparent.

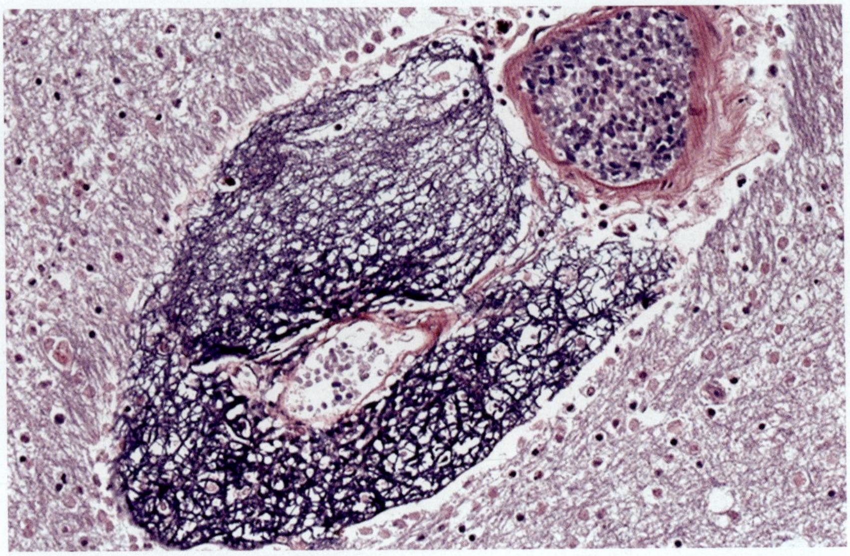

Figure 9-27

ACUTE HEMORRHAGIC LEUKOENCEPHALITIS

Perivascular fibrin deposits are accentuated with phosphotungstic acid-hematoxylin (PTAH) staining.

patients with ADEM is good, with complete neurologic recovery in 50 percent after an illness 1 to 3 weeks in duration. Significant neurologic impairment, however, remains in about one quarter of patients. It may be difficult to distinguish some of these cases from the first stage of MS of early onset. About one quarter of patients die of disease. The prognosis of patients with AHL is poor, with most patients having a rapidly fatal course.

HEREDITARY DEMYELINATING DISEASES

Hereditary demyelinating, or *"dysmyelinating," diseases* are conditions in which normal myelin cannot be formed or maintained. These rare conditions are known most commonly as *leukodystrophies*. In recent years, the genetic defects underlying most of these diseases have been pinpointed, allowing a combined clinical, neuroradiologic, biochemical, and molecular genetic diagnosis to be made for most affected patients.

In general, these are diseases of children that have characteristic inheritance patterns, ages of onset, neurologic signs and symptoms, neuroradiologic findings, and biochemical abnormalities. Many of the leukodystrophies, however, have atypical forms, including forms that affect adults and without typical inheritance patterns. It is these latter atypical forms that are most likely to undergo brain biopsy. Nonetheless, it is rare for patients affected with these conditions to have brain biopsies. As a result, most of the known neuropathology relates to autopsy findings and, for some entities, peripheral nerve biopsy findings.

As with other demyelinating diseases, these conditions feature the loss of myelin with the relative preservation of axons. Most affect the white matter in a diffuse manner, without creating focal mass-like lesions. Because these are usually chronic, longstanding illnesses, evidence of active demyelination, such as lipid-laden macrophages, may be scant. The unique features of these entities are discussed in chapter 12. While some of these diseases have characteristic pathologic findings (e.g., extensive Rosenthal fibers in Alexander disease or giant cells in Krabbe disease), the rare biopsied cases are not clinically, biochemically, or genetically typical (hence the need for biopsy), and it is unlikely that classic histopathologic findings will be found.

"SECONDARY" DEMYELINATING DISEASES

The entities described in this chapter are "primary" demyelinating conditions in the sense that the primary pathologic changes are related to preferential myelin loss. Each of these conditions presumably has a unique etiology, although the causes of the common, nonhereditary demyelinating diseases have not yet been elucidated. Other demyelinating diseases are more clearly "secondary" in nature, since the demyelination occurs as a response to a defined inciting event. The histologic evidence of demyelination may be identical to that observed in the entities discussed in this chapter: myelin loss, relative preservation of axons, reactive gliosis, myelin-laden macrophages. Further pathologic or clinical examination, however, should reveal specific etiologies or related conditions. For example, progressive multifocal leukoencephalopathy (see chapter 6) features plaque-like regions of myelin loss, but should feature the additional pathologic findings of enlarged, basophilic oligodendrocytes, as well as giant, bizarre astrocytes and immunohistochemical or ultrastructural evidence of viral particles. Another infectious disease that may produce plaque-like lesions is herpes zoster encephalitis; however, these sharply demarcated lesions may show considerable axonal loss as well as vasculitic changes. Primary CNS lymphoma (see chapter 15), particularly in the setting of prior steroid therapy, may be histologically indistinguishable from primary acute demyelinating disease; only clinical follow-up with rebiopsy upon recurrence yields the correct diagnosis (13,14). Widespread arteriolar sclerosis (see chapter 5) can result in pervasive white matter attenuation resembling demyelination.

REFERENCES

1. Adams RD, Kubik CS. The morbid anatomy of the demyelinative diseases. Am J Med 1952;12:510-546.
2. Sobel RA, Moore GW. Demyelinating diseases. In: Love S, Louis DN, Ellison DW, eds. Greenfield's neuropathology. London: Hodder Arnold; 2008.
3. Cree BA, Goodin DS, Hauser SL. Neuromyelitis optica. Semin Neurol 2002;22:105-122.
4. Nesbit GM, Forbes GS, Scheithauer BW, Okazaki H, Rodriguez M. Multiple sclerosis: histopathologic and MR and/or CT correlation in 37 cases at biopsy and three cases at autopsy. Radiology 1991;180:467-474.
5. Lucchinetti C, Bruck W, Rodriguez M, Lassmann H. Distinct patterns of multiple sclerosis pathology indicates heterogeneity on pathogenesis. Brain Pathol 1996;6:259-274.
6. Lucchinetti C, Bruck W, Parisi J, Scheithauer BW, Rodriguez M, Lassmann H. Heterogeneity of multiple sclerosis lesions: implications for the pathogenesis of demyelination. Ann Neurol 2000;47:707-717.
7. McDonald WI, Compston A, Edan G, et al. Recommended diagnostic criteria for multiple sclerosis: guidelines from the International Panel on the diagnosis of multiple sclerosis. Ann Neurol 2001;50:121-127.
8. Zagzag D, Miller DC, Kleinman GM, Abati A, Donnenfeld H, Budzilovich GN. Demyelinating disease versus tumor in surgical neuropathology. Clues to a correct pathological diagnosis. Am J Surg Pathol 1993;17:537-545.
9. Annesley-Williams D, Farrell MA, Staunton H, Brett FM. Acute demyelination, neuropathological diagnosis, and clinical evolution. J Neuropathol Exp Neurol 2000;59:477-489.
10. Youl BD, Kermode AG, Thompson AJ, et al. Destructive lesions in demyelinating disease. J Neurol Neurosurg Psychiatry 1991;54:288-292.
11. Peterson K, Rosenblum MK, Powers JM, Alvord E, Walker RW, Posner JB. Effect of brain irradiation on demyelinating lesions. Neurology 1993;43:2105-2112.
12. Paydafar D, de la Monte SM. Case Records of the Massachusetts General Hospital. Weekly clinicopathological exercises. A 50-year-old woman with multiple sclerosis and an enlarging frontal-lobe mass. Case 12-1997. N Engl J Med 1997;336:1163-1171.
13. Alderson L, Fetell MR, Sisti M, Hochberg F, Cohen M, Louis DN. Sentinel lesions of primary CNS lymphoma. J Neurol Neurosurg Psych 1996;60:102-105.
14. Kepes JJ. Large focal tumor-like demyelinating lesions of the brain: intermediate entity between multiple sclerosis and acute disseminated encephalomyelitis? A study of 31 patients. Ann Neurol 1993;33:18-27.
15. O'Connor P, Canadian Multiple Sclerosis Working Group. Key issues in the diagnosis and treatment of multiple sclerosis. An overview. Neurology 2002;59:S1-33.
16. Tenembaum S, Chamoles N, Fejerman N. Acute disseminated encephalomyelitis: a long-term follow-up study of 84 pediatric patients. Neurology 2002;59:1224-1231.
17. Garg RK. Acute disseminated encephalomyelitis. Postgrad Med J 2003;79:11-17.

10 DEMENTIA

Brain biopsy is only rarely performed to establish a histologic diagnosis of a dementing illness, primarily because many of the dementing disorders are slowly progressive neurodegenerative diseases for which clinical history, neurologic examination, laboratory studies, and noninvasive procedures have a high degree of diagnostic accuracy. Biopsies are typically performed in the setting of atypical presentation or more rapidly progressing dementia (1). The prion diseases are the most common processes that are suspected in the setting of rapidly progressive dementia. For them, tissue-based studies, which combine standard histologic examination, immunohistochemical studies, and Western blotting, form the basis of a definitive diagnosis.

Although neuropathologic examination of surgical specimens is rarely called for in the evaluation of a patient with a well-recognized neurodegenerative disease, the diagnostic features of these disorders may be observed by pathologists as "incidental findings" when surgery is performed for other reasons (such as for resection of tumors or vascular malformations or in the setting of trauma). Because the neuropathologic diagnostic criteria for these entities are often based upon autopsy evaluation of the full nervous system in combination with clinicopathologic correlation, definitive diagnosis of these neurodegenerative diseases cannot be proffered from a surgical specimen. Nonetheless, it is essential for pathologists to recognize the underlying pathology of these diseases and to be able to convey their findings in an accurate manner. Indeed, the specific pathologic findings of a neurodegenerative disease may greatly narrow diagnostic possibilities for the cause of dementia in a patient with an atypical clinical presentation.

When pathologic findings of a neurodegenerative disease are present in a neurosurgical specimen, this information needs to be communicated to the relevant physicians involved in the patient's care. As mentioned above, the presence of histopathologic abnormalities may not meet the established criteria for rendering one of these diagnoses, but it does strongly support other clinical evidence. It should be remembered, however, that the presence of an underlying neurodegenerative disease does not preclude the coexistence of another process.

While all surgical specimens are handled with universal precautions, the unique pathogenic mechanism of prion diseases results in a need for special handling of cases in which these are considered to be part of the differential diagnosis. For this reason, all cases of rapidly progressive dementia, typically considered as those with a course of several months or even up to 1 year duration, should be handled with appropriate precautions, as described below. At the same time, the presence of spongiform pathology may be found by a pathologist on a brain biopsy specimen from a patient in whom the diagnosis of prion disease had not been previously considered. When this happens, prompt communication with the neurosurgical and neurology services is essential in order to allow for appropriate and rapid decontamination or disposal of surgical instruments.

GENERAL DIAGNOSTIC APPROACH

Dementia is formally defined by the presence of memory impairment along with at least one other type of cognitive deficit. There must be a change from the baseline level of neurologic function and must be severe enough to limit the person's normal functions. While many dementing illnesses are not currently amenable to therapeutic intervention, the purpose of a biopsy is often to exclude the possibility of an atypical presentation of a treatable disorder. When confronted with a biopsy in a patient with rapidly progressive dementia, the pathologist must include prion diseases in the differential diagnosis. This has significant implications for tissue handling and diagnostic evaluation.

Clinical Features

The details of the clinical history, laboratory findings, and imaging studies complement the morphologic interpretation of the histologic findings from brain biopsy. When brain biopsy is performed for the purpose of evaluating a nonfocal progressive neurologic decline, possibly reversible conditions, such as metabolic abnormalities or toxic/drug-induced states, have typically already been excluded. Parameters that can be informative and contributory toward a diagnosis, both in a positive and negative sense, include peripheral markers of inflammatory processes (sedimentation rate, C-reactive protein levels, angiotensin-converting enzyme [ACE] levels), markers of particular diseases (in particular, evidence of autoimmune thyroiditis), and evidence of systemic neoplasia.

Radiologic Findings

Neuroimaging studies can contribute to the diagnosis of neurodegenerative disease on brain biopsy in two ways. Imaging abnormalities, if present, guide tissue sampling, within limits of safety. More importantly, the combination of pathologic findings, which can suggest but not absolutely diagnose many of the neurodegenerative diseases, and imaging findings can be informative.

Gross Findings

These diseases are typically encountered by pathologists in small biopsy specimens, either stereotactically directed needle biopsies or open biopsies. Given this, the gross examination is limited in the information it can yield. When brain tissue appears firmer than expected, there is often reactive gliosis.

Intraoperative Diagnosis

As the majority of these diseases require detailed morphologic and immunohistochemical studies to render the appropriate diagnosis, intraoperative consultation has a small role. The most common settings in which frozen section evaluation is requested are cases in which the differential diagnosis includes vasculitides or encephalitides. In these situations, frozen sections are used to indicate the appropriateness of immunosuppressive therapies, although sampling that results in false negative interpretation is a problem.

Microscopic Findings

While the specific microscopic appearance of distinct entities is considered below, it is possible to group those disorders that may present with dementia or related symptoms by the overall pattern of histologic changes. These can be characterized as 1) inclusion/aggregates, 2) inflammatory lesions, and 3) spongiform lesions. Although these distinctions are not absolute, they do represent the major patterns of pathologic findings. Many of the neurodegenerative diseases are marked by the presence of intracellular and/or extracellular protein aggregates, in the form of inclusion bodies or deposits. The recognition of these abnormal structures, typically in association with reactive gliosis but without inflammatory cell infiltrates, prompts subsequent investigation with other staining methods. In contrast, the disorders in which inflammation is present include vasculitides, infectious processes, and paraneoplastic conditions, for which the characterization of the immune response and the detection of underlying pathogens would be the appropriate next steps in determining etiology, guiding therapy, and predicting prognosis. Finally, the presence of spongiform change, even in the absence of a history of rapidly progressive dementia, should prompt consideration of prion diseases. Again, this particular histologic pattern guides subsequent immunohistochemical, biochemical, and molecular studies.

Immunohistochemical Findings

Diagnosing this group of diseases involves a combination of standard morphologic examination with special stains and immunohistochemical approaches. In addition to the use of antibodies directed against disease-specific antigens, such as beta-amyloid (Aβ), tau, alpha(α)-synuclein, and PrP^{sc} (pathologic prion protein), there is also a role for less specific markers of the diseased brain such as glial fibrillary acidic protein (GFAP) and CD68 for evidence of astrocytic or microglial reactions, respectively.

Ultrastructural Findings

With the exception of the viral encephalitides and some of the metabolic diseases, there is little role for ultrastructural studies in the diagnostic evaluation of dementia. For this reason, fixation of tissue for potential use in electron microscopy is usually of low priority. If adequate amounts of tissue are available, as from an open biopsy procedure, then some small tissue samples may be fixed in this manner. These samples are not processed for ultrastructural analysis until light microscopic evaluation has been completed.

Laboratory and Molecular Findings

Auxilliary methods (in particular, Western blotting) provide a critical complement to pathologic examination in the evaluation of potential prion diseases. In order to employ these methods effectively, frozen tissue is needed. For this reason, the approach to cases of rapidly progressive dementing illnesses that come to biopsy should include, if possible, the allocation of small portions of tissue for snap freezing. Because the procedures necessary for preparation of samples for Western blotting in the potential presence of prion disease require the use of biosafety precautions that exceed those available in most settings, these studies are often performed in reference laboratories or in research settings.

Treatment and Prognosis

The absence of effective therapies for neurodegenerative diseases and their characteristically relentless downwardly progressive nature provide two of the arguments against the use of brain biopsy in the evaluation of dementia. Because some of these diseases have heritable forms, there may be implications for other family members. Thus, appropriate procedures need to be followed in the acquisition and subsequent distribution of genetic information.

DEPOSITS AND INCLUSIONS

Many of the neurodegenerative diseases require broader examination of the brain than is available through a surgical biopsy in order to meet currently accepted criteria for definitive diagnosis. Nevertheless, the presence of the certain types of structural abnormalities can suggest that one of these disorders may represent the basis for the patient's neurologic symptoms. Many of the neurodegenerative diseases have protein aggregation as a common etiology, and as a result have characteristic morphologically identifiable abnormalities. Just as these abnormalities are markers of the underlying biologic changes in the brain, they should also stand as signposts for the pathologist; they may not identify a final destination (the diagnosis), but should send the pathologist and other physicians in the correct direction toward that diagnosis.

Plaques

Plaques are roughly spherical, extracellular deposits that occur in gray matter structures, including the cerebral cortex. The most common disease in which they occur is Alzheimer disease (AD), but they may also be found in some forms of prion disease, as well as in the rare entities of familial British dementia (FBD) and familial Danish dementia (FDD). In all of these disorders, plaques have a predominant component of a single aggregated peptide that has significant beta-pleated sheet structure and binds amyloid-specific compounds such as Congo red and thioflavin. The outer portion of a plaque (beyond the amyloid core), depends, in part, on the type of disease; the florid plaques of variant Creutzfeldt-Jakob disease are surrounded by spongiform change, while the plaques in AD typically have a collection of dystrophic, tortuous and thickened neurites around them.

Plaques are recognizable on routine hematoxylin and eosin (H&E)-stained sections because of their refractile centers and the disruption of the surrounding neuropil (fig. 10-1). In general, the highly refractile cores of lesions from AD are irregularly contoured and lumpy (fig. 10-2), while those of prion diseases are more likely to have fine, radially disposed fibrils. Depending on the plane of section and the size of the amyloid core in relationship to the neuritic response, the plaques of AD may appear predominantly as round islands of neuropil with an abnormal consistency, sometimes with scattered dystrophic neurites that are visible even on routine staining (fig. 10-3). Plaques of AD, FBD, and FDD are also well demonstrated with silver impregnation techniques, particularly the Bielschowsky and Gallayas methods (fig. 10-4). Immunohistochemistry for Aβ highlights plaques of AD (fig. 10-5); other peptides are found in FBD and FDD. Recognition, or suspicion, of the presence of plaques in a brain biopsy should prompt the application of additional staining methods to characterize them. In addition, there should

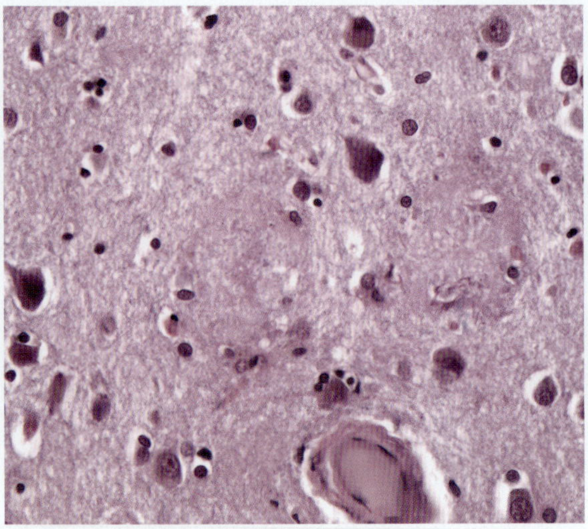

Figure 10-1

PLAQUES

The two plaques present in this field disrupt the texture of the neuropil.

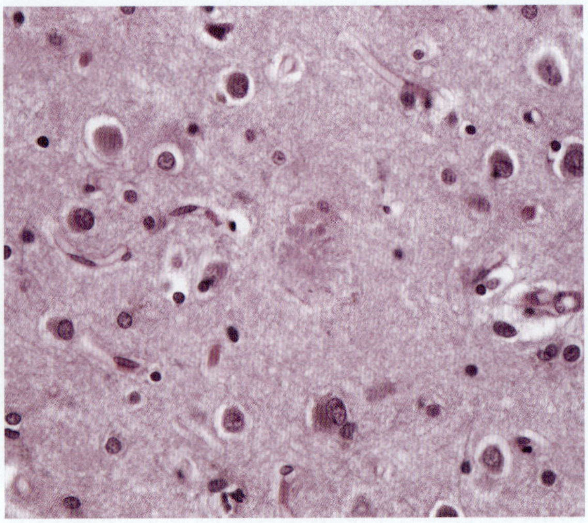

Figure 10-2

PLAQUES

The irregular amyloid core of a plaque in Alzheimer disease is seen as refractile material.

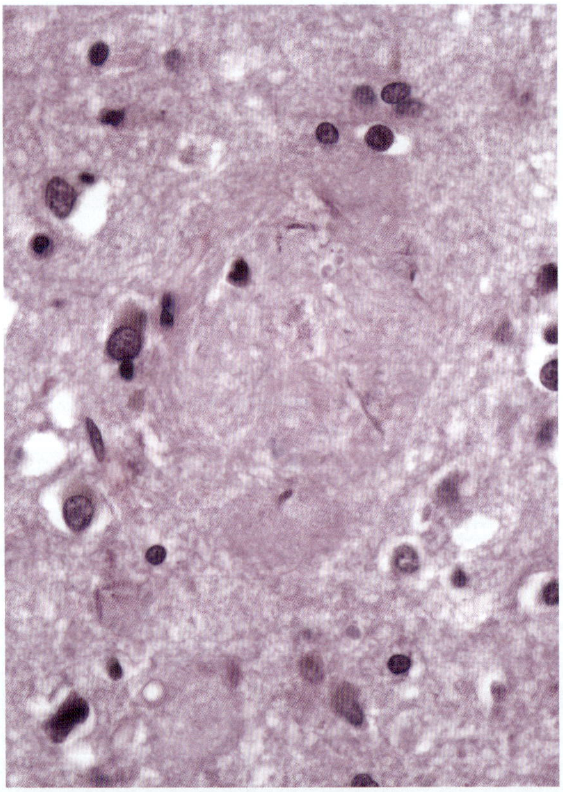

Figure 10-3

DYSTROPHIC NEURITES

Thickened and mildly tortuous neurites are present around plaques.

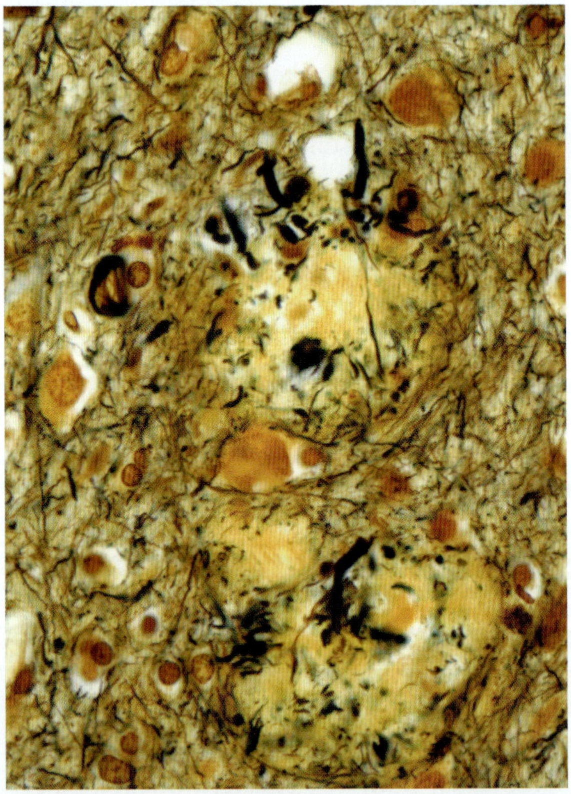

Figure 10-4

PLAQUES

Silver staining highlights plaques as well as the dystrophic neurites (Bielschowsky silver impregnation).

be a search for the appropriate accompanying histologic findings of these diseases (tangles for AD, FBD, and FDD; spongiform change for prion diseases).

Tangles and Other Tau Immunoreactive Deposits

Tangles are filamentous aggregates primarily composed of hyperphosphorylated isoforms of tau, a microtubule-binding protein. In many diseases, this form of tau pathology is referred to as *neurofibrillary tangles*, while in other diseases abnormal deposits of tau can be found in glial cells. Normal tau is associated with the microtubule skeleton of axons; pathologic tau is redistributed into the somatic and dendritic compartments of neurons and is hyperphosphorylated in the disease state. The bundles of filaments are recognizable within neurons on routine H&E staining as mildly basophilic strand-like structures that typically extend from the neuronal cell body into the proximal portion of the apical dendrite (fig. 10-6). Another pattern that is commonly seen is the *globose tangle*, in which the meshwork of fibrils enwraps the neuronal nucleus (fig. 10-7). Tangles often outlive the neurons in which they form, and remain as markers of neuronal cell death. When seen with H&E staining, these "ghost tangles" are often less basophilic and less compact than their intracellular counterparts (fig. 10-8).

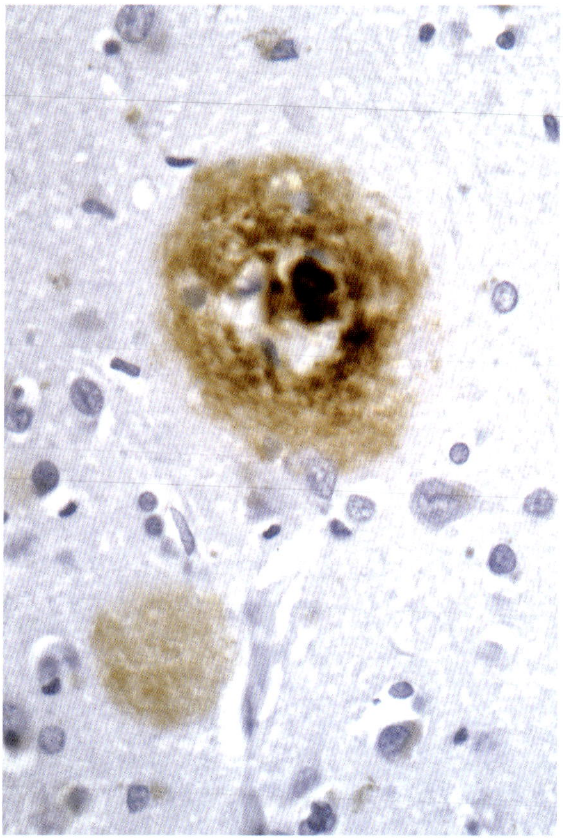

Figure 10-5

PLAQUES

The parenchymal deposits, but not the majority of dystrophic neurites, are highlighted by immunohistochemistry for beta-amyloid (Aβ).

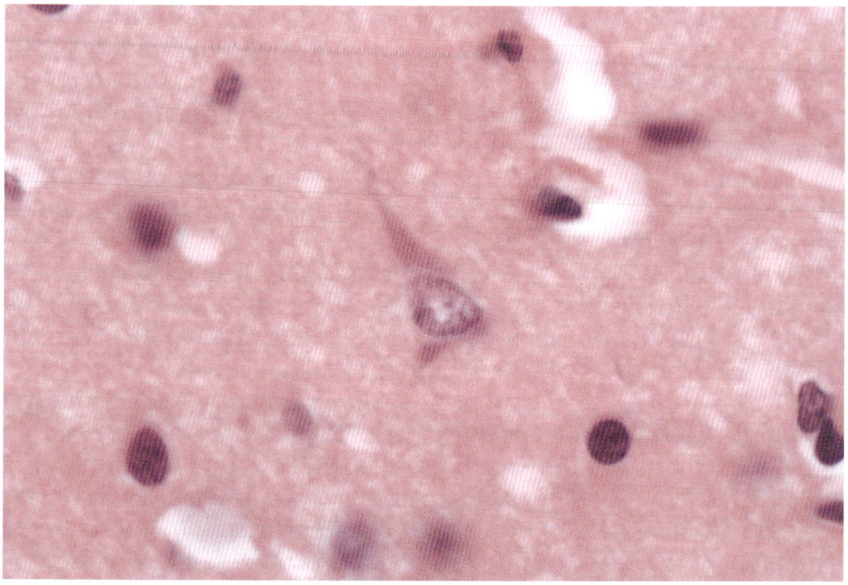

Figure 10-6

TANGLES

The basophilic fibrils of a tangle are visible in this neuron, and extend into the apical dendrite.

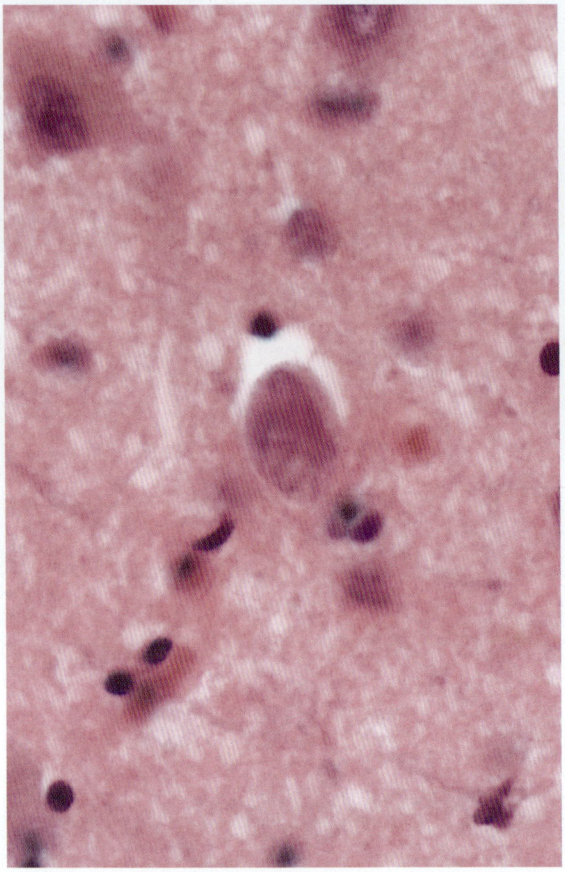

Figure 10-7

TANGLES

In globose tangles, the fibrils wrap around the nucleus of the neuron.

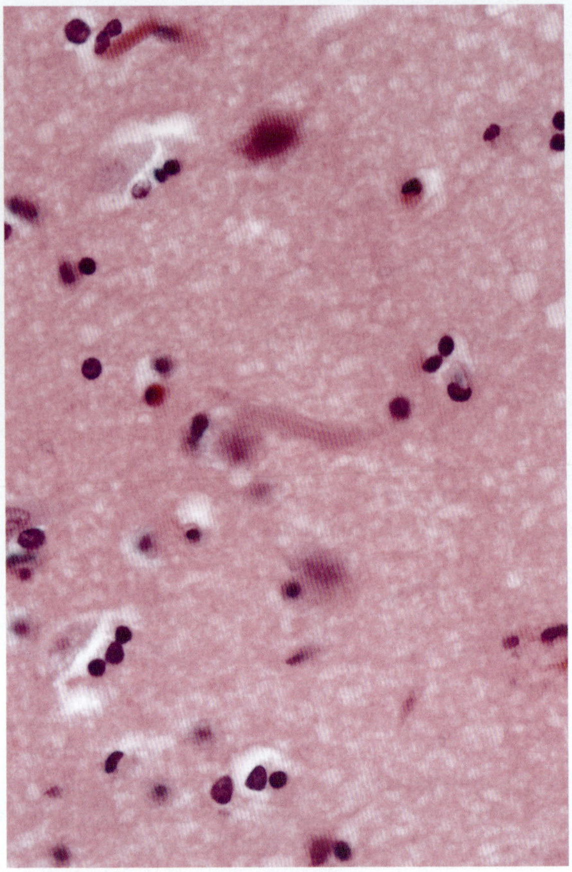

Figure 10-8

TANGLES

After the death of a tangle-bearing neuron, the insoluble fibrils may remain in the neuropil as a "ghost" tangle.

The presence, or suspicion, of tangles on H&E-stained specimens should prompt the application of additional investigative methods to evaluate the biopsy further. Tangles are well demonstrated with a variety of methods, including various silver impregnation methods (most commonly, Bielschowsky or Gallayas) (fig. 10-9), fluorescence microscopy after thioflavin staining (fig. 10-10), or immunostaining for tau (fig. 10-11). Tau is encoded by a gene (*MAPT*) with an alternatively spliced transcript; there are six possible isoforms, with the most important distinction being between those that do or do not contain exon 10 (1a). As this exon encodes one of the microtubule-binding domains, forms of the protein that contain this sequence have four such domains (often referred to as 4 repeat [4R] tau) while those without it have only three such repeats (3R tau).

Unlike plaques, which suggest the presence of a limited range of neurodegenerative diseases, tangles may be found in a wide range of diseases (Table 10-1), although AD is the most common context in which they are recognized. When both plaques and tangles are identified in a brain biopsy, the presence of AD should be strongly suspected.

When tangles are identified in the absence of plaques, several other entities are added to the neuropathologic differential diagnosis, although the possibility of AD inadequately sampled by the surgical specimen remains. Diseases that are collectively termed *tauopathies* are marked by the presence of tangles or other tau-containing inclusions. Among these are the various forms of frontotemporal dementia, sometimes linked to mutations in the *MAPT* gene, which codes

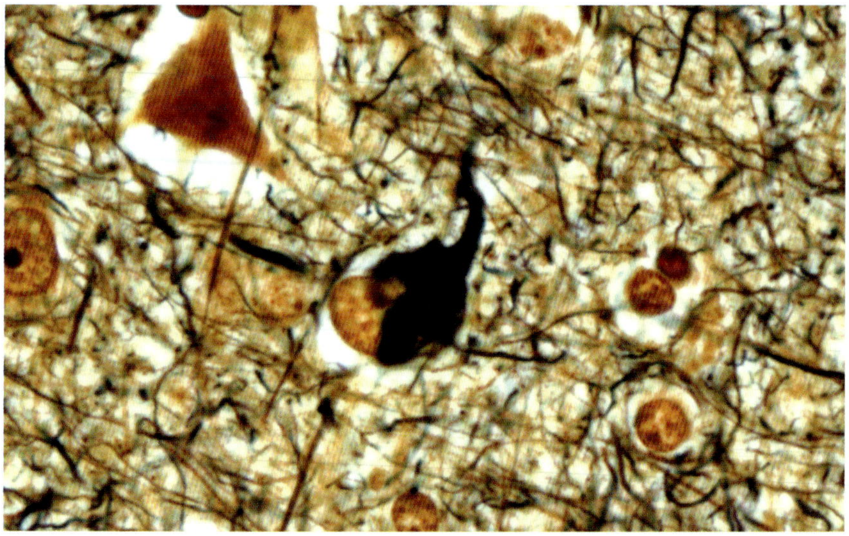

Figure 10-9

TANGLES

Silver staining is an excellent technique for demonstrating a tangle-bearing neuron (Bielschowsky silver impregnation).

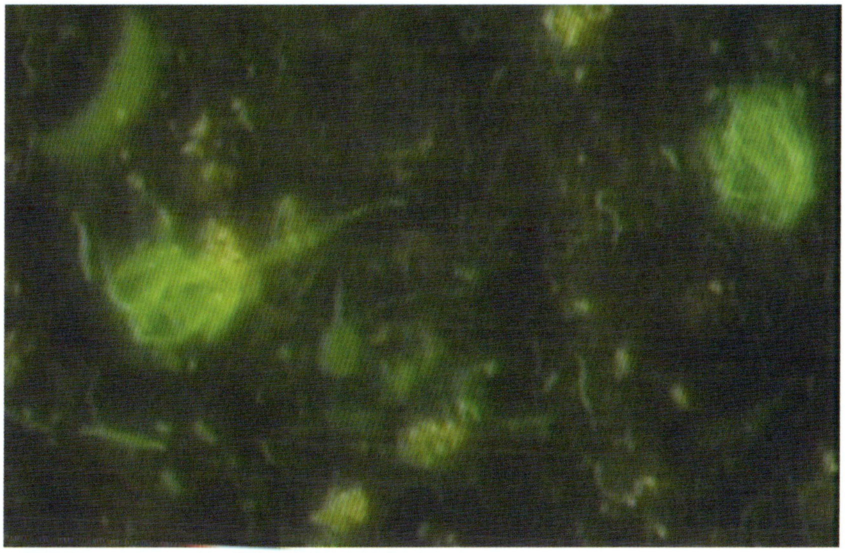

Figure 10-10

TANGLES

After treatment with thioflavin S, tangles can be detected by fluorescence microscopy. Plaques are also present.

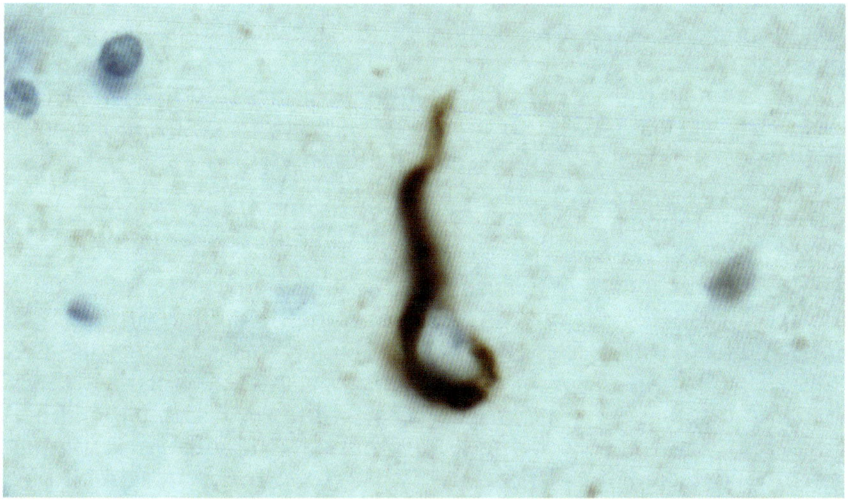

Figure 10-11

TANGLES

The major protein component of a tangle is tau (immunohistochemistry for tau).

Table 10-1

CONDITIONS IN WHICH NEUROFIBRILLARY TANGLES MAY BE OBSERVED

Alzheimer disease (AD)
Frontotemporal dementia(s) (FTD)
Progressive supranuclear palsy (PSP)
Corticobasal degeneration (CBD)
Subacute sclerosing panencephalitis (SSPE)
Prion diseases (selected mutations)
Dementia pugilistica
Parkinsonian-dementia complex of Guam
Postencephalitic parkinsonism
Niemann-Pick disease type C
Familial British Dementia (FBD)
Familial Danish Dementia (FDD)

for tau, along with progressive supranuclear palsy and corticobasal degeneration. These two disorders have specific patterns of neurofibrillary tangle distribution, in addition to specific clinical presentations and courses.

Apart from the presence of neuronal tau pathology (neurofibrillary tangles), there are typical forms of tau deposits associated with glial cells. These include: *astrocytic plaques* (fig. 10-12), in which a collection of astrocytic processes form a plaque resembling the dystrophic neurites of a plaque but lacking the central core of amyloid; *tufted astrocytes* (fig. 10-13), in which individual astrocytes have a stellate pattern of surrounding processes containing aggregated tau which may be demonstrated with silver stains or by immunostaining for tau, and *coiled bodies* (fig. 10-14), in which curved fibrils of tau are present in the perisomatic region of oligodendrocytes. As discussed below, the relative abundance of these various forms of glial tau pathology can help to discriminate between progressive supranuclear palsy and corticobasal degeneration.

In addition to tangles, there are several other forms of recognizable pathologic inclusions and structures that can be identified on H&E stains, and are highlighted by the application of many of the same methods used to search for tangles and related abnormalities. Pick bodies, one of the pathologic hallmarks of Pick disease, a frontotemporal dementia, are neuronal intracytoplasmic inclusions that are spherical and slightly basophilic (fig. 10-15). They are often detected best with silver impregnation techniques (Bielschowsky but not Gallayas method highlights Pick bodies) and by immunostaining for tau or ubiquitin among routinely available methods. The distribution of these inclusions, the presence of concomitant forms of pathology, and the immunophenotype of these lesions help distinguish them from other forms of homogeneous cytoplasmic inclusions.

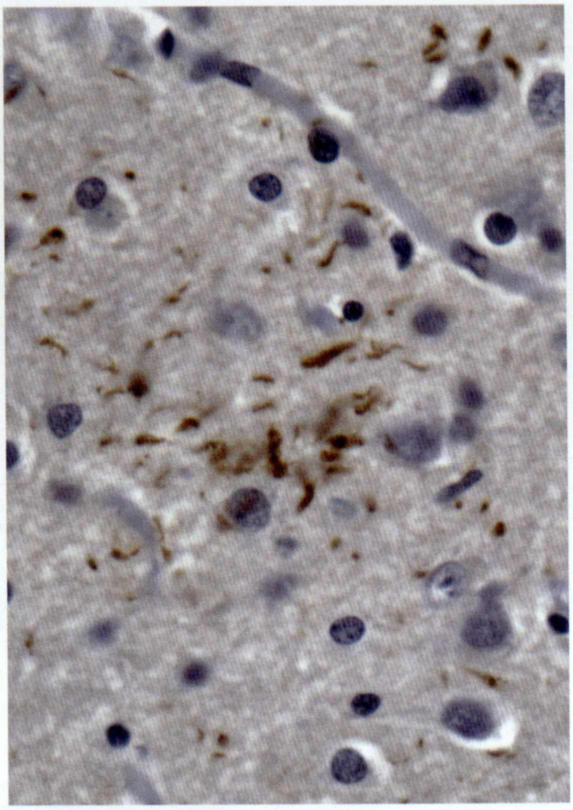

Figure 10-12

ASTROCYTIC PLAQUES

Tau-containing processes of multiple glial cells are directed toward a central area of the neuropil (immunohistochemistry for tau).

Lewy Bodies and Other Alpha-Synuclein Immunoreactive Deposits

Neuronal intracytoplasmic inclusions, which may initially raise the possibility of Pick bodies, may be found in a variety of other diseases. While many pathologists are familiar with *Lewy bodies,* the glassy, eosinophilic, laminated spherical inclusions found in the substantia nigra in Parkinson disease (fig. 10-16), the comparable

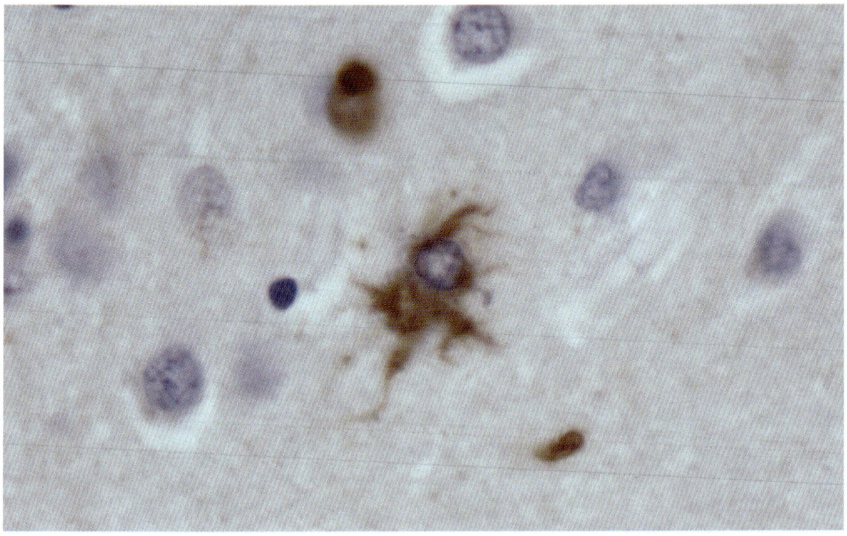

Figure 10-13

TUFTED ASTROCYTE

Tau-containing processes of an astrocyte resemble tangle-bearing dystrophic neurites (immunohistochemistry for tau).

Figure 10-14

COILED BODY

Tau-containing inclusion in an oligodendrocyte (immunohistochemistry for tau).

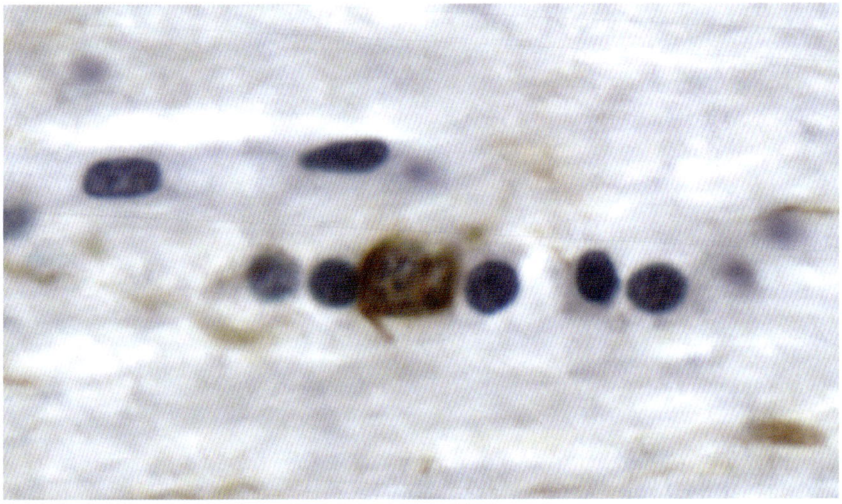

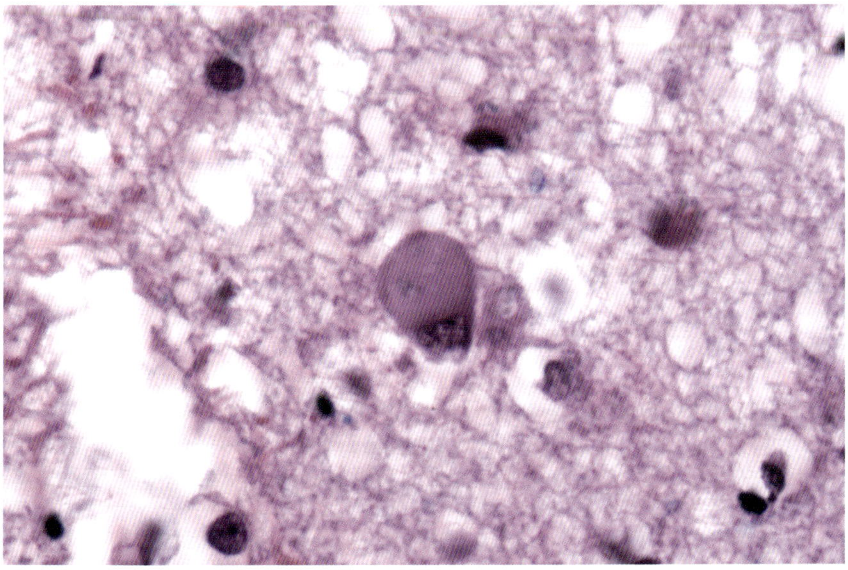

Figure 10-15

PICK BODY

A round cytoplasmic inclusion is one of the hallmarks of Pick disease.

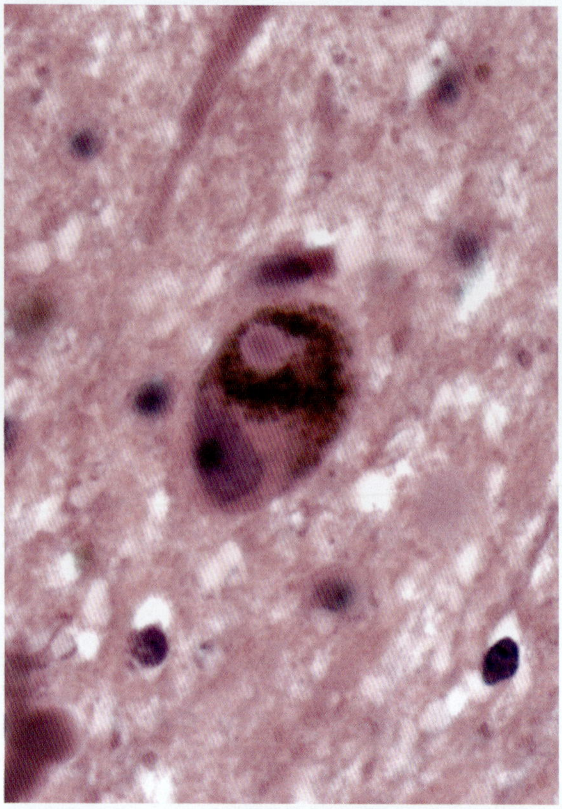

Figure 10-16

LEWY BODY

A classic Lewy body is in the substantia nigra in a case of Parkinson disease.

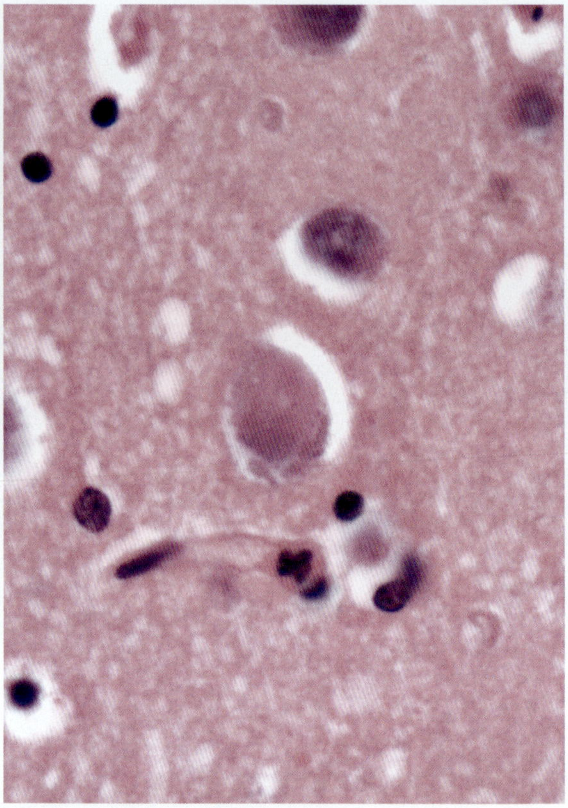

Figure 10-17

LEWY BODY

A cortical Lewy body is less distinct than those found in the brain stem.

lesions that may be found in cerebral cortex as well as other brain regions are often less distinct. Cortical Lewy bodies are typically found in the cytoplasm of neurons in deeper cortical layers, and are spherical, mildly glassy masses which are often poorly defined relative to the surrounding cytoplasm (fig. 10-17). They are often difficult to appreciate apart from a discrete region of cytoplasmic homogeneity. Occasionally, cortical Lewy bodies have the characteristic appearance of brain stem Lewy bodies. Unlike Pick bodies, cortical Lewy bodies are not stained by silver methods, but are routinely identified by immunostaining either for ubiquitin or the more specific α-synuclein. Because cortical Lewy bodies are often accompanied by striking superficial vacuolization of the cerebral cortex, the identification of the latter pathology (although not specific in itself) may prompt a more aggressive hunt for these structures.

In addition to inclusions in the form of Lewy bodies, immunostaining for α-synuclein may reveal two other types of structural abnormalities: one related to diseases with cortical Lewy bodies and the other not. Abnormal neurites (known as Lewy neurites) that contain increased amounts of α-synuclein are often present in certain brain regions in combination with Lewy bodies. Unlike the dystrophic neurites associated with plaques in AD, these are not identified consistently with either silver methods or by the presence of tau. They are mostly found in noncortical structures, mostly in the hippocampus in area CA2.

In contrast to these α-synuclein-containing lesions that are associated with Lewy body diseases, this same protein is the most specific marker of the inclusions found in multiple system atrophy. The marker is commonly recognized as *glial cytoplasmic inclusions* that occur in

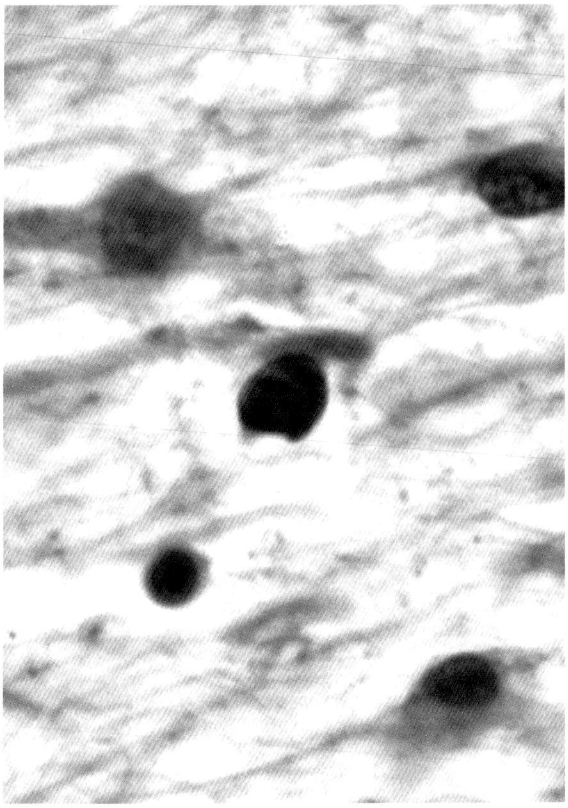

Figure 10-18

GLIAL CYTOPLASMIC INCLUSIONS

These α-synuclein-containing inclusions are found in the white matter in multiple system atrophy (immunohistochemistry for α-synuclein).

oligodendrocytes (fig. 10-18). This particular form of α-synuclein immunoreactive pathology can also be visualized with silver impregnation techniques and by immunostaining against ubiquitin. Because the clinical presentation and radiologic findings of multiple system atrophy usually allow for an accurate diagnosis or for a differential diagnosis in which there is no role for brain biopsy, these inclusions are typically only seen by surgical pathologists as incidental findings.

Ubiquitin Immunoreactive Deposits

It should be clear from the preceding discussions that immunohistochemistry with antibodies for ubiquitin has the potential to identify a wide range of the disease-specific inclusions associated with many of the dementing neurodegenerative diseases. At the same time, the breadth of the type of inclusions that can be identified by staining for ubiquitin has the disadvantage of lacking specificity. For this reason, it can be usefully applied, often in parallel with appropriate silver methods, as a screening method when evaluating biopsies performed for the evaluation of dementia. It is less useful when attempting to perform follow-up examination after a routinely stained biopsy raises suspicion of a particular type of structural abnormality.

Other Immunologically Identified Deposits

A variety of specific abnormal inclusions, typically associated with protein aggregation in the setting of mutations in the corresponding gene, have been described in dementing or other neurodegenerative diseases. These are often found in the context of familial disorders and are typically analyzed in the context of autopsy neuropathology, and thus fall outside of the field of surgical neuropathology.

CLASSIC NEURODEGENERATIVE DISEASES

As discussed above, each neurodegenerative disease features a stereotyped pattern of degeneration of sets of neurons across the central nervous system (CNS), often in combination with a characteristic set of pathologic inclusions or deposits. The fact that the distribution of the lesions forms a prominent portion of the diagnostic criteria shifts the diagnosis of these entities out of the realm of surgical neuropathology (2). Nonetheless, while neuronal loss and reactive gliosis often appear similar regardless of the underlying disease, the specific types of inclusions or deposits allow the pathologist to suggest the presence of these diseases. This possibility can then be evaluated in the context of the clinical, laboratory, and radiographic findings.

Alzheimer Disease

Definition. *Alzheimer disease* (AD) is the most common of the neurodegenerative diseases causing dementia. The disease is characterized by a slow, relatively smooth, progressive loss of cognitive functions. It has an increasing clinical incidence with age, affecting approximately 1 percent of the population at age 60 but rising to nearly 40 percent by age 80. Pathologic findings are thought to develop well in advance of significant clinical deficits, and may be seen in younger patients.

General Comments. The pathologic hallmarks of AD, which form the basis of the diagnosis, are plaques and tangles, which occur in combination with neuronal loss (3–5). The distribution of these lesions in the brain forms the basis for making the diagnosis of AD and determining the likelihood that a patient's underlying dementia is associated with the pathologic findings. Estimates of clinical diagnostic accuracy of AD range upwards of 90 percent (6); the relatively rare cases in which the disease is rapidly progressive or in which age of onset is unusual are more likely to provoke a diagnostic biopsy as part of the evaluation. Onset before the age of 50 should raise the possibility of a familial form of the disease, associated with mutations in one of the genes whose proteins are associated with AD pathogenesis (7).

Clinical Features. AD most often presents with forgetfulness and other memory disturbances, and with progression, other symptoms such as language deficits, loss of mathematical skills, and loss of learned motor skills join the list of cognitive deficits. With the passage of time, usually over the course of 10 years of more, patients may become incontinent, mute, and unable to walk.

Radiologic Findings. Standard imaging studies reveal that these neurologic deficits are matched by progressive and extensive cortical atrophy, enlargement of the temporal horn of the lateral ventricle, and associated loss of volume in mesial temporal lobe structures (hippocampus, entorhinal cortex, and amygdala) (fig. 10-19) (8–10). Methods for direct imaging of Aβ deposits are developing rapidly and are likely to enter clinical practice shortly (11,12).

Gross Findings. Although no alterations are evident in small biopsies, cortical atrophy may be observed when larger portions of brain are resected. This can be difficult to appreciate, however, when the underlying cause for resection is associated with cerebral edema. In the setting of the widespread cerebral atrophy of AD, patients with space-occupying lesions can develop larger masses with fewer symptoms than in younger individuals.

Intraoperative Diagnosis. The pathologic hallmarks of AD can be seen on frozen section, although confirmation of the composition of the plaques and tangles typically requires additional studies.

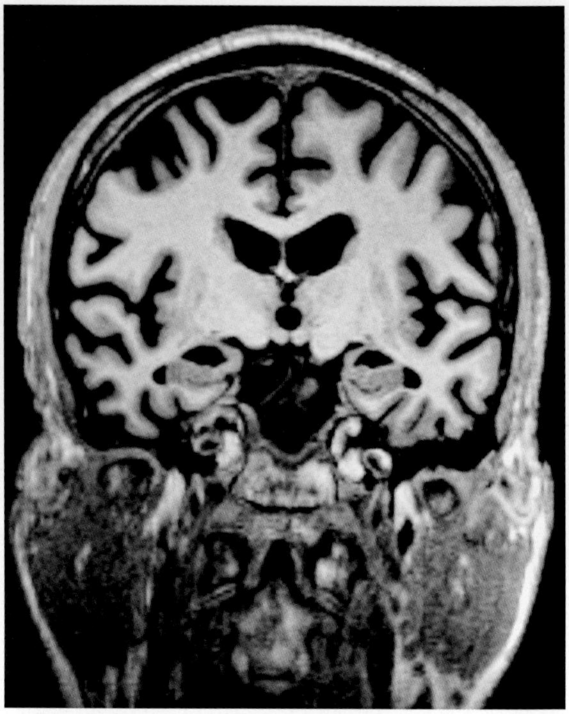

Figure 10-19

ALZHEIMER DISEASE

Magnetic resonance imaging (MRI) demonstrates loss of volume from mesial temporal lobe structures and expansion of the temporal horn of the lateral ventricle. (Courtesy of Dr. B. Dickerson, Boston, MA.)

Microscopic Findings. The two findings that suggest the presence of AD on brain biopsy may be found on routine H&E-stained sections. They are then confirmed by both special staining and immunostaining (3).

Neuritic plaques are recognizable by their disruption of the normal texture of the neuropil (fig. 10-20). These are spherical lesions with diameters ranging from 20 to 200 µm, based around a core of refractile amyloid. In any given histologic section, however, the amyloid may not be present. This amyloid, which is composed of the 40 to 42 amino acid peptide Aβ, can also be found in the walls of leptomeningeal and cortical vessels as cerebral amyloid angiopathy. Plaques may have evident abnormally thickened and tortuous neuritic processes around them, along with reactive gliosis and microglia.

Although plaques can be detected with H&E stains, their presence can be better demonstrated (or confirmed) by special stains. For

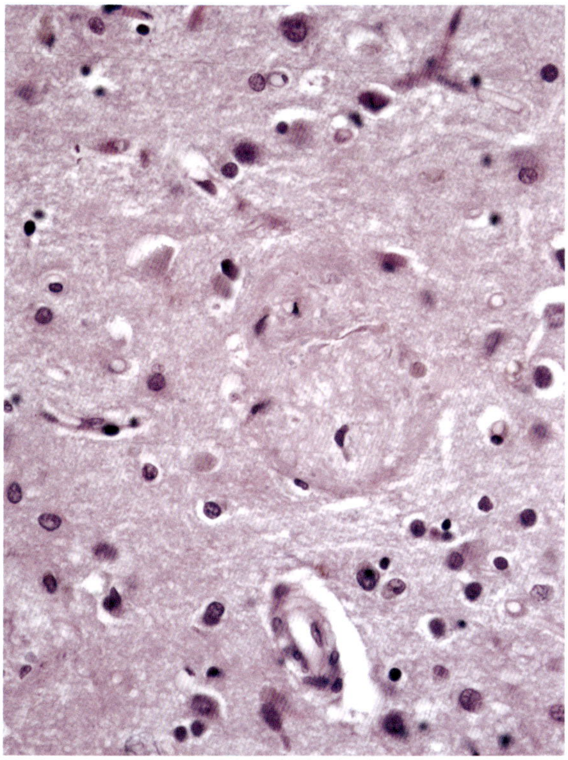

Figure 10-20

ALZHEIMER DISEASE

Plaques can be seen on routine sections because they disrupt the normal texture of the neuropil.

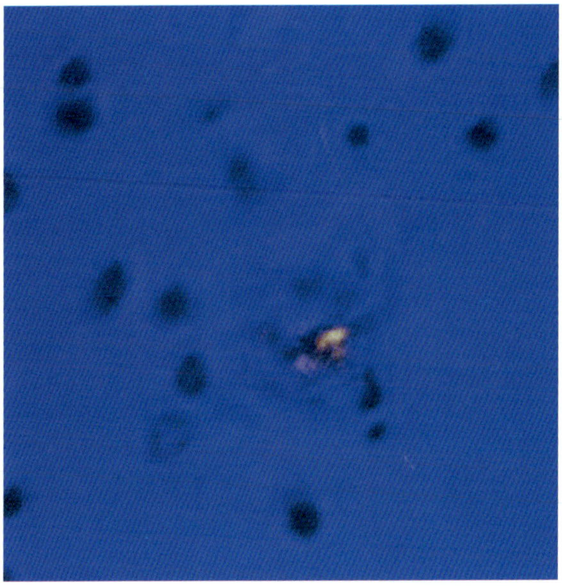

Figure 10-21

ALZHEIMER DISEASE

Plaque cores are birefringent after staining with Congo red.

those lesions in which an amyloid core is present, Congo red staining combined with the demonstration of birefringence highlights the lesions (fig. 10-21). Thioflavin S staining with fluorescence microscopy can also highlight the plaques cores (fig. 10-22). Although technically more difficult, methods such as modified Bielschowsky or Gallayas silver impregnation have greater sensitivity than H&E or Congo red staining, in part because they are not specific for amyloid cores (fig. 10-23).

In contrast to neuritic plaques, *diffuse plaques* are characterized by the deposition of Aβ without the formation of amyloid or the elicitation of a strong neuritic response. Because of these features, these lesions are best demonstrated by immunohistochemistry directed against Aβ (fig. 10-24) or by the Bielschowsky method (fig. 10-25).

In some familial forms of AD linked to some mutations in the *PS1* gene, there are large plaques which can be recognized with H&E stains and immunohistochemistry against Aβ (fig. 10-26).

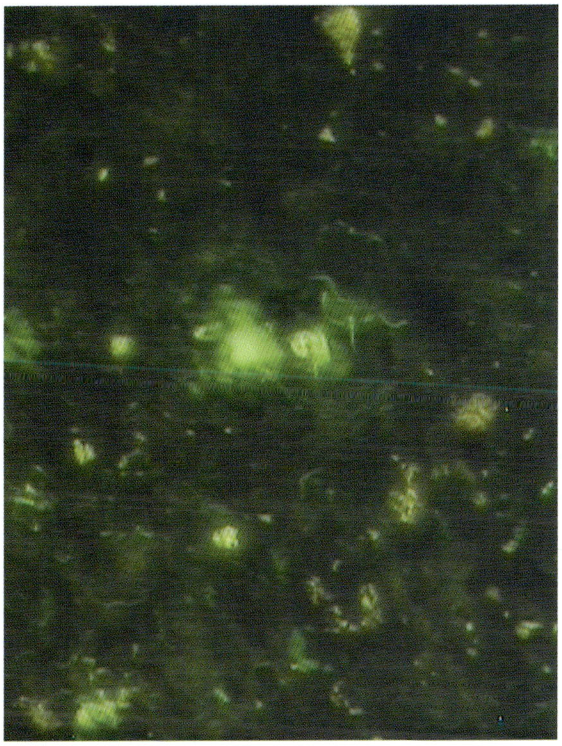

Figure 10-22

ALZHEIMER DISEASE

Plaques are easily recognized with fluorescence microscopy after staining with thioflavin S.

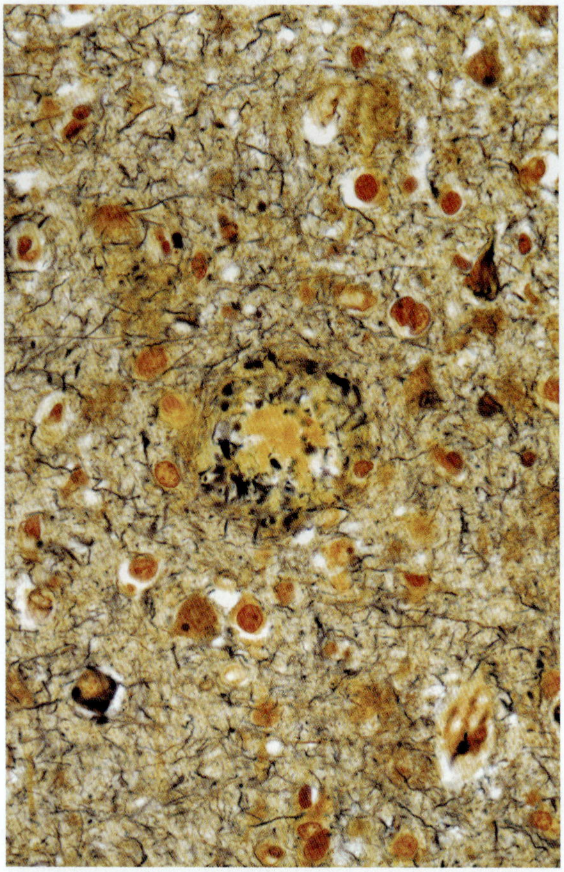

Figure 10-23

ALZHEIMER DISEASE

The neuritic reaction around plaques and the plaque core are highlighted with silver stains (Bielschowsky silver impregnation).

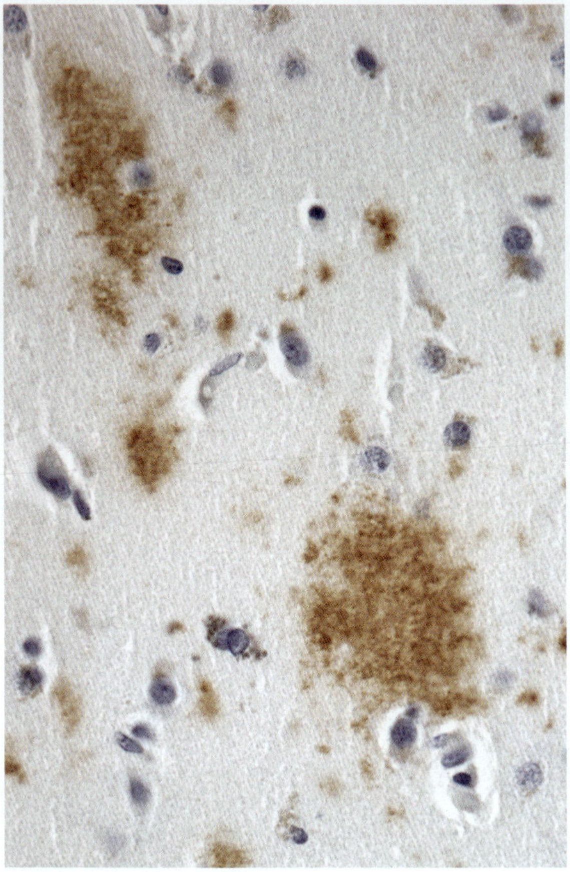

Figure 10-24

ALZHEIMER DISEASE

Diffuse plaques are stained with immunohistochemistry for Aβ.

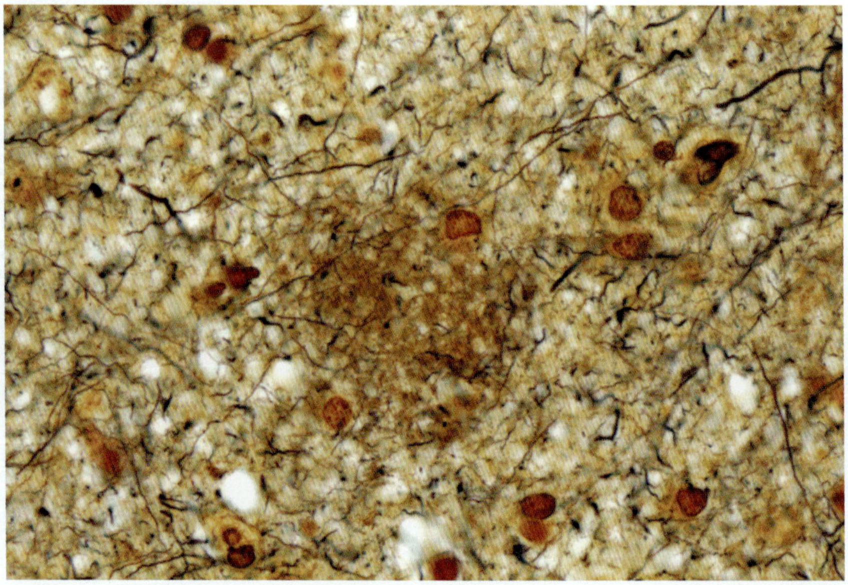

Figure 10-25

ALZHEIMER DISEASE

Diffuse plaques are seen with silver staining (Bielschowsky silver impregnation).

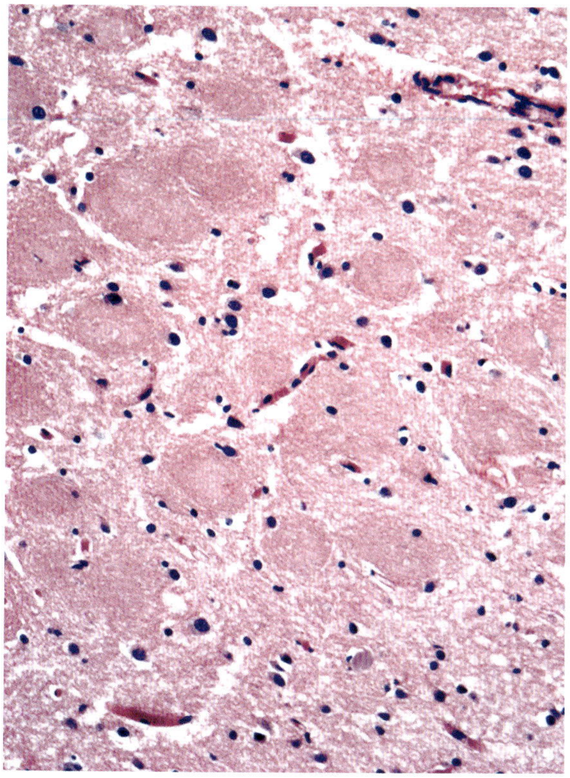

Figure 10-26

ALZHEIMER DISEASE

Large deposits of Aβ form "cotton wool" plaques, without visible central amyloid cores.

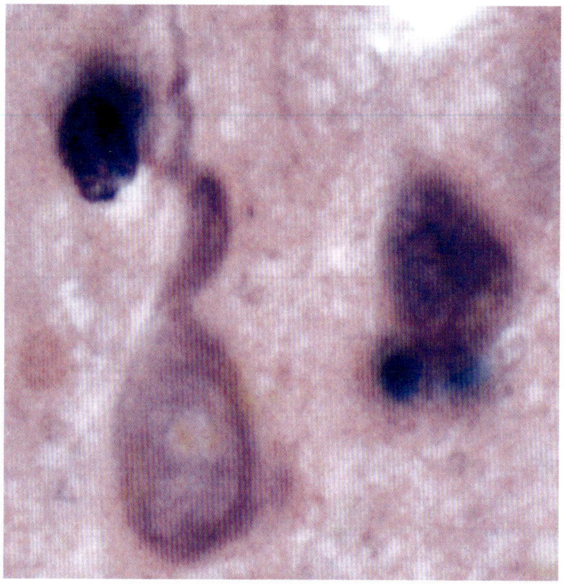

Figure 10-27

ALZHEIMER DISEASE

Tangles are seen within neurons.

These have been termed *cotton wool plaques*, have relatively little amyloid formation or neuritic response, and are predominantly composed of Aβ42 (13–17). Plaques with this morphology may be found in the setting of sporadic AD, where they are associated with more typical lesions (18). In the *PS1*-mutation linked form of early onset AD with cotton wool plaques, spastic paraplegia has been a common clinical finding in addition to the dementia.

The other hallmark lesion of AD is the *neurofibrillary tangle*. Tangles, primarily composed of the microtubule-associated protein tau, are recognizable as mildly basophilic bundles of elongated fibrils. These inclusions begin as intracellular lesions and are often oriented from the cell body toward the apical dendrite (fig. 10-27). The fibrils of a tangle may form a basket weave pattern around the nucleus, and then are termed globose tangles. When the neuron containing a tangle dies, the tangle often persists in the extracellular space. These ghost tangles, which have been likened to the tombstones of dead neurons, gradually become less basophilic and more difficult to detect with H&E staining (fig. 10-28). Thioflavin S staining and visualization with fluorescence microscopy can demonstrate the presence of tangles. As with plaques, appropriate silver methods, such as Bielschowsky or Gallayas, are excellent means to confirm the presence of tangles (fig. 10-29). Particularly with the modified Bielschowsky impregnation techniques, extracellular tangles tend to have a golden color as compared with the black staining of intracellular tangles and the dystrophic neurites of neuritic plaques.

As mentioned above, cerebral amyloid angiopathy is a common finding in the setting of AD (19–21). Attempts to demonstrate the presence of vascular amyloid with Congo red or thioflavin S staining (or immunostaining as mentioned below) often highlight the pathologic lesions of AD in addition to confirming the presence of vascular pathology.

Immunohistochemical Findings. Because the pathologic hallmarks of plaques and tangles have specific peptide/proteins as their dominant components, specific antibodies directed against these molecules play a role in the demonstration

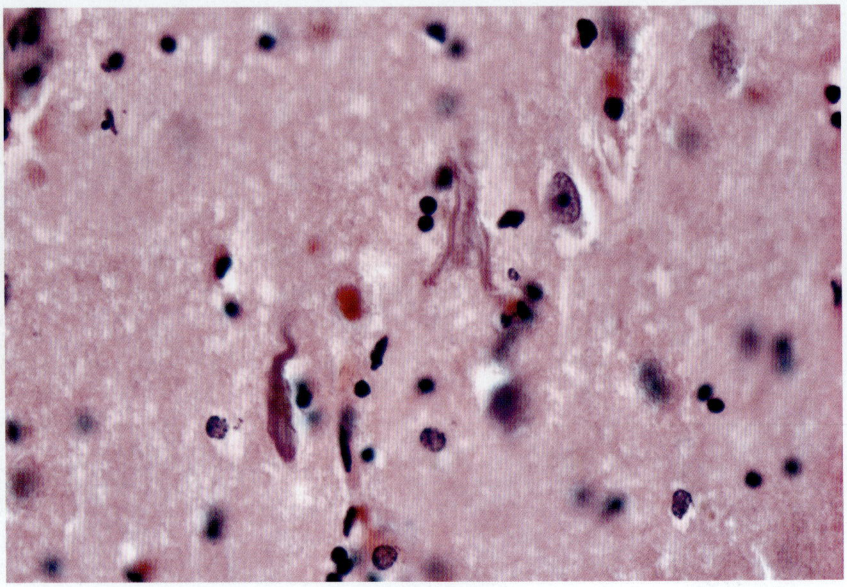

Figure 10-28

ALZHEIMER DISEASE

Extracellular tangles may be found after the death of the neuron.

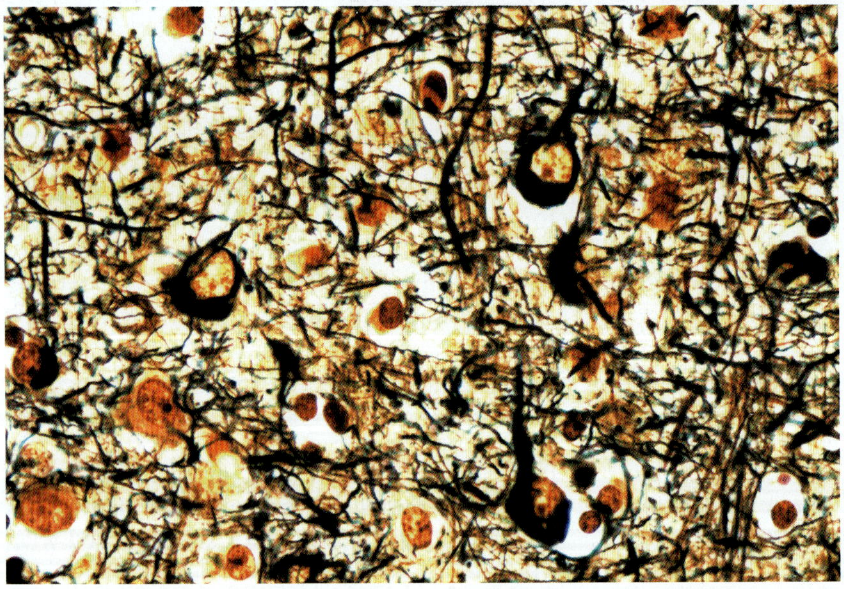

Figure 10-29

ALZHEIMER DISEASE

Tangles are well demonstrated with silver impregnation methods (Bielschowsky silver impregnation).

of these disease-related abnormalities. Plaques, both diffuse and neuritic, are well demonstrated by immunostaining with antibodies directed against epitopes of Aβ. With anti-Aβ immunohistochemistry, diffuse plaques appear as regions of staining across the neuropil, but lack the dense cores of neuritic plaques (fig. 10-30). There is generally only minimal staining of the dystrophic neurites for Aβ. Antibodies that are specific for different isoforms of Aβ (most commonly the 40 and 42 amino acid forms of the peptide) will show distinct patterns. Staining for Aβ40 highlights deposits in vessels of cerebral amyloid angiopathy as well as neuritic plaques, while staining for Aβ42 marks both neuritic and diffuse plaques. Various other proteins have been identified as components of plaques; however, none are useful as targets for diagnostic studies.

The major protein component of tangles is the microtubule-associated protein, tau. This protein can exist in multiple isoforms, which are functionally distinguished by the presence of either three (3R) or four (4R) copies of the

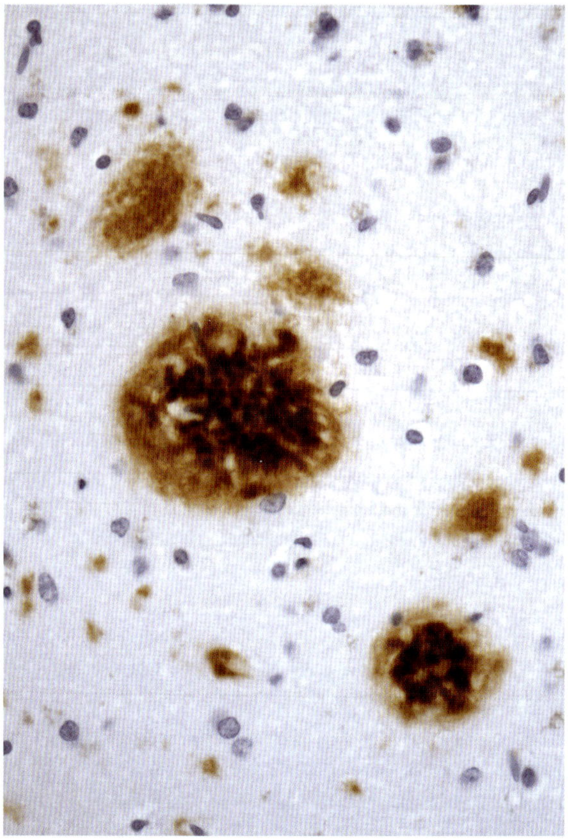

Figure 10-30

ALZHEIMER DISEASE

Plaque cores as well as diffuse plaques contain Aβ deposits (immunohistochemistry for Aβ).

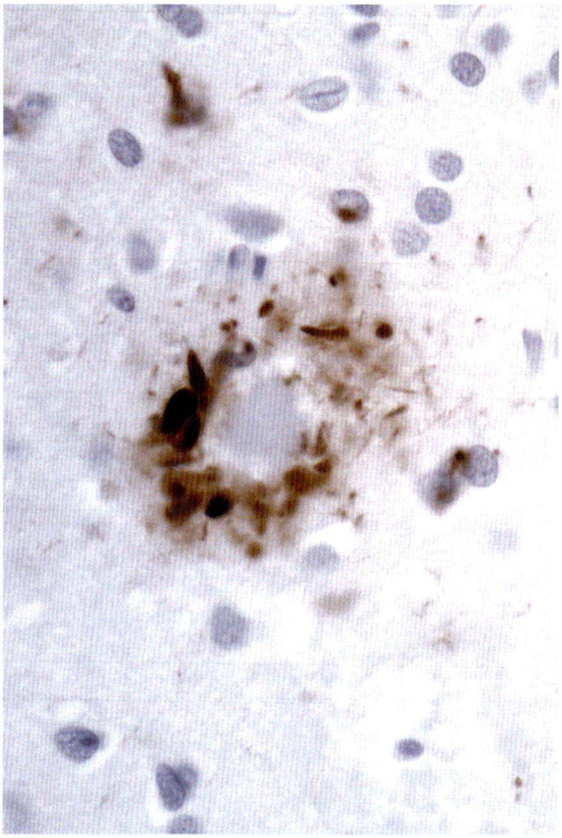

Figure 10-31

ALZHEIMER DISEASE

Dystrophic neurites around plaques contain abnormal tau, just as in tangles (immunohistochemistry for tau).

microtubule-binding domain (1). The normal physiologic distribution of tau is associated with microtubules in the axon. As part of the pathologic process of tangle formation, the protein undergoes redistribution toward the somatodendritic compartment, takes on a new set of conformations, acquires an increased number of phosphorylations (hyperphosphorylation), and acquires the paired helical filament structure that can be seen by electron microscopy. For these reasons, tangles, both within neurons and free in the neuropil, can be demonstrated immunohistochemically with antibodies against epitopes of phosphorylated tau or conformation-specific epitopes (fig. 10-31). Because the dystrophic neurites that are found in neuritic plaques have undergone similar alterations in their cytoskeleton, antibodies against tau also highlight this component of such plaques (fig. 10-32).

As both plaques and tangles represent accumulations of normal proteins in abnormal conformations or aggregations, there is often a high level of ubiquitination in these lesions. Both plaques and tangles can be demonstrated with antibodies against ubiquitin; however, the lack of specificity of this approach, as well as the typically high level of nonspecific background staining, makes it less effective than the use of specific antibodies for the diagnosis of AD.

Laboratory and Molecular Findings. Advances in the understanding of the pathogenesis of AD have come, in large part, from dissection of the genetic forms of AD. The finding of plaque and tangle pathology in tissue from someone younger than age 50 should raise the possibility of a familial form of AD. The three gene loci that have been defined to date are the genes for amyloid precursor protein (APP;

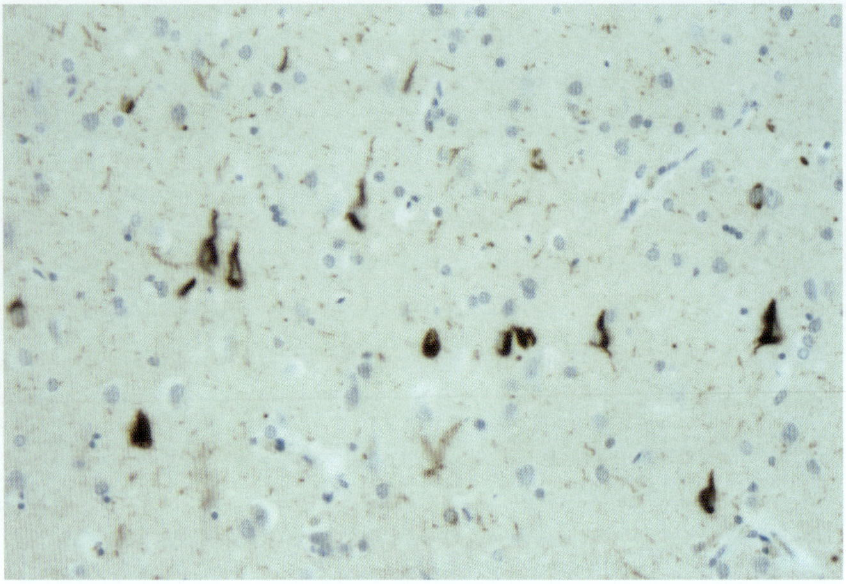

Figure 10-32

ALZHEIMER DISEASE

Tangles are strongly immunoreactive for tau.

chromosome 21), presenilin-1 (PS1; chromosome 14) and presenilin-2 (PS2; chromosome 1) (7). The gene for tau has not been found to be a locus for mutations causing AD, despite the prominence of tau pathology in the disease. As is considered below, mutations in the gene encoding tau are associated with forms of frontotemporal dementia, where the pathologic findings include tangles but not plaques. The definition of sensitive and specific biomarkers from the cerebrospinal fluid (CSF) and plasma continues to evolve, both for clinical use and as potential surrogate markers in studies of therapies (22–24).

Differential Diagnosis. As with many of these neurodegenerative diseases, the currently accepted diagnostic criteria for AD preclude establishing a diagnosis on the basis of a surgical pathology specimen, although, in the correct clinical setting, the suspicion can be high. The full consideration of these lesions as diagnostic of the disease requires histologic access to multiple brain regions (as is possible at autopsy) (25–27). In addition to sampling a range of neocortical sites as well as the entorhinal cortex, hippocampus, and amygdala, there is a requirement to assess the brain for other pathologic changes, which may have contributed to the dementia.

Several approaches to diagnostic criteria are currently used, which focus on plaques, tangles, or both. The *Consortium to Establish a Registry for Alzheimer Disease (CERAD) criteria* were developed with an emphasis on the burden of plaques across multiple cortical regions, and are now implemented using silver methods or immunohistochemistry with antibodies directed toward Aβ (3). The *Braak and Braak staging system* for tangles is based on the observation that these lesions have a relatively stereotyped pattern of progressive involvement of specific brain regions (based on sampling of a large number of cases rather than on actual serial observations on individual brains) (28). This staging is most commonly implemented with either appropriate silver impregnation techniques or immunostaining for tau. The approach of these two methods has been combined recently with the *National Institute on Aging (NIA)-Reagan criteria* (27,29–32), which provides an estimate of the likelihood that AD pathology caused dementia, although situations in which there is discrepancy between the severities of the two types of lesion are not addressed.

As should be clear from this discussion, the presence of plaques and tangles in a surgical specimen is not sufficient to make a diagnosis of AD. Whether the presence of low numbers of these two types of pathologic structures represents an early preclinical stage of AD or a variant of aging (so-called pathologic aging) remains a point of significant controversy (30,33). When both types of lesion are present in a surgical specimen, however, the potential disease process is most consistent with AD, at some stage in its development. As imaging methods are developed that can detect Aβ at potentially preclinical stages, this apparent discrepancy between clinical and pathologic findings may be better resolved (11,12).

Head trauma has been demonstrated to result in increased levels of tissue Aβ, and the deposition of this peptide in the form of diffuse plaques (34). This can occur relatively rapidly after the episode of head injury. When associated with repetitive trauma, as in the setting of dementia pugilistica, tangles are present as well (35).

There have been a few families described in which the histologic findings resemble AD (amyloid deposition in the brain parenchyma with neuritic response to plaques, as well as tangles and vascular amyloid) yet the deposited amyloid is distinct. On a morphologic basis, these diseases, familial British dementia (FBD) (36,37) and familial Danish dementia (FDD) (38), can be best separated from AD by immunohistochemistry, since the amyloid is derived from a different protein than APP and will not stain for Aβ (39). These disorders also have clinical contexts that usually set them apart from AD. FDD begins with cataracts and ocular hemorrhages when patients are in their late 20s, often resulting in blindness. After one to two decades, these are followed by hearing loss and cerebellar ataxia. Psychiatric symptoms and dementia follow toward the end of the course of the disease. FBD is a disorder in which the combination of memory loss, cerebellar ataxia, and spastic paraplegia are common (40). The disease typically begins around age 48, with a 10-year course that eventually evolves to a persistent vegetative state. Because of the overlapping symptoms and evidence of a familial disorder, FBD does show similarity to some of the PS1-linked forms of familial AD associated with spastic paraplegia.

When tangles are present in a surgical specimen without evidence of plaques or amyloid deposition, there are several possible lines of interpretation. First, it is possible that the limited sampling of a neurosurgical specimen has not provided the pathologist with the other pathologic hallmarks of AD-related pathology, as discussed above. It is also essential to recognize, however, that tangles are by far the less specific of the lesions observed in AD; given this promiscuity, the finding of tangles in a brain biopsy should be reported only as an observation rather than as the basis of a diagnosis.

Dementia with Lewy Bodies

Definition. *Dementia with Lewy bodies* (DLB) is a neurodegenerative disorder characterized by the presence of Lewy bodies in neurons of various cortical structures (41). There is a strong relationship with Parkinson disease and AD, both clinically and pathologically (42–48).

General Comments. The identification of Lewy bodies in the dopaminergic neurons of the substantia nigra and other brain stem structures as the pathologic substrate of Parkinson disease preceded the recognition of DLB as a pathologically and clinically related entity. When the inclusions were originally described in the context of a disease, it was felt to be a cortical-specific process. Over time, it has become clear than the development of Lewy bodies and related forms of α-synuclein pathology lies along a continuum. Given this, the most recently developed classification and staging schemes (which can only be applied in the setting of an autopsy evaluation of the brain) are directed at the distribution and abundance of these inclusions (42,44).

There is an additional complicating relationship between the presence of Lewy bodies and AD. While the literature does not suggest that these inclusions are a pathologic component of the disease process in AD, there are several lines of evidence that have bound these forms of pathology together. When examining the cerebral cortex of individuals with DLB, the frequency with which plaques and tangles are also observed exceeds that which would be suspected simply on the basis of chance. Conversely, in the amygdala of patients with clinically and pathologically diagnosed AD, Lewy bodies are common, being present in a third to nearly all cases (49,50). Similarly, they have been identified in the brains of members of kindreds with familial AD associated with mutations in the *APP* gene. Finally, a portion of the α-synuclein protein, the major component of Lewy bodies, can be found in association with plaque cores in AD (51–54). For all of these reasons, controversy existed previously as to whether DLB was a dementing illness independent of AD or whether it represented a variant form of AD pathology. With the current understanding of the associated brain stem α-synuclein pathology that is found with DLB, this question has become less pertinent.

Clinical Features. A consensus set of diagnostic criteria for DLB have been developed (46–48). While DLB is often considered as a dementing illness, the presenting cognitive changes often show attentional and frontal executive deficits that are larger than memory disturbances. With time, deficits in all domains are typically observed. Additional clinical features that contribute to the suspicion of the diagnosis include unpredictable fluctuations in the severity of the deficits, complaints of visual hallucinations, parkinsonian symptoms, falls, and marked neuroleptic sensitivity.

Radiologic Findings. There are no specific abnormalities on imaging studies that are diagnostic of DLB. Given the relative preservation of memory function in the disease and the relatively low burden of pathologic findings in the hippocampus, there may be less evidence of atrophy in the medial temporal lobe on structural magnetic resonance imaging (MRI) studies.

Microscopic Findings. There are four major histologic hallmarks of DLB: Lewy bodies, both classic and cortical; Lewy neurites; and cortical vacuolation. Notably, however, only the first three of these have specificity for this disorder. Classic Lewy bodies (55), which are relatively rare in structures that are represented in neurosurgical specimens but are found in brain stem nuclei such as substantia nigra, locus ceruleus, dorsal motor nucleus of the vagus, as well as in the nucleus basalis of Meynert, are neuronal cytoplasmic inclusions (fig. 10-33). They are eosinophilic inclusions, with a darker staining core and a halo of lighter, less dense staining. They can be laminated and are typically round, ranging from 10 to 30 μm, and there may be multiple bodies within a single cell.

Cortical Lewy bodies are also cytoplasmic neuronal inclusions, but lack the biphasic appearance of the classic type (56–58). Instead, these inclusions are more vaguely defined areas of mild eosinophilic staining in the cytoplasm, often toward the smaller end of the size spectrum (10 to 20 μm diameter) (fig. 10-34). They are predominantly distributed in the deeper layers of the cortex. As considered above, cortical Lewy bodies can be difficult to identify

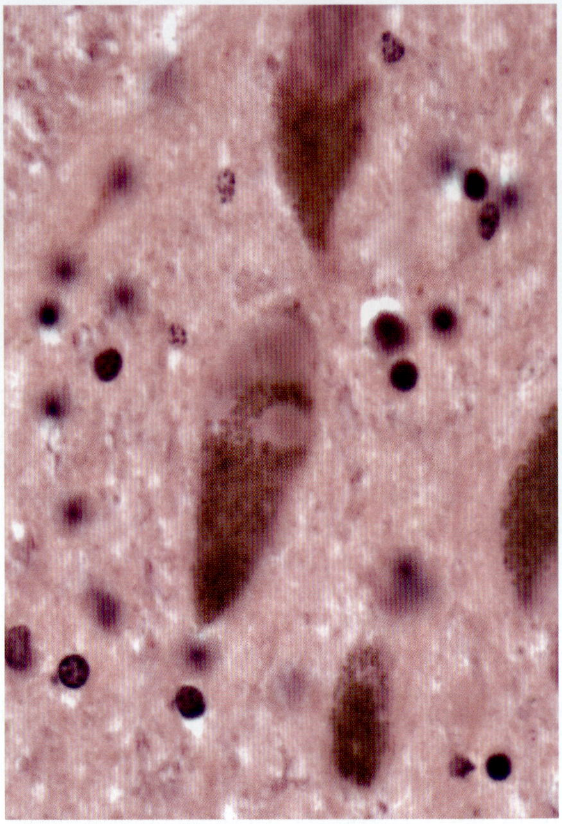

Figure 10-33

LEWY BODY DISEASE

Brain stem Lewy bodies are often laminated and can be multiple within a neuron.

without the application of immunostaining for either ubiquitin or α-synuclein. Depending on the stage of the disease (see below), these may be found predominantly in limbic structures such as cingulate or insular cortices, or in other association areas.

A separate finding, primarily in the hippocampus, in the CA2 region, as well as in brain stem nuclei and deep gray matter, is the presence of Lewy neurites, which are dystrophic neuronal processes that are highlighted by immunohistochemistry against α-synuclein (fig. 10-35) (59,60). The presence and distribution of these structures form part of one of the recently proposed systems for staging DLB (42).

The final pathologic hallmark of DLB is the presence of spongiform change in the upper cortical layers (typically layers I to II) (61). This is found as a continuous band of vacuolization of the neuropil, most prominently in the medial temporal lobe (fig. 10-36). The distribution, continuity of the change, and clinical context help to distinguish it from the changes found in prion diseases.

Immunohistochemical Findings. When classic Lewy bodies are present, they can be easily recognized; additional staining methods are of use only to confirm that the inclusions contain α-synuclein. In contrast, since cortical Lewy bodies can be difficult to recognize on routine H&E-stained sections, the use of immunohistochemistry has greatly increased the ability to detect these inclusions. The diagnostic use of antiubiquitin immunostaining, in fact, has facilitated the recognition of the lesions to the point that there has been an increased incidence of the neuropathologic diagnosis of DLB among patients with movement or memory disorders. With the identification of α-synuclein as the major component of the Lewy body, the use of antibodies directed against this protein has increased the specificity of the immunologic identification of these lesions (fig. 10-37). Additionally, Lewy neurites require immunohistochemistry directed against α-synuclein.

The application of immunohistochemical staining for the increased detection and quantification of cortical Lewy bodies was an important step toward the development of the two currently used systems for describing and grading DLB (46). While the older system,

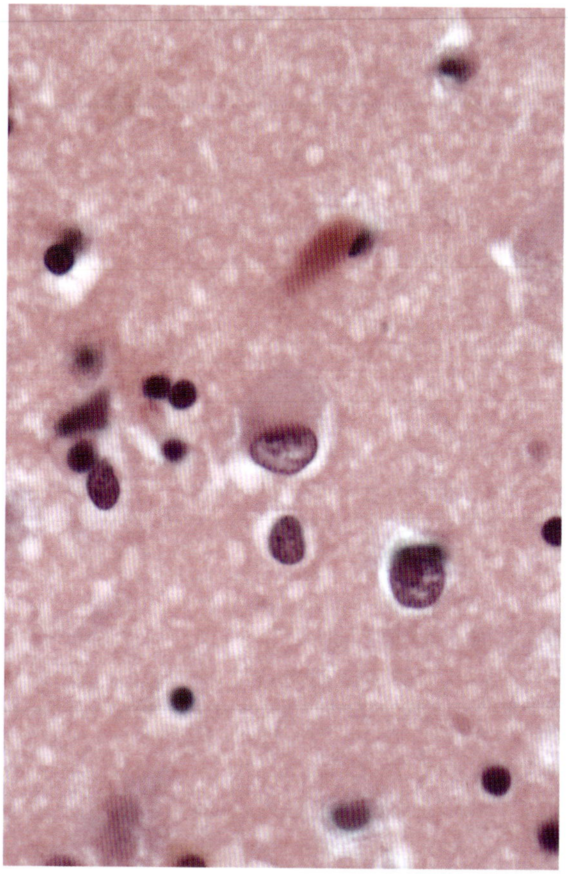

Figure 10-34

LEWY BODY DISEASE

Cortical Lewy bodies may be difficult to detect in H&E-stained sections.

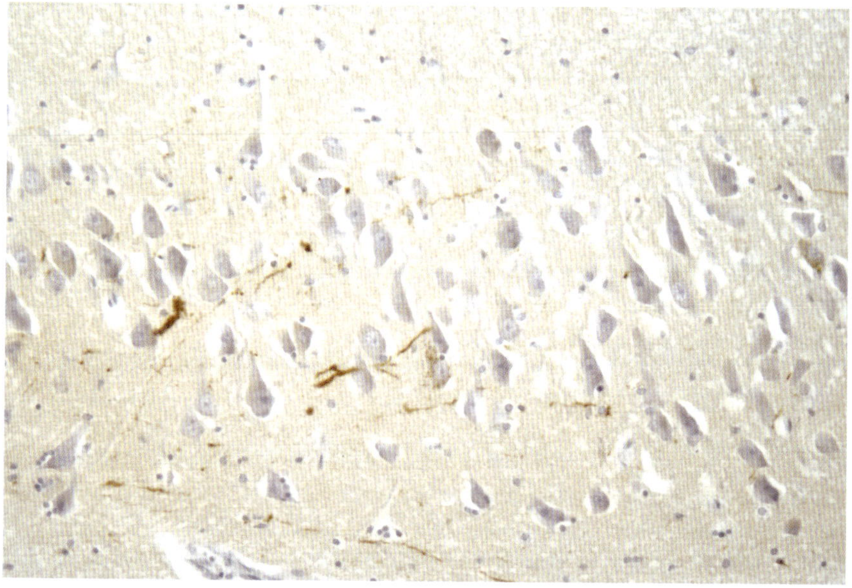

Figure 10-35

LEWY BODY DISEASE

Lewy neurites can be seen in area CA2 of the hippocampus (immunohistochemistry for α-synuclein).

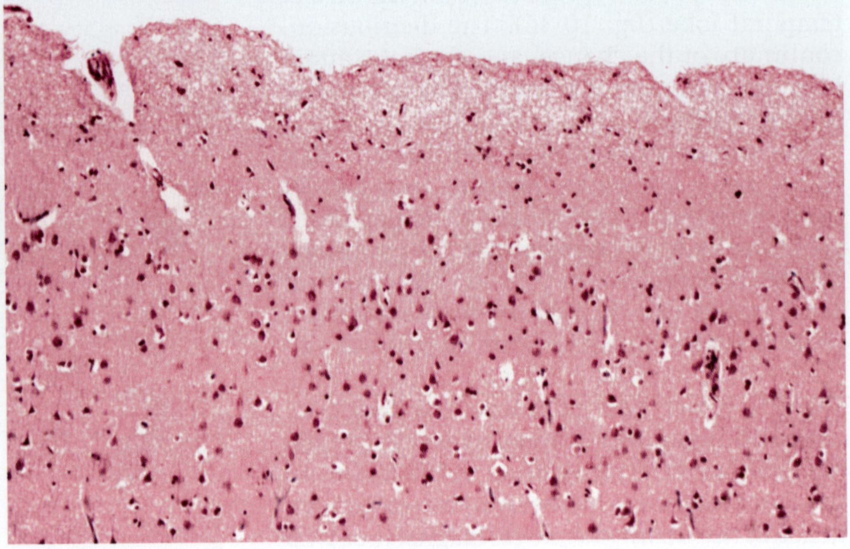

Figure 10-36

LEWY BODY DISEASE

Superficial spongiotic change is common in the mesial temporal lobe.

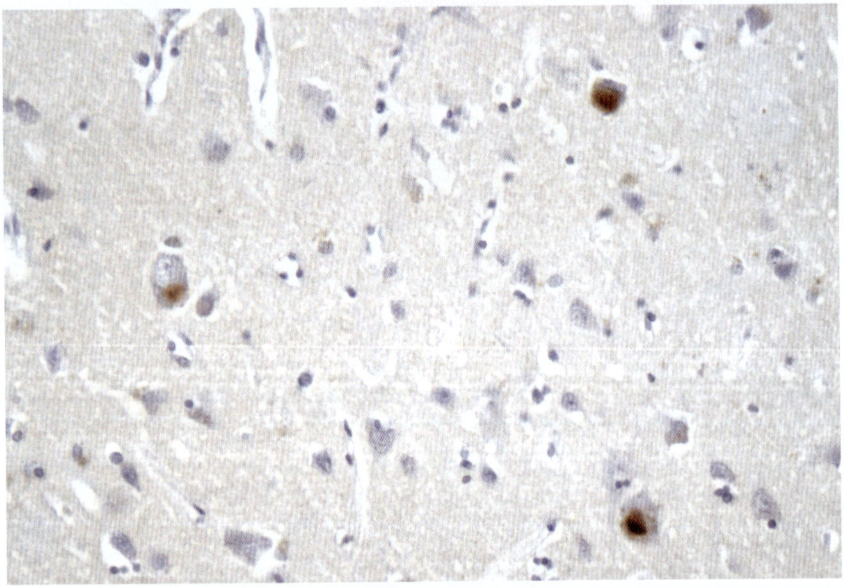

Figure 10-37

LEWY BODY DISEASE

Lewy bodies are well highlighted by immunostaining for α-synuclein.

which is still more widely used, is based on immunohistochemistry directed against ubiquitin, it is widely accepted that staining for α-synuclein has higher specificity. Given that surgical pathology specimens do not sample all of the required regions and may not even sample the carefully specified Brodmann areas used in this classification scheme, there is limited applicability of these systems to brain biopsies. Nevertheless, as with the other neurodegenerative diseases, the examination of a small portion of the brain can be put into the probable context of the remainder of the CNS because of the observed stereotypic pattern of progression of involvement in DLB.

The *Newcastle criteria* were developed to describe the distribution of cortical Lewy bodies based on their abundance in a series of distinct cortical regions (46). It is a classification scheme, and not a set of diagnostic criteria. Depending on the abundance of the Lewy bodies in different regions, the disease may be considered as either brain stem only, limbic (also called transitional), or cortical. The specifics of quantification are less important than the recognition that the disease tends to progress from the brain stem, through limbic structures (cingulated gyrus, insular cortex, parahippocampal gyrus), and then to higher cortical association areas (prefrontal cortex, superior parietal lobule, superior temporal gyrus).

This same sense of progression underlies the more recently described *staging system of α-synuclein pathology* (including Lewy bodies and Lewy neurites), which defines a progression from various brain stem structures through higher gray matter regions and on to the cerebral cortex (42,44). In this system, involvement of the substantia nigra (as is found in Parkinson disease) falls near the midpoint of the stages of progression (3/6). Again, it is not possible to apply this system to a small biopsy, or even a large cortical resection, but the understanding of the orderly progression of Lewy bodies and Lewy neurites across the brain allows the pathologist to suggest the severity of the disease elsewhere. It remains essential, however, to remember two caveats to this: 1) while these evaluations of the progression of pathology are based on a large number of patients with DLB, not every brain will conform to these guidelines; 2) there may also be a dissociation between the presence of pathology and evidence of clinical symptoms (that is, not every individual with Lewy bodies in the substantia nigra will have parkinsonian symptoms).

Differential Diagnosis. Two aspects of the pathology of DLB raise important questions when first examining a brain biopsy: the presence of the associated superficial spongiotic change and the presence of the inclusions. The first of these may suggest several additional possibilities, including artifact, edema, or prion disease. Clues that help the pathologist to associate this spongiotic change with DLB include the uniformity of the vacuolization (in contrast to the typically uneven distribution found in prion diseases), the restriction to the superficial cortical layers including layer I (which is usually spared in edema, ischemia, and prion disease), and the presence of Lewy bodies.

When confronted with an inclusion in a neuron that raises the possibility of cortical Lewy bodies, the differential diagnosis includes the variety of other neuronal cytoplasmic spherical inclusions. The most commonly considered other entity would be a Pick body, followed by rare disorders. The identity of an inclusion as a cortical Lewy body should be straightforward through the application of immunostaining against α-synuclein. It is also important to ensure that corpora amylacea are not mistaken for neuronal inclusions, although these will be nonreactive with the various antibody-based methods.

Tauopathies

General Comments. *Tauopathies* are a group of diseases united by the common thread of pathologic inclusions containing tau (62). Although this aspect of the pathologic findings is shared, the diseases include a range of clinical presentations, including dementias and movement disorders. For none of them is a single microscopic finding an adequate basis for rendering a specific diagnosis. There is need for clinicopathologic correlation and for an understanding of the distribution of the pathologic findings across the brain (in a manner not accessible to the surgical pathologist) (62,63). What is important for the pathologist evaluating a brain biopsy is to recognize the type of inclusion and to be able to suggest the possibility of an underlying neurodegenerative disease. Once again, however, none of these diseases are processes for which brain biopsy plays a role in the diagnostic evaluation; rather, they are seen by the pathologist as potentially unexpected abnormalities when a patient undergoes surgery for another indication. For this reason, these diseases are discussed as a group rather than as specific entities.

Clinical and Radiologic Findings. *Dementias.* The dementing illnesses under consideration here are those in which tau pathology, usually, but not always in the form of tangles and in the absence of Aβ deposits, represents the common alteration (62,63). The relevant diseases to be considered include frontotemporal dementia with parkinsonism linked to the gene for tau (*MAPT*) (64), frontotemporal dementia (63), and Pick disease (65). These diseases, on the basis of their prominent frontal lobe involvement, often have predominant behavioral components during the earlier stages of presentation. While involving the temporal lobes, there is usually a relative sparing (at least early in the disease) of hippocampal structures, and thus there is often preferential involvement of language over memory. Reflecting the anatomic distribution of these processes with a preference for the frontal

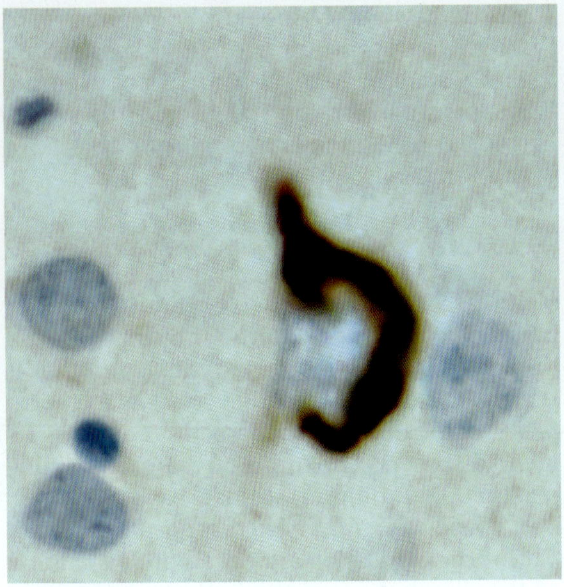

Figure 10-38

TAUOPATHY

Immunohistochemistry for tau highlights the tangle.

and temporal lobes, imaging studies confirm the lobar nature of the cortical atrophy. When seen pathologically in the absence of clinical data, these diseases are often referred to as *frontotemporal lobar degenerations* (FTLD).

Movement Disorders. In contrast to other tauopathies, *progressive supranuclear palsy* (PSP) (66) and *corticobasal degeneration* (CBD) (67) both begin with movement disorders, with frontal lobe signs such as behavioral abnormalities and dementia coming later in the course of the disease. With PSP, early signs typically include falls as well as postural instability. There are signs of parkinsonism, and the disorder is often termed one of the "Parkinson plus" syndromes. One of the traditionally considered diagnostic hallmarks of the disease, although not always present at presentation, is impaired downward gaze; symptomatically this may present with difficulty walking down steps. Because much of the burden of pathology in PSP lies in the deep gray structures and the brain stem, standard structural imaging studies are less contributory to this diagnosis than for others, except to exclude other disease processes.

CBD also has a varied presentation, but most often begins with unilateral (or at least strikingly asymmetric) motor symptoms, typically some combination of apraxia, dystonia, and rigidity. With time and progression of the disease, symptoms become bilateral and are associated with frontal lobe cognitive impairment. Structural imaging makes a minor contribution to the diagnosis, again except through exclusion of other processes.

Microscopic Findings. *Dementias*. In FTD caused by mutations in the tau gene, tangles as well as other forms of tau pathology may be seen. There is a moderate degree of correlation between the type of mutation present and the distribution of pathologic tau; in general, point mutations are associated with predominantly neuronal deposits, while splice mutations show evidence of tau deposits in both neurons and glia. Deposits may be recognized either by immunostaining for tau or through a variety of silver methods, including Bodian, Bielschowsky, or Gallayas. The inclusions in neurons sometimes take the form of well-recognized tangles, either extending out into the dendrite or in a predominantly perinuclear location (fig. 10-38). Various cases have been reported in which the abnormal tau forms a sharply defined perinuclear ring (fig. 10-39) (68). Several of the mutations causing this disease are associated with homogeneously staining cytoplasmic inclusions, and are reminiscent of Pick bodies.

Glial tau pathology may take several forms, all of which overlap partially with the findings in the other tauopathies. Inclusions in oligodendrocytes usually take the form of coiled bodies, in which the abnormal protein wraps around the nucleus and extends out into a cytoplasmic process (fig. 10-40). Two forms of astrocyte pathology may also be found (tufted astrocytes and astrocytic plaques), which are discussed below in the context of movement disorders, in which they form a more critical diagnostic component.

In contrast to the fibrillary nature of these tangles and related inclusions, the characteristic pathologic hallmark of Pick disease is the presence of smooth spherical cytoplasmic inclusions in neurons (fig. 10-41). These inclusions may be recognized on routine H&E staining because of their sharp demarcation from the adjacent cytoplasm and their mildly basophilic nature. They may be identified with some (Bodian or

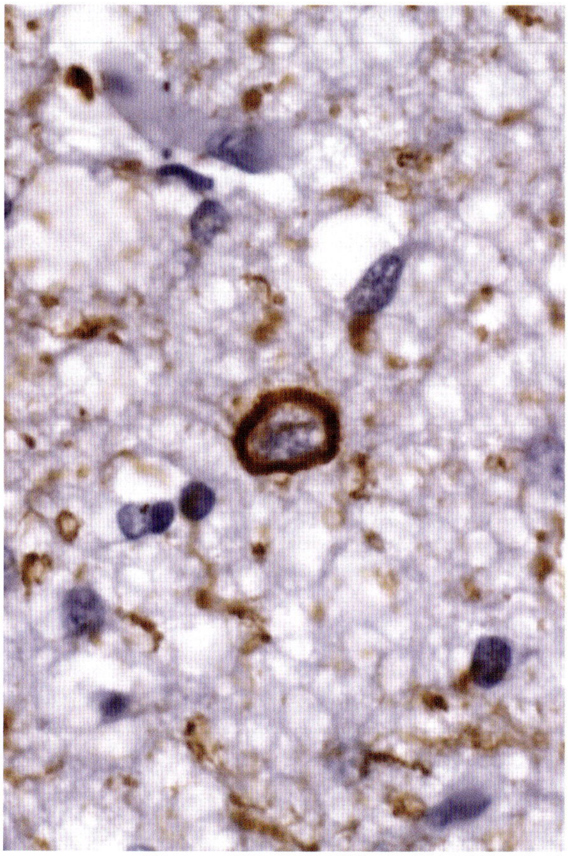

Figure 10-39

TAUOPATHY

Perinuclear rings of tau deposition rather than the more classic tangle are seen in some cases (immunohistochemistry for tau).

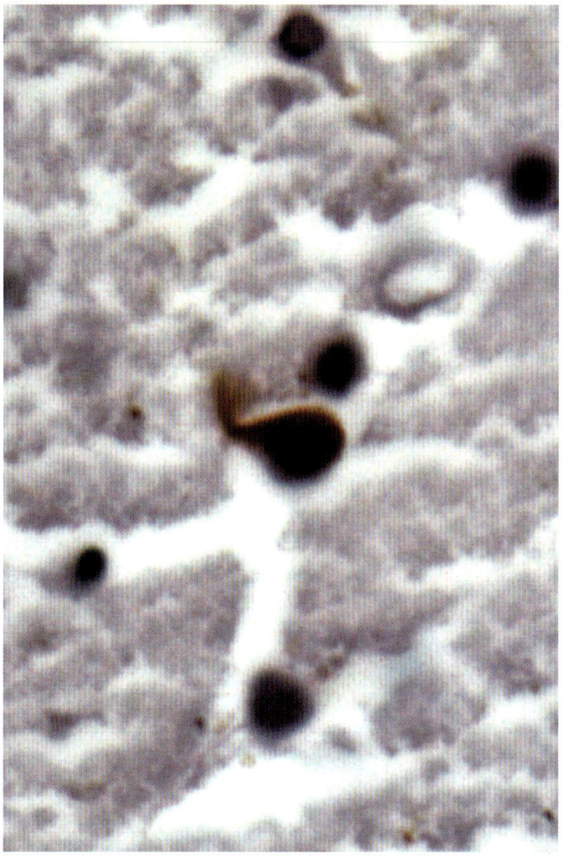

Figure 10-40

COILED BODY

A tau-containing inclusion is in an oligodendrocyte in the white matter (immunohistochemistry for tau).

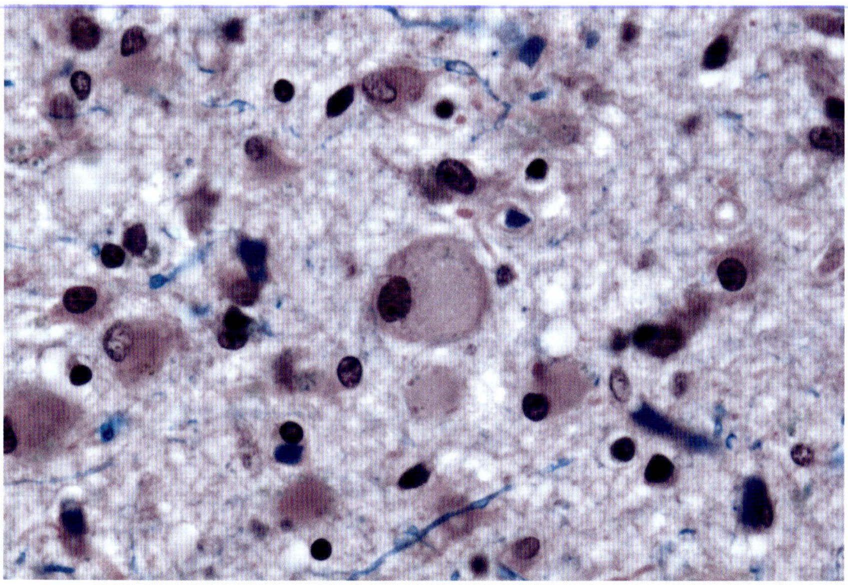

Figure 10-41

PICK DISEASE

Pick bodies are cytoplasmic, round, well-defined inclusions (Luxol fast blue-H&E stain).

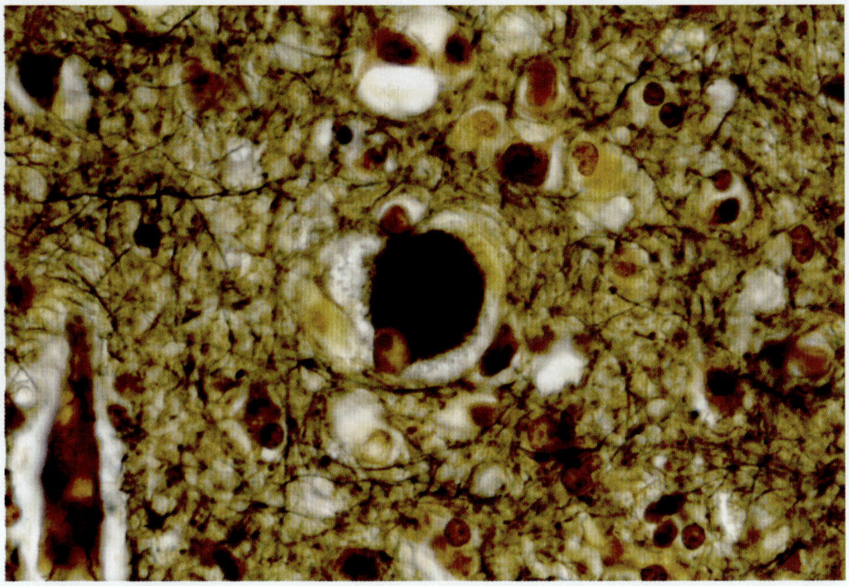

Figure 10-42

PICK DISEASE

Pick bodies are well demonstrated with silver methods (Bielschowsky silver impregnation).

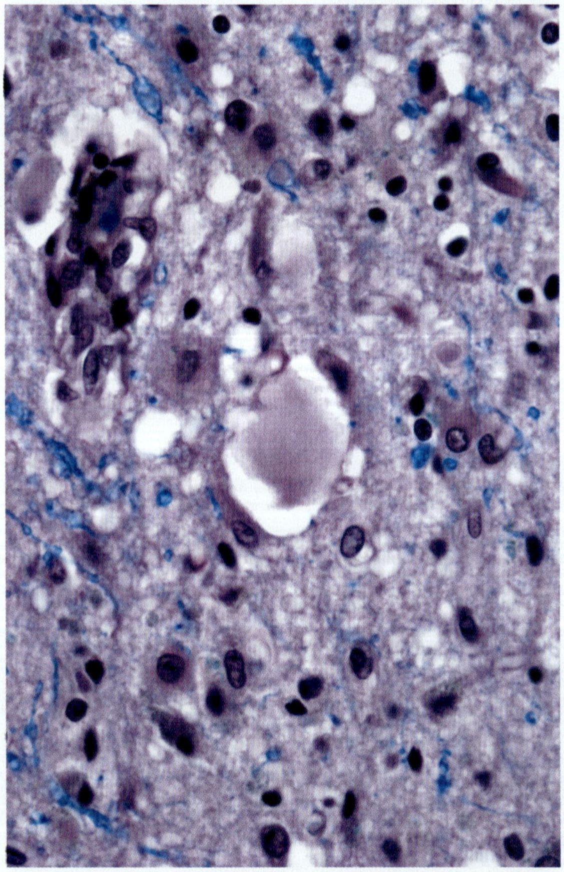

Figure 10-43

PICK DISEASE

The swollen neurons are termed Pick cells (Luxol fast blue-H&E stain).

Bielschowsky) silver methods (fig. 10-42), as well as with immunohistochemical methods. The swollen neurons, often termed "Pick cells," may be more abundant than the Pick bodies (fig. 10-43). Often associated with these inclusions is severe spongiform change of the cortex (figs. 10-44, 10-45).

Movement Disorders. The two disorders under consideration here, PSP and CBD, may be difficult to distinguish even when numerous brain areas are available, such as at autopsy evaluation. The burden of neuronal tau pathology in the cerebral cortex is relatively mild in these diseases; in fact, it is the distribution of neuronal tangles in deep gray and brain stem structures that contributes in large part to the distinctions between these entities. Between them, CBD typically carries a greater level of tau pathology in the cortex (69), and is thus more likely to be recognized by a surgical pathologist. It is nonetheless possible to identify several other aspects of these diseases that allow a pathologist to suggest one over the other. Although only recently recognized as being present, it is the abundance and patterns of glial pathology that may provide a clue (70–74). Oligodendroglial inclusions in the form of coiled bodies may be found in both disorders, although they are often more abundant in CBD (fig. 10-46).

The better discriminating form of pathology is associated with astrocytes. In PSP, the pathology takes the form of a "tufted astrocyte" in

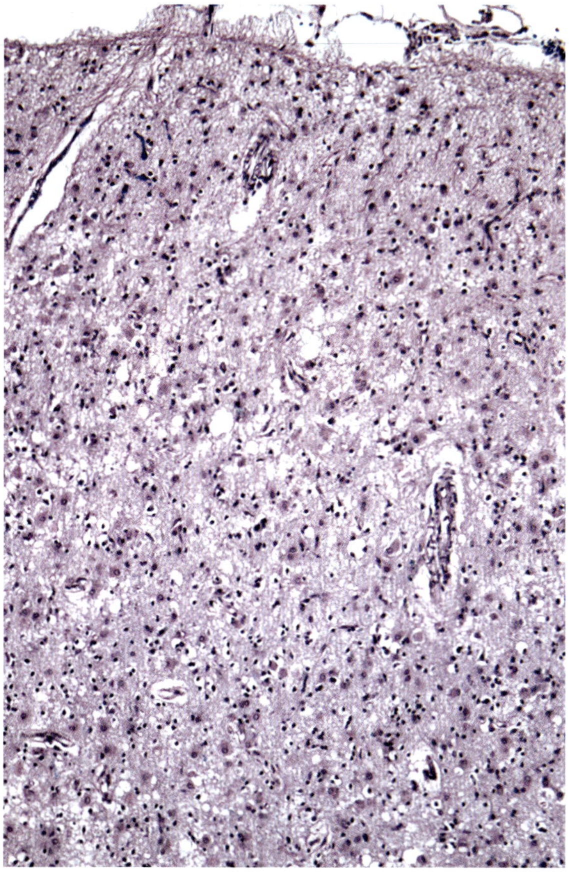

Figure 10-44

PICK DISEASE

Severe spongiosus of the cerebral cortex accompanies the disease.

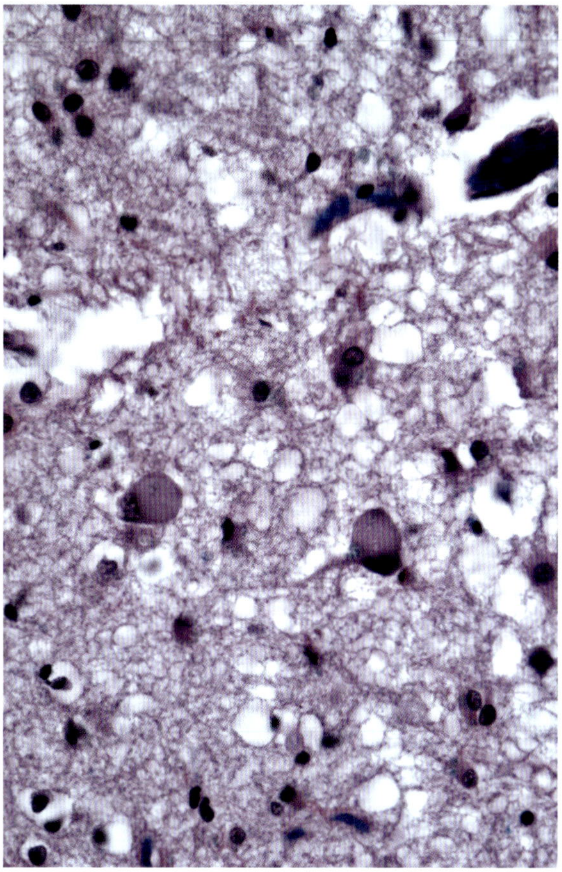

Figure 10-45

PICK DISEASE

The combination of Pick bodies and spongiosus is the hallmark of severe cases.

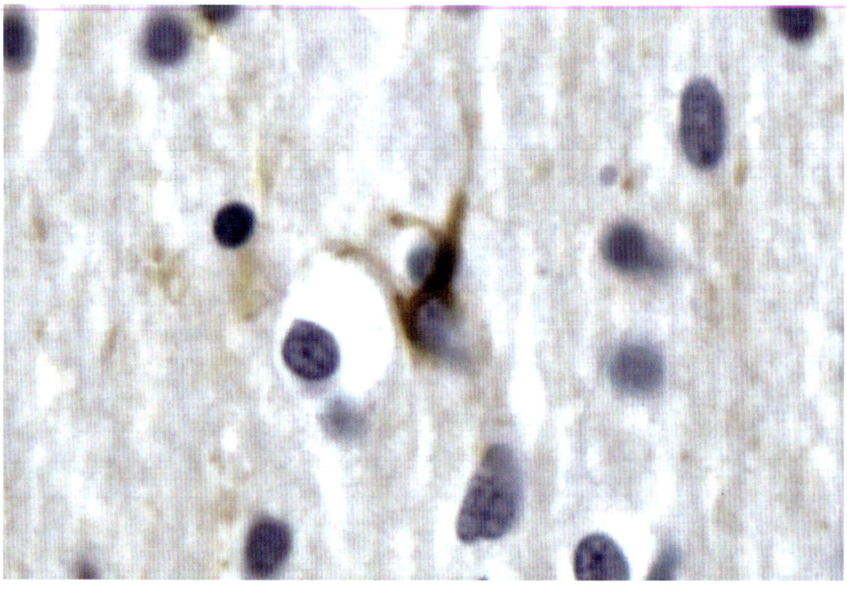

Figure 10-46

CORTICOBASAL DEGENERATION

Coiled bodies are tau-containing inclusions in oligodendrocytes.

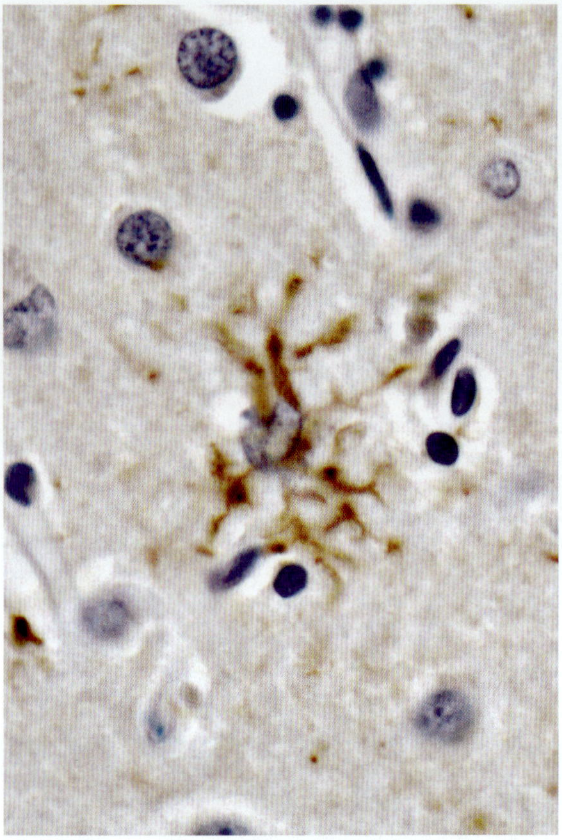

Figure 10-47

PROGRESSIVE SUPRANUCLEAR PALSY

Tufted astrocytes have processes filled with tau.

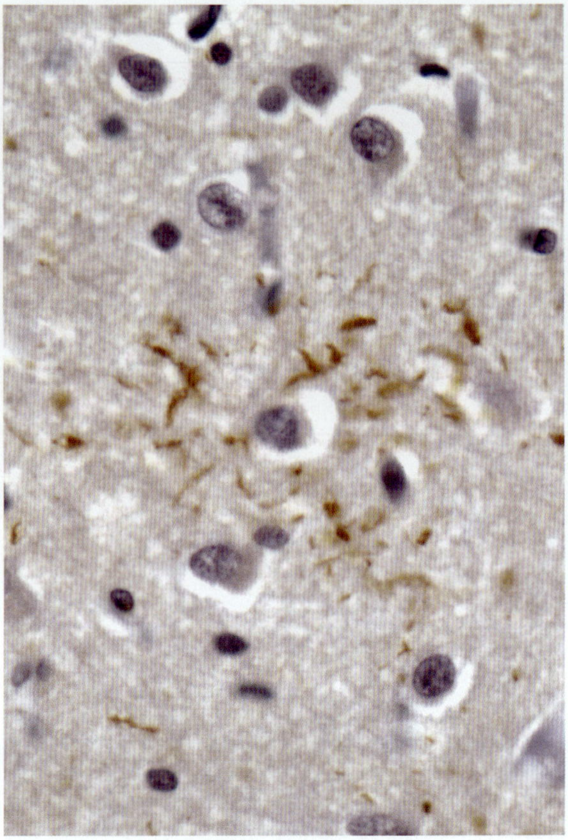

Figure 10-48

CORTICOBASAL DEGENERATION

Astrocytic plaques are highlighted by immunohistochemistry for tau, with multiple cells contributing processes to the lesion.

which many processes of a single astrocyte stain for tau, giving rise to a glial nucleus surrounded by small tufts of immunoreactivity (fig. 10-47). In contrast, CBD tends to show "astrocytic plaques" in which the immunoreactivity is found in small astrocytic processes from many cells all projecting toward a central point (fig. 10-48).

Immunohistochemical Findings. All of the inclusions that define these diseases contain tau protein. As considered above, the pathologic forms of tau are often hyperphosphorylated at many of the potential sites for post-translational modification. Many of the commercially available antibodies directed against tau do not discriminate between these diseases. Antibodies specific for tau phosphorylated at residue Ser262 typically do not recognize the lesions of Pick disease. Similarly, the antibody Alz50, which recognizes conformationally defined epitopes on tau inclusions in AD, can be useful because it recognizes fewer of the tangles found in these other diseases.

Apart from studies based on tau, other immunohistochemical methods may differentiate these diseases. In particular, the balloon neurons that are often part of the histologic phenotype of CBD may be highlighted by staining for phosphorylated neurofilaments or for αB-crystallin (figs. 10-49, 10-50).

Laboratory and Molecular Findings. Although important for research investigations, none of the molecular studies of tau protein or genetic studies of the corresponding gene (*MAPT*) plays a role in diagnostic evaluation of brain biopsies. Nonetheless, frozen tissue acquired at the time of a biopsy may be useful for these studies. In general, those cases of

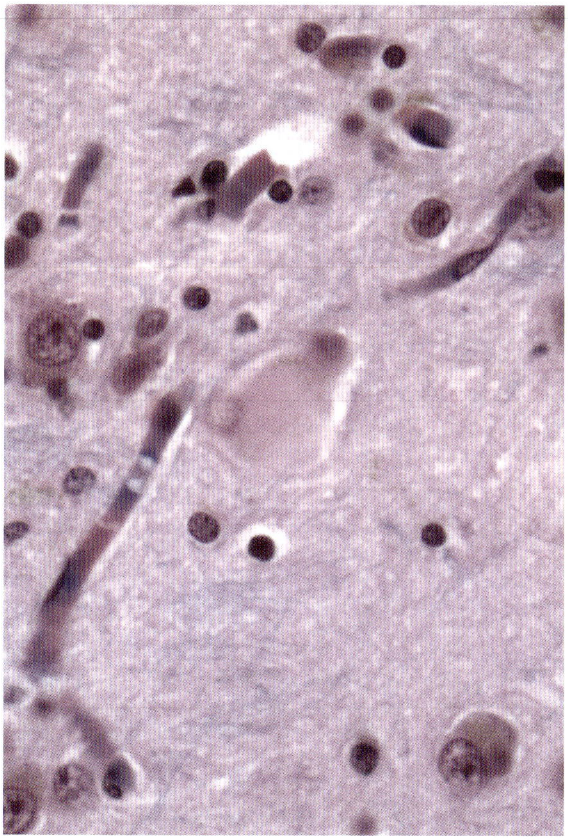

Figure 10-49

CORTICOBASAL DEGENERATION

Ballooned neurons are seen in the cortex (Luxol fast blue-H&E stain).

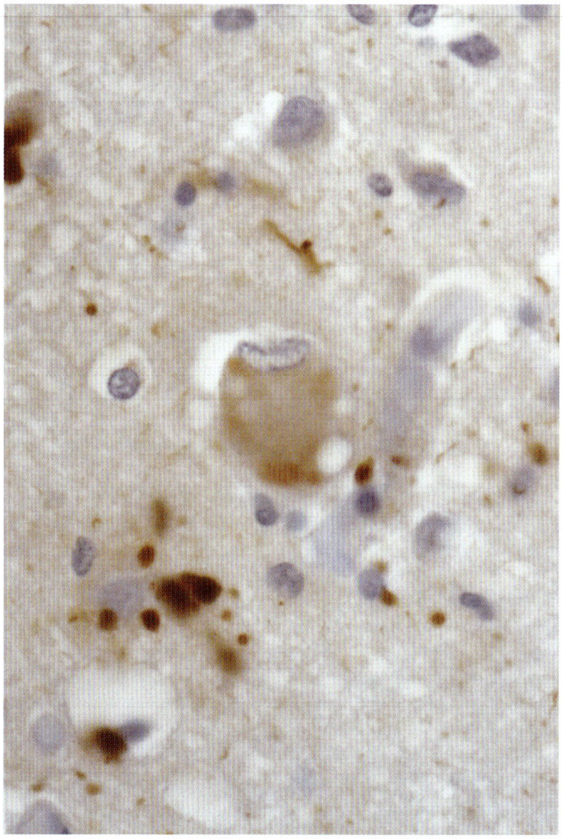

Figure 10-50

CORTICOBASAL DEGENERATION

Detection of ballooned neurons is facilitated by immunohistochemistry for αB-crystallin.

frontotemporal dementia with a strong family history or early age of onset are more likely to be associated with mutations in the gene encoding tau. While many of these mutations are associated with alterations that affect the splicing of one of the microtubule-binding domains (exon 10), the existence of point mutations associated with comparable phenotypes requires that extensive sequencing be performed in order to exclude the possibility of a familial form of the disease (75,76). Western blotting for tau isoforms is performed after appropriate extractions designed to solubilize, at least in part, the tau protein associated with tangles or other inclusions. While most tauopathies are characterized by the presence of both 3R- and 4R-containing isoforms of tau in the inclusions, Pick bodies have the distinction of being associated with primarily 3R tau (77).

Differential Diagnosis. As mentioned above, none of these forms of tauopathy can be diagnosed solely on a sample obtained at brain biopsy. What is more important for the pathologist examining a specimen is to recognize the presence of the pathology, partially characterize it, and attempt to place it in clinical context. The discrimination between these various forms of tau requires additional clinical investigations and diagnosis is likely confirmed only at the time of eventual autopsy. When evaluating a biopsy in which tau pathology has been noted, it remains essential to ensure that, for the sample available, there is no evidence of AD through rigorous exclusion of the presence of any form of amyloid deposits. The possibility of coincident diseases remains a potential point of confusion for the pathologist as well as for others involved in the patient's care.

Treatment and Prognosis. As with the majority of the neurodegenerative diseases, there is currently no significant disease-modifying therapy. These are all progressive disorders in which the symptoms increase in severity over time, with a relentless course, often over several years, before reaching an endpoint of severe disability and death. Recognition of tau pathology in the context of a strong family history of a neurodegenerative disease, on the other hand, would suggest a role for clinical genetic consultation in the care of the patient and extended family.

Argyrophilic Grain Disease

Definition. *Argyrophilic grain disease* (AGD) is a pathologic process, often diagnosed in demented individuals at autopsy, that is characterized by numerous, small silver-positive deposits in the neuropil, typically in the entorhinal cortex and other anterior medial temporal lobe structures (78–84).

General Comments. AGD was originally described in the context of demented subjects who were felt to lack evidence of another disease process, and the deposition of the silver-positive grains was believed to be the substrate for the dementia. There remains some ambiguity as to whether the pathologic findings of AGD have a well-defined clinical correlate. More recent studies have begun to emphasize the behavioral aspects of the clinical presentation. Structurally, the lesions seen in AGD are comprised of more 4R than 3R tau, and the pathologic abnormalities are found more often in the context of PSP and CBD than AD.

Clinical Features. As mentioned above, AGD was first considered to be a dementing illness because it was described in the context of a series of subjects who had been given a clinical diagnosis of probable AD. With increasing awareness of the entity, retrospective clinicopathologic studies have suggested that personality changes, problems in impulse or behavioral control, or lability may precede memory disturbances (85). AGD may also be observed in the brain of an individual without evidence of neurologic dysfunction (79,83). In fact, in some series of unselected autopsies, the incidence of the pathology is comparable to that observed in dementia brain banks (79).

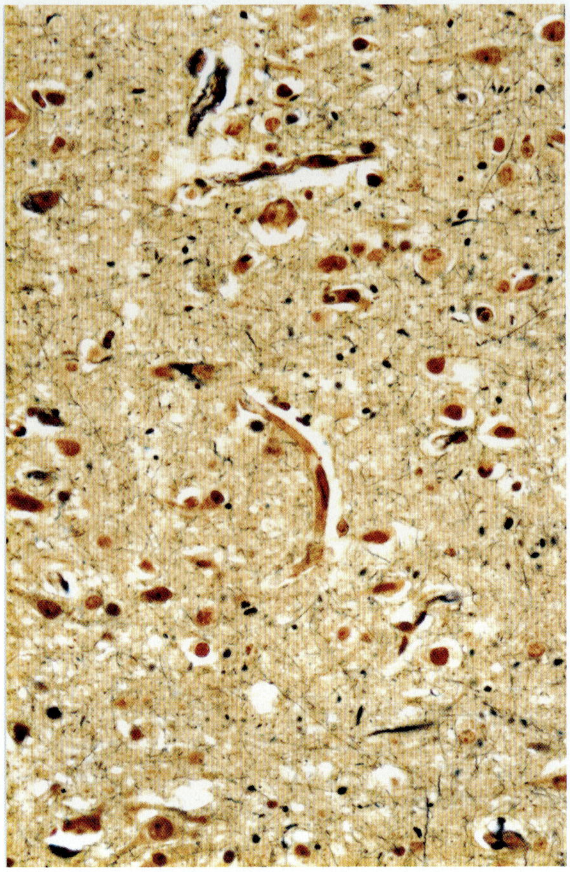

Figure 10-51

ARGYROPHILIC GRAIN DISEASE

The silver-positive small inclusions are scattered throughout the neuropil (Bielschowsky silver impregnation).

Microscopic Findings. As the name suggests, the stereotypic inclusions of AGD are highlighted with appropriate silver impregnation techniques, most optimally Gallayas, but also Bielschowsky methods. Small, comma-shaped, silver-positive grains or inclusions are present in the more superficial layers of the entorhinal cortex (fig. 10-51).

Immunohistochemical Findings. The silver-positive abnormalities that give rise to the name AGD are comprised of tau, but not all tau-immunoreactive neuropil granules are truly part of AGD. As with the inclusions of other forms of tauopathy, the grains contain hyperphosphorylated tau (fig. 10-52). There is a predominance of 4R tau over 3R, a feature that is shared with PSP and CBD (80).

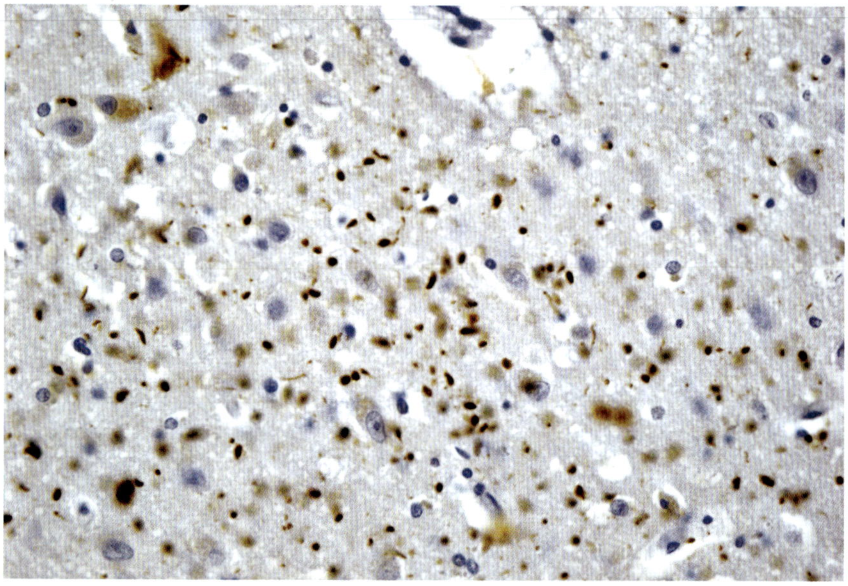

Figure 10-52

ARGYROPHILIC GRAIN DISEASE

Many of the silver-positive grains also contain tau (immunohistochemistry for tau).

Differential Diagnosis. The presence, in the correct anatomic location, of silver-positive deposits in the neuropil of the anterior temporal lobe is a defining feature of AGD (83). Unlike many of the other diseases considered in this chapter, there is no need for clinical correlation to render the diagnosis.

Treatment and Prognosis. No treatment is known for AGD. Given the uncertainty as to the clinical correlates of the pathologic findings, it is not even possible to make useful predictive statements regarding the clinical course, particularly given that it can be difficult to judge the current clinical condition based on the presence of the pathologic findings.

OTHER INCLUSION BODY DISEASES

It is clear from the ever-expanding neuropathology literature that a wide variety of other proteins may accumulate in neurons—most commonly because of rare mutations, and associated with the formation of inclusion bodies—and be associated with neurodegenerative disease (86). One pattern of pathology involves the presence of ubiquitin-positive inclusions which are negative for tau and associated with frontotemporal dementia (87). These inclusions can be observed in the setting of motor neuron disease (amyotrophic lateral sclerosis [ALS]) or in the absence of clinical and pathologic evidence of ALS. In many of these situations, the inclusions also contain TDP-43, a DNA binding protein that normally shows diffuse nuclear staining (88,89). While most of these inclusions occur in the cytoplasm of neurons, the presence of intranuclear inclusions suggests the presence of mutations either in the gene for progranulin (90,91) or in valosin-containing protein (92–94).

There remain forms of frontotemporal degeneration in which the inclusions are positive only for ubiquitin, among the standard battery of stains. Such cases often require detailed clinicopathologic correlations, extensive neuroanatomic mapping of abnormalities, and biochemical analyses. Among the proteins that have been found in such disease inclusions are neuroserpin (95–97), the intermediate-size subunit of neurofilament (98–101), and others that remain to be determined (102,103).

PRION DISEASES

Definition. *Prion diseases* are disorders associated with rapidly progressive dementia, spongiform change in the brain, and a unique underlying disease mechanism (104–108). The most common of these diseases is *Creutzfeldt-Jakob disease* (CJD), which can exist in sporadic (sCJD), familial (fCJD), and iatrogenic (iCJD) forms. Recently, a new variant form of the disease (vCJD) has emerged (109) that is associated with a related disorder in cattle (bovine spongiform encephalopathy). Other diseases of humans in this category include *fatal familial insomnia*

(FFI) (110–115), *fatal sporadic insomnia* (FSI), (114,116–118), *Gerstmann-Straussler-Scheinker syndrome* (GSS), a specific type of fCJD with a distinct clinical presentation) (119–122), and *kuru*, seen in the past among the Fore people of New Guinea (123,124).

Because of the currently untreatable nature of prion diseases, as well as the relentless natural history of these disorders, biopsy is primarily indicated when the differential diagnosis includes other, potentially treatable, entities. Because of the unusual requirements for instrument decontamination, a previously unsuspected diagnosis (or even potential diagnosis) of prion disease mandates rapid interaction with other clinical services caring for the patient as well as with institutional infection control staff (125).

General Comments. Prion diseases have a unique set of pathogenetic mechanisms, which underlie the different modes of transmission and have implications for biosafety and tissue handling (104). Current understanding of the diseases emphasizes the central role of the prion protein (PrP), a normal cellular protein encoded by the *PRNP* gene. Conformational alteration of PrP from its normal form (PrP^{c}) to its pathologic form (PrP^{res} or PrP^{sc} or PrP^{CJD} [named alternatively for the property of relative proteinase K resistance, the disease of sheep known as scrapie, or CJD]; the term PrP^{sc} will be used here) is associated with the development of disease. This conformational change is associated with a series of structural alterations in the protein: loss of α-helical domains and appearance of β-sheet conformation, propensity to aggregate and form fibrils, and acquisition of relative resistance to proteinase K. The familial forms of prion disease are linked to various mutations in the *PRNP* gene, and are presumed to accelerate this conformational change.

While prion diseases of animals, in particular, scrapie in sheep, have been known for many years, the appearance of a new disease in cattle (bovine spongiform encephalopathy [BSE]) in the 1980s lead to a great awareness of these diseases. As a result of the surveillance programs put in place in response to the appearance of BSE, the development of a new prion disease in humans (vCJD) was recognized in the mid-1990s (109). These diseases have had significant public health and economic implications.

An alternative name for prion disease is *transmissible spongiform encephalopathy*, a term that highlights the spongiform nature of the neuropathologic findings as well as the transmissible nature of the diseases. Transmission, as first demonstrated for kuru and then for CJD, can be done using brain extracts. The active infectious component required for transmission is the altered form of PrP, probably in the form of aggregates. This property played an important role in the development of our scientific understanding of prion disease biology, and continues to be important for iatrogenic forms of the disease as well as vCJD.

Given the capacity of the abnormal protein to transmit the disease, prion diseases must be considered as a type of infectious disease. Unlike other pathogens, for which fixation by normal methods eliminates infectivity, PrP^{sc} is resistant to inactivation by formalin fixation (126). Similarly, standard autoclaving does not eliminate infectivity. For these reasons, an understanding of the methods required to inactivate this infectivity is required for safe specimen handling and to minimize personnel exposure.

Because of the current public health concerns regarding vCJD, a series of prion disease pathology surveillance centers have been developed under the aegis of appropriate governmental institutions. Many of the specialized studies that contribute to the diagnosis of prion diseases are most appropriately performed in these laboratories. This is particularly true of those that require the handling of tissue that has not been treated with formic acid in order to inactivate the infectious agents.

Clinical and Radiologic Findings. *CJD.* CJD has an overall incidence of approximately 1 case/million population and is most characteristically a disease of individuals in the seventh and eighth decades of life. The most typical clinical presentation of CJD is rapidly progressive dementia, with clear deterioration over the course of months. The time course from presentation to death, which is usually preceded by deterioration to the point of unresponsiveness, is less than a year for nearly all patients. It is the pace of this decline that sets the clinical presentation of CJD apart from other neurodegenerative diseases such as AD. In cases of CJD, the neurologic examination may progress almost on a daily basis, and this relentless and rapid accumulation of deficits often allows for a diagnosis to be rendered with a high level of confidence. In addition to the cognitive impairment, other common neurologic deficits that accompany the progression of CJD include myoclonus, visual abnormalities, cerebellar dysfunction (typically manifest as ataxia), extrapyramidal dysfunction, and akinetic mutism.

Several laboratory studies can increase the probability of a clinical diagnosis of CJD. Measurement of CSF levels of the chaperone protein 14-3-3 has a role in the diagnosis of prion disorders, although a negative result does not exclude the disease (127–130). While neuroimaging studies have a primary role in the exclusion of other potential causes for rapid impairment of cognition, there is recent evidence that diffusion-weighted (DWI) MRI can be helpful in the diagnosis of CJD (fig. 10-53) (131,132). While not present in all cases of CJD, periodic synchronized sharp waves on electroencephalogram (EEG), often triphasic, are considered to be highly specific for the disease. The combination of imaging studies, 14-3-3 levels, and EEG findings have a high degree of diagnostic specificity and sensitivity, although serial measurements may be required.

When considering the possibility of CJD, issues such as family history (relevant for fCJD) need to be assessed. Similarly, the best established risk factor for iCJD is exposure to pituitary hormone therapy in the pre-recombinant protein era (133). Other documented forms of iCJD have been associated with neurosurgical instruments and some types of dural grafts.

vCJD. Unlike the presentation of other forms of CJD, vCJD is usually a disease of younger individuals, with a peak in the mid-20s (109,133–135). Several additional features serve to distinguish vCJD on clinical grounds: prominent psychiatric symptoms that are present from onset and may precede neurologic deficits by 6 months and complaints of pain or painful dyesthesias. These are eventually joined by dementia and ataxia. The overall clinical course is somewhat slower than for other forms of CJD. The EEG changes that characterize CJD are not found in this form of the disease. There is, however, a characteristic bilateral bright signal on fluid-attenuated inverse recovery (FLAIR) imaging in the posterior thalamus (136).

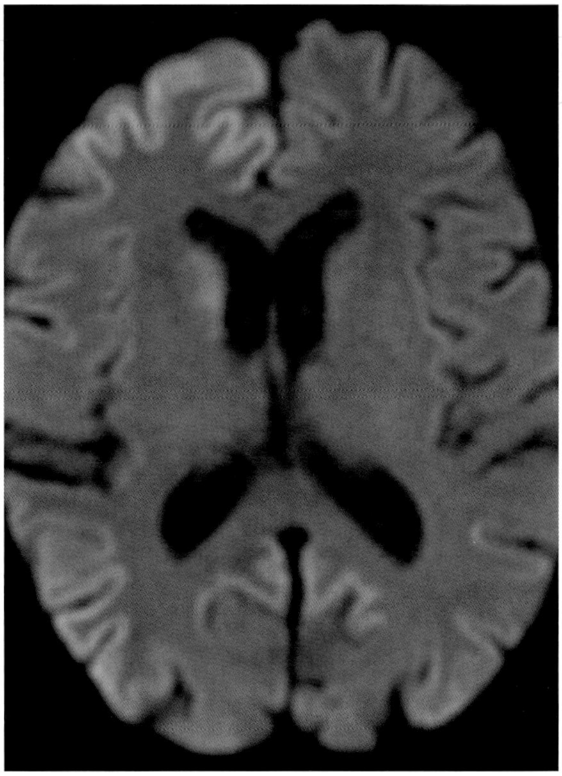

Figure 10-53

PRION DISEASE

Diffusion-weighted magnetic resonance imaging (MRI) shows abnormalities in the cerebral cortex as well as in the caudate.

While exposure to BSE is currently considered to be the major risk factor for vCJD, a few cases of vCJD developed in individuals who received blood transfusions from a donor who went on to develop vCJD (137). The actuarial implications of this potential route of transmission are difficult to assess; however, the consequences for blood donor exclusion rules have been significant (138).

Given these characteristic clinical and additional diagnostic findings, there is a relatively small role for biopsy in the diagnosis of prion diseases. Most biopsies that yield positive evidence of prion disease, either morphologic or biochemical, are performed with some suspicion of the disease as part of the preoperative differential diagnosis. The most common settings in which biopsies are performed are during the early stages of the disease (before the full flavor of the disease has become evident) and in cases where the disease does not follow the stereotypical pattern. This is most common when the tempo is slower than otherwise expected for CJD. In these settings, the biopsies are indicated to exclude other diseases, but are done with attention to the possibility of CJD. There are occasions, however, when the differential diagnosis may not include prion diseases, but is rather focused on diagnostic possibilities such as vasculitis or more typical forms of encephalitis. When the diagnosis of prion disease is suggested from a biopsy, it is incumbent upon the pathologist to contact clinical services rapidly in order to allow for appropriate infection control measures to be taken with regard to neurosurgical instruments (125).

With the demonstration that the lymphoid tissues (including tonsils) accumulate pathologic forms of PrP in vCJD, sampling of this material can provide a diagnosis without need to resort to brain biopsy (139–144). This approach, however, is not fruitful for other forms of prion disease, and it has been pointed out that sampling tissue other than the brain precludes detection of mimics of vCJD (145).

Gross Findings. Biopsies for prion disease are performed as either needle biopsies with stereotactic guidance or as small open cortical biopsies. There are no specific alterations in the gross appearance of the brain tissue. In situations of longstanding disease, there may be significant gliosis, leading to thinning of the cortical ribbon, a subtle yellow discoloration, and slightly firmer than normal consistency, although these changes are unlikely to be appreciated in a core biopsy.

Intraoperative Diagnosis. Given the potentially infectious nature of the tissue in prion diseases as well as the requirements for adequate inactivation and cleaning (see below), there is no role for frozen section or smear preparation in diagnosis. If the preoperative clinical differential diagnosis includes forms of prion disease, it is contraindicated to perform either of these types of evaluation.

There may be situations in which the possibility of prion disease does not constitute part of the preoperative differential diagnosis and frozen sections are performed. When this happens, the diagnostic feature of the diseases, the presence of spongiform change in gray matter, is not recognizable on frozen sections. The only likely finding will be gliosis. There is no inflammatory infiltrate associated with prion diseases, either in the parenchyma or around blood vessels.

It is important, however, for the pathologist to evaluate the biopsy specimen at the time of surgery in order to make tissue allocation decisions. Given the role of Western blotting for diagnosis confirmation and classification, tissue should be frozen unless there are severe limitations on the available material (146). This is particularly true in the early stages of the disease, when the histologic changes may be more subtle and focal yet biochemical measures reveal the disease.

Most laboratories that perform the specialized diagnostic Western blotting for detection of prion diseases request 0.5 g of tissue as a diagnostic sample, although as little tissue as a single stereotactic core biopsy can be used if that is all that is available. This material should be frozen at -70°C, if possible.

Special consideration must be given to the method of fixation prior to processing. Tissue for standard processing should first be fixed in 10 percent buffered formalin for 24 hours; if a large specimen has been received, it should be cut to yield slabs of 3 mm or less. Once initial fixation has occurred, the tissue should be treated with formic acid for 1 hour (126). This is then followed by an additional 24 hours of formalin fixation prior to processing. These steps require a delay relative to standard brain biopsy turn-around time, which should be understood and anticipated by the physicians involved in the patient's care.

Microscopic Findings. *CJD.* The most striking and specific pathologic finding in the various forms of CJD (including sCJD, fCJD, and iCJD) is spongiform change. Spongiform change is typically patchy, involving some gyri while sparing adjacent ones, especially in the early stages of the disease (fig. 10-54). Even in advanced cases at the time of autopsy, it is common to find uninvolved regions of cerebral cortex in close proximity to heavily spongiform regions. This uneven nature of the abnormality can result in histologically equivocal biopsies. The spongiform pathology is characterized by the presence in the gray matter of small bubbles that give a partially transparent appearance to the neuropil (figs. 10-55, 10-56). This process begins as vacuoles within neurons,

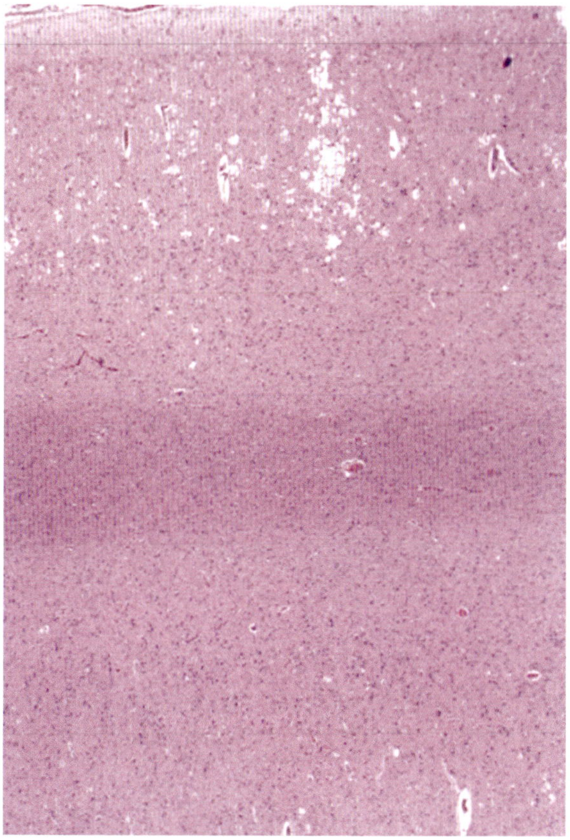

Figure 10-54

PRION DISEASE

The patchy distribution of spongiform change can result in failure to detect the histologic abnormalities in a small biopsy.

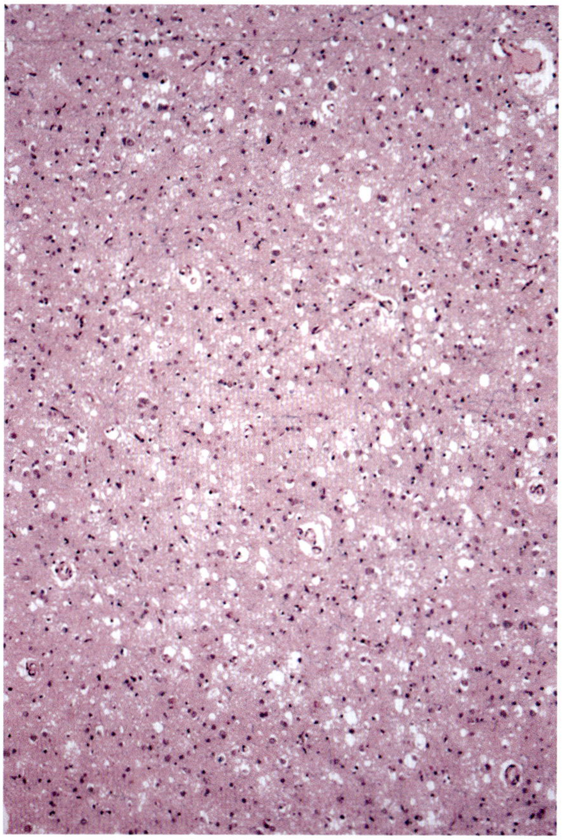

Figure 10-55

PRION DISEASE

Spongiform changes are often most evident in the deeper layers of cortex (Luxol fast blue-H&E stain).

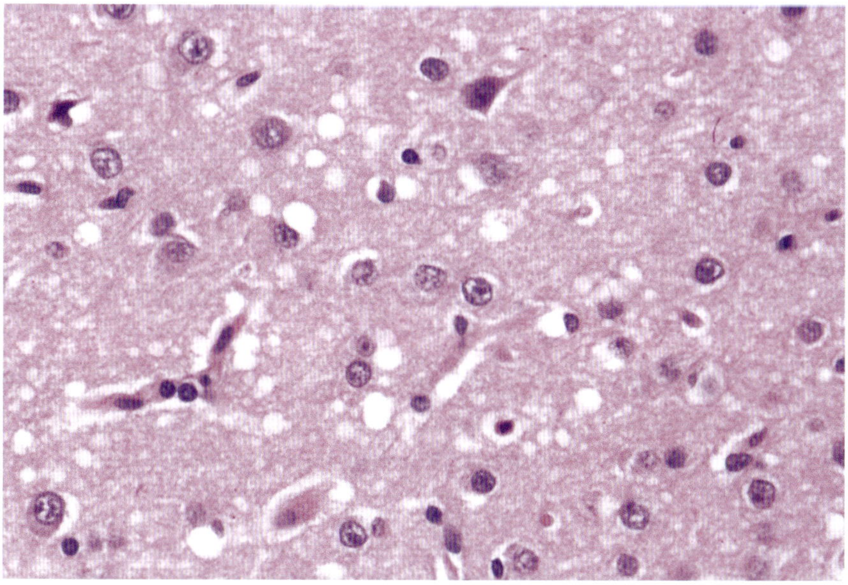

Figure 10-56

PRION DISEASE

Abundant vacuoles form the primary histologic hallmark of the disease.

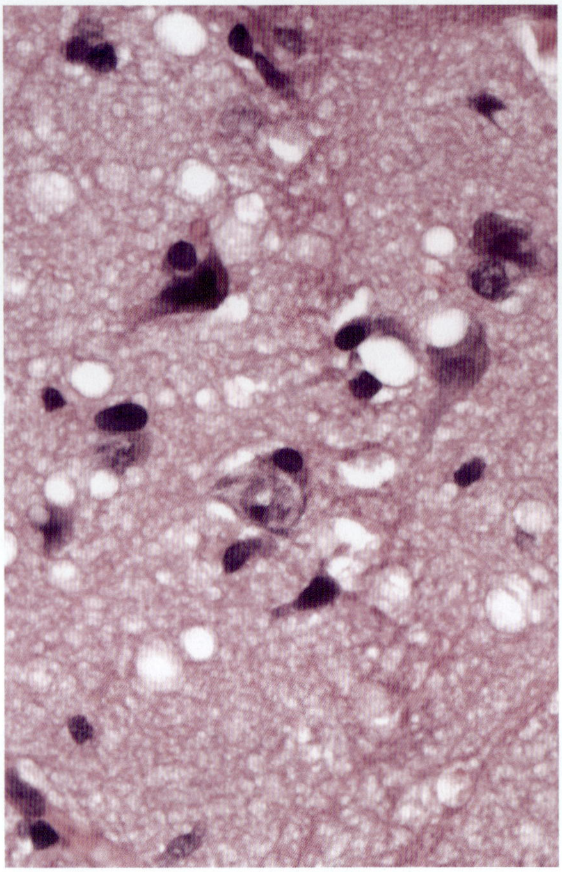

Figure 10-57

PRION DISEASE

Vacuoles can sometimes intrude on the nucleus of a neuron.

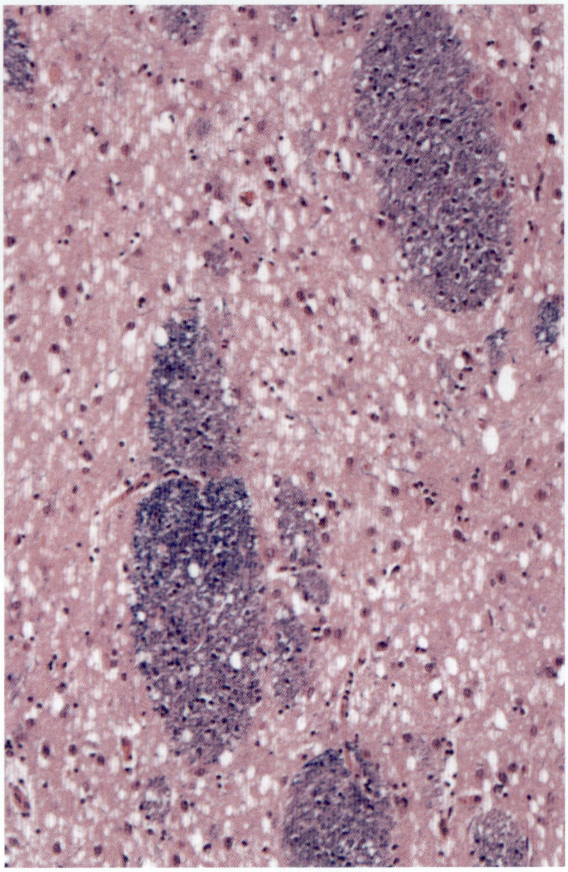

Figure 10-58

PRION DISEASE

When the striatum is involved, the changes are more diffuse than in the cortex (Luxol fast blue-H&E stain).

both in the cell body and in dendrites, and it is occasionally possible to identify vacuoles that impinge on the nucleus of neurons (fig. 10-57). If spongiform change is present in the striatum, the involvement is more homogeneous yet spares the white matter (fig. 10-58).

Within the cerebral cortex, spongiform change often occurs more toward the deeper layers, in contrast to the superficial spongiosus found in Lewy body disease or with aging. Associated with this change in the deeper cortical layers, there is usually gliosis at the gray-white junction, sometimes even in advance of the spongiform pathology. As the disease progresses, significant neuronal loss becomes evident. Even in the absence of spongiform change by standard light microscopy, biopsies can be diagnostic through the application of immunohistochemical or biochemical methods (see below). When examining a biopsy, it is advantageous to determine the specificity of the spongiform process for gray matter by comparison with the white matter in the specimen. This can be particularly helpful with biopsies of the striatum, where the penetrating bundles of myelinated fibers are surrounded by gray matter (fig. 10-59).

In a minority of cases of CJD, particularly in some familial forms, plaques of PrP^{sc} are deposited in the brain, typically in the cerebellar cortex (fig. 10-60), but occasionally in the cerebral cortex (147–149). These are round deposits with fibrillar radiating spicules visible under light microscopy. These deposits, often termed "kuru plaques," can be stained by the periodic acid–Schiff (PAS) as well as methods for the detection of amyloids. They are not immunoreactive for

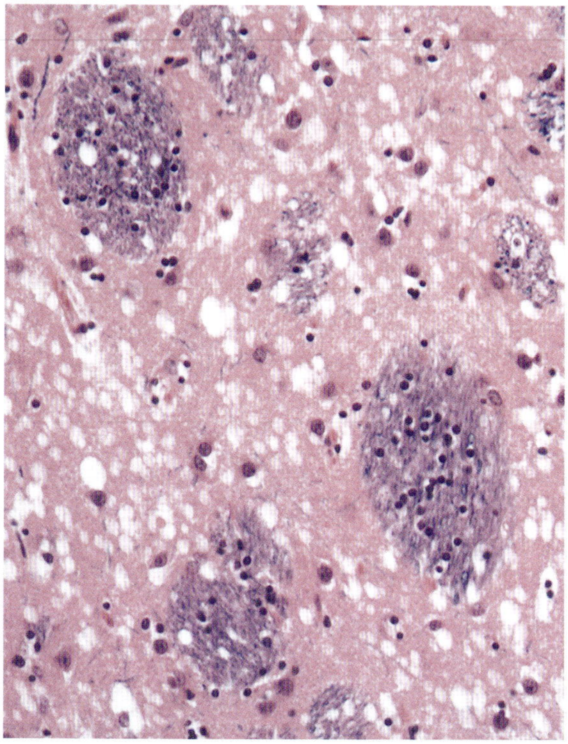

Figure 10-59

PRION DISEASE

Gray and white matter are mixed in the striatum, providing an internal control for potential processing and handling artifacts (Luxol fast blue-H&E stain).

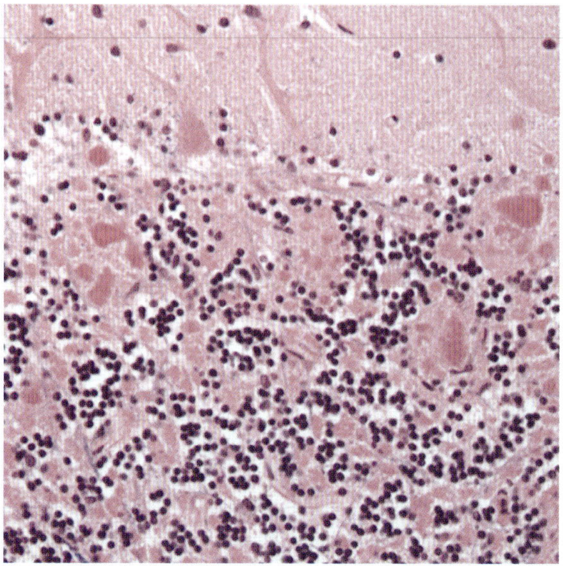

Figure 10-60

PRION DISEASE

Plaques of amyloid containing PrP^{sc} can be found in the cerebellum in some patients.

the Aβ peptide of AD and cerebral amyloid angiopathy; rather, they stain with methods for the detection of PrP^{CJD} in tissue.

vCJD. The most characteristic hallmark of vCJD is the presence of extensive numbers of cortical and cerebellar plaques ("florid plaques") (figs. 10-61, 10-62) (134,135). The appearance of individual plaques is similar to the cerebellar kuru plaques that may be found in sCJD. They may occur in clusters and tend to be located in the deep layers of the cortex, although these features may be difficult to appreciate on limited biopsy material. While there is usually not extensive spongiform change in the cerebral cortex, it is present around the plaques, a pattern that is not prominent with kuru plaques (fig. 10-63). Spongiform change is often most evident in the striatum, while the posterior thalamus, which has a characteristic imaging abnormality that can contribute to the diagnosis, commonly shows neuronal loss and gliosis.

Immunohistochemical Findings. To perform immunohistochemical staining for pathologic forms of PrP, it is necessary to remove the immunoreactivity of the remaining PrP^{c} in the tissue. To be able to detect all of the different patterns of PrP^{res}, a combination of hydrated autoclaving with treatment by formic acid or other agents that recover the antigenicity masked by formalin fixation has been adopted (146). Alternatively, it is possible to perform "tissue blots" with transfer of histologic sections to an appropriate carrier membrane, which allows extensive proteinase K digestion prior to immunostaining (150). This latter method is more commonly applied in research settings, primarily because it uses approaches that are not part of the standard repertoire of diagnostic laboratories. For either of these approaches, given that they fall outside of the methods used in the immunohistochemical evaluation of other types of pathology specimens, central reference laboratories are used.

Several distinct patterns of immunoreactivity for PrP^{sc} have been described, and these can generally be found in combinations in a given case at autopsy; in the limited tissue of a brain biopsy, however, a single pattern typically

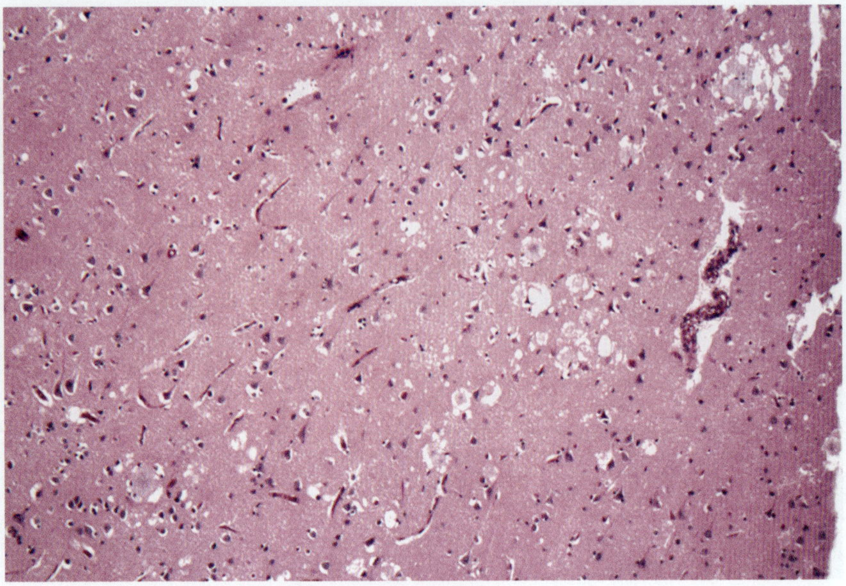

Figure 10-61

VARIANT CREUTZFELDT-JAKOB DISEASE

The cerebral cortex contains foci of spongiform change, often surrounding plaques.

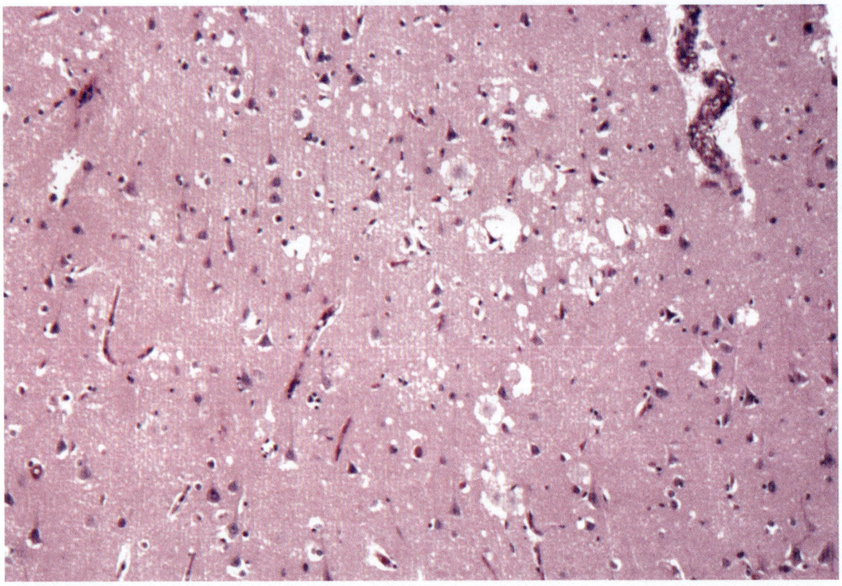

Figure 10-62

VARIANT CREUTZFELDT-JAKOB DISEASE

The presence of numerous plaques in the cerebral cortex is one of the hallmarks of this disorder.

dominates (146). The most commonly observed pattern is "synaptic," with diffuse punctuate granular staining filling regions of neuropil. While evident in the cerebral cortex, it may be more prominent in the cerebellum, where it highlights the synaptic complexes in the granular cell layer (fig. 10-64).

The other patterns of staining that may be observed in cases of sCJD, fCJD, and iCJD are perivacuolar, perineuronal, and plaque-like. The perivacuolar pattern is most commonly observed in the setting of severe spongiform change, as seen in very late stages of the diseases (which are only rarely biopsied). Plaque-like immunoreactive deposits do not all correspond to recognizable kuru plaques, and may be found in some cases extending into the subcortical white matter.

In keeping with the distinctive histologic findings of vCJD, there is a corresponding pattern of immunohistochemical staining that marks this form of the disease: florid plaques and staining of the plaques and the surrounding vacuoles (fig. 10-65). In only this form of the disease, PrP^{sc} immunoreactivity can be demonstrated in lymphoid tissues, including tonsil, lymph nodes, and spleen (139,141–144).

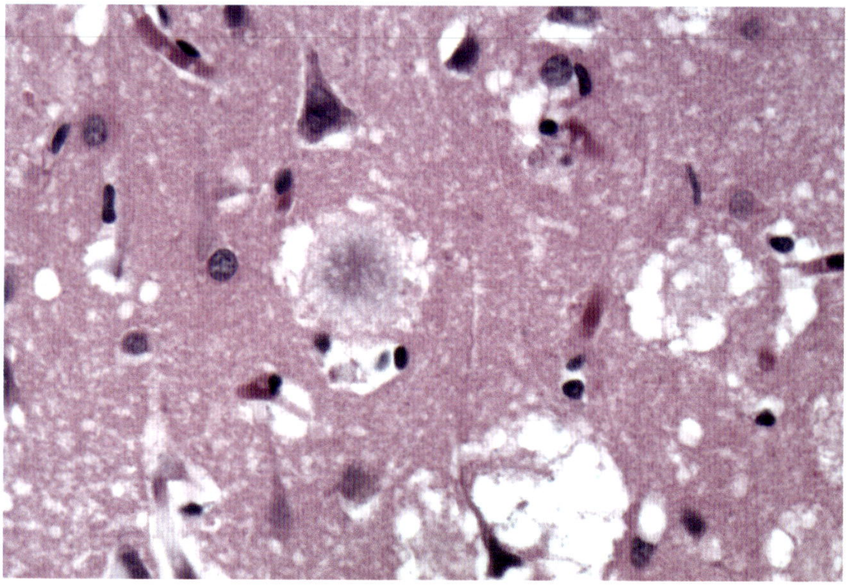

Figure 10-63

VARIANT CREUTZFELDT-JAKOB DISEASE

The plaque sits in the center of severe spongiform change. (Higher power of fig. 10-62.)

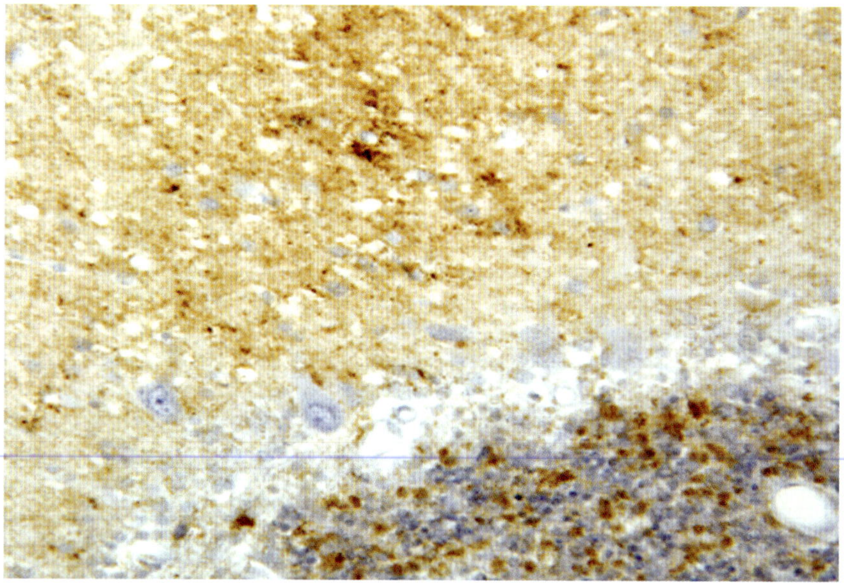

Figure 10-64

PRION DISEASE

The synaptic pattern of PrP^{sc} immunohistochemical staining.

Ultrastructural Findings. Although electron microscopy has been used in the past in attempts to understand the structural origins of the vacuoles that mark the pathologic finding in prion diseases, there is currently no role for this approach in the diagnosis of these disorders.

Laboratory and Molecular Findings. The detection of PrP^{sc} is best performed by Western blot analysis. This method is based on the relative proteinase K resistance of PrP^{sc} compared to PrP^{c}. Because of the biohazards involved in the tissue handling, these studies are most appropriately performed in centralized laboratories with developed expertise. The essential approach is to prepare a tissue homogenate from frozen unfixed tissue. This is then subjected to a partial proteinase K digestion, which eliminates the normal PrP^{c} from the homogenate while only partially cleaving the PrP^{res}. When these homogenates are then examined by Western blotting using antibodies against PrP, the resistant protein is detected.

Classification of the forms of PrP is based, in part, on the pattern of glycosylation, as the PrP protein may be modified by the addition of sugar chains at either one or two specific

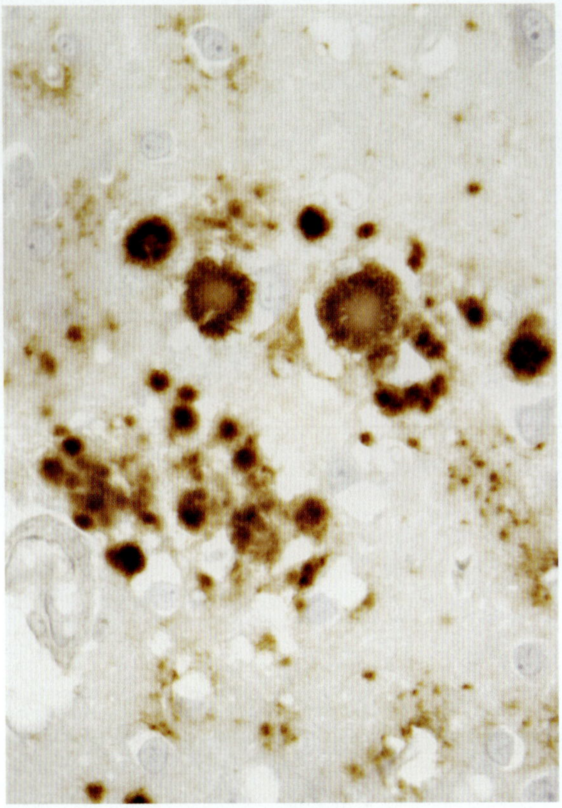

Figure 10-65

VARIANT CREUTZFELDT-JAKOB DISEASE

Immunohistochemical staining for PrP^{sc} is concentrated in the plaques and surrounding vacuolated neuropil.

amino acid residues, resulting in unglycosylated, monoglycosylated, and diglycosylated forms (104–106,146). The other major variation in the pattern of PrP^{res} is found in the length of the protein after proteinase K treatment. The type 1 pattern results in a longer protein fragment, associated with cleavage closer to the N-terminal; the type 2 pattern reflects a fragment approximately 15 amino acids shorter. These differences are highlighted on Western blotting after the combination of proteinase K digestion and enzymatic deglycosylation.

There is a role for sequencing of the *PRNP* gene in all cases of prion disease for several reasons. First, the proper classification of cases of CJD, which has clear relevance for public health and epidemiology, depends on the recognition of familial forms of the disease, especially those which were previously unsuspected. In addition to the various mutations that have been identified as causal for fCJD, there is a polymorphic site at codon 129 at which each copy of the *PRNP* gene may contain either methionine (M) or valine (V) (104–106,146). Homozygosity at codon 129 is associated with an increased risk for sporadic CJD and for pituitary hormone replacement therapy-related iCJD. Most strikingly, nearly every symptomatic case of vCJD recognized to date has occurred in an MM homozygote.

Differential Diagnosis. When evaluating a biopsy with possible spongiform change, the most critical role for the pathologist is to distinguish between true spongiform change and other causes of similar pathologic changes. The most common concern is that tissue handling and poor fixation have led to artifacts that resemble the specific spongiform changes of prion disease. True pathologic spongiform change of prion disease is best distinguished from artifact by demonstrating that the abnormality is restricted to the gray matter, it does not affect adjacent white matter, there is a mild reactive gliosis present, and some vacuoles involve neuronal cell bodies. Cerebral edema can also lead to mild spongiform change, but this is typically uniform across the thickness of the cerebral cortex rather than showing the asymmetric and uneven distribution both across the cortical thickness and along its length seen in prion diseases. Another feature of the vacuolation observed in prion diseases is the variation in the size of the vacuoles, with some extending fully through the thickness of the tissue and thus appearing empty; other vacuoles have some residual tissue visible. The most striking aspect, which is only sometimes clearly observable in biopsies, is that vacuoles are visible within the perinuclear cytoplasm of larger neurons. While the other vacuoles in neuropil are located within the neuronal processes, these somatic vacuoles may conspicuously indent the nucleus.

In general, the application of the full battery of the above-described methods may result in a positive diagnosis of prion disease with minimal ambiguity. The use of Western blotting methods to confirm the presence of proteinase K-resistant PrP in a biopsy sample, even in the absence of recognizable spongiform change, allows for an unequivocal diagnosis. If this method of molecular confirmation is not available, most commonly because CJD represents an unexpected diagnosis and no tissue was frozen at the time of surgery, then it becomes essential to combine immunohistochemical evidence of abnormal PrP with the presence of spongiform change. The use of these methods is considered appropriate, if available, if prion disease is suspected but the biopsy fails to show either spongiform change or another pathologic process.

Treatment and Prognosis. Unfortunately, no effective therapeutic interventions currently exist for these disorders. Affected individuals typically show rapid and continual progression of symptoms, eventually reaching a severely disabled state with minimal interaction with their environment and caregivers. The search for biologically active molecules that can disrupt the propagation of prions in experimental systems continues to move forward, and it is possible that such agents will enter the clinical repertoire soon.

Rendering a diagnosis of a prion disease in a member of a family with a history an autosomal dominant inherited neurodegenerative disease raises the possibility that the mutation lies in the *PRNP* gene. Such mutations can be searched for after obtaining the appropriate permissions. Consideration of screening for the detection of the mutation in family members needs to be done in collaboration with experienced genetic counselors, particularly since there are no methods to prevent disease onset or to treat it once it begins.

Biosafety Concerns. Consideration of the full complement of issues surrounding infection control and decontamination methods appropriate for prion diseases is outside the scope of this chapter and well described elsewhere (125). However, some pertinent aspects require comment: methods used in most settings for cleaning and decontamination are not adequate to eliminate infectious prions from potentially contaminated instruments and surfaces. In general, exposure to sodium hydroxide (2N) or sodium hypochlorite (bleach, at a concentration of 20,000 ppm available chlorine) for 1 hour inactivates prions. In addition to the instruments and working surfaces, solutions that were in contact with tissue (such as the formalin used for fixation steps prior to formic acid treatment) also must be appropriately handled. While formalin can be decontaminated by the use of bleach, this is a highly exothermic reaction and can result in even greater safety concerns. Fluids may also be disposed by absorption with a nonreactive material followed by incineration as hazardous material.

SUBACUTE SCLEROSING PANENCEPHALITIS

Definition. *Subacute sclerosing panencephalitis* (SSPE), which is sometimes referred to as *Dawson encephalitis* in the older literature, is a slowly progressive disorder associated with measles virus infection, and is distinct from the rapidly progressive measles encephalitis. SSPE is associated with a persistent defective measles virus infection. The slow yet relentless progression of the disease is attributed, in part, to the ability of the defective virus to elude immune clearance.

General Comments. With the introduction of widespread childhood immunization for measles, much of the burden of the disease has shifted to the developing world. It continues to be observed in other settings, however, either in immigrant populations or in individuals who may have had previously unrecognized infection by measles prior to the delivery of the vaccine. There is no association of SSPE with the viral strains used in the preparation of the vaccine. Additionally, as increasing numbers of individuals have elected not to have their children participate in recommended vaccination programs, there may be a reappearance of the disease.

Clinical Features. The development of SSPE is associated with having had a measles infection in early life, typically before the age of 2 years. There is usually a several year delay between the initial infection and the onset of symptoms of SSPE, so the disease usually begins in mid-childhood; nonetheless, cases have been observed in adults, including during pregnancy.

While several staging systems have been proposed for the clinical findings of SSPE, there are several characteristic aspects of the earlier stages of presentation, including behavioral changes with loss of skills and cognitive function. This is usually followed by the development of myoclonus and loss of motor function. With time, there is loss of cortical function with unresponsiveness, mutism, and eventual coma. The disease progresses over several years, with a mean of approximately 2 years (151,152). Patients who have more aggressive disease deteriorate in just months (153–155). EEG abnormalities are common during the course of the illness, and are most typically burst-like periodic paroxysmal discharges (156,157).

Gross Findings. When large samples of tissue are examined, the striking finding is marked gliosis in the white matter, typically associated with a slight yellowish discoloration. The white matter of individuals dying of SSPE is markedly firm or sclerotic. Because of the widespread distribution of pathology by the end stages of the illness, much of the white matter takes on this rubbery consistency.

Intraoperative Diagnosis. The inflammatory nature of the pathology of SSPE can be appreciated on frozen section, along with gliosis. Because these are the less specific components of the pathologic findings, they do not usually establish a diagnosis. When the possibility of SSPE is considered in the preoperative differential diagnosis, it is appropriate to retain some frozen tissue to be used, if necessary, as a source of RNA for reverse transcriptase-polymerase chain reaction (RT-PCR) investigations. Also, some antibodies directed against measles virus proteins for immunohistochemistry perform best with frozen tissue. Since the differential diagnosis often includes other viral encephalitides, and because there can be a potential role for electron microscopy in the evaluation of a biopsy suspicious for SSPE, tissue should be fixed for ultrastructural studies if the size of the biopsy allows.

Microscopic Findings. Inflammatory infiltrates are the primary hallmark of SSPE, with lymphocytes found in the meninges, in the brain parenchyma, and around blood vessels (fig. 10-66). The severity of the inflammation usually is inversely proportional to the duration of the illness. As this component of the pathology declines over time, there is a corresponding increase in the level of reactive gliosis (fig. 10-67). In the end stages of the illness, the gliosis predominates. Within the inflammatory infiltrates, there is a predominance of CD4-positive T cells in the perivascular component, with B cells present in the parenchyma (158).

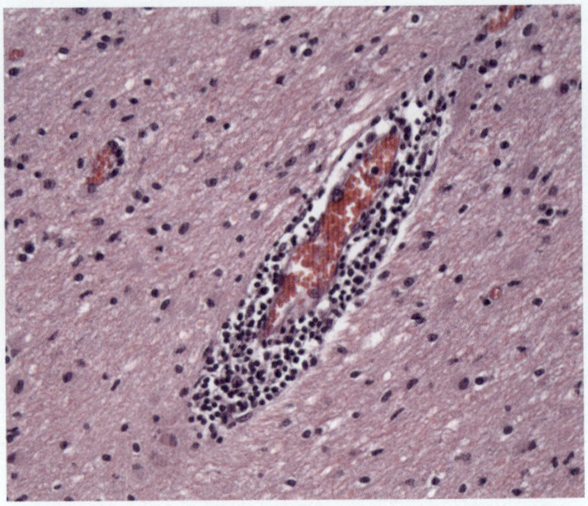

Figure 10-66

SUBACUTE SCLEROSING PANENCEPHALITIS

Inflammation, including microglial activation, can be profound.

Viral cytopathic changes may be present, although their distribution in the brain is often uneven, resulting in failure to detect them on biopsy samples. When present, they are characterized by their intranuclear location, glassy eosinophilic staining, and crisp borders (fig. 10-68). These changes often have the appearance of Cowdry type A inclusions, characterized by being single, moderate to large, intranuclear, eosinophilic accumulations surrounded by a clear halo. Evidence of neuronal death is also present; sometimes microglial nodules are found, but more often the slow tempo of the disease results in a diffuse gliosis associated with decreased numbers of neurons. In addition to neurons, oligodendrocytes may be infected by the defective measles virus, and this contributes to the white matter damage and demyelination seen with the disease (159).

Neurofibrillary tangles are sometimes present, particularly in cases of longer duration, and may be the clue that helps discriminate this diagnosis from others in which gliosis and a diffuse inflammatory cell infiltrate are present. The tangles often involve the cortical neurons and contain tau and paired helical filaments, similar to the tangles of AD. While coincident pathology might be considered, the absence of plaques and the age of the patient are normally enough to eliminate this consideration. Although there is poor correlation between viral proteins and the presence of tangles, there may be a relationship between tangles and the viral genome (160).

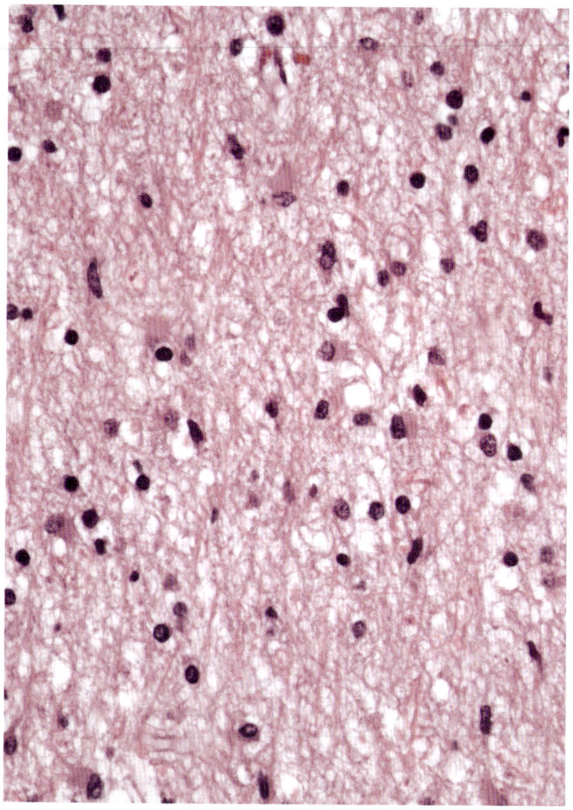

Figure 10-67

SUBACUTE SCLEROSING PANENCEPHALITIS

Marked gliosis in the white matter gives rise to the firm consistency of the brain.

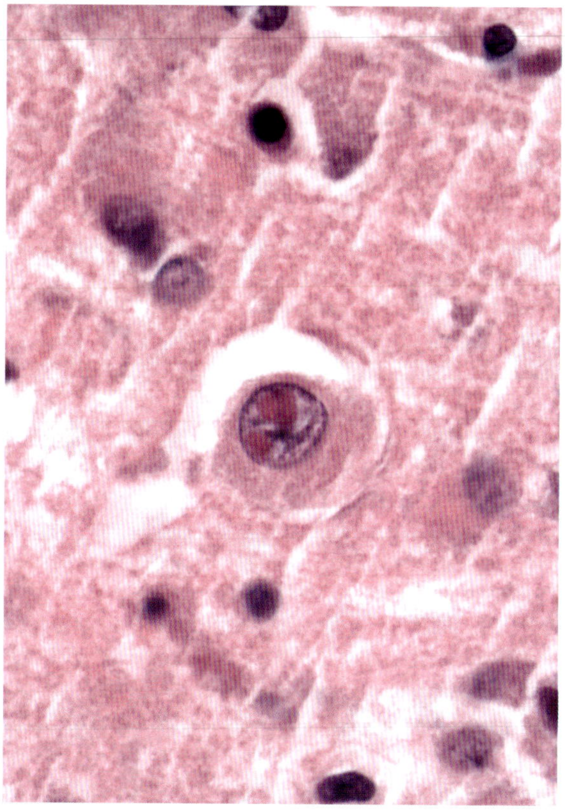

Figure 10-68

SUBACUTE SCLEROSING PANENCEPHALITIS

Neurons may show viral nuclear inclusions.

Immunohistochemical Findings. Appropriate antibodies can detect many of the components of the pathology of SSPE. The most specific of these are the antibodies directed against components of the measles virus that highlight inclusions or demonstrate the presence of viral proteins in the absence of recognizable inclusions (161). It is often possible to demonstrate the presence of measles virus in some inflammatory cells within the brain as well, a finding that has been suggested to reflect a potential route of virus across the blood brain barrier. The other major role for immunohistochemical studies in the setting of a brain biopsy from a young individual with neuronal loss, gliosis, and an inflammatory infiltrate is to identify the presence of tangles. This is most appropriately done with antibodies against tau, but can also be approached in a less specific manner using antibodies against ubiquitin.

The inflammatory cell infiltrate, the microglial reaction, and the astrocytic reaction can all be highlighted with appropriate immunohistochemical techniques. Results from such studies, however, only serve to confirm findings on routine staining, and while consistent with a diagnosis of SSPE, are not adequate to allow a definitive diagnosis.

Ultrastructural Findings. Because SSPE is a viral disease, significant efforts have been directed at the demonstration of the presence of viral particles within cells of the brain. It is sometimes possible to demonstrate the presence of viral particles within neurons and oligodendrocytes, although the yield is low (162). Given the evolving ability to confirm the presence of virus through immunologic and PCR-based methods, the role of ultrastructural studies is diminishing.

Laboratory and Molecular Findings. The identification of the histologic features of SSPE in a biopsy should trigger the examination of serum and CSF titers of antibodies directed against the measles virus, as well as other viruses as appropriate controls. Methods exist for the detection of viral RNA by in situ hybridization (161,163). In addition, RT-PCR assays may contribute to the diagnosis of SSPE, although these are more commonly used in epidemiologic studies for the evaluation of viral subtypes (164,165).

Differential Diagnosis. When viral inclusions or evidence of viral RNA or protein is observed, then the diagnosis may be established on pathologic grounds alone. While many of the findings of SSPE are nonspecific, the constellation of the generic findings of neuronal loss in the cortex and demyelination in the subcortical white matter, both associated with gliosis, microglial proliferation, and inflammatory cell infiltrates, should raise the possibility of SSPE. Usually, only the inflammatory process with evidence of cell injury is observed, and the differential diagnosis continues to include other infectious processes as well as paraneoplastic syndromes. When tangles are found in addition to the other morphologic findings, and the age of the patient and the disease tempo argue against the presence of a neurodegenerative disease, then the index of suspicion is increased. Similar pathology has been associated with other viruses on rare occasions, but whether the pathogenesis of such cases is similar to that of SSPE is not clear (166,167).

Treatment and Prognosis. To date, attempts to provide therapeutic intervention to reverse acquired deficits from SSPE have been disappointing. Interferon-alpha, either alone or in combination with antiviral agents, may stabilize patients or slow the rate of disease progression (168). In the absence of any intervention, the natural history of the disease is marked by continued deterioration leading to death. If there is a possibility of minimizing subsequent progression once intervention is begun, then there is a need for diagnosis at the early stages of the disease, perhaps with an increased role for brain biopsy.

INFLAMMATORY AND IMMUNE-MEDIATED DISEASES

The majority of inflammatory processes that involve either the brain or its supporting structures (meninges or cerebral vasculature) have distinct presentations that allow them to be separated from neurodegenerative diseases, and are therefore discussed elsewhere. A few entities, however, may enter the differential diagnosis when a patient with a possible neurodegenerative disease comes to brain biopsy. In general, these processes are characterized by a diffuse inflammatory cell infiltrate, predominantly associated with gray matter. They are often associated with disease processes elsewhere in the body, such as neoplasms, and successful treatment of neurologic symptoms may depend, in part, on the treatment of this underlying disease. Alternatively, manipulation of the immune system (either through immunosuppression or plasmapheresis) may be of some benefit.

Paraneoplastic Syndromes

Definition. *Paraneoplastic syndromes* are combinations of neurologic symptoms that are associated with the presence of a neoplasm elsewhere in the body. They represent "action at a distance," and must be distinguished from direct effects such as metastases or compression syndromes.

General Comments. There have been significant recent advances in the identification of antibodies that often recognize antigens within the nervous system and that are commonly associated with specific tumor types and with specific clinical presentations. The recognition of the well-characterized clinical syndromes such as cerebellar degeneration, opsoclonus-myoclonus, subacute sensory neuronopathy, and limbic encephalitis, coupled with the ability to screen for paraneoplastic antibodies, has drastically reduced the need for brain biopsy in nearly all cases of these diseases. This is particularly true for those syndromes such as opsoclonus-myoclonus that have no recognizable pathologic substrate. In fact, a recent consensus report on the diagnostic criteria for paraneoplastic neurologic syndromes does not include brain biopsy as part of the decision tree (169). Thus, these disease processes are most likely to be encountered by a pathologist when other entities dominate the differential diagnosis. A study based on 4 years of serum submissions to a reference laboratory (approximately 60,000 specimens) revealed a less than 1 percent yield when screening for antibodies associated with paraneoplastic syndromes (170). This study also indicated that there was a stronger correlation between antibody profile and tumor type than between either of these parameters and specific paraneoplastic syndromes.

Clinical Features. Paraneoplastic syndromes are characterized by a relatively rapid (on the order of months) progression of neurologic symptoms that are referable to the anatomic structures involved (171). Because of the time course, these disorders are usually easily distinguished from strokes and classic neurodegenerative diseases. The most common entities in the differential diagnosis are vasculitis, encephalitis, and occasionally, prion diseases. For this reason, paraneoplastic syndromes should be considered by the pathologist when biopsies are performed for these indications. In some settings, the distinction between the histologic findings of a paraneoplastic syndrome and some of these other diseases (most commonly, viral encephalitis) is difficult and it is incumbent upon the pathologist to raise the possibility of such a diagnosis to direct subsequent clinical testing.

Two major clinical presentations are considered in the scope of this chapter, one rather narrow and the other extremely broad. *Paraneoplastic cerebellar degeneration* is, within the CNS, the only commonly observed syndrome in which there is stereotypic anatomic involvement. In this form of paraneoplastic syndrome, there is Purkinje cell death and, therefore, clinical evidence of cerebellar dysfunction, typically involving a combination of ataxia, dysarthria, and nystagmus. This paraneoplastic syndrome is also most likely to precede the detection of the underlying malignancy. When the disease has had the unfortunate opportunity to progress significantly, cerebellar atrophy may be seen on structural imaging studies.

The other category of paraneoplastic syndrome that may come to biopsy, and which is considerably more pleotropic, is the *encephalomyelitides*. These are most commonly gray matter processes and, depending on the areas involved, have different clinical presentations (172,173). Several well-recognized subtypes have been described, including "limbic encephalitis," in which the brunt of pathology occurs in the medial temporal lobe structures and clinical symptoms often include progressive dementia and new onset of seizures. When a similar process involves the brain stem, combinations of cranial nerve nuclei deficits as well as changes in consciousness and alertness predominate. If there is widespread cortical involvement, the accumulated deficits in multiple cognitive arenas may lead to a differential diagnosis that includes prion disease. Often a combination of these CNS manifestations is accompanied by a similar pathologic process involving the sensory ganglia. This combination of a CNS deficit that can be localized to gray matter and a sensory neuronopathy characteristically leads to the clinical recognition of the disease as a paraneoplastic process.

Intraoperative Diagnosis. As discussed above, brain biopsies are rarely performed in order to establish a diagnosis of paraneoplastic disease. There are no specific findings on the frozen section or smear preparation that allow for a definitive diagnosis. When a biopsy comes from a patient with paraneoplastic encephalomyelitis, the characteristic histologic findings (if present at all) are likely to be scant chronic inflammation, microglial reaction, astrocytosis, and neuronal loss. These findings may be seen on frozen section and should be reported descriptively, as they may reflect a variety of disease processes.

Microscopic Findings. The histopathologic findings are nonspecific and are associated with the presumed immune attack on the neurons, based in part on the presence of antineuronal antibodies and secondary changes (174). In most cases, paraneoplastic cerebellar degeneration is characterized by the loss of Purkinje cells, with significant preservation of other neuronal components of the cerebellar cortex. Bergmann gliosis, an astrocytic reaction at the interface of the granule cell layer and the molecular layer that is seen in all processes associated with Purkinje cell loss, is often present. There are typically no microglial reactions and no parenchymal inflammation, although scant lymphocytic infiltrates may be found in the leptomeninges. Given the often uneven distribution of the Purkinje cells in standard histologic sections, demonstration of Purkinje cell loss may be facilitated through the use of an appropriate silver impregnation method (Bielschowsky or Bodian). Normally, the cell body of

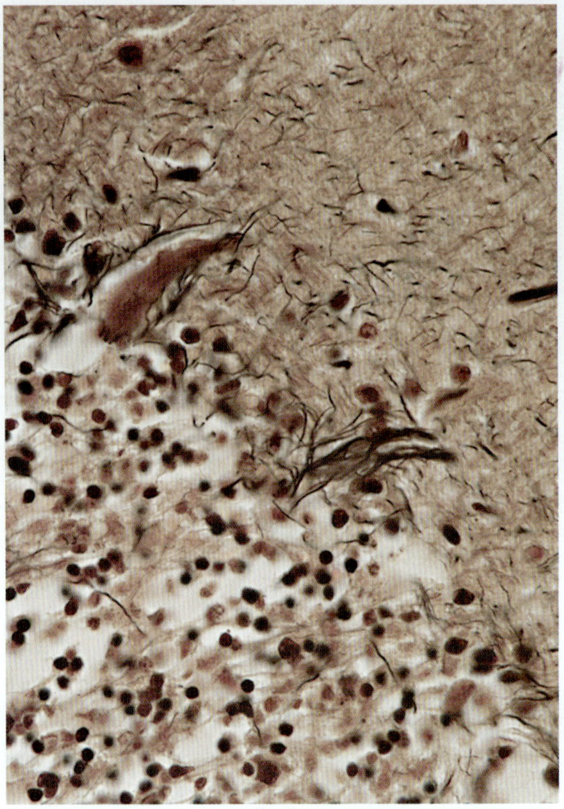

Figure 10-69

PARANEOPLASTIC SYNDROMES

Purkinje cell loss is highlighted by staining the processes of basket cells (Bielschowsky silver impregnation).

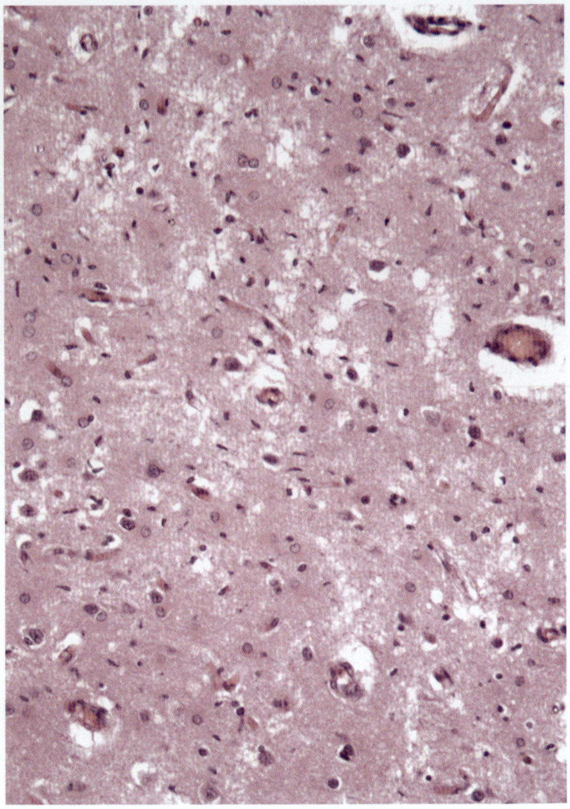

Figure 10-70

PARANEOPLASTIC SYNDROMES

Microglial proliferation in the cortex is observed.

a Purkinje cell is enmeshed in the silver-positive processes of a basket neuron; if Purkinje cells are lost, the basket neuron processes usually remain intact and the recognition of "empty baskets" increases confidence in establishing Purkinje cell dropout (fig. 10-69).

While the encephalomyelitis forms of paraneoplastic syndromes share the feature of neuronal loss, they differ by the prominence of the inflammatory reaction (fig. 10-70). Neuronal loss is associated with both reactive astrocytes as well as microglia; the latter may be present as scattered cells or in the form of microglial nodules (fig. 10-71). The inflammatory infiltrate is present in a perivascular distribution, often involves blood vessels in the meninges as well as in the gray matter, and may be focally intense. Even though the disorder is usually associated with the presence of neuronal antibodies, the infiltrate often contains a mixture of B and T cells.

Immunohistochemical Findings. Evaluation of biopsies can be facilitated through the use of appropriate markers for neurons (NeuN), reactive astrocytes (GFAP), microglia (CD68), and lymphocytes (CD3 and CD20). Importantly, the definition of new types of paraneoplastic syndrome–associated antibodies is driven by the availability of serum from affected patients. Such sera can be used, after appropriate purification of immunoglobulin fractions, as reagents for screening tissue homogenates through Western blotting or brain sections through immunohistochemistry. Attempts to demonstrate the presence of antibody deposited on neurons in the biopsy tissue from affected individuals are nearly always unsuccessful and for this reason are unlikely to contribute to the diagnosis of a paraneoplastic syndrome.

Laboratory and Molecular Findings. While screening for paraneoplastic syndrome–associated antibodies is usually performed prior to

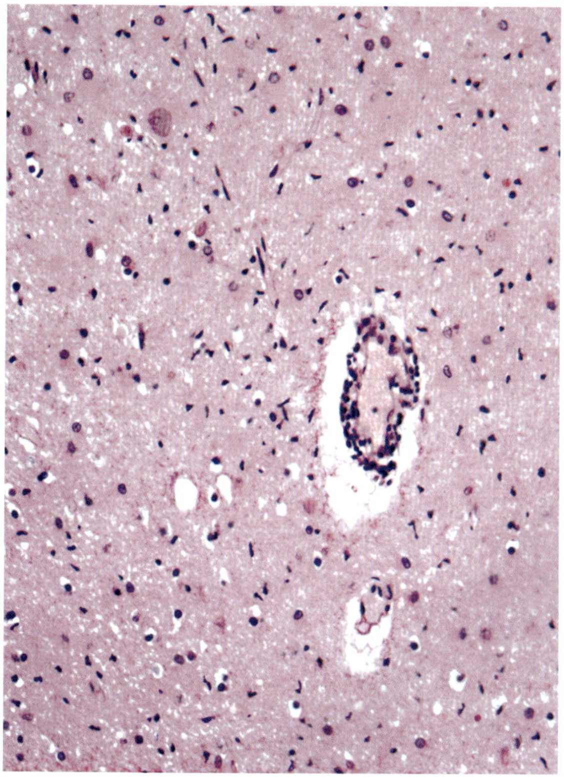

Figure 10-71

PARANEOPLASTIC SYNDROMES

Neuronal loss with microglial nodules and perivascular inflammatory cell infiltrates are part of the histologic picture.

brain biopsy, there may be situations in which the findings on a biopsy suggest this diagnosis and studies are instituted subsequently. Recent studies suggest that broad screening is appropriate, rather than narrowly focused studies that would be based on presumptive correlations between tumor type, neurologic syndrome, and antibody type (170).

Differential Diagnosis. The histologic finding of cerebellar degeneration as a portion of a paraneoplastic syndrome may be difficult to distinguish morphologically from that associated with a mild ischemic insult, given the relative sensitivity of Purkinje cells to hypoxic/ischemic injury. The clinical history should allow for discrimination between these two entities.

A more significant problem is differentiating paraneoplastic encephalomyelitis and viral encephalitis. Both show some element of neuronal loss, gliosis, microglial reaction sometimes with microglial nodules, and perivascular inflammation. Although not absolute, the absence of viral cytopathic features, the absence of hemorrhage and necrosis, and the presence of B cells within the inflammatory infiltrate suggest paraneoplastic syndrome. A combination of clinical history, other aspects of the clinical exam, and ancillary studies, including screening for paraneoplastic antibodies as well as for evidence of a viral infection, may be needed to decide between these two possibilities. There are situations in which the diagnosis remains uncertain, despite the presence of striking pathologic findings on brain biopsy.

Treatment and Prognosis. The primary therapeutic opportunity for the treatment of paraneoplastic syndromes lies in the treatment of the underlying malignancy. There may be additional benefit from immunosuppression, but even though the presence of antibodies against neuronal antigens is a diagnostic feature of these diseases, there is little effect of plasmapheresis on the course of those syndromes with prominent CNS symptoms.

Other Inflammatory Processes

There are a variety of other disease processes in which the brain is involved by a noninfectious inflammatory process. The majority of these present with evidence of a mass lesion, either in the parenchyma or associated with the meninges, and these are discussed elsewhere. Consideration is limited here to those situations in which the clinical presentation is primarily in the form of an encephalopathy. With the alterations in consciousness that accompany this clinical condition, brain biopsy may be performed.

Hashimoto Encephalopathy. Originally described several decades ago (175), this syndrome has recently received more attention as it often has a clinical course comparable to a prion disease yet is responsive to appropriate therapy. With increasing recognition, clinical identification of the process has improved and, for this reason, biopsies are less likely to be encountered in the future. The characteristic finding of the syndrome is relatively rapidly progressive encephalopathy, often accompanied by other neurologic findings including seizures, stroke-like episodes, and even myoclonus, and elevated levels of circulating antithyroid antibodies

(176). There does not appear to be a strong relationship between the neurologic deficits and the level of thyroid function. The additional characteristic feature of the syndrome is the remarkable response to steroid therapy.

Pathologic findings are minimal apart from the presence of a scant perivascular infiltrate. The antithyroid antibodies do not appear to be pathogenic in this syndrome; recently, several potential target antigens in the brain were identified through analysis of sera from patients with Hashimoto encephalopathy (177,178). The combination of circulating antibodies against neuronal antigens and encephalopathy indicates that this process should be considered a variation of paraneoplastic syndrome, a suggestion that may draw strength from some overlap of antigens (177,179).

Nonvasculitic Autoimmune Inflammatory Meningoencephalitis (NAIM). This disorder, which may be related to the inflammatory processes discussed above and with more classic vasculitides and other inflammatory brain diseases, was originally described as a clinical syndrome rather than as a pathologic pattern of injury (180). As with Hashimoto encephalopathy, NAIM is a rapidly progressing syndrome of cognitive impairment, worsening over the course of months, although without myoclonus or seizures. Some of the reported patients with NAIM have had evidence of either antithyroid antibodies or other forms of autoimmune disease (Sjögren syndrome). In NAIM there is elevated intrathecal immunoglobulin (Ig)G synthesis, which is not seen in the competing diagnoses.

There is little histologic description of this entity available, in large part because the disorder is rapidly responsive to steroids. The reports that are available suggest that there is a mixture of T and B cells in the perivascular infiltrate, but no evidence of vascular wall injury, as the name would imply (180,181). Whether NAIM is distinct from the other inflammatory processes that can affect the brain and cause rapidly progressive neurologic deterioration is not yet clear. Given the steroid responsiveness of the neurologic deficits in these individuals, as in those with Hashimoto encephalopathy, recognition of the pathologic findings should prompt a therapeutic trial, if such an exercise has not been completed prior to brain biopsy.

METABOLIC DISORDERS

Most metabolic disorders, either associated with defects in synthesis or metabolism of molecules critical for brain function, have stereotypical presentations and are rarely confused with neurodegenerative diseases (see chaper 14). For these reasons and because of the increasing availability of biochemical and genetic tests that allow these diagnoses to be made in the absence of brain biopsy, it is rare to encounter these entities in surgical neuropathology specimens. Biopsy is most commonly performed in the setting of an adult-onset degenerative disease after the exclusion of more likely candidates through application of other less invasive approaches.

When these entities enter into the differential diagnosis, it is important that the site of the biopsy be guided by clinical and radiologic information to ensure the highest diagnostic yield. For example, when adult-onset neuronal ceroid lipofuscinosis (Kuf disease) is under consideration, then adequate sampling of gray matter is required; in contrast, when leukodystrophy with axonal spheroids is considered in a patient with a frontal lobe syndrome, sampling of the affected white matter is essential.

In order to ensure that appropriate diagnostic studies are performed, it is advisable (if tissue amounts allow) to fix tissue for electron microscopy and to freeze material for biochemical and genetic studies. Ideally, these special procedures should be performed on both gray and white matter.

VASCULAR DISEASES

Several forms of vascular disease may present with a clinical history of declining cognitive function. The definition of the clinical spectrum of the vascular forms of dementia continues to evolve; however, several distinct disease processes may produce an unclear enough clinical course to prompt a brain biopsy. These include entities for which therapeutic interventions exist (most prominently, vasculitis), or that have implications for subsequent care (cerebral amyloid angiopathy and Binswanger disease), or that are genetic diseases with implications for other family members (CADASIL). While these disorders are covered in more detail elsewhere in this volume (see chapter 6), several general comments are appropriate here.

Vasculitis

Various findings from laboratory studies, including imaging of the cerebral vasculature, can suggest the presence of vasculitis (168). Despite this, meningeal and brain biopsy is sometimes performed in order to obtain a firm tissue diagnosis prior to the use of immunosuppressive agents as therapy. Because physicians caring for the patient are often waiting for the results of a brain biopsy in order to initiate therapy, frozen sections are often requested. The presence of vascular wall damage with associated inflammation can be detected on frozen section; however, the patchy nature of the disease process may well result in a false negative finding on a limited sample at frozen section. It is necessary to assess the value of the trade-off between a rapid return of information with the introduction of artifact in tissue freezing. This difficult balance can often be solved by the use of rapid processing of fixed tissue to provide evaluation of paraffin-embedded sections in an extremely timely manner.

When attempting to assess a biopsy performed for the evaluation of an uneven process, such as vasculitis, it is often advantageous to place individual tissue fragments into separate cassettes. While this results in a marginal increase in laboratory volume for processing, embedding, sectioning, and staining, there is a strong advantage in being able to perform step sectioning to look for vasculitic involvement independently on each tissue fragment.

Cerebral Amyloid Angiopathy with Inflammation

It is well established that *cerebral amyloid angiopathy* (CAA) is a major risk factor for lobar hemorrhage, but there are other clinical presentations that may be associated with this vascular disease. A distinct clinical presentation has been described in which the dominant neurologic findings are progressive cognitive impairment, sometimes associated with seizures, and radiologic evidence of multiple, small cortical and white matter infarcts. The dominant pathologic finding is an inflammatory reaction to the vascular amyloid. While giant cells are common in these lesions, suggesting granulomatous angiitis of the nervous system, there is a strong correlation between the inflammatory reaction and the amyloid burden, suggesting that the amyloidosis is the primary lesion in this disease. As described by different groups, there may either be true vasculitis with fibrinoid necrosis of the vessel wall (183) or primarily inflammatory perivascular infiltrates with scattered giant cells (184). Whether these represent distinct stages along a continuum is not currently clear.

Hypertension/Binswanger Disease

Clinical findings and imaging studies are fully adequate to provide for a diagnosis of hypertensive cerebrovascular disease. While the definitions and criteria of vascular cognitive impairment and vascular dementia are still in evolution and reflect a complex mixture of underlying etiologies (large territory infarcts, small vessel cortical lesions, white matter changes) (185–187), the need to assess this etiology of dementia is rarely an indication for brain biopsy. Arteriolar sclerosis, with vascular wall hyalinosis in the white matter, is associated with rarefaction of the surrounding white matter and hemosiderin accumulation in perivascular macrophages. Binswanger disease remains a poorly defined entity of cognitive impairment associated with diffuse white matter volume loss associated with severe and diffuse arteriolar sclerosis. It may represent one end of the spectrum of multi-infarct dementia.

CADASIL

CADASIL (cerebral autosomal dominant arteriopathy with subcortical infarcts and leukoencephalopathy) is a genetic form of cerebrovascular disease linked to mutations in the *Notch3* gene. It is associated with vascular wall thickening and destruction, as well as white matter injury (188–190). The combination of family history and imaging studies often leads to a diagnosis without the need of a brain biopsy. The need to proceed to brain biopsy to seek the pathologic hallmark of this disease (granular osmophilic material) in the basement membrane of blood vessels has been reduced by the identification of these findings in vessels of other tissues, including skin and muscle (191–195).

REFERENCES

1. Warren JD, Schott JM, Fox NC, et al. Brain biopsy in dementia. Brain 2005;128(Pt 9):2016-2025.

1a. Lee VM, Goedert M, Trojanowski JQ. Neurodegenerative tauopathies. Annu Rev Neurosci 2001;24:1121-1159.

2. Dickson D, ed. Neurodegeneration: the molecular pathology of dementia and movement disorders. Basel: ISN Neuropath Press; 2003.

3. Mirra SS, Hart MN, Terry RD. Making the diagnosis of Alzheimer's disease. A primer for practicing pathologists. Arch Pathol Lab Med 1993;117:132-144.

4. Selkoe DJ. Alzheimer's disease: genes, proteins, and therapy. Physiol Rev 2001;81:741-766.

5. Selkoe DJ, American College of Physicians, American Physiological Society. Alzheimer disease: mechanistic understanding predicts novel therapies. Ann Intern Med 2004;140:627-638.

6. Knopman DS, Boeve BF, Petersen RC. Essentials of the proper diagnoses of mild cognitive impairment, dementia, and major subtypes of dementia. Mayo Clin Proc 2003;78:1290-1308.

7. Bertram L, Tanzi R. Genetics of Alzheimer's disease. In: Dickson D, ed. Neurodegeneration: the molecular pathology of dementia and movement disorders. Basel: ISN Neuropath Press; 2003:40-46.

8. Dickerson BC, Sperling RA. Neuroimaging biomarkers for clinical trials of disease-modifying therapies in Alzheimer's disease. NeuroRx 2005;2:348-360.

9. Jack CR Jr, Shiung MM, Weigand SD, et al. Brain atrophy rates predict subsequent clinical conversion in normal elderly and amnestic MCI. Neurology 2005;65:1227-1231.

10. Killiany RJ, Gomez-Isla T, Moss M, et al. Use of structural magnetic resonance imaging to predict who will get Alzheimer's disease. Ann Neurol 2000;47:430-439.

11. Klunk WE, Engler H, Nordberg A, et al. Imaging brain amyloid in Alzheimer's disease with Pittsburgh compound-B. Ann Neurol 2004;55:306-319.

12. Klunk WE, Lopresti BJ, Ikonomovic MD, et al. Binding of the positron emission tomography tracer Pittsburgh compound-B reflects the amount of amyloid-beta in Alzheimer's disease brain but not in transgenic mouse brain. J Neurosci 2005;25:10598-10606.

13. Crook R, Verkkoniemi A, Perez-Tur J, et al. A variant of Alzheimer's disease with spastic paraparesis and unusual plaques due to deletion of exon 9 of presenilin 1. Nat Med 1998;4:452-455.

14. Houlden H, Baker M, McGowan E, et al. Variant Alzheimer's disease with spastic paraparesis and cotton wool plaques is caused by PS-1 mutations that lead to exceptionally high amyloid-beta concentrations. Ann Neurol 2000;48:806-808.

15. Steiner H, Revesz T, Neumann M, et al. A pathogenic presenilin-1 deletion causes abberrant Abeta 42 production in the absence of congophilic amyloid plaques. J Biol Chem 2001;276:7233-7239.

16. Tabira T, Chui H, Nakayama H, Kuroda S, Shibuya M. Alzheimer's disease with spastic paresis and cotton wool type plaques. J Neurosci Res 2002;70:367-372.

17. Verkkoniemi A, Kalimo H, Paetau A, et al. Variant Alzheimer disease with spastic paraparesis: neuropathological phenotype. J Neuropathol Exp Neurol 2001;60:483-492.

18. Le TV, Crook R, Hardy J, Dickson DW. Cotton wool plaques in non-familial late-onset Alzheimer disease. J Neuropathol Exp Neurol 2001;60:1051-1061.

19. Gilbert JJ, Vinters HV. Cerebral amyloid angiopathy: incidence and complications in the aging brain. I. Cerebral hemorrhage. Stroke 1983;14:915-923.

20. Vinters HV, Gilbert JJ. Cerebral amyloid angiopathy: incidence and complications in the aging brain. II. The distribution of amyloid vascular changes. Stroke 1983;14:924-928.

21. Vonsattel JP, Myers RH, Hedley-Whyte ET, Ropper AH, Bird ED, Richardson EP Jr. Cerbral amyloid angiopathy without and with cerebral hemorrhages: a comparative histological study. Ann Neurol 1991;30:637-649.

22. Blennow K, Vanmechelen E. CSF markers for pathogenic processes in Alzheimer's disease: diagnostic implications and use in clinical neurochemistry. Brain Res Bull 2003;61:235-242.

23. Blennow K, Vanmechelen E, Hampel H. CSF total tau, Abeta42 and phosphorylated tau protein as biomarkers for Alzheimer's disease. Mol Neurobiol 2001;24:87-97.

24. Irizarry MC. Biomarkers of Alzheimer disease in plasma. NeuroRx 2004;1:226-234.

25. Khachaturian ZS. Diagnosis of Alzheimer's disease. Arch Neurol 1985;42:1097-1105.

26. Duyckaerts C, Dickson DW. Neuropathology of Alzheimer's disease. In: Dickson DW, ed. Neurodegeneration: the molecular pathology of dementia and movement disorders. Basel: ISN Neuropath Press; 2003:47-65.

27. Consensus recommendations for the postmortem diagnosis of Alzheimer's disease. The National Institute on Aging, and Reagan Institute Working Group on Diagnostic Criteria for the Neuropathological Assessment of Alzheimer's Disease. Neurobiol Aging 1997;18:S1-2.

28. Braak H, Braak E. Neuropathological staging of Alzheimer-related changes. Acta Neuropathol (Berl) 1991;82:239-259.
29. Hyman BT, Trojanowski JQ. Consensus recommendations for the postmortem diagnosis of Alzheimer disease from the National Institute on Aging and the Reagan Institute Working Group on diagnostic criteria for the neuropathological assessment of Alzheimer disease. J Neuropathol Exp Neurol 1997;56:1095-1097.
30. Jellinger KA, Bancher C. Neuropathology of Alzheimer's disease: a critical update. J Neural Transm Suppl 1998;54:77-95.
31. Newell KL, Hyman BT, Growdon JH, Hedley-Whyte ET. Application of the National Institute on Aging (NIA)-Reagan Institute criteria for the neuropathological diagnosis of Alzheimer disease. J Neuropathol Exp Neurol 1999;58:1147-1155.
32. Wisniewski HM, Silverman W. Diagnostic criteria for the neuropathological assessment of Alzheimer's disease: current status and major issues. Neurobiol Aging 1997;18:S43-50.
33. Knopman DS, Parisi JE, Salviati A, et al. Neuropathology of cognitively normal elderly. J Neuropathol Exp Neurol 2003;62:1087-1095.
34. Ikonomovic MD, Uryu K, Abrahamson EE, et al. Alzheimer's pathology in human temporal cortex surgically excised after severe brain injury. Exp Neurol 2004;190:192-203.
35. Schmidt ML, Zhukareva V, Newell KL, Lee VM, Trojanowski JQ. Tau isoform profile and phosphorylation state in dementia pugilistica recapitulate Alzheimer's disease. Acta Neuropathol (Berl) 2001;101:518-524.
36. Rostagno A, Tomidokoro Y, Lashley T, et al. Chromosome 13 dementias. Cell Mol Life Sci 2005;62:1814-1825.
37. Vidal R, Frangione B, Rostagno A, et al. A stop-codon mutation in the BRI gene associated with familial British dementia. Nature 1999;399:776-781.
38. Vidal R, Revesz T, Rostagno A, et al. A decamer duplication in the 3' region of the BRI gene originates an amyloid peptide that is associated with dementia in a Danish kindred. Proc Natl Acad Sci U S A 2000;97:4920-4925.
39. Revesz T, Ghiso J, Plant G, Holton J, Frangione B. Inherited amyloidoses and neurodegeneration: familial British dementia and familial Danish dementia. In: Dickson DW, ed. Neurodegeneration: the molecular pathology of dementia and movement disorders. Basel: ISN Neuropath Press; 2003:380-385.
40. Mead S, James-Galton M, Revesz T, et al. Familial British dementia with amyloid angiopathy: early clinical, neuropsychological and imaging findings. Brain 2000;123(Pt 5):975-991.
41. Ince PG, McKeith IG. Dementia with lewy bodies. In Dickson DW, ed. Neurodegeneration: the molecular pathology of dementia and movement disorders. Bsael: ISN Neuropath Press; 2003:188-199.
42. Braak H, Del Tredici K, Rub U, de Vos RA, Jansen Steur EN, Braak E. Staging of brain pathology related to sporadic Parkinson's disease. Neurobiol Aging 2003;24:197-211.
43. Braak H, Rub U, Jansen Steur EN, Del Tredici K, de Vos RA. Cognitive status correlates with neuropathologic stage in Parkinson disease. Neurology 2005;64:1404-1410.
44. Del Tredici K, Rub U, De Vos RA, Bohl JR, Braak H. Where does Parkinson disease pathology begin in the brain? J Neuropathol Exp Neurol 2002;61:413-426.
45. Geser F, Wenning GK, Poewe W, McKeith I. How to diagnose dementia with Lewy bodies: state of the art. Mov Disord 2005;20(Suppl 12):S11-20.
46. McKeith IG, Galasko D, Kosaka K, et al. Consensus guidelines for the clinical and pathologic diagnosis of dementia with Lewy bodies (DLB): report of the consortium on DLB international workshop. Neurology 1996;47:1113-1124.
47. McKeith IG, Perry EK, Perry RH. Report of the second dementia with Lewy body international workshop: diagnosis and treatment. Consortium on Dementia with Lewy Bodies. Neurology 1999;53:902-905.
48. McKeith IG, Dickson DW, Lowe J, et al. Diagnosis and management of dementia with Lewy bodies. Third report of the DLB consortium. Neurology 2005;65:26-27.
49. Kotzbauer PT, Trojanowsk JQ, Lee VM. Lewy body pathology in Alzheimer's disease. J Mol Neurosci 2001;17:225-232.
50. Popescu A, Lippa CF, Lee VM, Trojanowski JQ. Lewy bodies in the amygdala: increase of alpha-synuclein aggregates in neurodegenerative diseases with tau-based inclusions. Arch Neurol 2004;61:1915-1919.
51. Iwai A, Masliah E, Sundsmo MP, et al. The synaptic protein NACP is abnormally expressed during the progression of Alzheimer's disease. Brain Res 1996;720:230-234.
52. Iwai A, Masliah E, Yoshimoto M, et al. The precursor protein of non-A beta component of Alzheimer's disease amyloid is a presynaptic protein of the central nervous system. Neuron 1995;14:467-475.
53. Iwai A, Yoshimoto M, Masliah E, Saitoh T. Non-A beta component of Alzheimer's disease amyloid (NAC) is amyloidogenic. Biochemistry 1995;34:10139-10145.
54. Masliah E, Iwai A, Mallory M, Ueda K, Saitoh T. Altered presynaptic protein NACP is associated with plaque formation and neurodegeneration in Alzheimer's disease. Am J Pathol 1996;148:201-210.

55. Forno LS. Neuropathology of Parkinson's disease. J Neuropathol Exp Neurol 1996;55:259-272.
56. Dickson DW. Dementia with Lewy bodies: neuropathology. J Geriatr Psychiatry Neurol 2002;15:210-216.
57. Gomez-Tortosa E, Ingraham AO, Irizarry MC, Hyman BT. Dementia with Lewy bodies. J Am Geriatr Soc 1998;46:1449-1458.
58. Kosaka K. Diffuse Lewy body disease. Intern Med 1998;37:6-10.
59. Dickson DW, Ruan D, Crystal H, et al. Hippocampal degeneration differentiates diffuse Lewy body disease (DLBD) from Alzheimer's disease: light and electron microscopic immunocytochemistry of CA2-3 neurites specific to DLBD. Neurology 1991;41:1402-1409.
60. Dickson DW, Schmidt ML, Lee VM, Zhao ML, Yen SH, Trojanowski JQ. Immunoreactivity profile of hippocampal CA2/3 neurites in diffuse Lewy body disease. Acta Neuropathol (Berl) 1994;87:269-276.
61. Hansen LA, Masliah E, Terry RD, Mirra SS. A neuropathological subset of Alzheimer's disease with concomitant Lewy body disease and spongiform change. Acta Neuropathol (Berl) 1989;78:194-201.
62. Goedert M. Introduction to the tauopathies. In: Dickson DW, ed. Neurodegeneration: the molecular pathology of dementia and movement disorders. Basel: ISN Neuropath Press; 2003:82-85.
63. McKhann GM, Albert MS, Grossman M, Miller B, Dickson D, Trojanowski JQ. Clinical and pathological diagnosis of frontotemporal dementia: report of the Work Group on Frontotemporal Dementia and Pick's Disease. Arch Neurol 2001;58:1803-1809.
64. Ghetti B, Hutton M, Wszolek Z. Frontotemporal dementia and parkinsonism linked to chromosome 17 associated with tau gene mutations (FTDP-17 T). In: Dickson DW, ed. Neurodegeneration: the molecular pathology of dementia and movement disorders. Basel: ISN Neuropath Press; 2003:86-102.
65. Bergeron C, Morris H, Rossor MN. Pick's disease. In: Dickson DW, ed. Neurodegeneration: the molecular pathology of dementia and movement disorders. Basel: ISN Neuropath Press; 2003:124-131.
66. Hauw JJ, Agid Y. Progressive supranuclear palsy (PSP) or Steele-Richardson-Olszewski disease. In: Dickson DW, ed. Neurodegeneration: the molecular pathology of dementia and movement disorders. Basel: ISN Neuropath Press; 2003:103-114.
67. Dickson DW, Litvan I. Corticobasal degeneration. In: Dickson DW, ed. Neurodegeneration: the molecular pathology of dementia and movement disorders. Basel: ISN Neuropath Press; 2003:115-123.
68. Adamec E, Murrell JR, Takao M, et al. P301L tauopathy: confocal immunofluorescence study of perinuclear aggregation of the mutated protein. J Neurol Sci 2002;200:85-93.
69. Dickson DW. Neuropathologic differentiation of progressive supranuclear palsy and corticobasal degeneration. J Neurol 1999;246(Suppl 2):II6-15.
70. Dickson DW, Feany MB, Yen SH, Mattiace LA, Davies P. Cytoskeletal pathology in non-Alzheimer degenerative dementia: new lesions in diffuse Lewy body disease, Pick's disease, and corticobasal degeneration. J Neural Transm Suppl 1996;47:31-46.
71. Feany MB, Dickson DW. Neurodegenerative disorders with extensive tau pathology: a comparative study and review. Ann Neurol 1996;40:139-148.
72. Feany MB, Dickson DW. Widespread cytoskeletal pathology characterizes corticobasal degeneration. Am J Pathol 1995;146:1388-1396.
73. Feany MB, Mattiace LA, Dickson DW. Neuropathologic overlap of progressive supranuclear palsy, Pick's disease and corticobasal degeneration. J Neuropathol Exp Neurol 1996;55:53-67.
74. Feany MB, Ksiezak-Reding H, Liu WK, Vincent I, Yen SH, Dickson DW. Epitope expression and hyperphosphorylation of tau protein in corticobasal degeneration: differentiation from progressive supranuclear palsy. Acta Neuropathol (Berl) 1995;90:37-43.
75. Goedert M, Ghetti B, Spillantini MG. Tau gene mutations in frontotemporal dementia and parkinsonism linked to chromosome 17 (FTDP-17). Their relevance for understanding the neurogenerative process. Ann N Y Acad Sci 2000;920:74-83.
76. Goedert M, Jakes R. Mutations causing neurodegenerative tauopathies. Biochim Biophys Acta 2005;1739:240-250.
77. Buee L, Delacourte A. Comparative biochemistry of tau in progressive supranuclear palsy, corticobasal degeneration, FTDP-17 and Pick's disease. Brain Pathol 1999;9:681-693.
78. Jellinger KA. Dementia with grains (argyrophilic grain disease). Brain Pathol 1998;8:377-386.
79. Togo T, Cookson N, Dickson DW. Argyrophilic grain disease: neuropathology, frequency in a dementia brain bank and lack of relationship with apolipoprotein E. Brain Pathol 2002;12:45-52.
80. Togo T, Sahara N, Yen SH, et al. Argyrophilic grain disease is a sporadic 4-repeat tauopathy. J Neuropathol Exp Neurol 2002;61:547-556.
81. Tolnay M, Clavaguera F. Argyrophilic grain disease: a late-onset dementia with distinctive features among tauopathies. Neuropathology 2004;24:269-283.
82. Tolnay M, Monsch AU, Probst A. Argyrophilic grain disease. A frequent dementing disorder in aged patients. Adv Exp Med Biol 2001;487:39-58.

83. Tolnay M, Schwietert M, Monsch AU, Staehelin HB, Langui D, Probst A. Argyrophilic grain disease: distribution of grains in patients with and without dementia. Acta Neuropathol (Berl) 1997;94:353-358.
84. Tolnay M, Ghebremedhin E, Probst A, Braak H. Argyrophilic grain disease. In: Dickson DW, ed. Neurodegeneration: the molecular pathology of dementia and movement disorders. Basel: ISN Neuropath Press; 2003:132-136.
85. Ikeda K, Akiyama H, Arai T, Matsushita M, Tsuchiya K, Miyazaki H. Clinical aspects of argyrophilic grain disease. Clin Neuropathol 2000;19:278-284.
86. Lantos P. Other neurodegenerative disorders: introduction. In: Dickson DW, ed. Neurodegeneration: The molecular pathology of dementia and movement disorders. Basel: ISN Neuropath Press; 2003:378-379.
87. Cairns NJ, Bigio EH, Mackenzie IR, et al. Neuropathologic diagnostic and nosologic criteria for frontotemporal lobar degeneration: consensus of the Consortium for Frontotemporal Lobar Degeneration. Acta Neuropathol 2007;114:5-22.
88. Neumann M, Sampathu DM, Kwong LK, et al. Ubiquitinated TDP-43 in frontotemporal lobar degeneration and amyotrophic lateral sclerosis. Science 2006;314:130-133.
89. Cairns NJ, Neumann M, Bigio EH, et al. TDP-43 in familial and sporadic frontotemporal lobar degeneration with ubiquitin inclusions. Am J Pathol 2007;171:227-240.
90. Mackenzie IR. The neuropathology and clinical phenotype of FTD with progranulin mutations. Acta Neuropathol 2007;114:49-54.
91. Pickering-Brown SM. Progranulin and frontotemporal lobar degeneration. Acta Neuropathol 2007;114:39-47.
92. Forman MS, Mackenzie IR, Cairns NJ, et al. Novel ubiquitin neuropathology in frontotemporal dementia with valosin-containing protein gene mutations. J Neuropathol Exp Neuro 2006;65:571-581.
93. Guyant-Marechal L, Laquerriere A, Duyckaerts C, et al. Valosin-containing protein gene mutations: clinical and neuropathologic features. Neurology 2006;67:644-651.
94. Guinto JB, Ritson GP, Taylor JP, Forman MS. Valosin-containing protein and the pathogenesis of frontotemporal dementia associated with inclusion body myopathy. Acta Neuropathol 2007;114:55-61.
95. Davis RL, Holohan PD, Shrimpton AE, et al. Familial encephalopathy with neuroserpin inclusion bodies. Am J Pathol 1999;155:1901-1913.
96. Davis RL, Shrimpton AE, Holohan PD, et al. Familial dementia caused by polymerization of mutant neuroserpin. Nature 1999;401:376-379.
97. Kimber TE, Blumbergs PC, Rice JP, et al. Familial neuronal intranuclear inclusion disease with ubiquitin positive inclusions. J Neurol Sci 1998;160:33-40.
98. Cairns NJ, Zhukareva V, Uryu K, et al. Alpha-internexin is present in the pathological inclusions of neuronal intermediate filament inclusion disease. Am J Pathol 2004;164:2153-2161.
99. DeKosky ST, Ikonomovic MD. NIFID: a new molecular pathology with a frontotemporal dementia phenotype. Neurology 2004;63:1348-1349.
100. Cairns NJ, Grossman M, Arnold SE, et al. Clinical and neuropathologic variation in neuronal intermediate filament inclusion disease. Neurology 2004;63:1376-1384.
101. Armstrong RA, Kerty E, Skullerud K, Cairns NJ. Neuropathological changes in ten cases of neuronal intermediate filament inclusion disease (NIFID): a study using alpha-internexin immunohistochemistry and principal components analysis (PCA). J Neural Transm 2006;113:1207-1215.
102. Ishihara K, Araki S, Ihori N, Shiota J, Kawamura M, Nakano I. An autopsy case of frontotemporal dementia with severe dysarthria and motor neuron disease showing numerous basophilic inclusions. Neuropathology 2006;26:447-454.
103. Yokota O, Tsuchiya K, Terada S, et al. Basophilic inclusion body disease and neuronal intermediate filament inclusion disease: a comparative clinicopathological study. Acta Neuropathol 2007;115:561-575.
104. Collinge J. Molecular neurology of prion disease. J Neurol Neurosurg Psychiatry 2005;76:906-919.
105. Collins SJ, Lawson VA, Masters CL. Transmissible spongiform encephalopathies. Lancet 2004;363:51-61.
106. Gambetti P, Kong Q, Zou W, Parchi P, Chen SG. Sporadic and familial CJD: classification and characterisation. Br Med Bull 2003;66:213-239.
107. Prusiner SB. Shattuck lecture—neurodegenerative diseases and prions. N Engl J Med 2001;344:1516-1526.
108. Aguzzi A. Introduction to prion diseases. In: Dickson DW, ed. Neurodegeneration: the molecular pathology of dementia and movement disorders. Basel: ISN Neuropath Press; 2003:282-286.
109. Will RG, Ironside JW, Zeidler M, et al. A new variant of Creutzfeldt-Jakob disease in the UK. Lancet 1996;347:921-925.
110. Gambetti P, Petersen R, Monari L, et al. Fatal familial insomnia and the widening spectrum of prion diseases. Br Med Bull 1993;49:980-994.

111. Lugaresi E, Medori R, Montagna P, et al. Fatal familial insomnia and dysautonomia with selective degeneration of thalamic nuclei. N Engl J Med 1986;315:997-1003.
112. Lugaresi E, Tobler I, Gambetti P, Montagna P. The pathophysiology of fatal familial insomnia. Brain Pathol 1998;8:521-526.
113. Medori R, Tritschler HJ, LeBlanc A, et al. Fatal familial insomnia, a prion disease with a mutation at codon 178 of the prion protein gene. N Engl J Med 1992;326:444-449.
114. Montagna P, Gambetti P, Cortelli P, Lugaresi E. Familial and sporadic fatal insomnia. Lancet Neurol 2003;2:167-176.
115. Parchi P, Petersen RB, Chen SG, et al. Molecular pathology of fatal familial insomnia. Brain Pathol 1998;8:539-548.
116. Mastrianni JA, Nixon R, Layzer R, et al. Prion protein conformation in a patient with sporadic fatal insomnia. N Engl J Med 1999;340:1630-1638.
117. Parchi P, Capellari S, Chin S, et al. A subtype of sporadic prion disease mimicking fatal familial insomnia. Neurology 1999;52:1757-1763.
118. Scaravilli F, Cordery RJ, Kretzschmar H, et al. Sporadic fatal insomnia: a case study. Ann Neurol 2000;48:665-668.
119. Bugiani O, Giaccone G, Piccardo P, Morbin M, Tagliavini F, Ghetti B. Neuropathology of Gerstmann-Straussler-Scheinker disease. Microsc Res Tech 2000;50:10-15.
120. Ghetti B, Dlouhy SR, Giaccone G, et al. Gerstmann-Straussler-Scheinker disease and the Indiana kindred. Brain Pathol 1995;5:61-75.
121. Ghetti B, Tagliavini F, Giaccone G, et al. Familial Gerstmann-Straussler-Scheinker disease with neurofibrillary tangles. Mol Neurobiol 1994;8:41-48.
122. Hsiao K, Dlouhy SR, Farlow MR, et al. Mutant prion proteins in Gerstmann-Straussler-Scheinker disease with neurofibrillary tangles. Nat Genet 1992;1:68-71.
123. Gajdusek DC, Zigas V. Kuru; clinical, pathological and epidemiological study of an acute progressive degenerative disease of the central nervous system among natives of the Eastern Highlands of New Guinea. Am J Med 1959;26:442-469.
124. Gajdusek DC, Zigas V. Degenerative disease of the central nervous system in New Guinea; the endemic occurrence of kuru in the native population. N Engl J Med 1957;257:974-978.
125. WHO infection control guidelines for transmissible spongiform encephalopathies. Geneva: World Health Organization; 1999.
126. Brown P, Wolff A, Gajdusek DC. A simple and effective method for inactivating virus infectivity in formalin-fixed tissue samples from patients with Creutzfeldt-Jakob disease. Neurology 1990;40:887-890.
127. Castellani RJ, Colucci M, Xie Z, et al. Sensitivity of 14-3-3 protein test varies in subtypes of sporadic Creutzfeldt-Jakob disease. Neurology 2004;63:436-442.
128. Geschwind MD, Martindale J, Miller D, et al. Challenging the clinical utility of the 14-3-3 protein for the diagnosis of sporadic Creutzfeldt-Jakob disease. Arch Neurol 2003;60:813-816.
129. Lemstra AW, van Meegen MT, Vreyling JP, et al. 14-3-3 testing in diagnosing Creutzfeldt-Jakob disease: a prospective study in 112 patients. Neurology 2000;55:514-516.
130. Collins S, Boyd A, Fletcher A, et al. Creutzfeldt-Jakob disease: diagnostic utility of 14-3-3 protein immunodetection in cerebrospinal fluid. J Clin Neurosci 2000;7:203-208.
131. Murata T, Shiga Y, Higano S, Takahashi S, Mugikura S. Conspicuity and evolution of lesions in Creutzfeldt-Jakob disease at diffusion-weighted imaging. AJNR Am J Neuroradiol 2002;23:1164-1172.
132. Shiga Y, Miyazawa K, Sato S, et al. Diffusion-weighted MRI abnormalities as an early diagnostic marker for Creutzfeldt-Jakob disease. Neurology 2004;63:443-449.
133. Will RG. Acquired prion disease: iatrogenic CJD, variant CJD, kuru. Br Med Bull 2003;66:255-265.
134. Ironside JW. Pathology of variant Creutzfeldt-Jakob disease. Arch Virol Suppl 2000;16:143-151.
135. Ironside JW, McCardle L, Horsburgh A, Lim Z, Head MW. Pathological diagnosis of variant Creutzfeldt-Jakob disease. APMIS 2002;110:79-87.
136. Zeidler M, Sellar RJ, Collie DA, et al. The pulvinar sign on magnetic resonance imaging in variant Creutzfeldt-Jakob disease. Lancet 2000;355:1412-1418.
137. Llewelyn CA, Hewitt PE, Knight RS, et al. Possible transmission of variant Creutzfeldt-Jakob disease by blood transfusion. Lancet 2004;363:417-421.
138. WHO guidelines on transmissible spongiform encephalopathies in relation to biological and pharmaceutical products. Geneva: World Health Organization; 2003.
139. Bruce ME, McConnell I, Will RG, Ironside JW. Detection of variant Creutzfeldt-Jakob disease infectivity in extraneural tissues. Lancet 2001;358:208-209.
140. Frosh A, Smith LC, Jackson CJ, et al. Analysis of 2000 consecutive UK tonsillectomy specimens for disease-related prion protein. Lancet 2004;364:1260-1262.
141. Head MW, Ritchie D, Smith N, et al. Peripheral tissue involvement in sporadic, iatrogenic, and variant Creutzfeldt-Jakob disease: an immunohistochemical, quantitative, and biochemical study. Am J Pathol 2004;164:143-153.

142. Hill AF, Butterworth RJ, Joiner S, et al. Investigation of variant Creutzfeldt-Jakob disease and other human prion diseases with tonsil biopsy samples. Lancet 1999;353:183-189.
143. Hill AF, Zeidler M, Ironside J, Collinge J. Diagnosis of new variant Creutzfeldt-Jakob disease by tonsil biopsy. Lancet 1997;349:99-100.
144. Hilton DA, Sutak J, Smith ME, et al. Specificity of lymphoreticular accumulation of prion protein for variant Creutzfeldt-Jakob disease. J Clin Pathol 2004;57:300-302.
145. Zeidler M, Knight R, Stewart G, et al. Diagnosis of Creutzfeldt-Jakob disease. Routine tonsil biopsy for diagnosis of new variant Creutzfeldt-Jakob disease is not justified. BMJ 1999;318:538.
146. Parchi P, Giese A, Capellari S, et al. Classification of sporadic Creutzfeldt-Jakob disease based on molecular and phenotypic analysis of 300 subjects. Ann Neurol 1999;46:224-233.
147. Hayek J, Ulrich J. Kuru-plaques in Creutzfeldt-Jakob disease. Eur Neurol 1975;13:251-257.
148. Masters CL, Gajdusek DC, Gibbs CJ Jr. Creutzfeldt-Jakob disease virus isolations from the Gerstmann-Straussler syndrome with an analysis of the various forms of amyloid plaque deposition in the virus-induced spongiform encephalopathies. Brain 1981;104:559-588.
149. Miyazono M, Iwaki T, Kitamoto T, Kaneko Y, Doh-ura K, Tateishi J. A comparative immunohistochemical study of kuru and senile plaques with a special reference to glial reactions at various stages of amyloid plaque formation. Am J Pathol 1991;139:589-598.
150. Schulz-Schaeffer WJ, Tschoke S, Kranefuss N, et al. The paraffin-embedded tissue blot detects PrP(Sc) early in the incubation time in prion diseases. Am J Pathol 2000;156:51-56.
151. Miller C, Farrington CP, Harbert K. The epidemiology of subacute sclerosing panencephalitis in England and Wales 1970-1989. Int J Epidemiol 1992;21:998-1006.
152. Risk WS, Haddad FS. The variable natural history of subacute sclerosing panencephalitis: a study of 118 cases from the Middle East. Arch Neurol 1979;36:610-614.
153. Gagnon A, Bouchard RW. Fulminating adult-onset subacute sclerosing panencephalitis in a 49-year-old man. Arch Neurol 2003;60:1160-1161.
154. PeBenito R, Naqvi SH, Arca MM, Schubert R. Fulminating subacute sclerosing panencephalitis: case report and literature review. Clin Pediatr 1997;36:149-154.
155. Tamari H, Matsukura M, Matsuda I, Ueda K, Ohtsuka H. An acute variant of subacute sclerosing panencephalitis: an autopsy case report. Brain Dev 1981;3:87-91.
156. Yaqub BA. Subacute sclerosing panencephalitis (SSPE): early diagnosis, prognostic factors and natural history. J Neurol Sci 1996;139:227-234.
157. Yemisci M, Gurer G, Saygi S, Ciger A. Generalised periodic epileptiform discharges: clinical features, neuroradiological evaluation and prognosis in 37 adult patients. Seizure 2003;12:465-472.
158. Nagano I, Nakamura S, Yoshioka M, Kogure K. Immunocytochemical analysis of the cellular infiltrate in brain lesions in subacute sclerosing panencephalitis. Neurology 1991;41:1639-1642.
159. Allen IV, McQuaid S, McMahon J, Kirk J, McConnell R. The significance of measles virus antigen and genome distribution in the CNS in SSPE for mechanisms of viral spread and demyelination. J Neuropathol Exp Neurol 1996;55:471-480.
160. McQuaid S, Allen IV, McMahon J, Kirk J. Association of measles virus with neurofibrillary tangles in subacute sclerosing panencephalitis: a combined in situ hybridization and immunocytochemical investigation. Neuropathol Appl Neurobiol 1994;20:103-110.
161. McQuaid S, Isserte S, Allan GM, Taylor MJ, Allen IV, Cosby SL. Use of immunocytochemistry and biotinylated in situ hybridisation for detecting measles virus in central nervous system tissue. J Clin Pathol 1990;43:329-333.
162. Lewandowska E, Lechowicz W, Szpak GM, Sobczyk W. Quantitative evaluation of intranuclear inclusions in SSPE: correlation with disease duration. Folia Neuropathologica 2001;39:237-241.
163. McQuaid S, Allan GM. Detection protocols for biotinylated probes: optimization using multistep techniques. J Histochem Cytochem 1992;40:569-574.
164. Forcic D, Baricevic M, Zgorelec R, et al. Detection and characterization of measles virus strains in cases of subacute sclerosing panencephalitis in Croatia. Virus Res 2004;99:51-56.
165. Jin L, Beard S, Hunjan R, Brown DW, Miller E. Characterization of measles virus strains causing SSPE: a study of 11 cases. J Neurovirol 2002;8:335-344.
166. Guizzaro A, Volpe E, Lus G, Bravaccio F, Cotrufo R, Paolozzi C. Progressive rubella panencephalitis. Follow-up EEG study of a case. Acta Neurol (Napoli) 1992;14:485-492.
167. Weil ML, Itabashi H, Cremer NE, Oshiro L, Lennette EH, Carnay L. Chronic progressive panencephalitis due to rubella virus simulating subacute sclerosing panencephalitis. N Engl J Med 1975;292:994-998.

168. Gascon GG, International Consortium on Subacute Sclerosing Panencephalitis. Randomized treatment study of inosiplex versus combined inosiplex and intraventricular interferon-alpha in subacute sclerosing panencephalitis (SSPE): international multicenter study. J Child Neurol 2003;18:819-827. [Erratum in J Child Neurol 2004 May;19:342.]
169. Graus F, Delattre JY, Antoine JC, et al. Recommended diagnostic criteria for paraneoplastic neurological syndromes. J Neurol Neurosurg Psychiatry 2004;75:1135-1140.
170. Pittock SJ, Kryzer TJ, Lennon VA. Paraneoplastic antibodies coexist and predict cancer, not neurological syndrome. Ann Neurol 2004;56:715-719.
171. Bataller L, Dalmau J. Paraneoplastic neurologic syndromes. Neurol Clin 2003;21:221-247, ix.
172. Dropcho EJ. Neurologic paraneoplastic syndromes. J Neurol Sci 1998;153:264-278.
173. Gultekin SH, Rosenfeld MR, Voltz R, Eichen J, Posner JB, Dalmau J. Paraneoplastic limbic encephalitis: neurological symptoms, immunological findings and tumour association in 50 patients. Brain 2000;123(Pt 7):1481-1494.
174. Scaravilli F, An SF, Groves M, Thom M. The neuropathology of paraneoplastic syndromes. Brain Pathol 1999;9:251-260.
175. Brain L, Jellinek EH, Ball K. Hashimoto's disease and encephalopathy. Lancet 1966;2:512-514.
176. Chong JY, Rowland LP, Utiger RD. Hashimoto encephalopathy: syndrome or myth? Arch Neurol 2003;60:164-171.
177. Ochi H, Horiuchi I, Araki N, et al. Proteomic analysis of human brain identifies alpha-enolase as a novel autoantigen in Hashimoto's encephalopathy. FEBS Lett 2002;528:197-202.
178. Oide T, Tokuda T, Yazaki M, et al. Anti-neuronal autoantibody in Hashimoto's encephalopathy: neuropathological, immunohistochemical, and biochemical analysis of two patients. J Neurol Sci 2004;217:7-12.
179. Tojo K, Tokuda T, Yazaki M, et al. Paraneoplastic sensorimotor neuropathy and encephalopathy associated with anti-alpha-enolase antibody in a case of gastric adenocarcinoma. Eur Neurol 2004;51:231-233.
180. Caselli RJ, Boeve BF, Scheithauer BW, O'Duffy JD, Hunder GG. Nonvasculitic autoimmune inflammatory meningoencephalitis (NAIM): a reversible form of encephalopathy. Neurology 1999;53:1579-1581.
181. Josephs KA, Rubino FA, Dickson DW. Nonvasculitic autoimmune inflammatory meningoencephalitis. Neuropathology 2004;24:149-152.
182. Younger DS. Vasculitis of the nervous system. Curr Opin Neurol 2004;17:317-336.
183. Scolding NJ, Joseph F, Kirby PA, et al. Abeta-related angiitis: primary angiitis of the central nervous system associated with cerebral amyloid angiopathy. Brain 2005;128(Pt 3):500-515.
184. Eng JA, Frosch MP, Choi K, Rebeck GW, Greenberg SM. Clinical manifestations of cerebral amyloid angiopathy-related inflammation. Ann Neurol 2004;55:250-256.
185. Kalaria RN, Kenny RA, Ballard CG, Perry R, Ince P, Polvikoski T. Towards defining the neuropathological substrates of vascular dementia. J Neurol Sci 2004;226:75-80.
186. Roman GC, Sachdev P, Royall DR, et al. Vascular cognitive disorder: a new diagnostic category updating vascular cognitive impairment and vascular dementia. J Neurol Sci 2004;226:81-87.
187. Hachinski V, Iadecola C, Petersen RC, et al. National Institute of Neurological Disorders and Stroke-Canadian Stroke Network vascular cognitive impairment harmonization standards. Stroke 2006;37:2220-2241.
188. Dichgans M. CADASIL: a monogenic condition causing stroke and subcortical vascular dementia. Cerebrovasc Dis 2002;13(Suppl 2):37-41.
189. Kalaria RN, Viitanen M, Kalimo H, Dichgans M, Tabira T. The pathogenesis of CADASIL: an update. J Neurol Sci 2004;226:35-39.
190. Dichgans M, Mayer M, Uttner I, et al. The phenotypic spectrum of CADASIL: clinical findings in 102 cases. Ann Neurol 1998;44:731-739.
191. Ebke M, Dichgans M, Bergmann M, et al. CADASIL: skin biopsy allows diagnosis in early stages. Acta Neurol Scand 1997;95:351-357.
192. Mayer M, Straube A, Bruening R, et al. Muscle and skin biopsies are a sensitive diagnostic tool in the diagnosis of CADASIL. J Neurol 1999;246:526-532.
193. Ruchoux MM, Chabriat H, Bousser MG, Baudrimont M, Tournier-Lasserve E. Presence of ultrastructural arterial lesions in muscle and skin vessels of patients with CADASIL. Stroke 1994;25:2291-2292.
194. Ruchoux MM, Guerouaou D, Vandenhaute B, Pruvo JP, Vermersch P, Leys D. Systemic vascular smooth muscle cell impairment in cerebral autosomal dominant arteriopathy with subcortical infarcts and leukoencephalopathy. Acta Neuropathol (Berl) 1995;89:500-512.
195. Brulin P, Godfraind C, Leteurtre E, Ruchoux MM. Morphometric analysis of ultrastructural vascular changes in CADASIL: analysis of 50 skin biopsy specimens and pathogenic implications. Acta Neuropathol (Berl) 2002;104:241-248.

11 TRAUMA

The role of the surgical pathologist in classifying traumatic lesions is usually not integral to the immediate management of the patient, but may be important in establishing the cause and pattern of injury. Neurosurgical procedures may be necessary for the treatment of life-threatening traumatic lesions, especially the evacuation of epidural, subdural, and intraparenchymal hematomas and the resection of cerebral tissue damaged by contusions. The pathologist may be asked to establish the type of traumatic injury and, on occasion, consulted on potential medicolegal questions related to a case. Although the details of medicolegal evaluation are beyond the scope of this Fascicle, this chapter provides an approach to the proper classification of typically encountered traumatic lesions.

In the United States, traumatic injury to the brain and spinal cord is the leading cause of death for people between 1 and 45 years of age (1). Traumatic injury can be classified as either primary or secondary. Primary lesions result from mechanical forces, either focal or diffuse, that produce tissue deformation at the moment of the impact. Hemorrhages (epidural, subarachnoid, ventricular, and parenchymal), contusions, lacerations, and tears represent the spectrum of focal lesions. Diffuse lesions include traumatic axonal injury (also known as diffuse axonal injury), diffuse vascular injury, and brain swelling (2). Currently, subdural hemorrhage is included within diffuse injuries.

Secondary lesions typically develop as a complication of the primary injury. They are related to regional (infarct) or diffuse (anoxic-ischemic encephalopathy) circulatory disorders, infection, edema associated with internal and external herniations, and brain stem hemorrhage. In any given patient, however, such injuries rarely occur in isolation, but rather as a complex interplay of primary and secondary types of tissue damage. Nontraumatic initiating causes can also result in secondary trauma. For instance, primary vascular malformations may induce seizures, which could in turn lead to a fall or accident that results in brain contusion. Clinical and radiologic correlation is important to evaluate possible background etiologies. The entities discussed in this chapter—cerebral contusions, diffuse axonal injury, epidural and subdural hematomas—are therefore most often considered with the lesions discussed in the chapters on vascular diseases, infarcts, and hemorrhages (chapters 5 and 6).

CONTUSION

Definition. A *contusion* is a primary, focal, superficial hemorrhage related to a closed (nonpenetrating) head injury in which the meninges remain intact.

General Comments. Most contusions are postulated to result from contact injury (2). When a mechanical force is applied to the head, it causes an inward deformity of the skull that impacts on the crest of one or more cortical gyri. Contusions are frequently found in areas of the cerebral cortex that are in close contact with bony protuberances.

A blunt force impact to the head produces a contusion by two main mechanisms: a blow to the movable resting head or the moving head hitting a stationary object (e.g., a fall). Injury thresholds differ for the various structural components of the central nervous system (CNS). Contusions may be found throughout the entire CNS, including cerebrum, brain stem, particularly in the pons, cerebellum, and spinal cord. Cerebral contusions are more frequent in the frontal and temporal lobes; parietal and occipital lobe contusions are rare and usually associated with skull fractures and overlying lacerations. The most common sites for cerebral contusions are the frontal poles, orbital surfaces of frontal lobes, temporal poles, and lateral surface of temporal lobes.

Patterns of Contusions. Several contusion patterns are generally accepted (3).

Coup Contusions. These lesions are produced by focal vascular injury due to compressive (tensile) forces operating at the site of direct

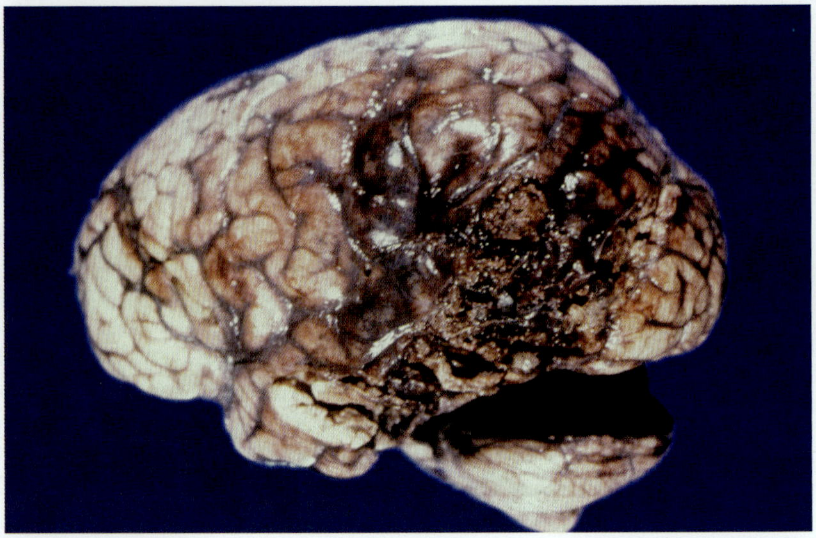

Figure 11-1

COUP CONTUSIONS

Hemorrhagic cortical contusions are present on the left temporal and parietal lobes. Head trauma occurred with a baseball bat.

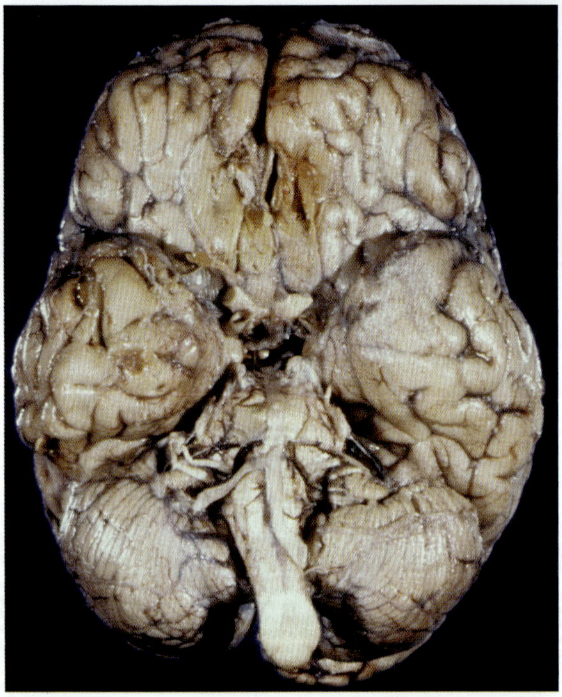

Figure 11- 2

CONTRECOUP CONTUSIONS

Old cortical contusions involve the gyrus rectus. The patient was an alcoholic with a history of falls.

impact. More specifically, this type of contact injury results from the negative pressure generated beneath an area of skull deformation that suddenly snaps back into place. Coup contusions result from an impact to the stationary head (e.g., a blow) (fig. 11-1).

Contrecoup Contusions. These injuries are located opposite to the site of impact. They occur when the moving head strikes a stationary object, as in a fall. When the back of the head is struck during a fall, contrecoup contusions are usually found on the frontal and temporal lobes, with few or no contusions on the occipital poles (figs. 11-2, 11-3).

Fracture Contusions. These contusions follow the lines of skull fractures (fig. 11-4).

Herniation Contusions. These lesions are found in the medial parahippocampal gyrus when displaced against the tentorium cerebelli or in the cerebellar tonsils when compressed through the foramen magnum during herniation events (fig. 11-5). These seldom come to the attention of the surgical pathologist.

Gliding "Contusions." These "contusions" correspond to hemorrhagic lesions of the cortex and white matter near the superior surfaces of the cerebral hemispheres (fig. 11-6). They tend to be bilateral and in close proximity to the pacchionian granulations along the superior sagittal sinus.

Diffuse axonal injury (DAI) often accompanies contusions and is thought to be induced by the rotational forces that produce shear injury. DAI is greatest in areas where the density difference is greatest. For this reason, approximately two thirds of such lesions occur at the gray-white matter junction. (While DAI represents an entity *sui generis*, when encountered in surgical pathology specimens, it is associated with other

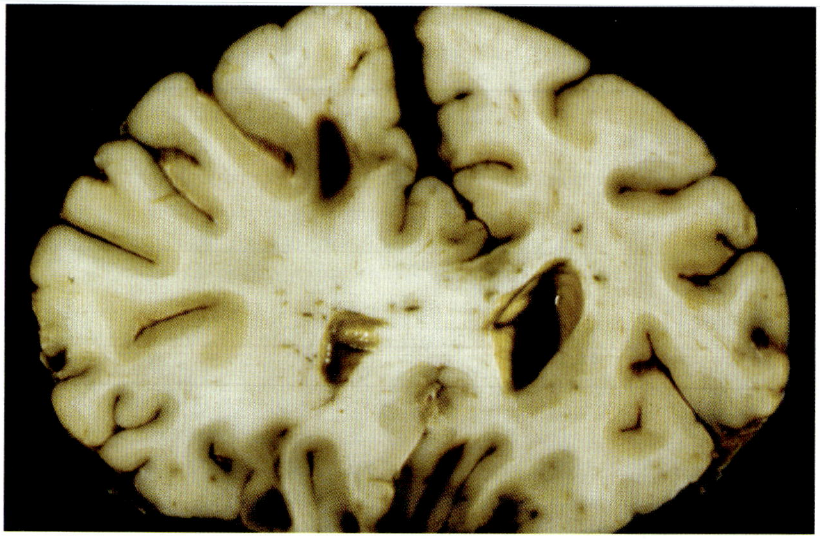

Figure 11-3

CONTRECOUP CONTUSIONS

Recent cortical contusions involve the orbital surfaces, and are associated with cerebral edema and herniation of the left cingulate gyrus. The patient, who fell on the top of his head, lived for 36 hours.

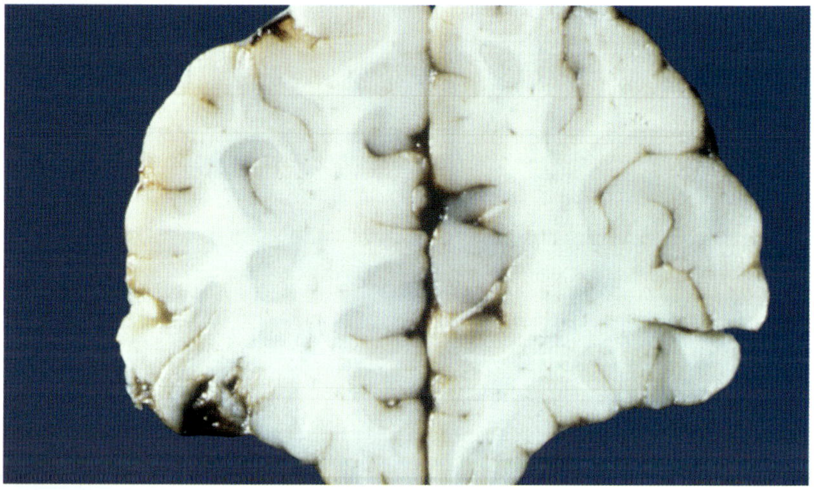

Figure 11-4

FRACTURE CONTUSION

Recent contusion of the left orbital gyri. A basilar fracture involves the anterior cranial fossa.

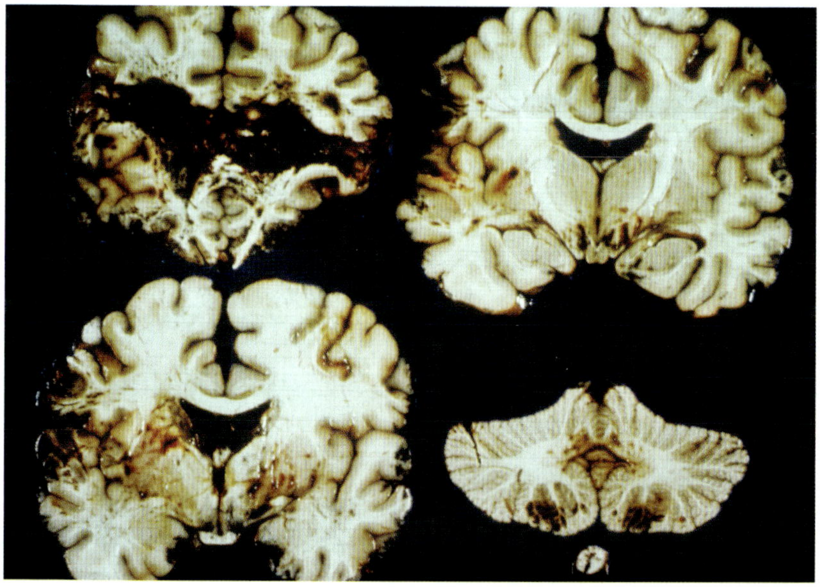

Figure 11-5

HERNIATION CONTUSIONS

Herniation contusions of the cerebellar tonsils are caused by a perforating gunshot wound of the frontal lobes.

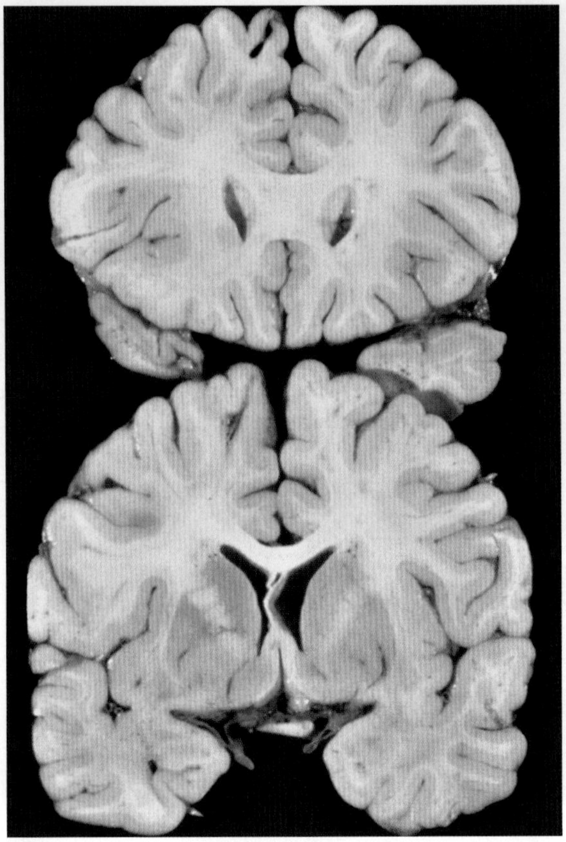

Figure 11-6

GLIDING CONTUSION

An old gliding contusion of the left superior frontal gyrus with cavitation involves the gray-white matter junction and subcortical white matter.

injuries. For this reason, it is discussed in the context of other entities below.)

The identification and classification of contusions require knowledge of the clinical history, type of impacting object, mode and location of impact, and presence or absence of fractures. Without this information, an accurate clinicopathologic correlation is not always possible and the role of the pathologist is limited to a general description of the lesion.

Clinical Features. The presence of recent or old contusions is de facto evidence of traumatic head injury. As noted, head injury is not a single entity but consists of many types of lesions that rarely occur in isolation. Accordingly, the number and extent of the lesions as well as the clinical presentation vary from case to case. Some individuals die suddenly at the time of the impact, while others experience a lucid interval between the time of injury and the development of symptoms and signs. Patients who have DAI generally experience an instantaneous loss of consciousness, and most patients remain in a persistent vegetative state, since brain stem function typically remains unaffected. Still, some contusions are asymptomatic and are discovered as an incidental finding at postmortem examination.

Different clinical features may be present at any given time during the evolution of a contusion, and it is not possible to describe a "classic" clinical picture or syndrome related to traumatic brain injury. The clinical severity of brain damage is commonly assessed by the Glasgow Coma Scale (GCS), which uses an aggregate score based on several parameters to measure functional impairment and level of consciousness, including eye movements, verbal responses, and motor responses (4). The Adelaide modification is available for children. The scores obtained with these two scales allow the classification of brain damage as mild (13 to15), moderate (9 to 12), or severe (3 to 8). There is essentially no correlation between the GCS and the underlying pathologic lesions. Thus, patients with the same GCS may have different pathologic lesions producing functional impairment, and the evolution of the distinct underlying lesions may result in different outcomes.

Radiologic Findings. Skull radiographs and neuroimaging studies are mandatory for the initial evaluation of the trauma patient. Skull radiographs remain the standard tool for the diagnosis of skull fractures. Computerized tomography (CT) scans and magnetic resonance imaging (MRI) are useful to detect contusions and other parenchymal and extraneural hemorrhagic lesions (fig. 11-7). The evolution of the contusion may be followed with serial neuroimaging. Other useful studies include magnetic resonance spectroscopy, which measures levels of metabolites like glutamate to provide a dynamic map of cerebral contusions, and diffusion magnetic resonance imaging and diffusion coefficient mapping, which demonstrate accumulation of edema fluid within necrotic tissue during the period 24 to 72 hours post-trauma (5). Perfusion magnetic resonance imaging may highlight abnormal regional cerebral blood flow in normal-appearing and contused brain (6).

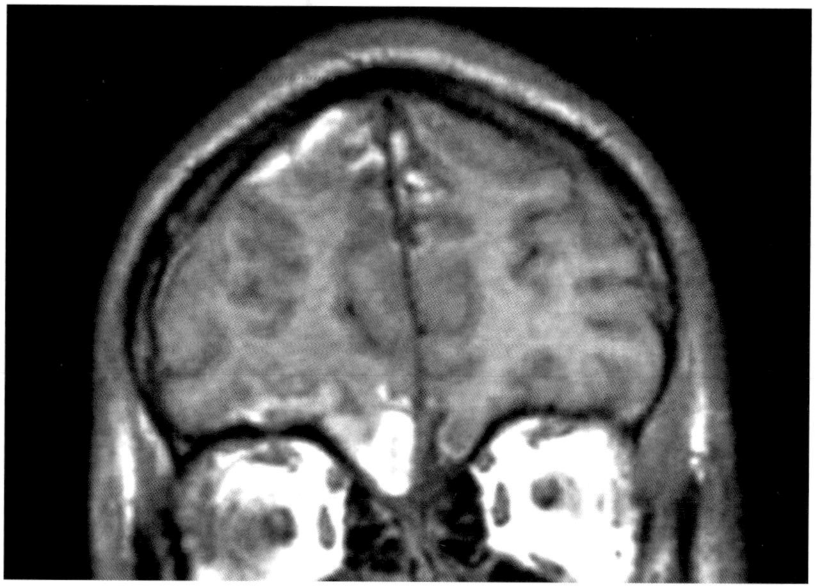

Figure 11-7

CORTICAL CONTUSIONS

There are mixed hemorrhagic and nonhemorrhagic cortical contusions of the frontal lobes, just above the cribriform plates, orbital roof, and planum sphenoidale. Small, poorly defined foci of hemorrhage are scattered throughout larger nonhemorrhagic zones of contusion.

At least half of the patients who have diffuse axonal injury have normal CT scans at presentation. Characteristic CT findings are petechial hemorrhages that are located at the gray-white matter junction, within the corpus callosum, and in the brain stem (fig. 11-8).

Gross Findings. Contusions are recognized as hemorrhagic lesions (bruises) on the superficial areas of the gyri. Cortical contusions are identified by the following cardinal features: location at the crest of the gyri, triangular shape with a wide base at the crest of the gyri and the point at the depth of the cortex or white matter, associated subarachnoid hemorrhage over the lesion, involvement of all cortical layers including the superficial molecular layer, and persistence of intact cortex in the depth of the gyri between two or more involved gyri (fig. 11-9) (3). In rare cases, contusions may be localized to the depth of the sulci.

The morphologic features of contusions evolve over time, depending on the length of survival. In cases of sudden death, hemorrhages are small, punctuate, or elongated, and may be confused with congested blood vessels. If the person survives several minutes, contusions are easily recognized by the columnar arrangement of hemorrhages perpendicular to the surface of the cerebral cortex (fig. 11-10). At 30 to 60 minutes, there may be hemorrhage within the adjacent white matter or hematoma formation, a phenomenon that more frequently occurs in alcoholic and hypertensive persons (fig. 11-11).

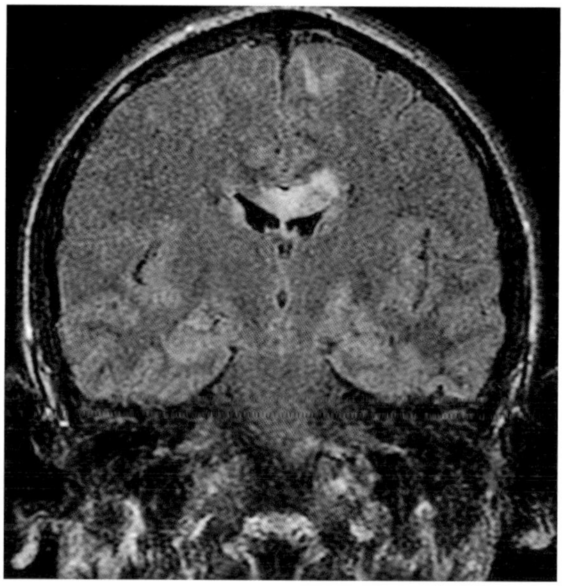

Figure 11-8

DIFFUSE AXONAL INJURY

Coronal fluid-attenuated inversion recovery (FLAIR) demonstrates a bright signal involving the body of the corpus callosum and subcortical white matter.

Over subsequent days, the color of the lesion changes to brown or orange. By 4 weeks, the lesion is a light brown color and by 6 weeks, a rust-brown color. Much later, as the necrotic tissue is ingested and removed by macrophages, the lesion becomes indented or cavitated (fig. 11-12). Cavitation is thought to occur after 6 months. Old, small contusions may be resorbed, without the formation of a cavity, and are identified as spots of yellow cortical discoloration.

The most commonly encountered area in DAI is the frontotemporal white matter at the gray-white matter interface. This site is followed in frequency by the posterior body and splenium of the corpus callosum, the caudate nuclei,

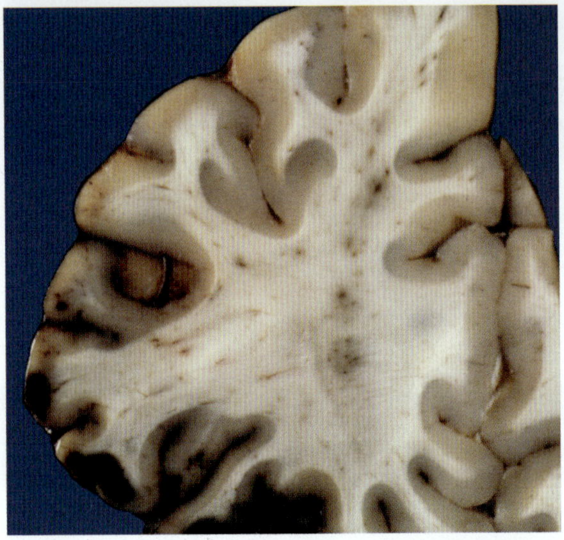

Figure 11-9

CORTICAL CONTUSIONS

Recent hemorrhagic contusions of inferior frontal and orbital gyri are triangular shaped, with their base at the crest of the gyri, and involve all cortical layers.

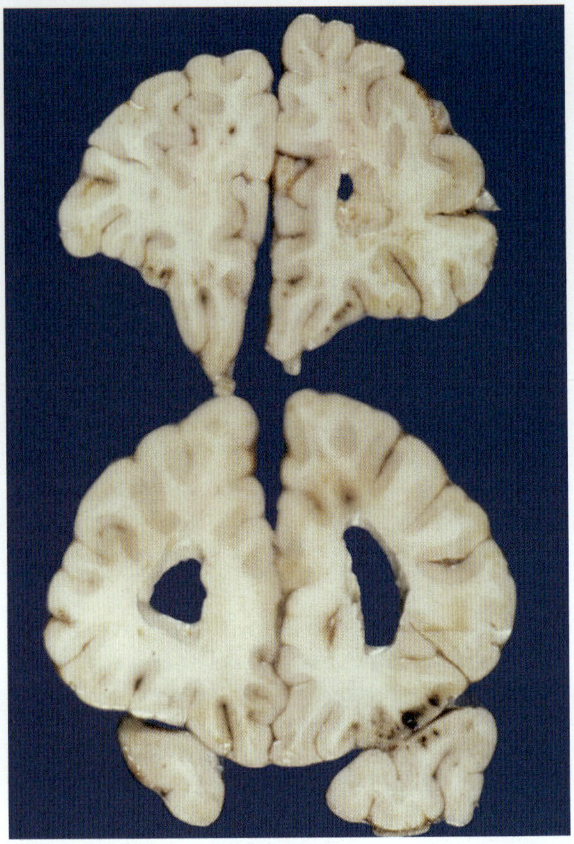

Figure 11-10

CORTICAL CONTUSIONS

The hemorrhages from the recent cortical contusions of the right orbital gyri and temporal pole have a columnar arrangement within the cortex. Survival was short after a motorcycle accident.

Figure 11-11

CORTICAL CONTUSIONS

Recent contusions are associated with hematoma formation.

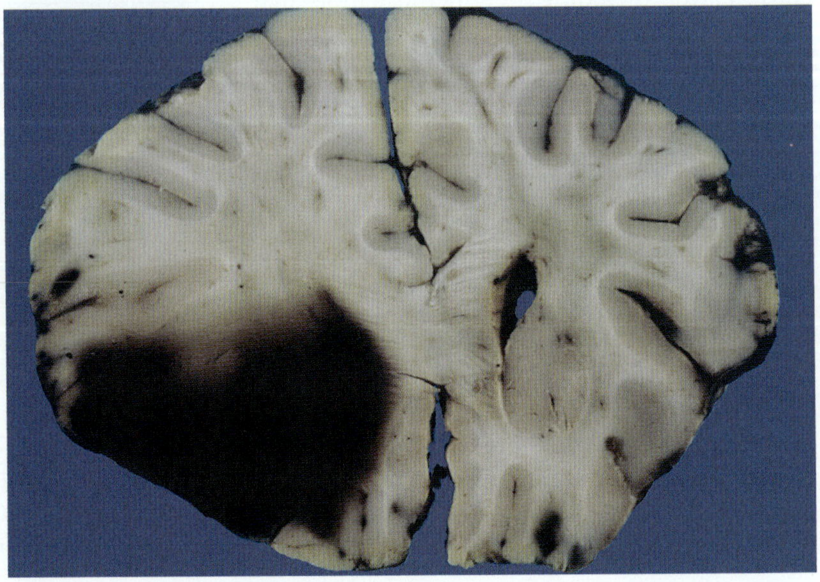

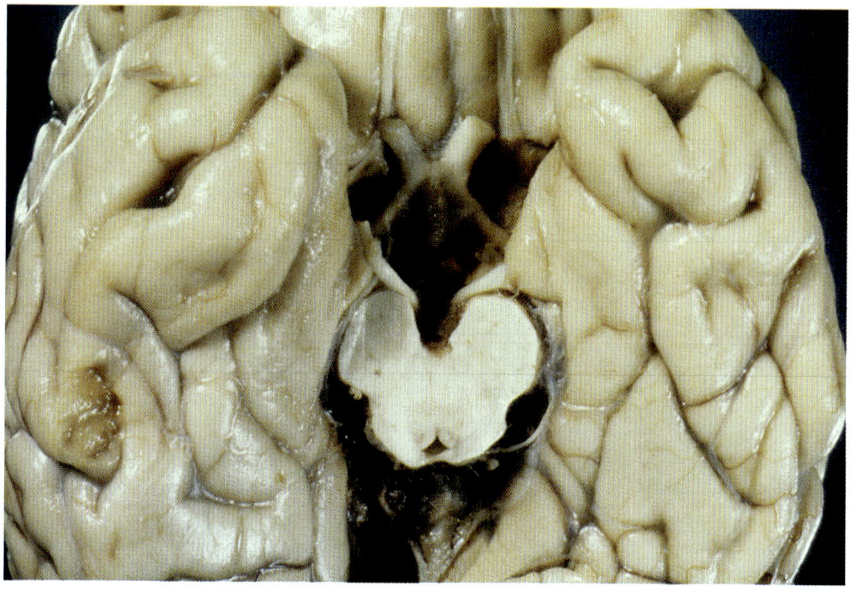

Figure 11-12

CORTICAL CONTUSION

An old contusion of right inferior temporal gyrus, with a cavity covered by the meninges, displays an orange color.

thalamus, tegmentum, and internal capsule. Acute lesions that are grossly visible are characterized by the presence of ovoid to elliptical single or multiple petechial hemorrhages, with the long axis parallel to the direction of the involved axonal tracts (fig. 11 -13) (7).

Microscopic Findings. Contusions have been studied in human tissues as well as in experimental trauma models. It is important to emphasize that one must exercise caution when extrapolating the data from experimental material to the precise age of evolution of the human lesions.

The microscopic features of cortical contusions involve cellular elements both intrinsic and extrinsic to the brain itself. In the acute phase, contusions are composed of a necrotic core, surrounded by a peripheral rim of ischemic non-necrotic tissue or a pericontusional zone. Apoptotic neurons with fragmented nuclei are present in the pericontusional zone, and apoptotic oligodendrocytes and astrocytes in the white matter (8–10).

The initial phase, which occurs within minutes after injury, is heralded by perivascular hemorrhages around small cortical veins and arterioles (3). Examination of the affected blood vessels may show tears within their walls. Expansion of these perivascular hemorrhages may be associated with edema, focal areas of tissue necrosis, and acute neuronal injury, similar to the changes described for cerebral infarct

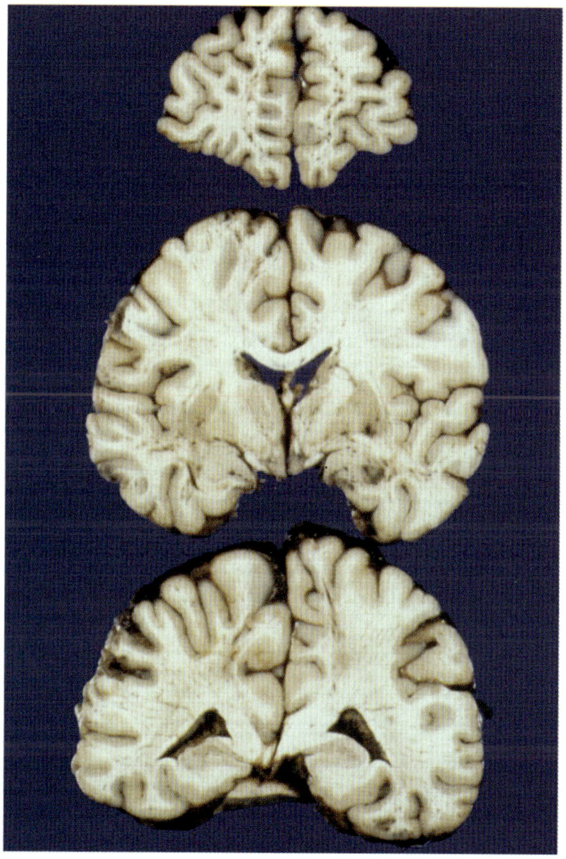

Figure 11-13

DIFFUSE AXONAL INJURY

Diffuse axonal injury is associated with recent petechial hemorrhages involving the cerebral white matter, corpus callosum, and deep gray matter.

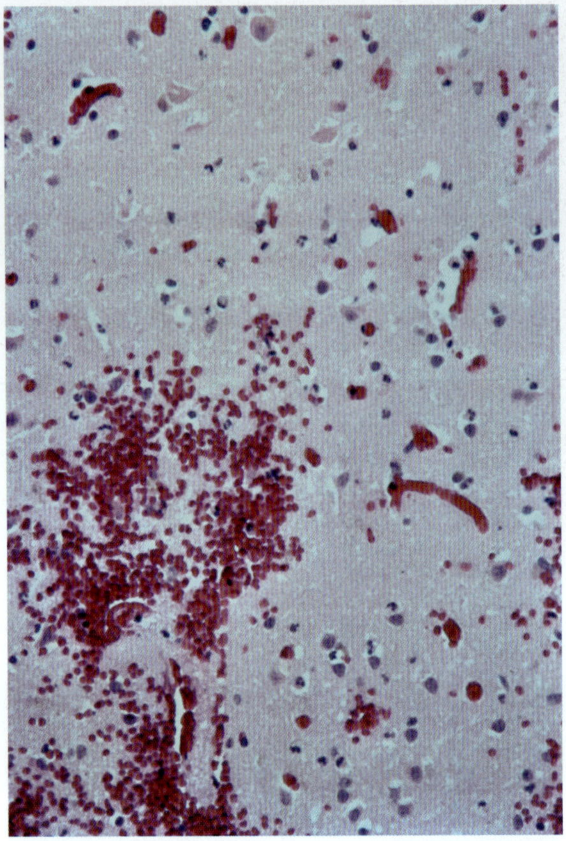

Figure 11-14

CORTICAL CONTUSION

The early phase of organization shows hemorrhages with intact erythrocytes and eosinophilic neurons.

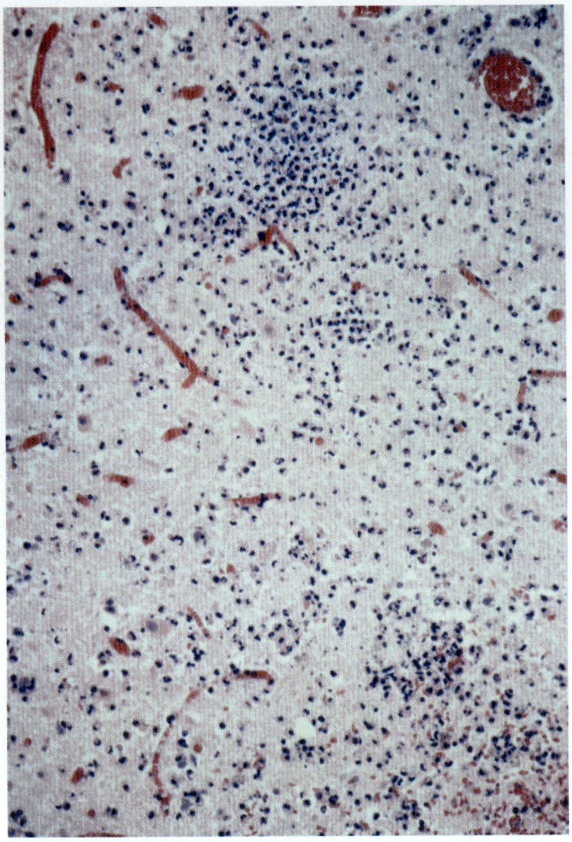

Figure 11-15

CORTICAL CONTUSION

The subacute phase of organization shows infiltration of necrotic tissue by neutrophils, lymphocytes, and macrophages.

and hemorrhage (fig. 11-14) (see chapter 5). Reactive astrocytes are present within 24 to 36 hours. Margination of neutrophils within vessels is identified by 24 hours. By 3 to 5 days, a subacute inflammatory response consisting of neutrophils and lymphocytes emerges, which is associated with macrophages and activated microglia (fig. 11-15) (11). During the next few days, necrotic tissue is removed by phagocytes. Small hemorrhages may be resorbed within 2 to 3 weeks leaving a cavity with scattered hemosiderin-laden macrophages (fig. 11-16); larger lesions may be resorbed after 6 to 12 weeks. At the periphery of the cavities, other features may be observed, including gliosis, proliferation of blood vessels, swollen axons, mineralized neurons, and hemosiderin-laden macrophages and astrocytes. In some cases, the only evidence of a traumatic lesion is the presence of hemosiderin-laden macrophages within the leptomeninges as an indication of focal subarachnoid hemorrhage associated with an old contusion.

DAI is recognized by the presence of axonal spheroids, also known as axonal retraction balls, which are sometimes associated with petechial hemorrhage; these axonal dilatations result from shearing injury and subsequent impaired axonal transport. Retraction balls are visible on routine hematoxylin and eosin (H&E)-stained sections as eosinophilic, round or oval masses, 5 to 40 μm in size (fig. 11-17).

Immunohistochemical Findings. Immunohistochemical preparations complement routine H&E stains in estimating the age of a contusion. Apoptotic neurons in pericontusional areas may express the apoptotic-related genes *p53*, *bcl-2*,

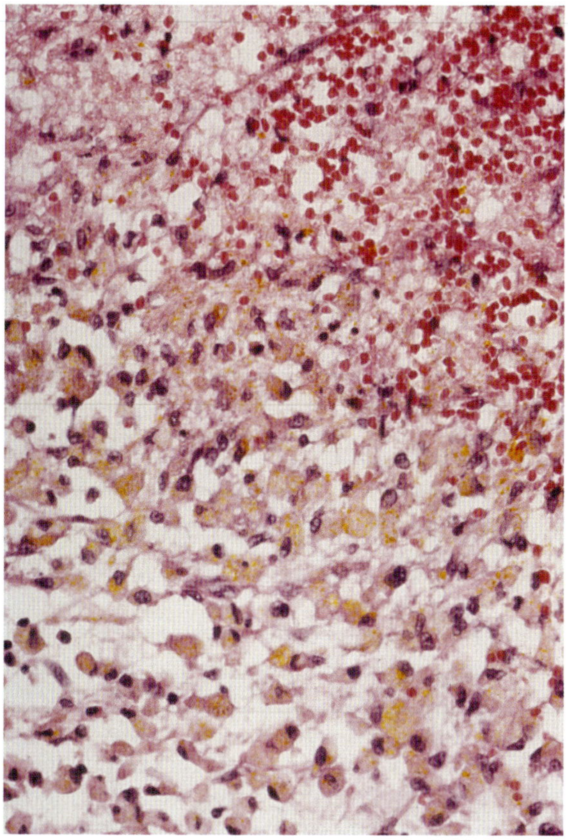

Figure 11-16

CORTICAL CONTUSION

At 37 days post-trauma, there is early cavitation with many hemosiderin-laden macrophages.

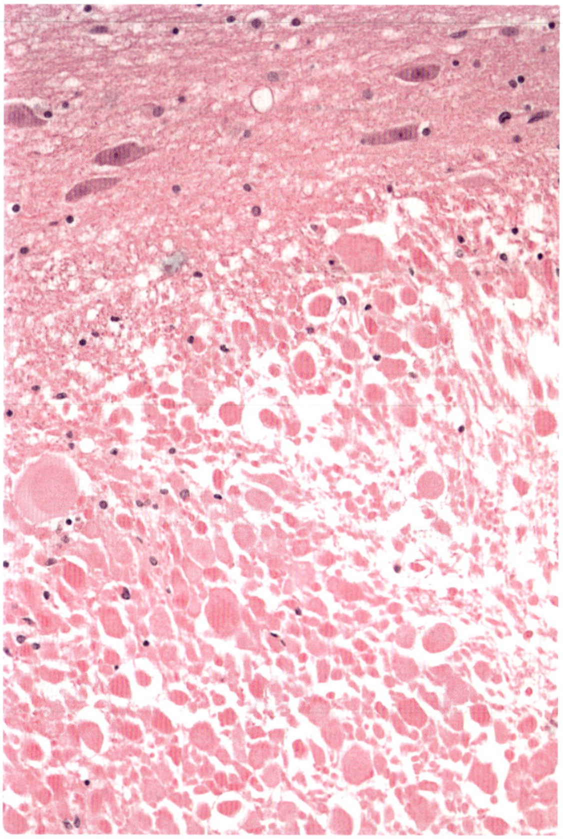

Figure 11-17

DIFFUSE AXONAL INJURY

Groups of spheroids of variable sizes are next to the large neurons of a brain stem cranial nucleus.

and *bax* (17). Such cells can be detected in contusions as early as 45 minutes after injury, tend to peak at 1 day postinjury, and persist for at least 22 days (12,13). Macrophages and activated microglia expressing the macrophage-related protein-8 (MRP-8) and MRP-14 are present after at least 72 hours. CD15-positive neutrophils are detectable after 10 minutes. Mononuclear cells express CD45 (leucocyte common antigen) at 1 day, CD3 at 2 days, and UCHL-1 at 3.7 days (14). The above immunohistochemical markers are largely restricted to investigational use and are not required or sufficient to determine the age of a contusion.

Both silver impregnation methods and beta-amyloid precursor protein (APP) immunohistochemical staining have proven useful in the pathologic identification of DAI lesions. APP immunostaining of damaged axons is more sensitive than silver impregnation for detecting early lesions (fig. 11-18).

Ultrastructural Findings. Ultrastructural studies of pericontusional tissues in humans have shown swelling of astrocytic processes and narrowing of microvascular lumens, which may contain erythrocytes and leucocytes (8). Endothelial cells may exhibit increased pinocytotic activity, swelling, and well-preserved tight junctions (15). The neuronal changes related to acute injury are similar to those seen in cerebral infarct.

Laboratory Findings. The diagnosis of brain injury is based on the combined evaluation of clinical, radiologic, and pathologic findings. Serological markers indicative of neuronal (neuron-specific enolase) and glial (S-100 protein)

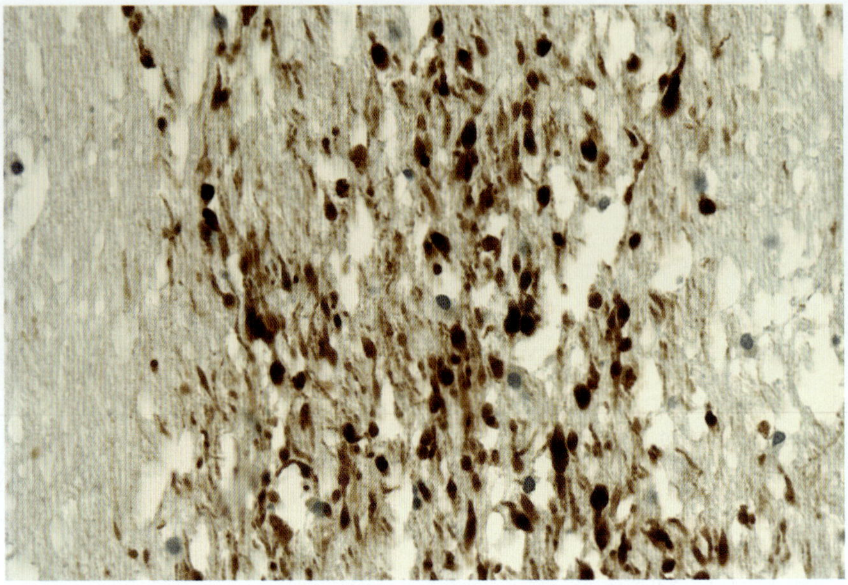

Figure 11-18

DIFFUSE AXONAL INJURY

Swollen axons are strongly immunoreactive for beta-amyloid precursor protein.

origin may be detected in the serum 1 to 3 days after traumatic brain injury (16).

Differential Diagnosis. The leading entity in the differential diagnosis of a cortical contusion is a hemorrhagic infarct associated with cortical petechia. On macroscopic examination, an infarct tends to follow a specific arterial territory. It involves the depth of the sulcus and may include the crest of the gyrus, while sparing the molecular layer. Contusions do not follow an arterial distribution, are usually restricted to the crest of the gyri, spare the depth of sulci, are triangular in shape with the base on the cortex, and are associated with subarachnoid hemorrhage. On the other hand, many cellular reactions relating to tissue response, including gliosis and inflammation, are common to both entities. On microscopic examination, the key differences include preservation of the external, molecular layer of the cerebral cortex in an infarct (as opposed to the compromise of all cortical layers by contusions) and the frequent presence of subarachnoid hemorrhage accompanying a contusion (fig. 11-19). The status of the molecular layer is best evaluated if sections are taken through the middle of the lesion, since the edges of this layer may be intact in both contusions and infarcts.

Treatment and Prognosis. Patients with cerebral contusions who develop edema, progressive elevation of intracranial pressure, mass effect, and clinical deterioration may require craniotomy and excision of necrotic tissue in an attempt to control the elevated intracranial pressure and clinical deterioration (5). Microscopic findings of apoptosis in tissue sections may herald a worse prognosis for patients with acute neurologic damage following traumatic brain injury (9). Some patients with expression of antiapoptotic bcl-2 have an improved outcome at the 6-month follow-up examination (17).

EPIDURAL HEMATOMA

Definition. *Epidural hematoma* (EDH) is an acute extravasation of blood between the inner table of the skull and the dural membrane, often associated with fractures and lacerations of the dural vessels, most often meningeal arteries and veins but occasionally a dural sinus.

General Comments. Although far less common than subdural hematoma, EDH is an acutely life-threatening complication of head injury, requiring immediate surgical intervention in the majority of cases. Two thirds of epidural hematomas are in the temporoparietal region and involve the middle meningeal artery. These lesions are typically limited by the firm attachment of the dura at the suture margins, but they may cross the midline, especially with superior sagittal sinus lacerations, and they also can bridge the supratentorial and infratentorial compartments, with tears along the torcula and transverse sinuses. Skull fractures occur in the majority of adults with EDH, but are less

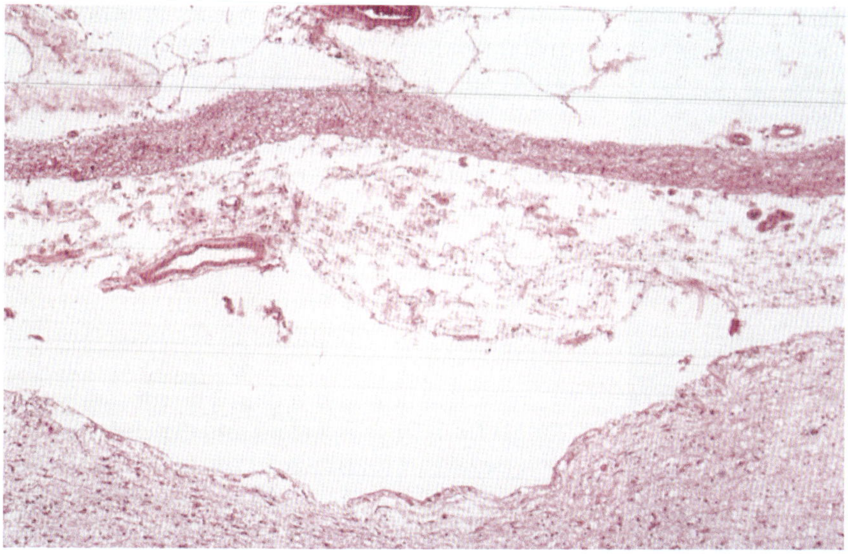

Figure 11-19

DIFFERENTIAL DIAGNOSIS OF CORTICAL CONTUSIONS

The cortical external molecular layer is preserved in an old cavitated infarct.

common in children because of the plasticity of the immature skull. In children, a posterior fossa location is most common. EDH associated with venous injuries tends to be smaller and associated with a more benign course, and in certain patients, may be treated nonsurgically. Spinal EDH also occurs, with the dorsal aspect of the thoracic or lumbar region involved. Unless otherwise indicated, most comments in this chapter are restricted to intracranial examples.

Clinical Features. EDH should be suspected in any individual who sustains craniocerebral trauma. The classic clinical presentation is that of a patient who experiences a "lucid interval" between the initial loss of consciousness at the time of impact; however, variable alterations in the level of consciousness have been described. Posterior fossa EDH can be associated with fulminating progression from minimal symptoms to death within minutes (18).

Radiologic Findings. Immediate, unenhanced CT scan is the diagnostic procedure of choice (fig. 11-20). EDH forms an extraaxial lenticular or biconvex homogeneous mass. Focal isodense or hypodense lesions indicate active bleeding. CT scan also has the capability of allowing visualization of the location, volume, and presence of mass effect and other significant signs of intracranial injury.

Gross and Microscopic Findings. EDH is a hematoma, or freshly clotted blood, that collects in the plane between the skull bone and the dura (fig. 11-21). As discussed below under Differential Diagnosis, microscopic examination is of primary importance in excluding other contributing causes.

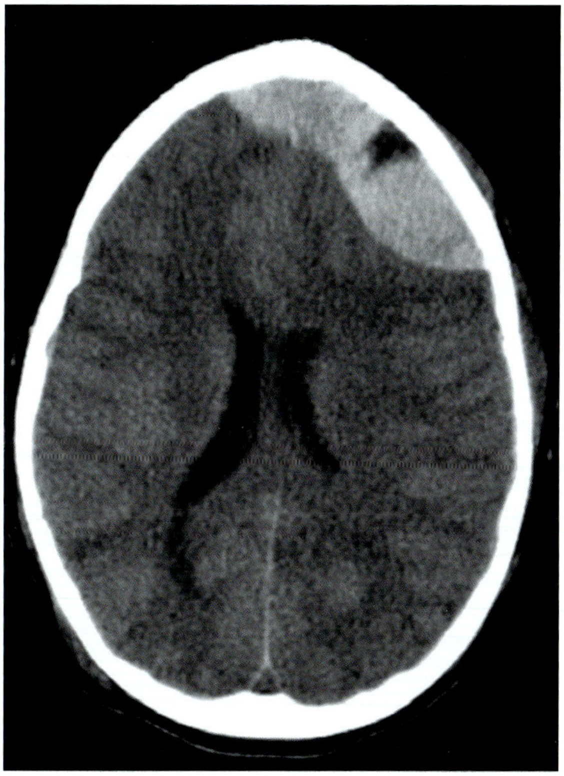

Figure 11-20

EPIDURAL HEMATOMA

A large frontal extraaxial mass is seen. The hematoma is biconvex and crosses the midline anteriorly.

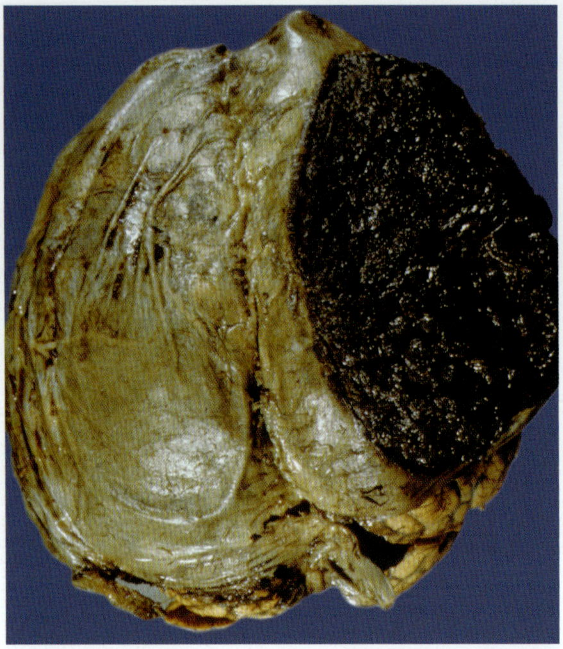

Figure 11-21

EPIDURAL HEMATOMA

Recent epidural hemorrhage over the cerebral convexities.

Ultrastructural, Immunohistochemical, and Laboratory Findings. Electron microscopy and immunohistochemistry have little place in the routine pathologic evaluation of EDH. No specific laboratory tests are required for the diagnosis of EDH. The determination of the coagulation status, however, is important in predicting patient outcome. Similar to other severe head injuries, which can result in disseminated intravascular coagulation due to the release of tissue thromboplastins, EDH can be associated with life-threatening hemodynamic instability.

Differential Diagnosis. Rarely, spontaneous (nontraumatic) epidural hematoma is ascribed to causes such as coagulopathies associated with other medical problems (disease states associated with dysfunctional platelets), infection, vascular malformations, or underlying malignant disease (19). As with all fresh hematoma specimens (see chapter 5), careful examination for coexisting pathologies should be undertaken, for example, to diagnose a previously unrecognized metastatic tumor.

Since the spinal epidural space is an already existing space, more processes occur here and enter the differential diagnosis. A number of inflammatory and vascular conditions may affect the spinal epidural space. These are discussed in chapter 8 and include extramedullary hematopoiesis and histiocytic lesions. Another rare condition that may mimic EDH is Foix-Alajouanine syndrome, which results from an arteriovenous (AV) fistula of the spinal dura mater (see chapter 6).

Treatment and Prognosis. In the majority of cases, EDH is a neurosurgical emergency that requires the placement of a burr hole and immediate evacuation and repair. The mortality rate ranges from 5 to 43 percent and depends on such diverse factors as the age of the patient (patients younger than 5 years and older than 55 years have an increased mortality rate), GCS, size of the hematoma, and the presence of associated subdural lesions. Not surprisingly, patients who present in deep coma have the worst prognosis. Patients over the age of 60 are less likely to develop EDH because the dura is strongly adherent to the inner table of the skull (18).

SUBDURAL HEMATOMA

Definition. *Subdural hematoma* (SDH) is a space-occupying collection of blood in the subdural space, which usually results from traumatic brain injury. Lacerated bridging veins pass from the surface of the brain to the dural sinuses.

General Comments. Bleeding into the subdural space may be associated with a thin-layered collection of blood without major clinical consequences, or with the formation of a life-threatening space-occupying hematoma that requires prompt surgical evacuation. Such bleeds result from traumatic and nontraumatic causes. Brain trauma is the leading cause of SDH: acute SDH is present in 25 percent of individuals who have sustained traumatic brain injury (1). Nontraumatic factors include coagulopathies, chronic alcohol abuse, chronic dialysis associated with the use of anticoagulants, rupture of a saccular aneurysm, and primary and metastatic neoplasms including meningioma, lymphoma, and metastatic carcinoma (20–22). Most traumatic SDHs are related to tears in bridging veins traveling in the subdural space of the frontoparietal region, parasagittal region, or base of the temporal lobe. A few cases may be related to lacerations of superficial cortical branches of the middle cerebral artery (23). Still others result from extension of a subarachnoid hemorrhage into the subdural space through a tear of the leptomeninges, laceration of the carotid and vertebral arteries or the vein of Galen where these vessels pass through the subdural space, and lacerations of cortical veins and arteries at the site of the contusion (3).

The time for accumulation of blood is variable: some hematomas develop rapidly, within minutes after the traumatic event, whereas others develop slowly in a multistep fashion. Blood moves freely within the subdural space and the hematoma may involve a single or several intracranial compartments. The majority are localized over the convexity of the cerebral hemispheres, extending from the frontal to the parietal, occipital, and temporal regions. Extension to the base of the brain may occur. Hematomas in the posterior fossa and along the cerebral interhemispheric fissure are rare.

In contrast to EDH, not all traumatic SDHs are associated with skull fractures and SDH may occur away from the site of the impact. Common traumatic events for the development of SDH include falls and blunt impacts. SDH is less common after traffic accidents. Some may develop after traumatic injuries not involving primarily the CNS. SDHs without impact are usually produced by inertial forces and are classified as diffuse traumatic lesions, such as occurs with the rotational movement of the head associated with sudden acceleration/deceleration. A SDH may be the only lesion in traumatic head injury (pure hematoma); however, other lesions, including bleeding at other sites and contusions, are often present.

Clinical Features. The clinical presentation depends on the size of the hematoma and the time it takes to develop. According to the clinical presentation, the hematoma is classified as acute, subacute, or chronic. Acute hematomas are associated with signs and symptoms that start within a few days of the injury. If the clinical presentation takes 2 to 3 weeks to develop, the hematoma is classified as subacute. Lesions older than 4 weeks are designated chronic hematomas. Chronic hematomas are usually not associated with a history of previous trauma, or they correspond to traumatic hematomas in which a period of recovery is followed by symptoms of increased intracranial pressure, which may be related to rebleeding.

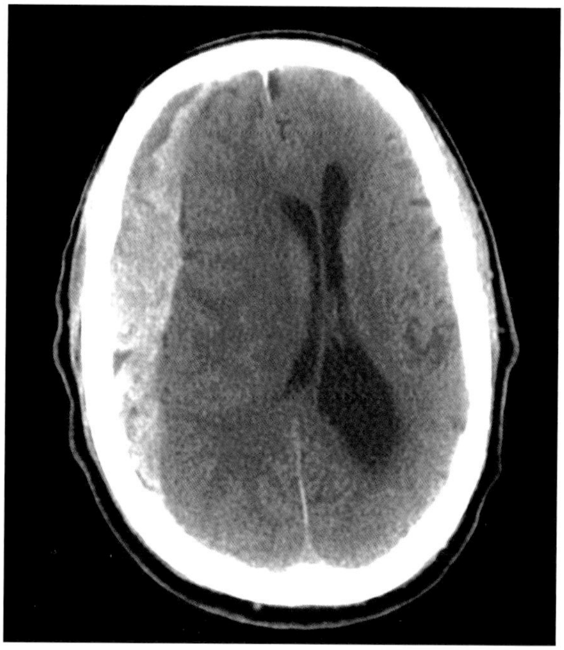

Figure 11-22

SUBDURAL HEMATOMA

This subdural hematoma features a crescentic hyperdense area overlying the right cerebral cortex, causing midline shift and subfalcine herniation.

Acute SDHs are unilateral in most cases; chronic hematomas are bilateral in 15 to 21 percent of cases (24). Risk factors for the development of a chronic subdural hematoma include hygromas and arachnoid cysts (24,25). Chronic hematomas are more frequent in the elderly, with an incidence of 7/100,000 for persons over 70 years of age (26).

As the hematoma enlarges, it tends to compress the brain and complications result from the shift of cerebral midline structures to the opposite site and from herniation. The clinical presentation of acute SDH may include an interval free of symptoms between the traumatic episode and the onset of headache, followed by confusion, loss of consciousness, and coma. The clinical presentation of chronic SDH is related to cognitive changes including confusion, dementia, behavioral changes, lethargy, sleep disturbances, and altered psychomotor activity (26).

Radiologic Findings. Neuroimaging findings should be correlated with the pathologic findings (fig. 11-22). Acute SDHs are hyperintense in comparison to brain structures on CT scan.

This is because of the presence of clotted blood during the first 7 to 10 days. As lysis of the blood clot progresses, the lesion reaches the subacute stage, and variable areas of intensity are seen on CT. Chronic SDHs are hypointense or isodense lesions on T1-weighted MRI and predominantly hyperintense on T2-weighted images. Localized dural enhancement may occur after gadolinium administration (27).

Gross Findings. Most surgical specimens are composed solely of fresh blood clot or, in the case of older lesions, fragments of organizing hematoma. Nonetheless, it is important to consider the known macroscopic changes that characterize the typical spectrum of SDH. Although these are best visualized at autopsy, the changes can be seen in fragmented surgical specimens as well.

The process of organization of a SDH is primarily related to the inner or meningeal layer of the dura. The leptomeninges do not participate in this reaction and there is no physiologic relationship between the hematoma and these membranes. Neurosurgeons may refer to the lesion as acute if it is composed of clotted blood (fig. 11-23), subacute if there is a mixture of clotted blood and fluid, and chronic if only fluid is present, but the pathologic spectrum of subacute and chronic SDH is wider, particularly at autopsy. Chronic SDH is usually encapsulated by a fibrous membrane, which is always present after 8 weeks. This membrane may cover the surface of the hematoma facing the leptomeninges, and in such cases, the lesion adheres to the dura (fig. 11-24). In other cases, the neomembrane extends over the entire circumference of the hematoma, which appears freely movable within the subdural space. As the organization of the hematoma progresses, the most prominent feature in the final stages is a neomembrane of variable thickness attached to the dura (fig. 11-25). Typically, the thicker aspect of the membrane is adjacent to the overlying dura mater. Areas of recent hemorrhage related to rupture of small vascular channels may be present as evidence of rebleeding, giving some chronic lesions a multicystic appearance. After 2 to 3 years, the neomembrane may be difficult to identify and the pathologist should focus attention on areas of brown or yellow discoloration on the dura; such cases are typically encountered at autopsy, rather than as surgical specimens.

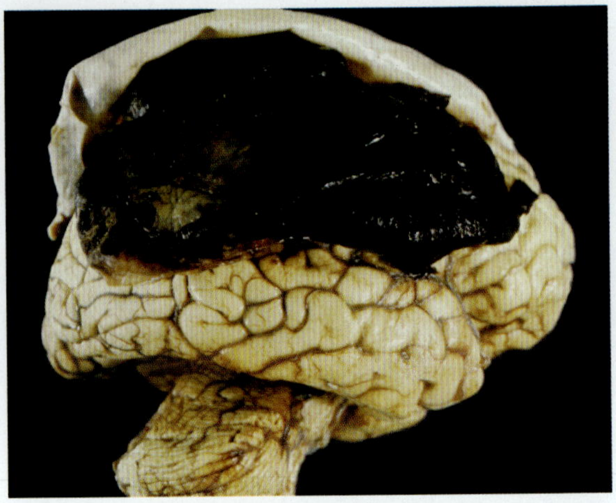

Figure 11-23

ACUTE SUBDURAL HEMATOMA

A nonencapsulated acute subdural hematoma.

At autopsy, when fresh or encapsulated hematomas are present, attempts are made to preserve the hematoma in situ and to sample the dura, the full thickness of the hematoma, and the capsule. For surgical specimens, this is not possible, but attempts at orientation of the fragments of subacute or chronic SDH should be undertaken. Enough representative sampling should be done to ensure adequate examination, for evaluation of the hematoma but, equally importantly, to rule out the presence of coexisting lesions (e.g., metastases).

Microscopic Findings. Organization of the hematoma starts with infiltration by inflammatory cells as well as proliferation of fibroblasts and vascular channels from the dural side of the lesion, which lead to the formation of granulation tissue and a fibrous neomembrane (3). Neutrophils are identified at around 14 hours (fig. 11-26). By 5 days, there are hemosiderin-laden macrophages, and the neomembrane shows a layer of 3 to 7 fibroblasts in thickness (fig. 11-27). The formation of granulation tissue with fibroblasts, delicate vascular channels, collagen deposition, macrophages, and inflammation is prominent in the next 10 to 20 days after the injury (fig. 11-28). During days 20 to 30, granulation tissue is replaced by compact fibrous tissue. Between days 30 and 90, an encapsulating membrane with abundant vascular channels and hemosiderin-laden macrophages is present (fig.11-29). Infiltration with

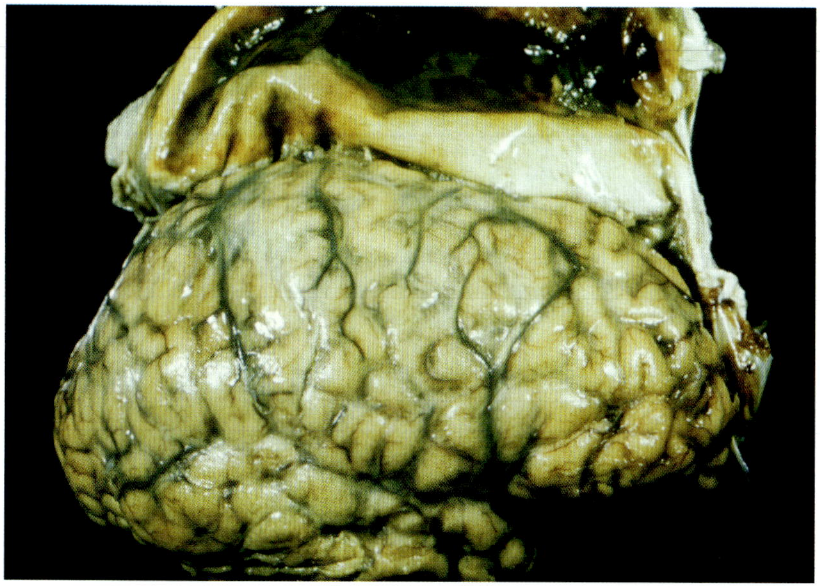

Figure 11-24

CHRONIC SUBDURAL HEMATOMA

A hematoma is encapsulated by a neomembrane attached to the meningeal surface of the dura.

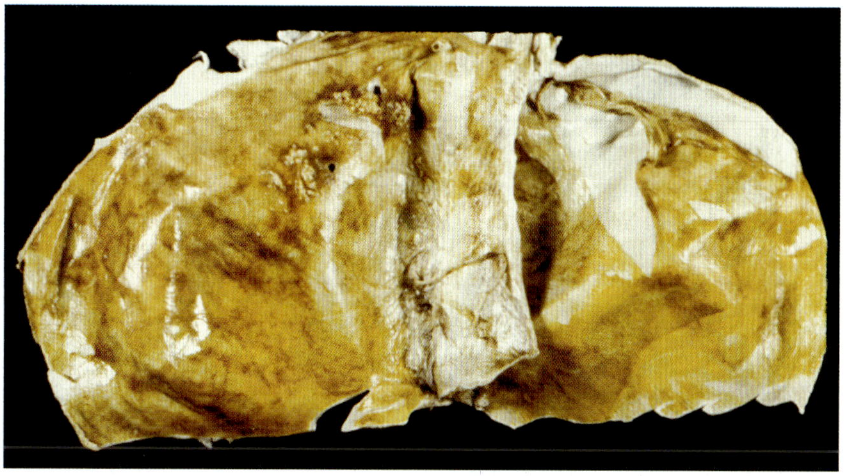

Figure 11-25

CHRONIC SUBDURAL HEMATOMA

Organized bilateral subdural hemorrhage with the formation of orange-brown neomembranes.

eosinophils in well-vascularized and hyalinized granulation tissue of the subdural membrane (often in the inner layer of the outer membrane) is common, especially in cases with a duration of more than 3 months (28). It is postulated that eosinophils may have an important role in the repair and healing processes of these membranes, and should not necessarily raise the index of suspicion for an infectious process. After 6 months, the membrane reaches its final stage and it is no longer possible to estimate the approximate age of the hematoma (fig. 11-30). Some hematomas undergo calcification.

Although detailed data exist, as discussed above, on the histologic changes that correlate with the age of the SDH, some of these estimates are based on experimental models. As a result, a precise determination of the age of an SDH based solely on microscopic findings is not reliable in surgical or autopsy material (fig. 11-31). Factors that limit this procedure include selective tissue sampling at surgery or during surgical pathology processing, intrinsic variability in organization rates, and the common loss of the relationship between the hematoma and the dura during surgical procedures or at the time of the autopsy.

Immunohistochemical Findings. Macrophage activity within an SDH may be demonstrated with immunohistochemistry for major histocompatability complex (MHC) class II antigens. Expression of these cellular markers differs between the dura and the hematoma

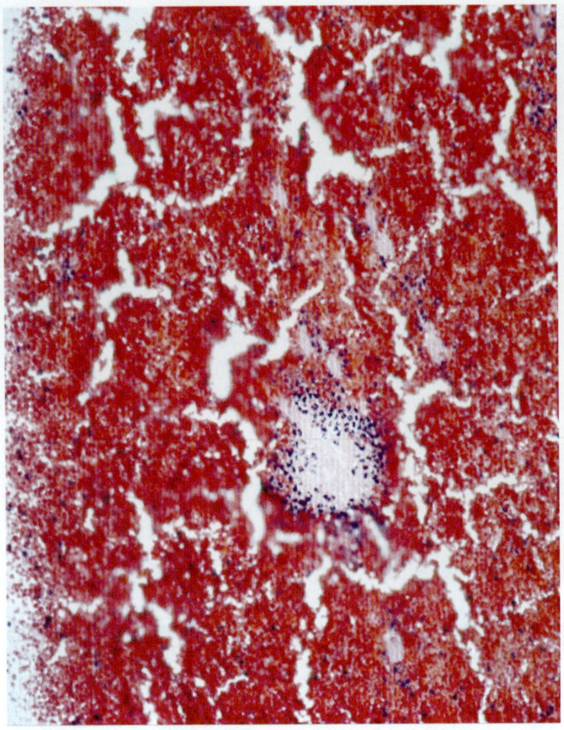

Figure 11-26

SUBDURAL HEMATOMA

A focus of neutrophils and fibrin in an 8-hour-old acute subdural hematoma.

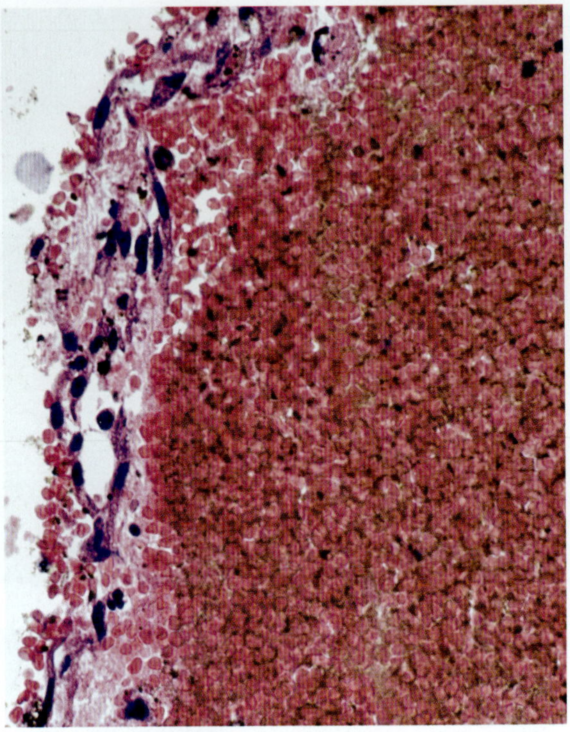

Figure 11-27

SUBDURAL HEMATOMA

A 4-day-old acute subdural hematoma. The formation of the neomembrane by fibroblastic and vascular proliferation is beginning.

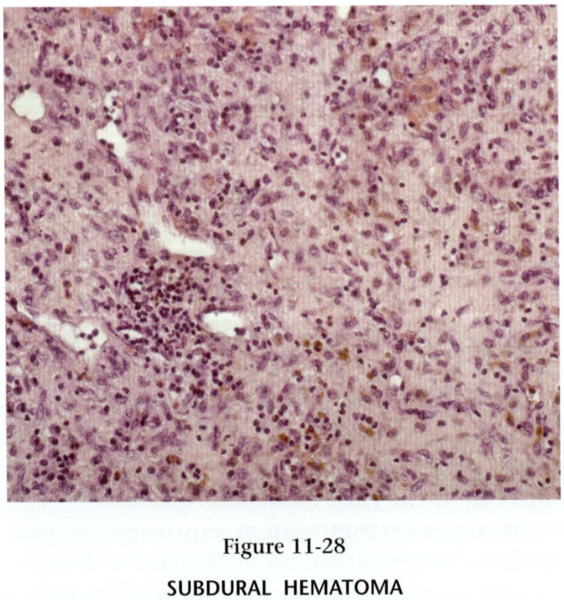

Figure 11-28

SUBDURAL HEMATOMA

Well-developed granulation tissue is seen in a 20-day-old subdural hematoma.

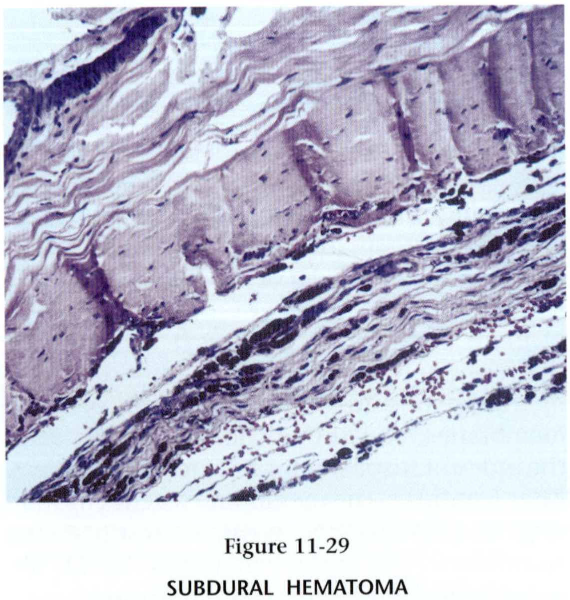

Figure 11-29

SUBDURAL HEMATOMA

The formation of a neomembrane comprised of fibrous tissue, delicate vascular channels, and hemosiderin-laden macrophages is seen in a chronic subdural hematoma at 60 days.

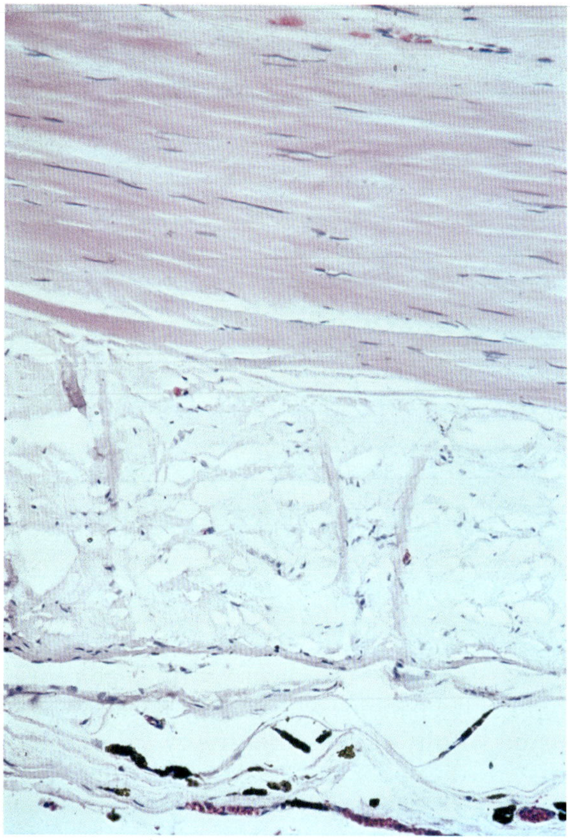

Figure 11-30

SUBDURAL HEMATOMA

An organized subdural hematoma that is older than 6 months shows a dense fibrous neomembrane and a few hemosiderin-laden macrophages.

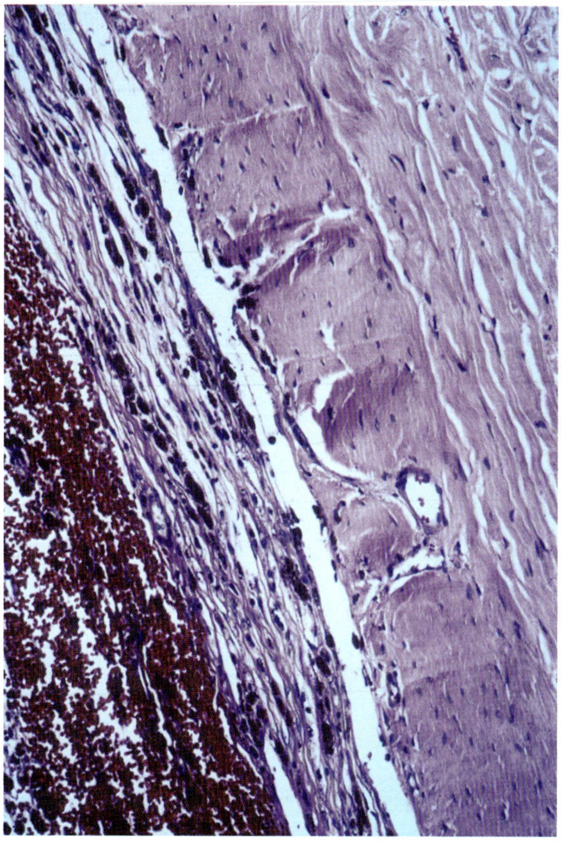

Figure 11-31

SUBDURAL HEMATOMA

An organized subdural hematoma with rebleeding has intact erythrocytes.

(29). MHC II antigen expression is usually localized to the inner surface of the dura, is detected within 24 hours after the injury, and is more prominent after 10 days. CD68 expression is usually present within the hematoma 24 to 48 hours post-trauma.

Ultrastructural Findings. The encapsulating membrane includes fibroblasts, mast cells, erythrocytes, platelets, eosinophils, and bundles of collagen fibrils. There are abundant blood vessels with endothelial cells exhibiting gap junctions and thin or absent basal lamina. The fragility of the vascular walls may be related to the appearance of the basal lamina or affected by secretion of plasminogen by the eosinophils (30).

Laboratory Findings. Coagulation abnormalities may underlie cases of chronic SDH, and may exacerbate all types of SDH. In addition, coagulation abnormalities have long been recognized in patients with existing head injuries, perhaps as a result of the release of thromboplastic materials by damaged brain tissue.

Differential Diagnosis. SDH with early granulation tissue formation may be confused with highly vascular or pigmented neoplasms. Granulation tissue usually shows cells with large, irregular, hyperchromatic nuclei, which may be interpreted as atypical neoplastic cells (fig. 11-32). Also, granulation tissue tends to be well vascularized, with channels of variable caliber and thickness. It may show mitoses, and hemosiderin that may resemble melanin. In such cases, a cautious diagnostic approach is advised to exclude primary or metastatic melanoma, choriocarcinoma, angiosarcoma, of metastatic poorly differentiated carcinomas. Stains for

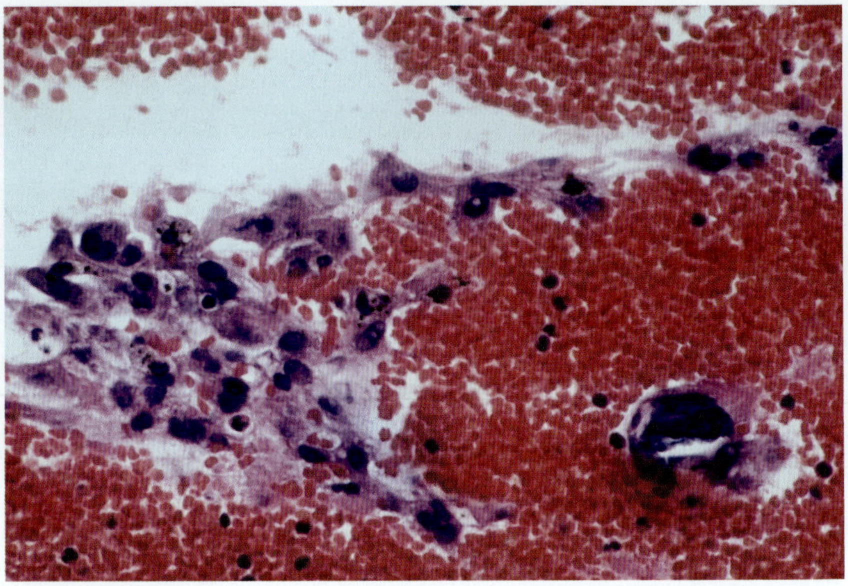

Figure 11-32

NUCLEAR CHANGES IN SUBDURAL HEMATOMA

Early granulation tissue formation shows nuclear changes simulating malignancy and mitosis.

iron and immunohistochemical markers for melanocytes, germ cells, and epithelial cells should be performed when doubt remains. CNS angiosarcomas are extremely rare and have distinctive histopathologic features. Inflammatory masses, such as those discussed in chapter 8, may resemble SDH, particularly in chronic SDH with prominent histiocytes. Extramedullary hematopoiesis may occur as a mass in the subdural space, but can be diagnosed by the characteristic hematopoietic elements (see chapter 8).

Treatment and Prognosis. Despite advances in the treatment of traumatic brain injury, the mortality rate for patients with acute SDH is 60 to 90 percent. This high mortality rate is related to the complications that accompany other lesions found with SDH including contusions, lacerations, subarachnoid hemorrhage, DAI, hypotension, and global ischemia. Intracranial hypertension is probably the main cause of global ischemia. A survival rate of 70 percent is reported in patients whose acute SDH was evacuated within 4 hours after injury (31). Factors that predict poor recovery include increasing age, an interval greater than 6 hours between fixed pupils and craniotomy, and compression of the basal cisterns (32).

Chronic SDH is one of the most common lesions treated by neurosurgeons. The extent of surgical treatment and the standard therapy are controversial. Treatment modalities include twist drill craniotomy, burr hole craniotomy, enlarged craniectomy, and extended craniotomy, with partial membranectomy and drainage in the last two procedures. Recurrence rates of 2.7 to 37.0 percent have been described with some of these approaches (33,34).

REFERENCES

1. Hlatky R, Valadka AB, Goodman JC, Robertson CC. Evolution of brain tissue injury after evacuation of acute traumatic subdural hematomas. Neurosurgery 2004;55:1318-1323.
2. Ellison D, Love S, Chimelli L, Harding BN, Lowe J, Vinters HV. Neuropatholgy, 2nd ed. Edinburgh: Mosby; 2004:241-269.
3. Lindenberg R. Trauma of the meninges and brain. In: Minckler J, ed. Pathology of the nervous system, Vol 2. New York: McGraw-Hill; 1971:1705-1764.
4. Teasdale G, Jennett B. Assessment of coma and impaired consciouness. A practical scale. Lancet 1974;2:81-84.
5. Katayama Y, Kawamata T. Edema fluid accumulation within necrotic brain tissue as a cause of the mass effect of cerebral contusion in head trauma patients. Acta Neurochir Suppl 2003;86:323-327.
6. Garnett MR, Blamire AM, Corkill RG, et al. Abnormal cerebral blood volume in regions of contused and normal appearing brain following traumatic brain injury using perfusion magnetic resonance imaging. J Neurotrauma 2001;18:585-593.
7. Adams JH, Jennett B, McLellan DR, et al. The neuropathology of the vegetative state after head injury. J Clin Pathol 1999;52:804-806.
8. Schroder ML, Muizelaar JP, Bullock MR, Salvant JB, Povlishock JT. Focal ischemia due to traumatic contusions documented by stable xenon-CT and ultrastructural studies. J Neurosurg 1995;82:966-971.
9. Nathoo N, Narotam PK, Agrawal DK, et al. Influence of apoptosis on neurological outcome following traumatic cerebral contusion. J Neurosurg 2004;101:233-240.
10. Raghupathi R, Graham DI, McIntosh TK. Apoptosis after traumatic brain injury. J Neurotrauma 2000;17:927-938.
11. Holmin S, Soderlund J, Biberfeld P, Mathiesen T. Intracerebral inflammation after human brain contusion. Neurosurgery 1998;42:291-298.
12. Hausmann R, Biermann T, Wiest I, Tubel J, Betz P. Neuronal apoptosis following human brain injury. Int J Legal Med 2004;118:32-36.
13. Smith FM, Raghupathi R, MacKinnon MH, et al. TUNEL-positive staining of surface contusions after fatal head injury in man. Acta Neuropathol (Berl) 2000;100:537-545.
14. Hausmann R, Kaiser A, Lang C, Bohnert M, Betz P. A quantitative immunohistochemical study on the time-dependent course of acute inflammatory cellular response to human brain injury. Int J Legal Med 1999;112:227-232.
15. Vaz R, Sarmento A, Borges N, Cruz C, Azevedo I. Ultrastructural study of brain microvessels in patients with traumatic cerebral contusions. Acta Neurochir (Wien) 1997;139:215-220.
16. Herrmann M, Jost S, Kutz S, et al. Temporal profile of release of neurobiochemical markers of brain damage after traumatic brain injury is associated with intracranial pathology as demonstrated in cranial computerized tomography. J Neurotrauma 2000;17:113-122.
17. Ng I, Yeo TT, Tang WY, Soong R, Ng PY, Smith D. Apoptosis occurs after cerebral contusions in humans. Neurosurgery 2000;46:949-956.
18. Rivas J, Lobato R, Sarabia R, Cordobes F, Cabrera A, Gomez P. Extradural hematoma: analysis of factors influencing the courses of 161 patients. Neurosurgery 1988;23:44-51.
19. Hayem G, Deutsch E, Roux S, Palazzo E, Grossin M, Meyer O. Spontaneous spinal epidural hematoma with spinal cord compression complicating plasma cell myeloma. A case report. Spine 1998;23:2432-2435.
20. Tomlin JM, Alleyne CH. Transdural metastasis from adenocarcinoma of the prostate mimicking subdural hematoma: case report. Surg Neurol 2002;58:329-331.
21. Goetz P, Lafuente J, Revesz T, Galloway M, Dogan A, Kitchen N. Primary low-grade B-cell lymphoma of mucosa-associated lymphoid tissue of the dura mimicking the presentation of an acute subdural hematoma. Case report and review of the literature. J Neurosurg 2002;96:611-614.
22. Tseng SH, Liao CC, Lin SM, Chen Y, Shun CT. Dural metastasis in patients with malignant neoplasm and chronic subdural hematoma. Acta Neurol Scand 2003;108:43-46.
23. Maxeiner H, Wolff M. Pure subdural hematomas: a postmortem analysis of their form and bleeding points. Neurosurgery 2002;50:503-508.
24. Lee KS, Bae WR, Yoon SM, Bae HG, Yun IG. Location of the chronic subdural haematoma: role of the gravity and cranial morphology. Brain Inj 2001;15:47-52.
25. Mori K, Yamamoto T, Horinaka N, Maeda M. Arachnoid cyst is a risk factor for chronic subdural hematoma in juveniles: twelve cases of chronic subdural hematoma associated with arachnoid cyst. J Neurotrauma 2002;19:1017-1027.
26. Machulda MM, Haut MW. Clinical features of chronic subdural hematoma: neuropsychiatric and neuropsycholgic changes in patients with chronic subdural hematoma. Neurosurg Clin N Am 2000;11:473-477.

27. Blitshteyn S, Mechtler LL, Bakshi R. Diffuse dural gadolinium MRI enhancement associated with bilateral chronic subdural hematomas. Clin Imaging 2004;28:90-92.
28. Golden J, Frim DM, Chapman PH, Vonsatttel JP. Marked tissue eosinophilia within organizing chronic subdural hematoma membranes. Clin Neuropathol 1994;13:12-16.
29. Al-Sarraj S, Mohamed S, Kibble M, Rezaie P. Subdural hematoma (SDH): assessment of macrophage reactivity within the dura mater and underlying hematoma. Clin Neuropathol 2004;23:62-75.
30. Loh JK, Howng SR. Electron microscopic study on the outer membrane of chronic subdural hematoma. Kaohsiung J Med Sci 1998;14:25-30.
31. Seelig JM, Beker DP, Miller JO. Traumatic acute subdural hematoma: major mortality reduction in comatose patients trated within four hours. N Engl J Med 1981;304:1511-1518.
32. Wijdicks EF. Uncal herniation in acute subdural hematoma: point of no return. Arch Neurol 2002;59:305.
33. Weigel R, Schmiedek P, Krauss JK. Outcome of contemporary surgery for chronic subdural haematoma: evidence based review. J Neurol Neurosurg Psychiatry 2003;74:937-943.

12 METABOLIC DISEASES

The metabolic diseases of the central nervous system (CNS) encompass a bewildering array of rare conditions. In general, these are diseases that begin in infancy or childhood, have characteristic clinical and laboratory findings, and are diagnosed on the basis of biochemical or genetic testing. In other words, these diseases are not usually encountered by diagnostic pathologists. But, importantly for the surgical pathologist, many of the diseases have atypical or adult variants that can pose diagnostic problems and that, on occasion, result in brain biopsies. In such situations, the surgical pathologist can play a key role in directing the subsequent diagnostic evaluation.

Because of the rarity of encountering metabolic diseases of the CNS in biopsy material, and since subsequent biochemical or genetic analyses are nearly always required for a firm diagnosis, the following chapter is organized primarily to guide the surgical pathologist in a general manner, with key features described for those metabolic diseases that have a greater likelihood of being biopsied. For additional information on the genetic basis of these conditions, the reader is referred to the online resource, Online Mendelian Inheritance in Man (OMIM; http://www.ncbi.nlm.nih.gov), which provides detailed, up-to-date information on all inherited diseases. Neuropathologic details can be found in reference texts (1).

Metabolic diseases are divided into those that primarily affect gray matter and those that primarily affect white matter or target specific organelles, such as lysosomes, mitochondria, or peroxisomes. In general, those that primarily affect gray matter target neurons, often causing the accumulation of material within neurons prior to their degeneration. Those that affect white matter are generally diseases that target myelin or glial cells, particularly oligodendroglia, and result in myelin degeneration. Some diseases affect both gray and white matter, and some diseases target other cell types, such as endothelial cells or macrophages. The neurologic signs and symptoms of gray matter disease differ from those of white matter disease, and neuroimaging helps determine preferential diseased sites. In many metabolic diseases, family history plays a key role in diagnosis. The clinical and radiologic features usually narrow a differential diagnosis to the point at which biochemical and/or genetic testing can be undertaken. For these reasons, only rarely are such lesions biopsied.

The pathologist should be in contact with the neurosurgeon and neurologist prior to the biopsy. Such interaction ensures that all three physicians understand the differential diagnosis and understand what tissues are needed for subsequent diagnostic approaches. Given the importance of sampling both gray and white matter and the importance of having enough tissue for standard histology, special stains, biochemical or genetic studies, and for electron microscopy, open biopsies are preferable to stereotactic needle biopsies.

GENERAL DIAGNOSTIC APPROACH

As emphasized above, nearly all metabolic diseases of the CNS present with characteristic clinical findings and are diagnosed with specific biochemical and genetic tests. Those uncommon metabolic diseases that are biopsied, are biopsied for other reasons, for instance, to evaluate the possibility of other diseases. In other words, the diagnosis of a neurologic metabolic disease based on a brain biopsy often comes as a surprise to the clinician. For this reason, the surgical pathologist needs to keep the possibility of metabolic disease in mind when evaluating brain biopsies for unusual neurologic conditions.

Many lysosomal and peroxisomal disorders affect the peripheral nervous system and visceral organs in addition to the CNS. As a result, most of these disorders can now be diagnosed using biochemical, ultrastructural, or molecular approaches to systemic tissues, without the need

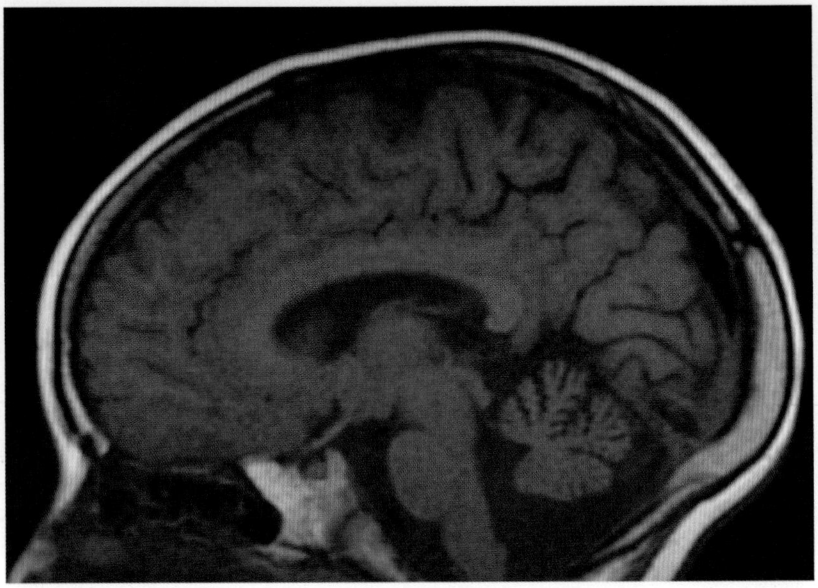

Figure 12-1

NEURONAL CEROID LIPOFUSCINOSIS

Magnetic resonance imaging (MRI) shows extensive gray matter atrophy, particularly of the cerebellum.

for a brain biopsy. Other affected and biopsied organs include skin, conjunctiva, peripheral blood, skeletal muscle, peripheral nerve, and rectum (2). In particular, the analysis of lymphocytes helps diagnose many lysosomal disorders and bone marrow biopsy is often diagnostic in Gaucher disease.

Clinical and Radiologic Findings

The characteristic clinical and radiologic findings of the most common and most commonly encountered neurologic metabolic diseases are covered in subsequent sections of this chapter. Those patients who undergo brain biopsy usually do not have the typical clinical features described in these sections. Rather, biopsied patients are usually older, either older children or adults, and have ill-defined combinations of neurologic problems. The diseases are divided into those that affect gray matter (fig. 12-1) and those that affect white matter structures (see fig. 12-15). Patients whose disease targets gray matter usually present with cognitive problems and seizures, whereas those with disease affecting white matter often present with cognitive problems coupled with motor or sensory impairment. Some conditions are restricted to involvement of the CNS, while others affect both the central and peripheral nervous systems, the latter resulting in signs and symptoms of a peripheral neuropathy.

Neuroimaging can readily distinguish gray and white matter abnormalities and, by doing so, can guide diagnoses. For example, in addition to demonstrating disease in the white matter, neuroimaging can show preferential involvement of parietooccipital white matter, which is typical of adrenoleukodystrophy. Some entities have particular neuroimaging findings, such as the increase in N-acetylaspartate noted in Canavan disease.

Gross Findings

Most diagnostic samples should come from open brain biopsies to allow for sufficient material for diagnosis, but sometimes a stereotactic biopsy is performed. Diagnostic macroscopic findings are not apparent in these specimens, but the gliosis that attends these conditions can give a firm quality to the tissue. In disorders that result in myelin loss, the normally bright white color of the normal white matter is lost, resulting in a tan color more similar to gray matter.

Intraoperative Diagnosis

There is no role for an intraoperative diagnosis of metabolic diseases, although it is useful for the pathologist to process the specimens immediately in the frozen section laboratory. Attempts should be made to avoid doing frozen sections, since this compromises the quality of subsequent sections from the formalin-fixed,

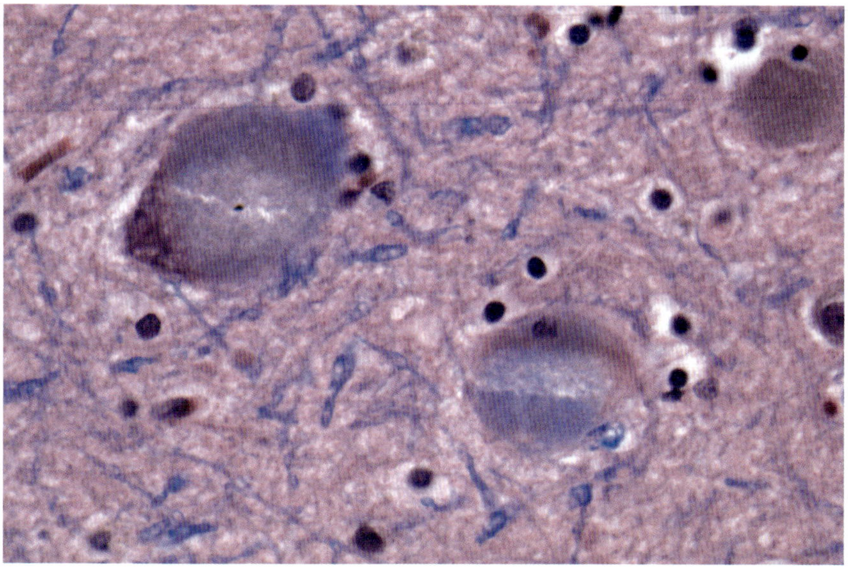

Figure 12-2

SANFILLIPO DISEASE

Marked "ballooning" of the neuronal cytoplasm is caused by storage material (Luxol fast blue-H&E stain).

paraffin-embedded material and intraoperative frozen sections will not affect the ongoing surgical procedure or the management of the patient over the subsequent days.

In most situations, in the setting of an unusual neurologic condition that includes metabolic disease in the differential diagnosis, the surgical pathologist should freeze small fragments of tissue for subsequent special stains and biochemical or genetic analysis and should reserve small fragments of tissue for electron microscopy. Because there can be substantial regional variability in severity of these processes, sampling from different regions of the biopsy is recommended.

Microscopic Findings

Metabolic diseases that affect the gray matter most often result in the storage of material in neurons, with an accentuation and sometimes "ballooning" of the neuronal cytoplasm (fig. 12-2). Indeed, ballooned neurons with granular cytoplasmic material are nearly diagnostic of neuronal storage diseases. Eventually, there is neuronal loss, with fewer and fewer remaining ballooned neurons. The ballooned neurons vary in size from relatively normal-sized neurons with storage material to markedly enlarged. Special stains such as hematoxylin and eosin (H&E), periodic acid–Schiff (PAS), Luxol fast blue, and Sudan red and black highlight the storage material. Frozen sections can be stained with acidic cresyl violet or toluidine blue to evaluate for metachromasia. Gliosis is a common accompanying feature.

In white matter diseases, the loss of myelin is seen with the Luxol fast blue stain, with relative preservation of axons with neurofilament immunohistochemistry or Bodian silver impregnation. Ingested myelin debris may be found in macrophages. Special stains such as PAS, cresyl violet, and Sudan black distinguish the myelin breakdown material. One means of separating the white matter diseases is into metachromatic and orthochromatic conditions, and into sudanophilic versus nonsudanophilic conditions. Some stains, particularly cresyl violet for demonstrating metachromasia, require frozen material. In some conditions, the myelin loss is attended by the loss of oligodendrocytes. Most white matter diseases also feature prominent reactive gliosis.

Some diseases have storage of material primarily in other cell types such as macrophages (Neimann-Pick disease [fig. 12-3]) or endothelial cells (Fabry disease). For all of these conditions, variability may be marked between different regions of brain. Some areas may have numerous ballooned cells while others feature neuronal loss and gliosis. The microscopic findings mentioned above are illustrated throughout this chapter.

Immunohistochemical Findings

With some exceptions, such as the workup of some neuronal ceroid lipofuscinoses, immunohistochemistry does not play a major

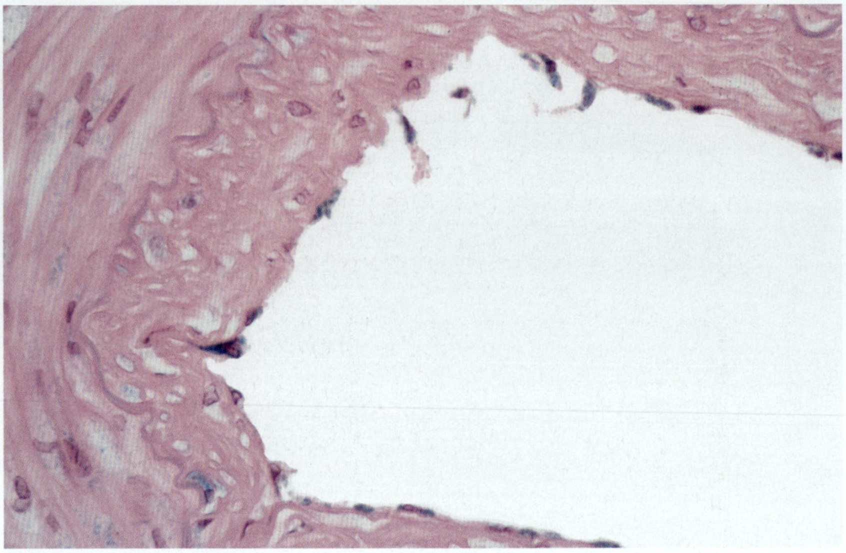

Figure 12-3

FABRY DISEASE

Blue storage material is in the vascular smooth muscle and endothelial cells (Luxol fast blue-hematoxylin and eosin [H&E] stain).

role in the evaluation or diagnosis of these metabolic conditions.

Ultrastructural Findings

Many of the metabolic diseases feature diagnostic inclusions that are visible on electron microscopy (3,4). For some diseases, the inclusions are similar among genetic variants, while in other diseases (such as the neuronal ceroid lipofuscinoses), the inclusions differ between the variants. For some of the metabolic conditions that affect the CNS, diagnostic ultrastructural changes can be found in other organs as well, including more easily biopsied organs like the skin. Given the potential diagnostic importance of ultrastructural analysis in these diseases, tissue should be preserved in appropriate fixative for electron microscopy in all brain biopsies that include the possibility of metabolic etiologies in the differential diagnosis.

Laboratory and Molecular Findings

The laboratory workup of metabolic diseases is complex, and the reader is referred to standard textbooks for details (3) as well as the OMIM website. Diagnostic workups involve a host of blood, cerebral spinal fluid (CSF), and urine tests as well as biochemical tests of frozen biopsied tissues and/or cultured skin fibroblasts or leukocytes. Molecular genetic diagnosis is typically directed to discovering germline DNA abnormalities, but mitochondrial DNA must also be investigated in particular clinical situations.

Differential Diagnosis

As discussed in the remainder of this chapter, the differential diagnosis of metabolic conditions is wide and varies depending on the specific disease. It is always important to bear in mind that these conditions are rarely biopsied for primary diagnosis in the setting of their typical presentations, but only in the setting of atypical presentations.

Treatment and Prognosis

Effective treatments are not available for most metabolic diseases, and most care relates to managing metabolic derangements and providing supportive care for the patient and family. In a few conditions, however, specific dietary interventions can alter the course of the neurologic deterioration. Otherwise, most patients follow a slowly progressive course, with worsening neurologic function, and death following years later.

NEURONAL STORAGE DISORDERS

The *neuronal storage disorders* feature the disruption of neuronal function because of the accumulation of storage materials. Storage typically results from defects in metabolic pathways that are primarily active in the neurons. The common histologic hallmark is the expansion of neuronal cytoplasm by granular material (figs. 12-2, 12-4). The distention varies from mild in most cases of neuronal ceroid lipofuscinosis to marked in some

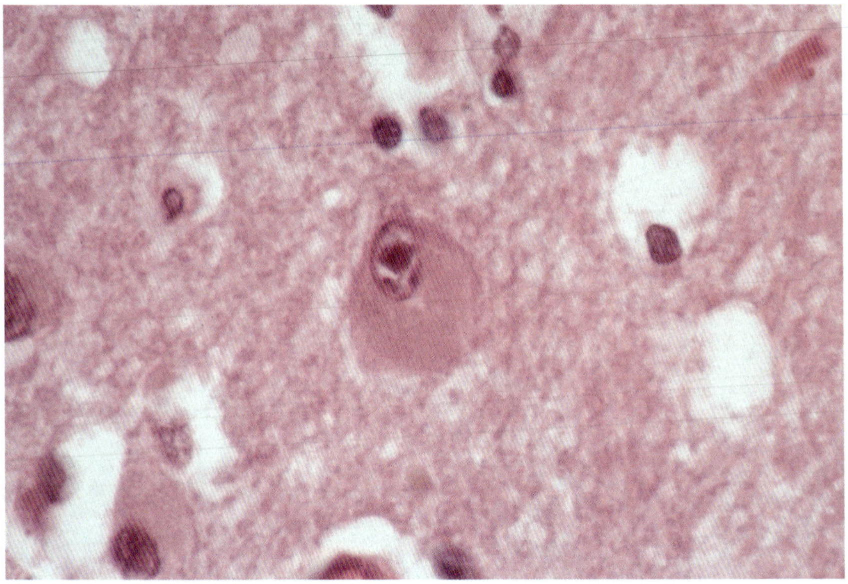

Figure 12-4

NEURONAL CEROID LIPOFUSCINOSIS

Moderate ballooning of the cytoplasm of a cortical neuron.

cases of Tay-Sachs disease; the latter situation results in ballooned cells. As the disease progress, however, there is increasing death of neurons and replacement of the cortex by gliosis.

Those rare cases biopsied for diagnostic purposes are likely to be in the early stages of disease and, therefore, one would expect to find distended neurons. In some conditions (e.g., Neimann-Pick and Gaucher diseases), there is a substantial macrophage component, with numerous macrophages stuffed with storage material present throughout the brain, particularly in the gray matter. For most of these conditions, however, the characteristic clinical, biochemical, and molecular features, often coupled with involvement of other organs (such as Gaucher disease), precludes the need for brain biopsy. As a result, for conditions such as Gaucher disease, documented brain biopsies are mostly restricted to the older literature (5). This section only discusses those diseases that have, albeit rarely, been documented on brain biopsy diagnosis in the last few decades.

Neuronal Ceroid Lipofuscinosis

The *neuronal ceroid lipofuscinoses* (NCL, also known as *Batten disease*) are a varied group of autosomal recessive, diverse conditions that present clinically as infantile, late-infantile, juvenile, and adult types. The reader is referred to other sources for details (4,6). At a biological level, however, their classification is more complex, since at least eight disease loci have been identified (*CLN1-CLN8*). Some of these genes have been identified, allowing for genetic diagnosis in some cases. In all cases, there is accumulation of ceroid lipofuscin (fig. 12-4), a poorly characterized material that most likely consists of many different compounds. Nonetheless, all NCLs demonstrate positivity for PAS, Sudan black, and Luxol fast blue (fig. 12-5) as well as yellow autofluorescence (fig. 12-6). In many of the variants, there are relatively specific ultrastructural findings and some immunohistochemical differences with regard to the storage material (4,6).

Infantile NCL (Haltia-Santavuori Disease). Infantile NCL occurs predominantly in Finland as a result of mutations in the *CLN1* gene (encoding palmitoyl protein thioesterase 1) on 1p32. Pathologic findings include marked cerebral atrophy and neuronal loss. The accumulated material stains immunohistochemically with antibodies to saposin (sphingolipid activating protein) A and saposin D (7). The ultrastructural presence of the accumulated material in granular osmiophilic deposits (GRODs) is diagnostic. GRODs are found in the remaining neurons.

Late Infantile NCL (Janksy-Bielschowsky Disease). This typically begins in children between 2 and 4 years of age, and is caused by mutations in the *CLN2* gene (encoding a lysosomal peptidase) on 11p15. Late infantile NCL is characterized pathologically by severe cerebral atrophy and by the ultrastructural finding of curvilinear bodies.

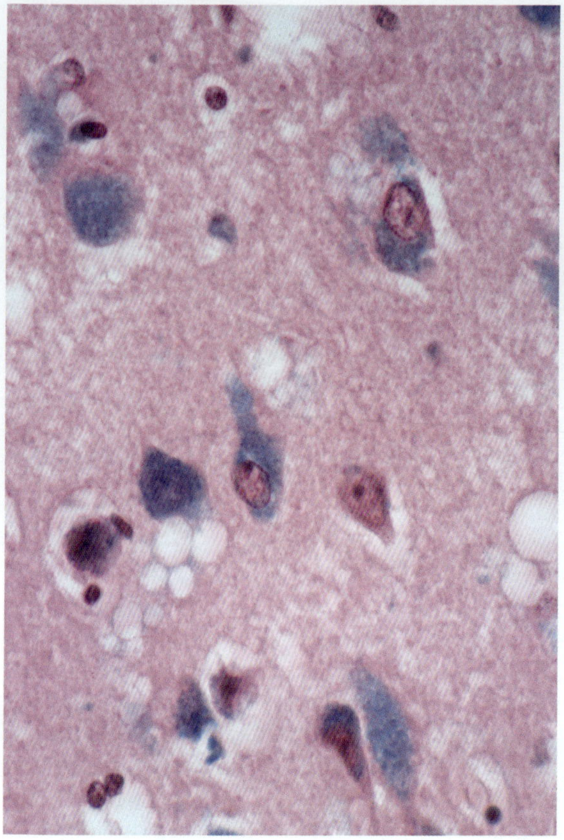

Figure 12-5

NEURONAL CEROID LIPOFUSCINOSIS

The stored material stains strongly with Luxol fast blue.

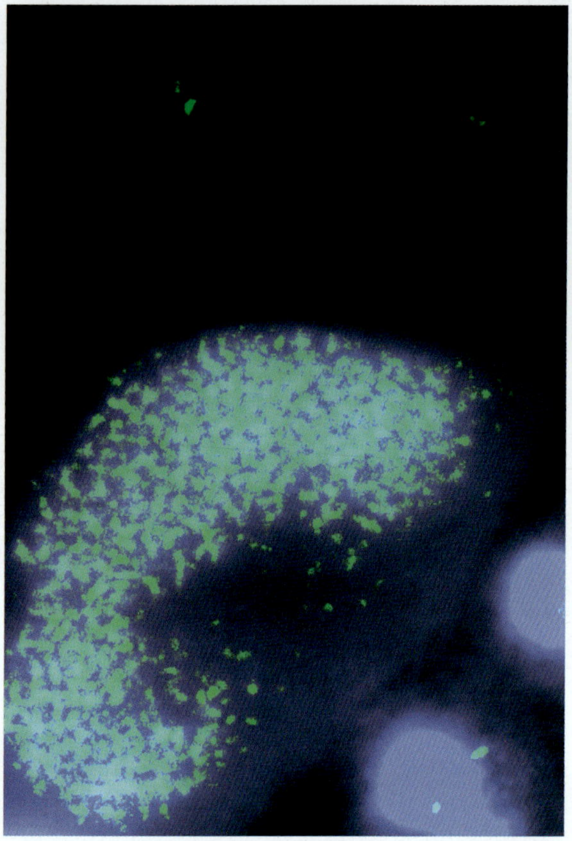

Figure 12-6

NEURONAL CEROID LIPOFUSCINOSIS

Autofluorescence of a cerebral cortical neuron.

On immunohistochemical analysis, the accumulated material stains with antibodies to subunit C of mitochondrial adenosine triphosphate (ATP) synthase (SCMAS) (4,8).

Juvenile NCL (Spielmeyer-Vogt-Sjogren-Batten Disease). This variant usually begins in the second half of the first decade of life and is related to mutations of the *CLN3* gene (encoding a highly conserved membrane protein of unknown function) on 16p12. In addition to marked cerebral atrophy and neuronal loss, there is accumulation of fingerprint bodies on ultrastructural analysis and immunopositivity for SCMAS. Of diagnostic importance, circulating lymphocytes may have a characteristic vacuolated appearance, with the vacuoles containing fingerprint bodies.

Adult NCL (Kufs Disease). This type is heterogeneous, with both autosomal recessive and dominant forms. A distinct gene has not been identified, although rare cases have been reported with defects in other *CLN* genes. Patients present with progressive myoclonus epilepsy or behavioral changes with dementia. Pathologically, there is cerebral atrophy with storage of ceroid lipofuscin; the storage material has features of many of the other NCLs, with ultrastructural findings including GRODs, curvilinear bodies, and fingerprint bodies, and with immunohistochemical findings including positivity for saposins and SCMAS.

There are a number of caveats regarding the diagnosis of NCL. As mentioned above, there are other forms of NCL, some of which have been mapped to particular gene loci and some that have not. A recent variant preferentially targeting the substantia nigra has been described, along with visceral deposition of storage material. The material was variably positive for SCMAS, but strongly positive for saposin D, and was ultrastructurally characterized by GRODs

(9). It is more likely that variants like this would be biopsied. The pathologist, therefore, must be aware of the light microscopic, special staining, immunohistochemical, and ultrastructural features of NCLs. Rare cases may present with clinical and imaging findings not suggestive of a metabolic disease and are therefore biopsied; for example, some adult cases present as psychiatric disease (10) and one had findings suggestive of a malignant glioma (11). In most cases, ultrastructural examination is of particular importance (12,13), and given the likelihood of storage material in other organs, biopsy of other sites is more common than biopsy of the CNS (14). Modern approaches to the morphologic diagnosis of NCL suggest that other preferred sites are skin, circulating lymphocytes (particularly in juvenile NCL), rectum, conjunctiva, and (less diagnostically) skeletal muscle and peripheral nerve (15).

Gangliosidoses

The gangliosidoses include *GM1 gangliosidosis* and *GM2 gangliosidosis*, both of which feature neuronal accumulation of gangliosides. GM1 gangliosidosis arises from defects in beta-galactosidase. It usually presents in infancy with neurologic decline and a macular cherry red spot, although later-onset cases occur, including some in adults. The adult cases may not have cherry red spots and more often present with extrapyramidal findings.

GM2 gangliosidosis includes classic *Tay-Sachs disease* as well as *adult-onset GM2 gangliosidosis*. GM2 gangliosidosis arises from defects in the subunits of hexosaminidase, with the gene for the alpha subunit (*HEXA*) on chromosome 15q23 and the gene for the beta subunit (*HEXB*) on chromosome 5q13. While classic Tay-Sachs disease presents in infancy with marked neurologic decline and a cherry red spot, the adult-onset cases most often present with signs and symptoms suggestive of motor neuron disease (such as amyotrophic lateral sclerosis), extrapyramidal conditions, or spinocerebellar degeneration.

The neuropathologic finding in all of the gangliosidoses is neuronal ballooning with storage material (fig. 12-7). The material stains weakly with PAS and Luxol fast blue, but is positive for acid phosphatase. On ultrastructural analysis, the distended neurons are typically filled with membranous cytoplasmic bodies (MCBs).

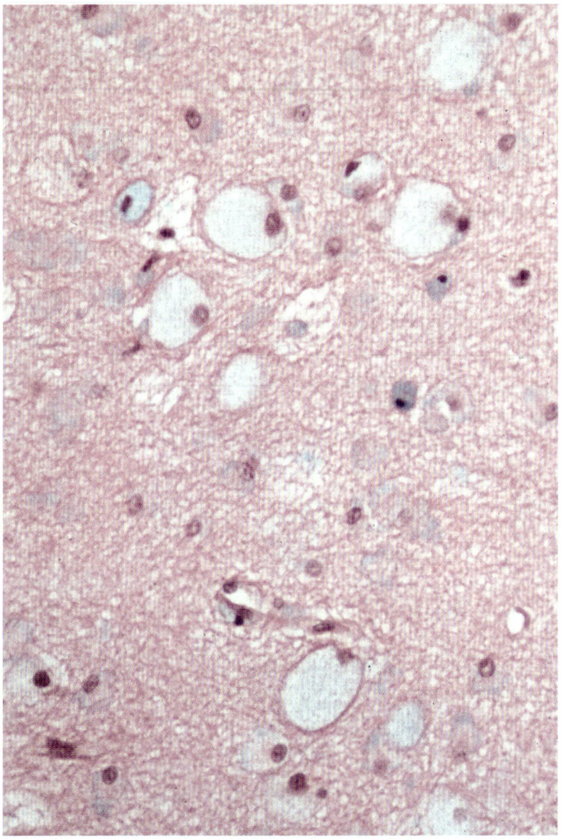

Figure 12-7

TAY-SACHS DISEASE

Ballooning of neuronal cytoplasm (Luxol fast blue-H&E stain).

For all of the gangliosidoses, brain biopsies are exceedingly rare (16–18), particularly now that biochemical and molecular diagnostic approaches are readily available. The brains of infants and children are never biopsied. There have been relatively few neuropathologic studies of adult-onset gangliosidoses, but it appears that cortical neurons are infrequently involved and that neuronal loss may be limited to the basal ganglia in GM1 gangliosidosis and to the thalamus, substantia nigra and other brain stem nuclei, and cerebellum in adult-onset GM2 gangliosidosis (19). On ultrastructural analysis, electron-dense heterogeneous conglomerates may be found alongside the more typical membranous cytoplasmic inclusions.

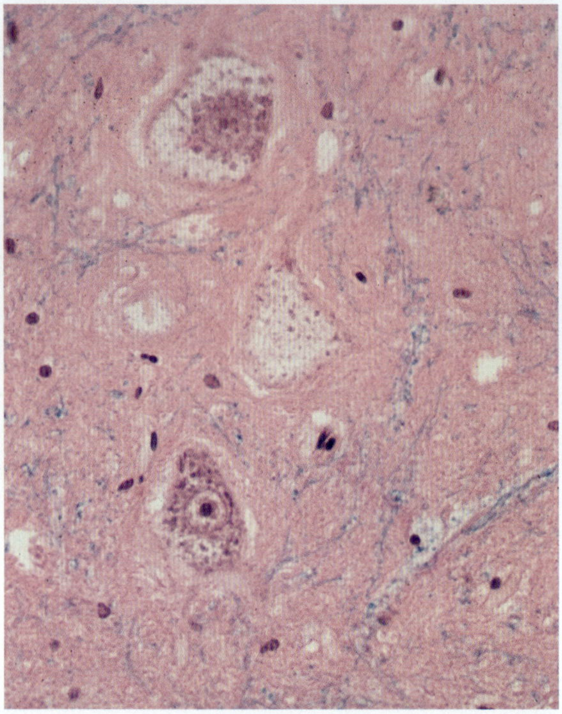

Figure 12-8

NIEMANN-PICK DISEASE

Storage material is seen in the anterior horn cells (Luxol fast blue-H&E stain)

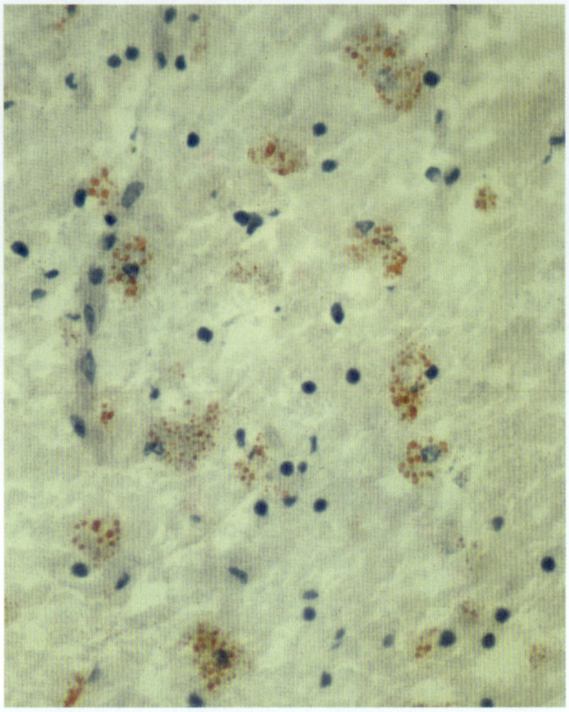

Figure 12-10

NIEMANN-PICK DISEASE

Numerous macrophages are highlighted with the oil red O stain.

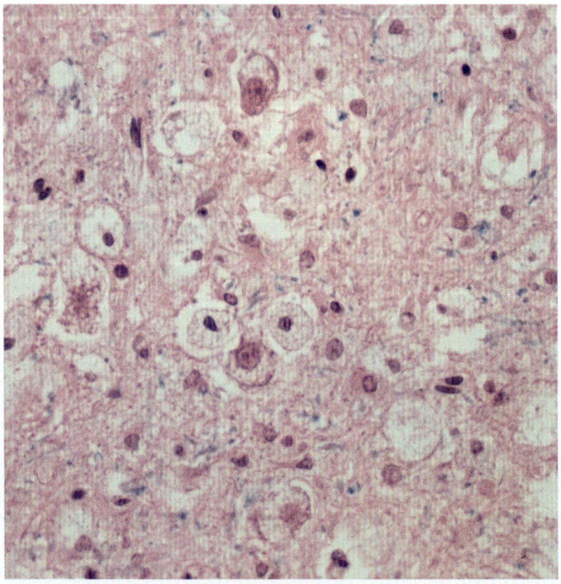

Figure 12-9

NIEMANN-PICK DISEASE

Storage material is present in macrophages and neurons (Luxol fast blue-H&E stain).

Niemann-Pick Disease

Niemann-Pick disease encompasses two sets of neurovisceral storage diseases, often termed Niemann-Pick types A and B and Niemann-Pick types C and D. Type A and B diseases are caused by defects in the gene encoding sphingomyelinase on 11p15; type A patients have neurologic disease, whereas type B patients only suffer from visceral storage. Classic Niemann-Pick type A presents in infancy with hepatosplenomegaly and neurologic decline.

The neuropathologic findings are those of ballooned neurons, but not often of the size seen in the gangliosidoses (fig. 12-8). In contrast to the gangliosidoses, there is conspicuous macrophage infiltration (figs. 12-9, 12-10). Some of the macrophages stain blue with the Giemsa or Wright stains (sea-blue histiocytes). The ultrastructural findings are nonspecific, with many different types of inclusions noted. Cerebral biopsies of classic Niemann-Pick disease have not been documented in the literature of the last few decades.

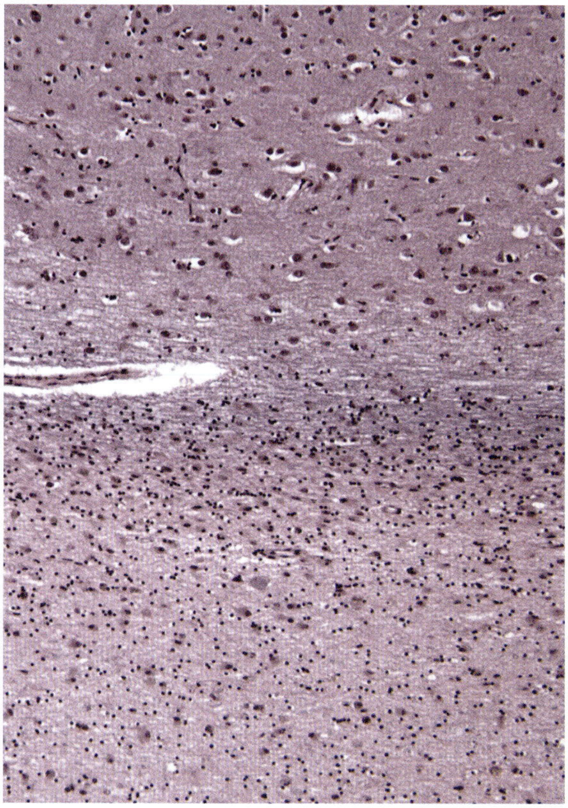

Figure 12-11

LEUKODYSTROPHY

A faint band of preserved subcortical U fibers overlies demyelinated cerebral white matter (Luxol fast blue-H&E stain).

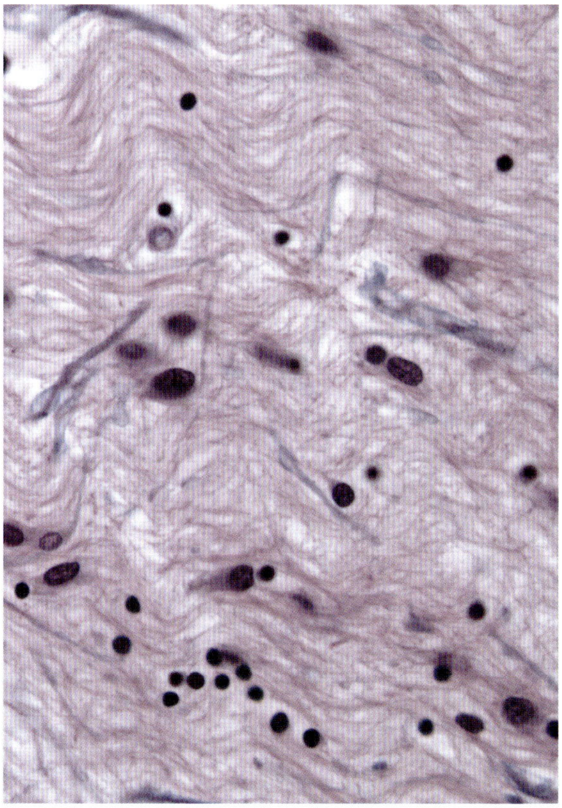

Figure 12-12

LEUKODYSTROPHY

Only rare axons have remaining myelin (Luxol fast blue-H&E stain).

Niemann Pick types C and D are entirely different diseases. Type C is more common, with type D restricted to Nova Scotia. Type C arises from mutations in the *NPC1* gene on 18q, which encodes a protein involved in cholesterol trafficking. Type C has a broad clinical phenotype, with onset later in childhood or adult life. Patients present sometimes with hepatic and sometimes with neurologic dysfunction; some patients present primarily with psychiatric problems. The likelihood of a patient with Niemann-Pick type C having a brain biopsy is exceedingly low, but could occur in the setting of late-onset disease with psychiatric symptoms or dementia in the absence of obvious hepatosplenic manifestations. Rare biopsies have been documented in such adult-onset cases (20).

The neuropathologic findings in type C include neuronal storage, with some preferential storage in deep gray nuclei and brain stem in later onset cases. On ultrastructural analysis, most of the inclusions are MCBs. There may also be conspicuous additional neuronal abnormalities, such as neuroaxonal spheroids in rapidly progressive cases and neurofibrillary tangles in slowly progressive cases.

LEUKODYSTROPHIES

The white matter disorders, or *leukodystrophies,* all involve a defect in the production or maintenance of myelin. Most affect the white matter diffusely, with some sparing the subcortical U fibers. Some cases, however, show more focal abnormalities on imaging studies and suggest a glioma, leading to biopsy (21). Special stains demonstrate loss of myelin (with Luxol fast blue staining) and relative preservation of axons (with neurofilament immunohistochemistry or Bodian silver impregnation), along with macrophages and gliosis (figs. 12-11–12-14).

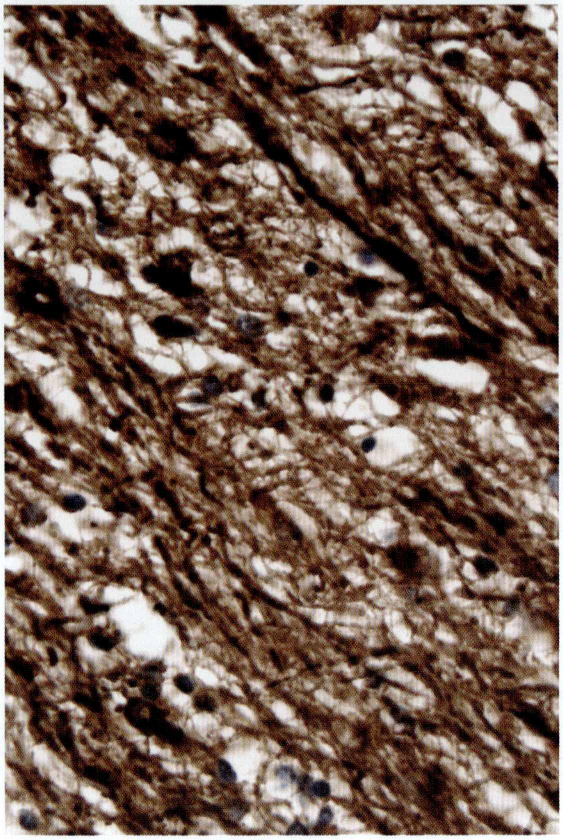

Figure 12-13

LEUKODYSTROPHY

Neurofilament immunohistochemistry demonstrates numerous intact axons.

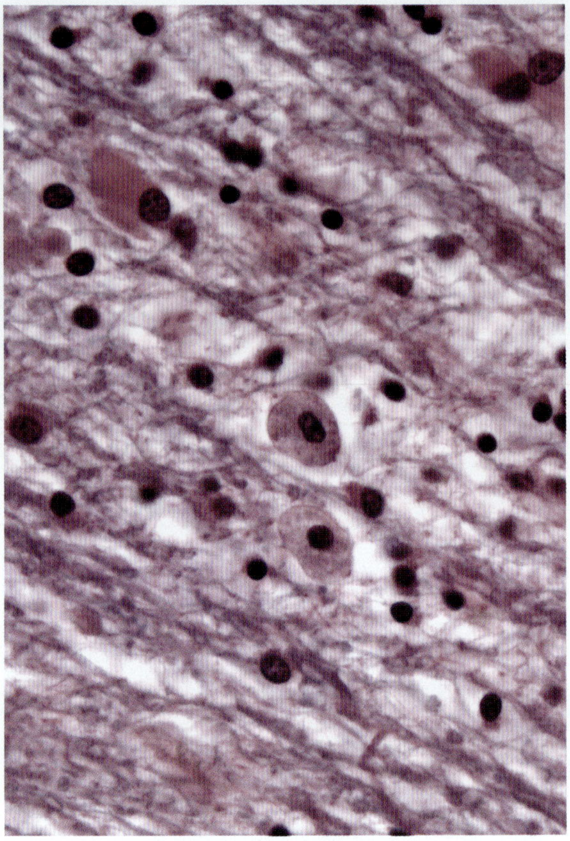

Figure 12-14

LEUKODYSTROPHY

Macrophages have myelin debris (Luxol fast blue-H&E stain).

Adrenoleukodystrophy and Adrenomyeloneuropathy

Adrenoleukodystrophy is an X-linked leukodystrophy resulting from mutations of the *ABCD1* (or *ALD1*) gene at Xq28, which encodes an ATP-binding cassette protein (subfamily D, member 1). Adrenoleukodystrophy usually presents in childhood. It primarily affects the cerebral hemispheres (fig. 12-15), cerebellum, and brain stem. *Adrenomyeloneuropathy* arises from mutations in the same gene, but presents in young adulthood with spinal cord and peripheral nerve disease.

In adrenoleukodystrophy, there is loss of myelin and oligodendrocytes, relative preservation of axons, and gliosis, but unlike most other leukodystrophies, this lesion shows a predilection for the parietal and occipital lobes (fig. 12-15) and is associated with more secondary corticospinal tract degeneration. Also, in distinction from most other leukodystrophies, there are extensive lymphocytic infiltrates (fig. 12-16). The inflammatory foci are most prominent at the edge of the demyelinated regions, that is, toward the more frontal reaches of the diseased white matter.

The lymphocytes are of both T- and B-cell lineage. Macrophages are numerous at the demyelinating edge as well (fig. 12-17), and these are PAS positive and sudanophilic (i.e., they stain with Sudan black). On ultrastructural analysis, these cells have elongated lamellar structures as well as lipid clefts that result from the accumulation of very long chain fatty acids, a characteristic of the disease. Sometimes the clefts are appreciated on light microscopy as a striation of the cytoplasm. (Identical material accumulates in the adrenal cortex and Leydig cells of the testis, and some cases of Addison disease arise from

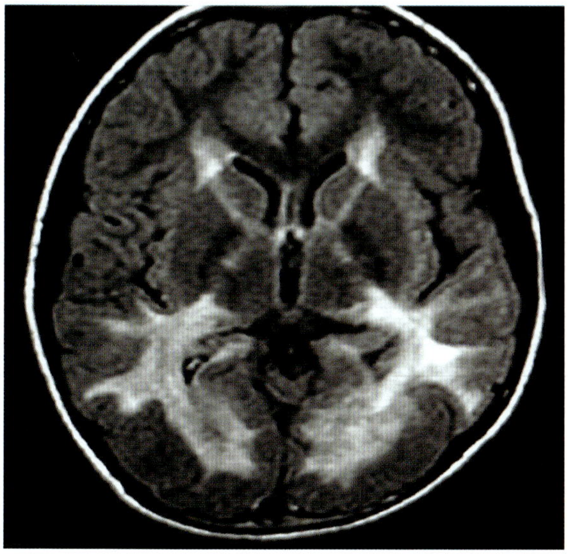

Figure 12- 15

ADRENOLEUKODYSTROPHY

Marked loss of parietooccipital white matter is seen on MRI.

mutations in the same gene.) Behind the advancing edge, in the parietooccipital lobes, there may be far less inflammation and macrophages and moderate axonal destruction, sometimes with cavitation of the white matter (fig. 12-18). The histologic changes in adrenomyeloneuropathy are similar, and cerebral lesions often accompany the spinal disease. *Neonatal adrenoleukodystrophy* is a distinct disorder that is autosomal recessive and due to a peroxisomal defect, but this variant is even more unlikely to be biopsied, and is not discussed here.

Occasionally, adrenoleukodystrophy has an acute onset in childhood (22) or in adulthood, with unusual features such as frontal lobe dementia (23). Although unlikely, such unusual presentations have the possibility of leading to biopsy of the brain (24–26) or other organs (27). Knowledge of how the biopsy site relates to the rostrocaudal spread of the disease on neuroimaging is important for interpretation. Biopsies

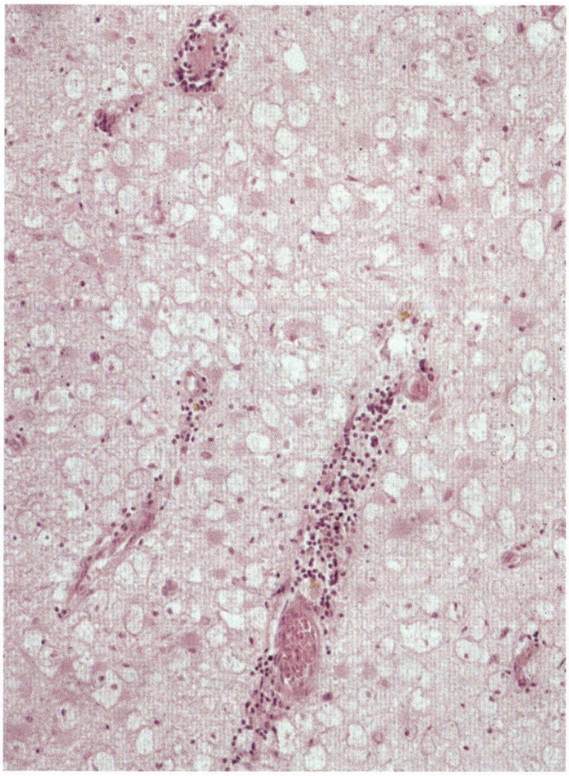

Figure 12-16

ADRENOLEUKODYSTROPHY

Perivascular lymphocytic cuffs are common in the actively demyelinating regions.

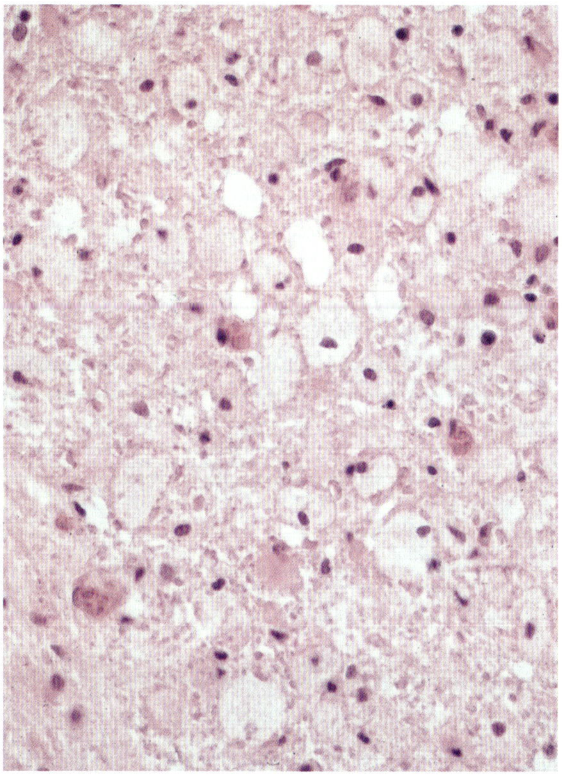

Figure 12-17

ADRENOLEUKODYSTROPHY

Numerous macrophages are present in the actively demyelinating regions.

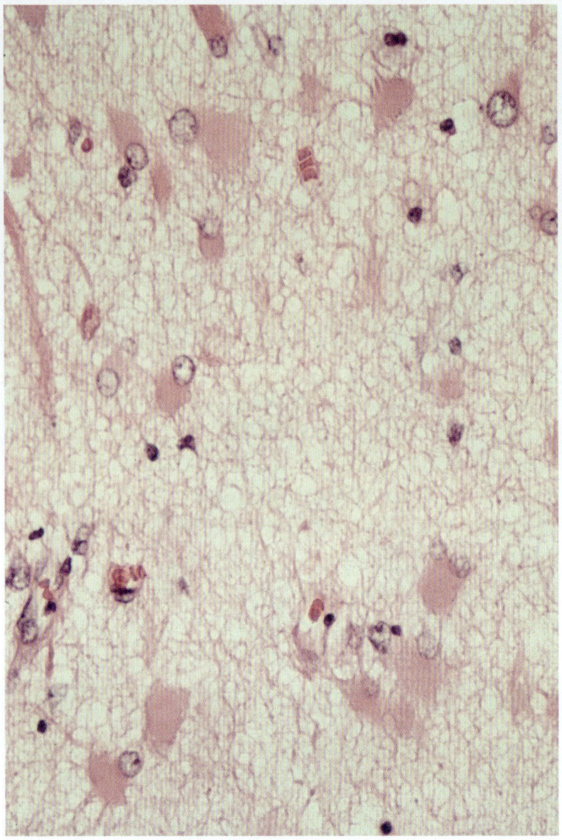

Figure 12-18

ADRENOLEUKODYSTROPHY

"Behind" the active zone is a region of marked myelin loss and gliosis.

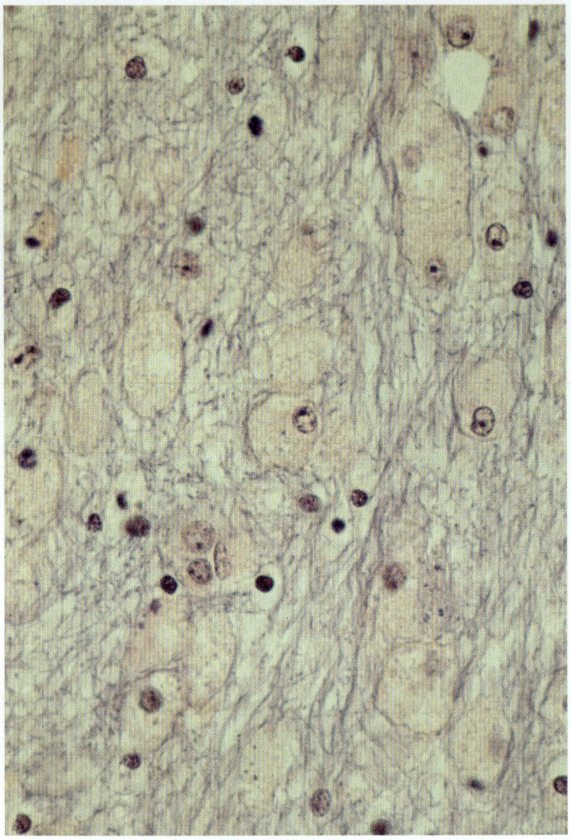

Figure 12-19

METACHROMATIC LEUKODYSTROPHY

Numerous macrophages have ingested myelin (Luxol fast blue-H&E stain).

obtained from near the leading edge may closely resemble standard acute demyelinating diseases, replete with chronic inflammation (see chapter 8). Correlation with the clinical course is necessary to make the distinction, although acute disseminated encephalomyelitis may have similar features.

Metachromatic Leukodystrophy

Metachromatic leukodystrophy is a set of autosomal recessive diseases, most resulting from alterations of the *ARSA* gene on 22q13, which results in defective arylsulfatase A activity. The leukodystrophy affects the central white matter diffusely, with some preference for the frontal lobes and some sparing of subcortical U fibers. There is loss of myelin, relative sparing of axons, and gliosis (fig. 12-19). The diagnostic histologic feature is the presence of metachromatic material in a variety of cell types. "Metachromasia" refers to the change in color of the storage material: when frozen sections are stained with acidic cresyl violet, the material is brown (fig. 12-20); when stained with toluidine blue, the material is pink. This contrasts with "orthochromasia" in which the color of the material is the expected color, and other leukodystrophies may be classified as orthochromatic leukodystrophies. The inclusions are PAS positive (fig. 12-21) and nonsudanophilic.

Electron microscopy demonstrates a variety of inclusions, including herringbone patterns and tuffstone inclusions, which are membrane-bound, electron-dense, granular structures specific to metachromatic leukodystrophy. The metachromatic material accumulates in many different cells of the CNS, including oligodendrocytes, macrophages, and some neurons. Metachromatic leukodystrophy also affects the

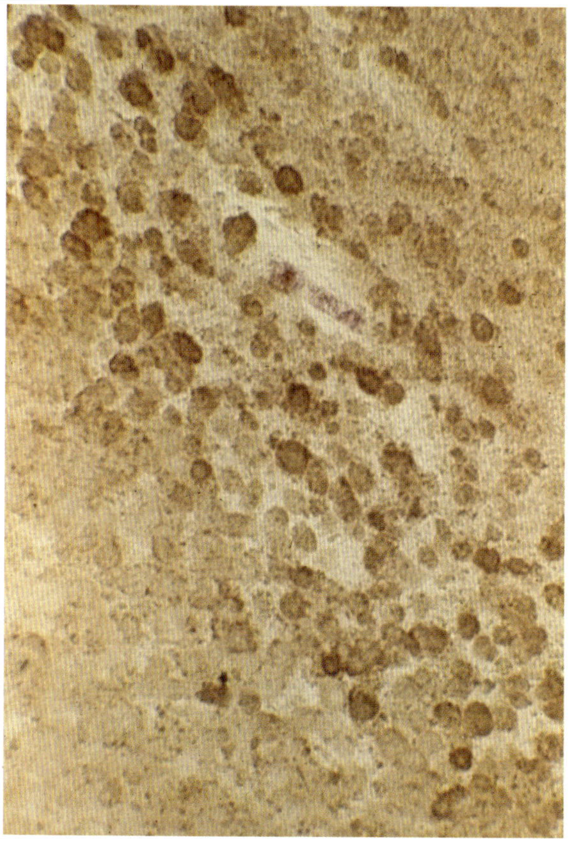

Figure 12-20

METACHROMATIC LEUKODYSTROPHY

Metachromasia is evident as brown material in the macrophages when stained with acidic cresyl violet.

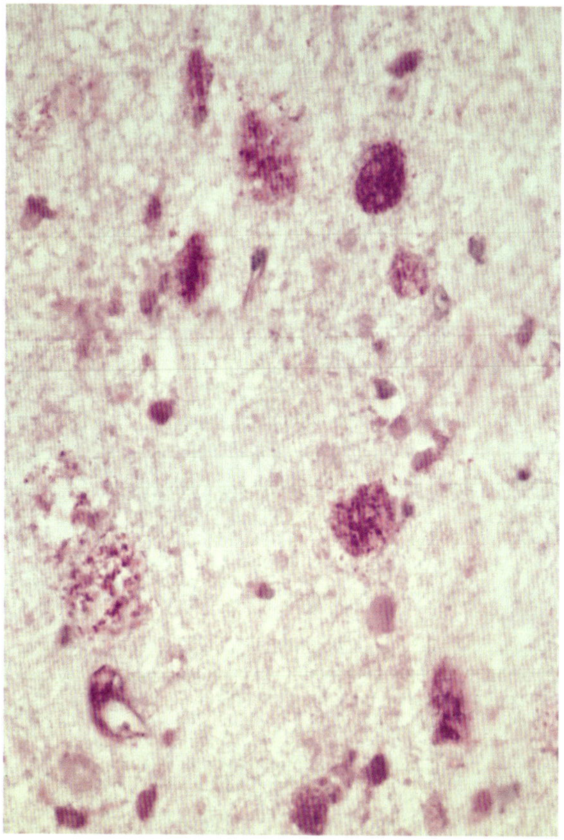

Figure 12-21

METACHROMATIC LEUKODYSTROPHY

The macrophages are periodic acid–Schiff (PAS) positive.

peripheral nervous system, often with marked peripheral neuropathy. Material accumulates in the Schwann cells of the peripheral nervous system and in systemic cells as well, such as macrophages in lymph nodes and spleen, renal tubules, bile ducts, the lining of the gall bladder, and the adrenal gland.

There are multiple metachromatic leukodystrophy variants that arise from different *ARSA* gene alterations: late infantile, juvenile, and adult forms; partial cerebroside sulfate deficiency; and pseudoarylsulfatase A deficiency. In addition, metachromatic leukodystrophy can arise in the setting of cerebroside sulfatase activator (saposin B) deficiency and in multiple sulfatase deficiency (in which patients have features of both a mucopolysaccharidosis and metachromatic leukodystrophy). Most diagnostically challenging are the adult forms of metachromatic leukodystrophy, since these typically present as psychiatric disease, often with a schizophrenia-like picture. Other patients with adult-onset disease present with pyramidal signs and a movement disorder, again posing an unusual clinical picture when combined with diffuse white matter abnormalities. These atypical presentations can, in rare instances, lead to biopsy (28). Still other patients present with an apparently isolated peripheral neuropathy (29) or with seizures (30).

Krabbe Disease

Krabbe disease, or *globoid cell leukodystrophy*, is an autosomal recessive disease of the white matter than affects infants. The molecular basis of the disease involves mutations in the *GALC* gene on 14q31, which result in a deficiency of galactocerebroside beta-galactosidase. The

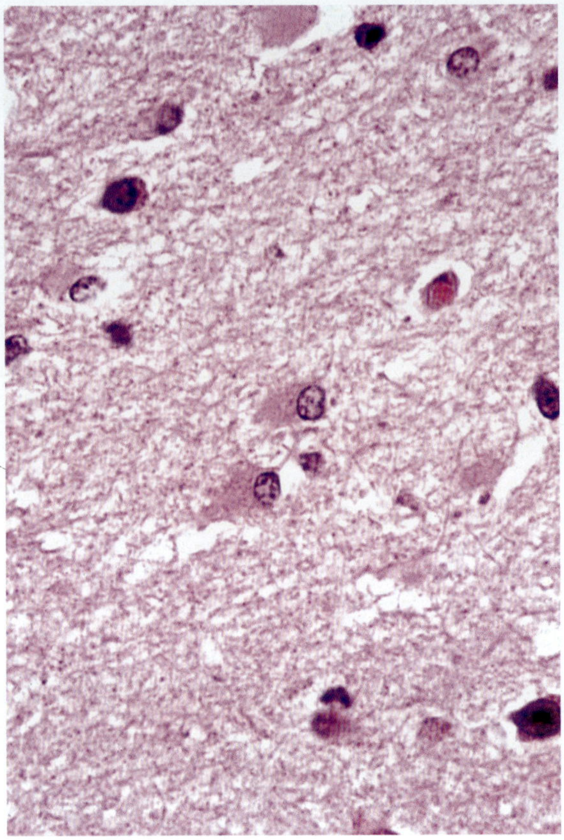

Figure 12-22

KRABBE DISEASE

The leukodystrophy is accompanied by gliosis and a marked loss of oligodendrocytes.

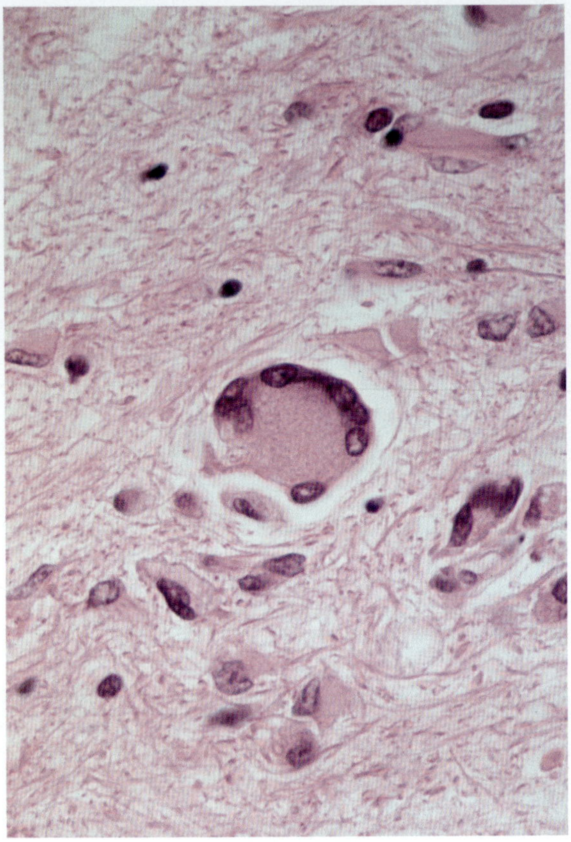

Figure 12-23

KRABBE DISEASE

Globoid cells have multiple nuclei and copious cytoplasm.

disease produces a diffuse leukodystrophy with sparing of the subcortical U fibers. In addition to the myelin loss, there is marked oligodendrocyte loss (fig. 12-22) and the pathognomonic presence of epithelioid and globoid cells. The latter are large, sometimes multinucleated, PAS-positive, "globoid" macrophages that often cluster around blood vessels (figs. 12-23, 12-24). These cells stain strongly for macrophage markers such as CD68, but it is their unique appearance that is most diagnostic. Ultrastructural studies show thin tubular structures with polygonal cross-sections within the cytoplasm of the globoid cells. Peripheral nerves can also be involved, with a demyelinating polyneuropathy and inclusions in Schwann cells and macrophages.

Rarely, Krabbe disease occurs in adults, affecting either the central or peripheral nervous system, or both. Patients have been reported with onset late in life, in the 8th decade, with a predilection for the parietooccipital white matter and the peripheral nervous system (31,32). Such late-onset cases do display *GALC* mutations, particularly a *GALC* genotype with one deleted and one polymorphic *GALC* activity-reducing allele (33). The 809G>A mutation may be particularly common in very late-onset cases (34). Magnetic resonance imaging (MRI) may demonstrate disease restricted to the pyramidal tracts in adult-onset cases (35), but magnetic resonance spectroscopy may not aid in the differential diagnosis (36).

Pelizaeus-Merzbacher Disease

Pelizaeus-Merzbacher disease is an X-linked disease of white matter that arises from mutations in the *PLP1* gene at Xq22. The mutations are more often duplication events than missense

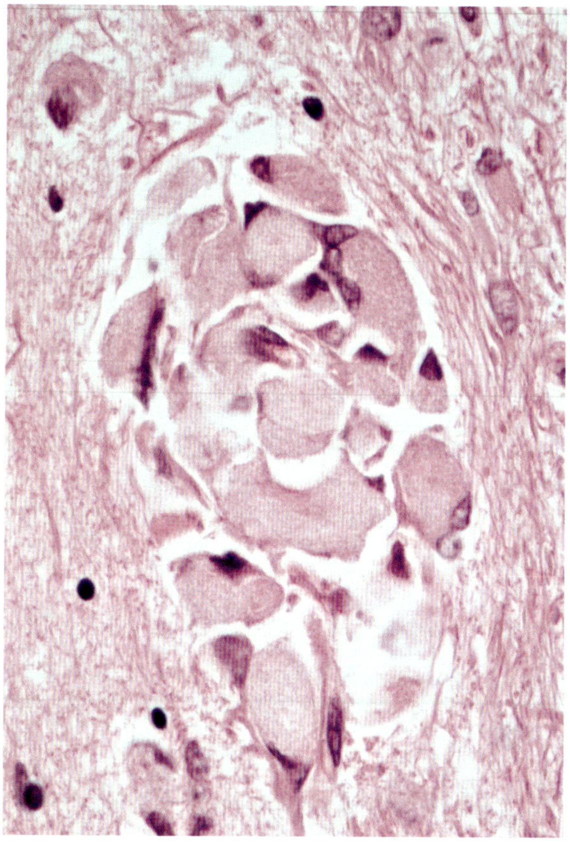

Figure 12-24

KRABBE DISEASE

Globoid cells often cluster around blood vessels.

Figure 12-25

PELIZAEUS-MERZBACHER DISEASE

A "tigroid" pattern of perivascular myelin preservation is observed after staining with Sudan black.

mutations (37), and such duplications can be detected using fluorescence in situ hybridization (FISH) (38,39). *PLP1* encodes a proteolipid protein, a major component of CNS myelin. Pelizaeus-Merzbacher disease affects males, with onset typically in infancy or childhood. Patients present with eye movement abnormalities, generalized movement disorders, pyramidal signs, and generalized neurologic decline.

The demyelination in Pelizaeus-Merzbacher disease has a characteristic appearance, with the preferential sparing of myelin around blood vessels. This spotted and linear appearance on myelin stains has been referred to as "tigroid" demyelination, and is relatively specific to the variants of Pelizaeus-Merzbacher (fig. 12-25), although it is also characteristic of Cockayne disease, a complex syndrome that includes brain and developmental abnormalities.

Variants of Pelizaeus-Merzbacher disease may follow an autosomal pattern of inheritance (40,41) and may present in older patients as dementia and a movement disorder (42–44). Female carriers may be affected and may present in adulthood (44). MRI sometimes reveals small foci of presumed myelin preservation, consistent with the tigroid pattern (42,43). Milder forms are more often caused by truncating or missense mutations (45). Certain forms of familial spastic paraplegia are allelic to Pelizaeus-Merzbacher disease and also result from mutations of the *PLP1* gene.

Alexander Disease

Alexander disease is a rare leukodystrophy that typically presents in infants as developmental delay and megalencephaly (46). The disease arises from de novo mutations in the *GFAP* gene

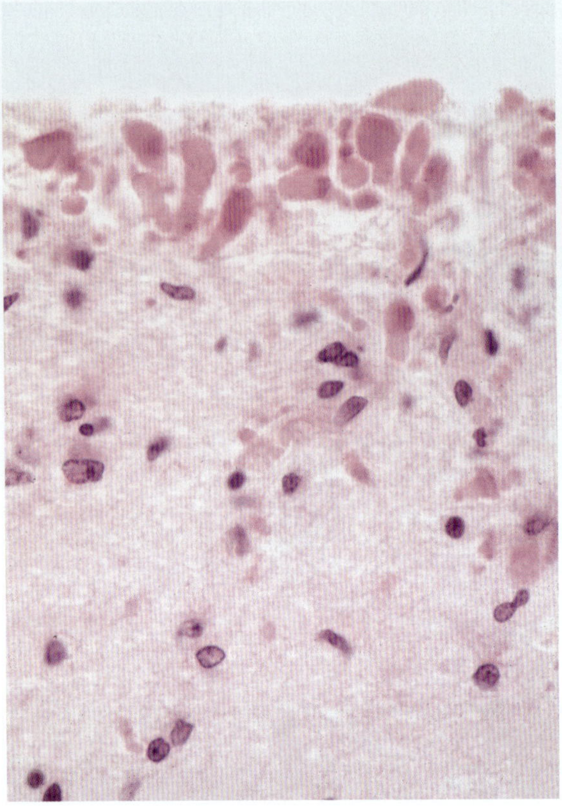

Figure 12-26

ALEXANDER DISEASE

Numerous Rosenthal fibers are present in the subpial region.

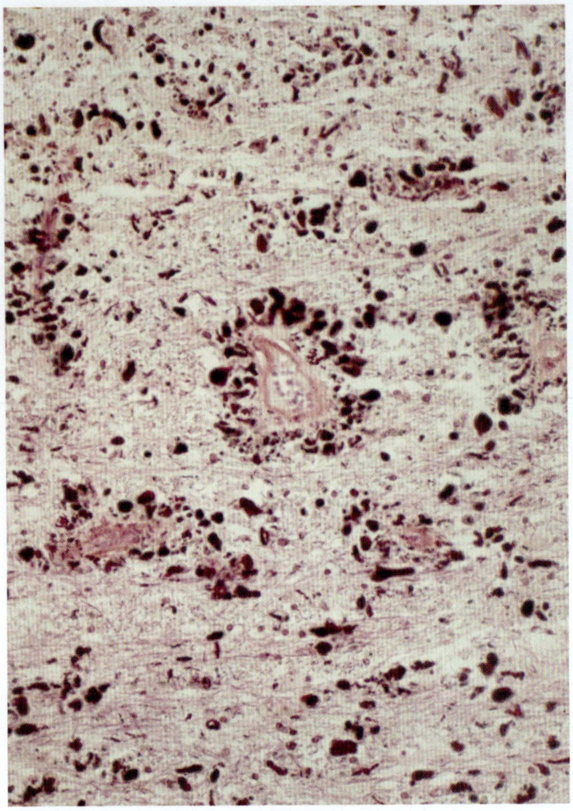

Figure 12-27

ALEXANDER DISEASE

The Rosenthal fibers are phosphotungstic acid-hematoxylin (PTAH) positive and cluster around blood vessels.

on 17q21 (47,48). There is a predilection for involvement of the frontal lobes, and rare cases with more focal abnormalities have also been reported (49).

This leukodystrophy is histopathologically unique since, in addition to gliosis, loss of myelin, and relative preservation of axons, there is extensive deposition of Rosenthal fibers. The Rosenthal material is distributed throughout both the gray and white matter (fig. 12-26), and is found in astrocyte foot processes, which leads to particular accumulation in subpial and perivascular regions (figs. 12-26, 12-27). The Rosenthal material found in Alexander disease has light microscopic, special staining, and ultrastructural characteristics that are identical to the material found in pilocytic astrocytomas and chronic gliosis. They stain brightly red and have a refractile appearance with the H&E stain, only show a periphery of labeling with glial fibrillary acidic protein (GFAP) but stain strongly for alpha-B-crystallin and ubiquitin. Special stains and immunohistochemistry, however, are not needed for identification.

The condition is seen rarely in adults. Some adult cases are hereditary and also result from *GFAP* mutations (50,51). These adults often have prominent bulbar signs and MRI may demonstrate marked loss in the pyramidal tracts. In other adults, however, typically in a nonhereditary setting, the abnormalities are more focal, and it has been debated whether this focal condition is the same as the usual Alexander disease or is an unusual gliotic reaction to another process (52,53). In some cases, brain biopsy may be performed (54,55). The large numbers of Rosenthal fibers will immediately raise the possibility of an unusual pilocytic astrocytoma, but careful examination fails to show any tumor cells or architectural

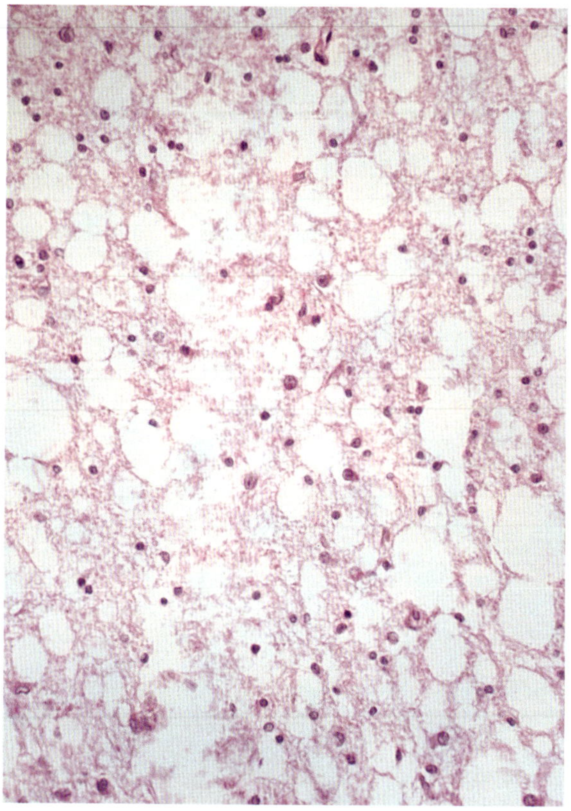

Figure 12-28

CANAVAN DISEASE

Vacuolar white matter changes are seen.

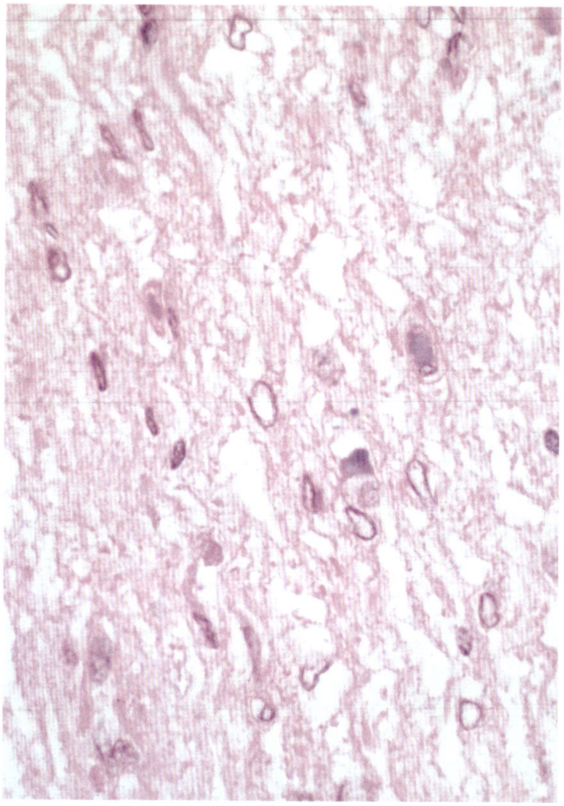

Figure 12-29

CANAVAN DISEASE

Alzheimer type 2 cells are characteristic.

features; rather, there is a dense accumulation of Rosenthal material within gliotic, but normally organized, cerebral cortex and underlying white matter. Nonetheless, in most biopsies from adults that feature large numbers of Rosenthal fibers, true Alexander disease does not enter the clinical differential diagnosis.

Canavan Disease

Canavan disease, also known as *van Bogart-Bertrand disease*, is an uncommon leukodystrophy that occurs primarily in young children of Ashkenazi Jewish descent, but which can occur in other ethnic backgrounds. The condition arises in the setting of mutations in the *ASPA* gene on 17p13, which encodes aspartoacylase. Most Ashkenazi descendants with the disease have characteristic mutations (56). The enzymatic defect results in high levels of N-acetylaspartic acid in the urine, which is useful in diagnosing the condition. Most patients present in infancy with megalencephaly, blindness, hypotonia, and severe developmental delay, although patients surviving to adulthood have been reported.

Most cases can now be diagnosed on the basis of biochemical and genetic testing, and magnetic resonance spectroscopy may show an increase in the N-acetylaspartate peak (57). Brain biopsy was used in the past for diagnosis (58). On brain biopsy, Canavan disease has some unique features: preferential involvement of subcortical U fibers and marked vacuolar change (fig. 12-28). There is also Alzheimer type II gliosis (fig. 12-29). On electron microscopy, the vacuoles seem to split myelin lamellae; irregular giant mitochondria may be present.

Vanishing White Matter Disease

Vanishing white matter disease, also known as *childhood ataxia with central hypomyelination*, is a recently described leukodystrophy sometimes associated with ovarian failure (59–62). The

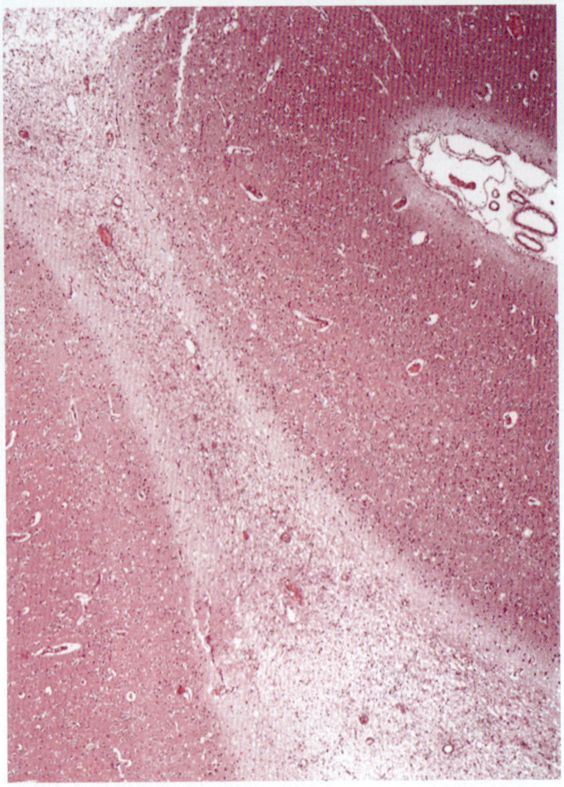

Figure 12-30

VANISHING WHITE MATTER DISEASE

The white matter is reduced in size and cavitated between the two cortical mantles.

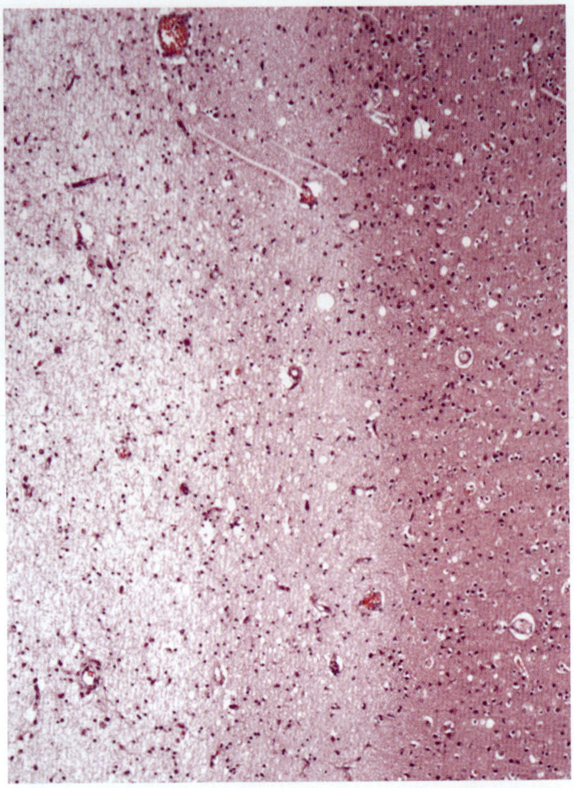

Figure 12-31

VANISHING WHITE MATTER DISEASE

There is a marked loss of white matter but a normal number of oligodendrocytes.

disease arises as a result of mutations in five related genes that encode subunits of the translation initiation factor eIF2B: *EIF2B1* on chromosome 12, *EIF2B2* on 14q24, *EIF2B3* on chromosome 1, *EIF2B4* on 2p23, or *EIF2B5* on 3q27. The disease overlaps clinically and genetically with *Cree leukoencephalopathy*, described in the Cree and Chippewa Indians (62). Vanishing white matter disease usually presents in children (63), but adults have been reported as well (64,65), including in presymptomatic stages (66,67). Biopsies have been performed in some patients (68). Patients present with neurologic deterioration, cerebellar ataxia, and spasticity, which worsen after minor infections or minimal head trauma.

The disease derives its name from the neuroimaging findings, in which the cerebral white matter gradually assumes the signal characteristics of CSF. Neuropathologic examination demonstrates a cavitating orthochromatic leukodystrophy (fig. 12-30), with marked myelin loss but sometimes with an apparent increase in the number of oligodendrocytes (fig. 12-31). The "foamy oligodendrocytes" seen in this condition (68) have an oligodendrocytic nucleus and homogeneously foamy to finely granular cytoplasm. Ultrastructural examination demonstrates numerous mitochondria as well as some myelin debris, accounting for the granularity of the cytoplasm (fig. 12-32). Although they have some light microscopic features of macrophages, the cells express oligodendrocytic genes and are not positive for macrophage markers such as CD68 (68).

Other Rare Leukodystrophies

A number of less well-characterized, sudanophilic, orthochromatic leukodystrophies have been reported in the literature. Given their relatively unusual clinical and imaging features and lack of diagnostic biochemical and/or molecular criteria, such entities may come to biopsy attention.

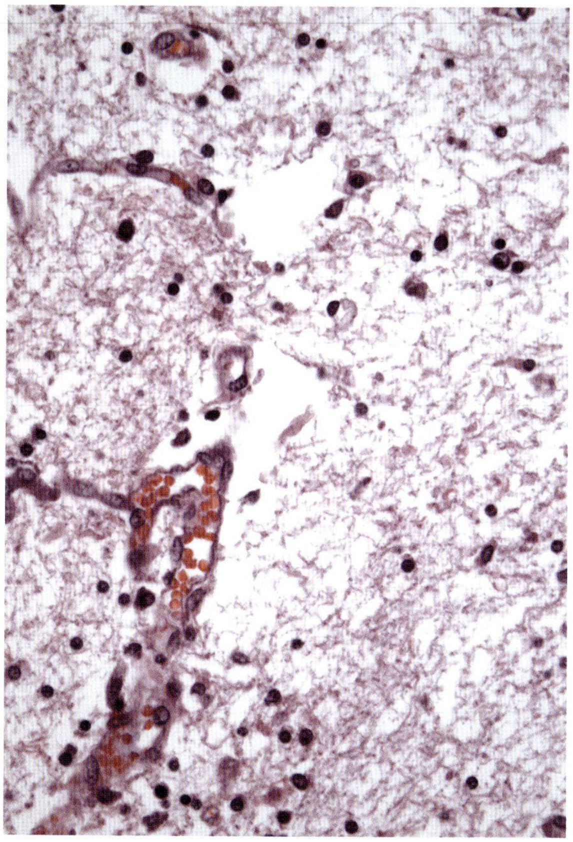

Figure 12-32

VANISHING WHITE MATTER DISEASE

Occasional foamy oligodendrocytes are seen.

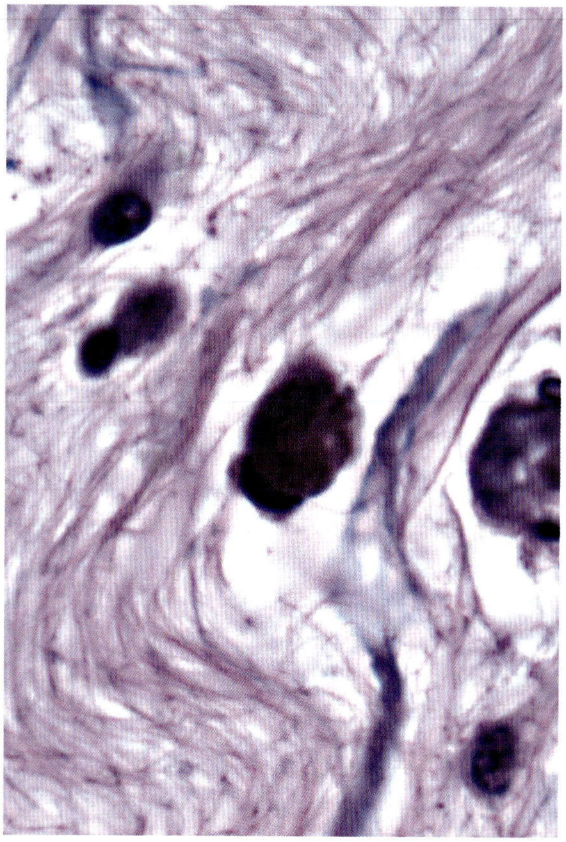

Figure 12-33

PIGMENTED LEUKODYSTROPHY

The macrophages contain brownish pigment (Luxol fast blue-H&E stain).

Orthochromatic pigmented leukodystrophy is a rare autosomal dominant condition that usually presents as a dementing illness in adults, accompanied by diffuse white matter changes (69,70). Biopsies have been performed on such patients to establish a diagnosis (71–73). In addition to the leukodystrophy, there is brown discoloration of the white mater that results from the deposition of pigment in glia and macrophages (fig. 12-33). The macrophages have an iron and lipid-rich pigment that is sudanophilic (fig. 12-34) and orthochromatic and that stains with PAS, Luxol fast blue, Fontana-Masson, and iron stains. There are electron-dense lysosomes with curvilinear and/or fingerprint profiles and ceroid-like material. Some of these cases display marked axonal spheroid accumulation (figs. 12-35, 12-36) and there is overlap between the pigmented and spheroid leukodystrophies (74). Hereditary cases that have predominant neuroaxonal spheroid

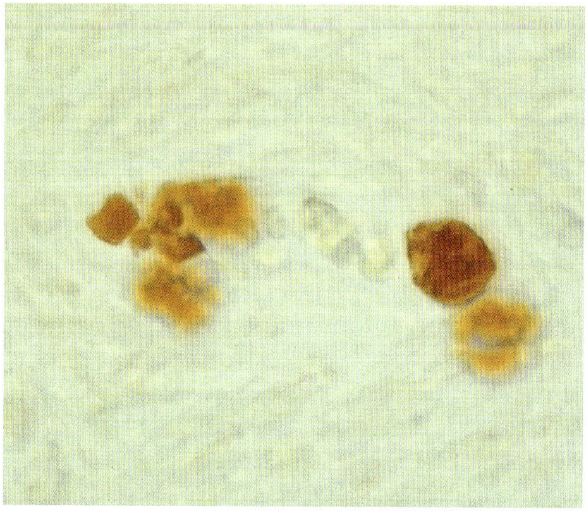

Figure 12-34

SUDANOPHILIC LEUKODYSTROPHY

The macrophages stain for Sudan red on frozen section.

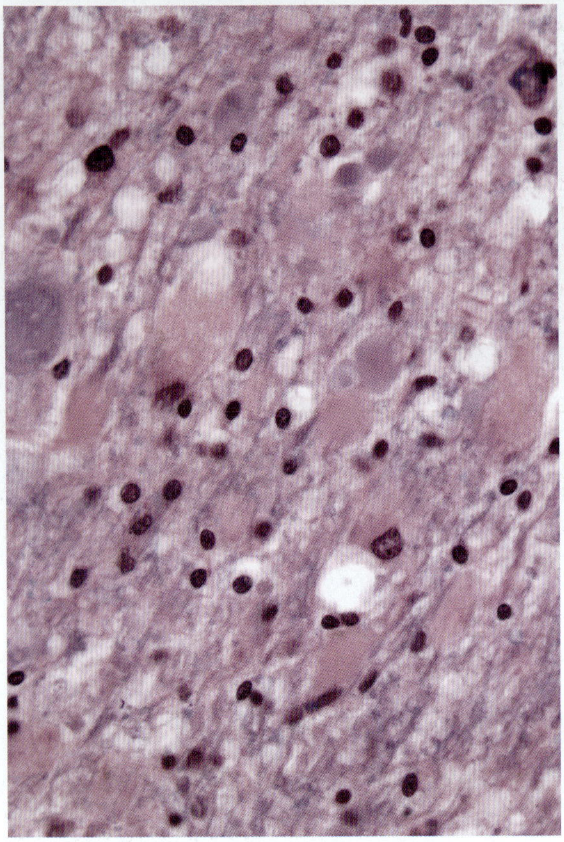

Figure 12-35

LEUKODYSTROPHY WITH SPHEROIDS

Many spheroids are noted along with loss of myelin (Luxol fast blue-H&E stain).

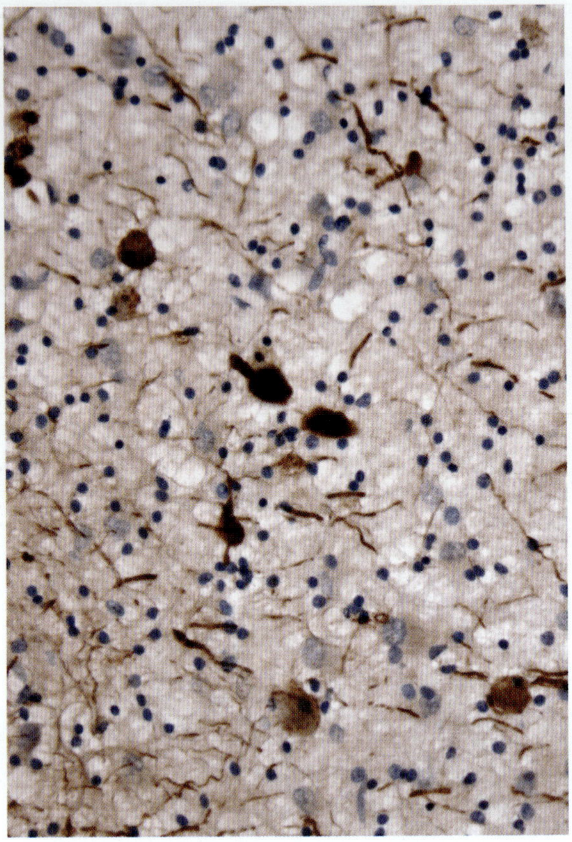

Figure 12-36

LEUKODYSTROPHY WITH SPHEROIDS

The spheroids are highlighted by immunohistochemistry for neurofilaments.

formation have been termed *hereditary diffuse leukoencephalopathy with spheroids* (75).

Megalencephalic cystic leukoencephalopathy (*megalencephalic leukoencephalopathy with subcortical cysts*) presents with macrocephaly in the first year of life, followed by a relatively slow neurologic decline characterized by spasticity, ataxia, and seizures over a few years (76–78). This rare disease appears to be autosomal recessive (79) and due to mutations in the *MLC1* gene on 22q (80,81). Neuroimaging reveals diffuse white matter abnormalities with cystic degeneration primarily affecting the temporal and parietal lobes (82,83). Because of the unusual clinical and radiologic features, biopsies have been performed (77,78). The pathologic findings include spongiform changes with oil red O-positive macrophages; splitting of myelin lamellae and associated vacuoles is seen ultrastructurally.

A leukodystrophy has been reported with onset as psychiatric disease in adults that features sudanophilic and PAS-positive macrophages clustered around blood vessels. Ultrastructural analysis demonstrates stacks of straight or curvilinear paired membranes within angulate lysosomes, which may indicate abnormal glycolipid accumulation (84). Other leukodystrophies have now been described on the basis of clinical and radiologic features, but remain poorly understood at a pathologic level. A leukoencephalopathy that is accompanied by atrophy of the basal ganglia and cerebellum occurs in infants and follows a variable course that includes movement disorders (61,85). Another leukoencephalopathy, characterized by slowly progressive ataxia and spasticity beginning in childhood, features brain stem and spinal cord involvement along with spectroscopic evidence of elevated white matter lactate levels (61,86). Other rare hereditary or metabolic diseases feature a leukoencephalopathy, but most of these affect other organs (87). On the rare occasion that such entities require a tissue diagnosis, biopsies are performed on systemic organs rather than on the CNS.

MITOCHONDRIAL ENCEPHALOPATHIES

Mitochondrial diseases include numerous clinicopathologic entities, ranging from full-blown neurologic compromise in young children to rather mild phenotypes affecting other organs in adults. In nearly all diagnostic situations in which the possibility of a mitochondrial disorder arises, these diseases can be recognized on the basis of biochemical or genetic features, or biopsy of other organs such as skeletal muscle. Nonetheless, while biopsy of the CNS is usually not done, rare cases of mitochondrial cytopathy defy standard diagnostic approaches (88) and a cerebral biopsy is performed. Such biopsies sometimes demonstrate features of mitochondrial encephalopathy (89) and sometimes prove diagnostic of other diseases (90).

The mitochondrial disease that can create a scenario in which cerebral biopsy is considered is *mitochondrial encephalomyopathy with lactic acidosis and stroke-like episodes* (MELAS), since this condition can mimic strokes or other multifocal lesions in young adults. Neuroimaging during the acute stroke-like episodes shows findings highly suggestive of small embolic infarcts that are not confined to vascular territories; calcification of the basal ganglia may also be seen. MELAS arises secondary to mutations in mitochondrial *tRNA* genes, with 80 percent of patients having the *A3243G* mutation in the *tRNA* leucine gene (91). The disease typically presents in young adulthood with stroke-like episodes, seizures, dementia, and exercise intolerance. Lactic acidosis, a common feature of many mitochondrial disorders, is nearly always present. Neuropathologic examination shows histologic findings similar to those of small subacute infarcts, but these do not conform to vascular territories and the crests of gyri may be preferentially involved (fig. 12-37). Increased numbers of mitochondria and enlarged and irregularly shaped mitochondria have been noted in the adjacent cerebral vasculature. Mineralization of the cerebral parenchyma, particularly the basal ganglia, is common in MELAS and can be readily detected on neuroimaging. The remaining white matter often has a spongiform appearance, occasioned by edema within the myelin sheaths, a CNS feature common to many mitochondrial diseases (fig. 12-38). In an appropriate clinical setting, the presence of infarct-like lesions, mineralization, and/or spongiform changes on cerebral biopsy suggests a diagnosis of MELAS.

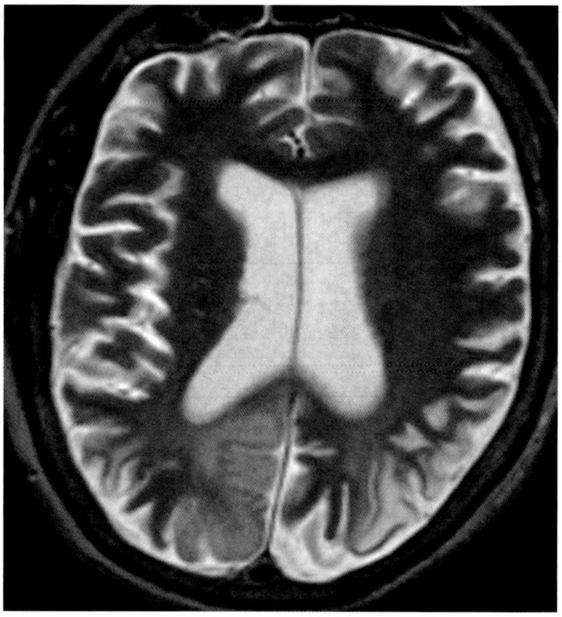

Figure 12-37

MELAS (MITOCHONDRIAL ENCEPHALOMYOPATHY WITH LACTIC ACIDOSIS AND STROKE-LIKE EPISODES)

MRI demonstrates white and gray matter abnormalities that do not conform to vascular territories.

OTHER METABOLIC DISEASES

Many other metabolic diseases affect the CNS. These include a host of other storage diseases as well as peroxisomal diseases for which precise biochemical or genetic features enable a diagnosis without resorting to CNS biopsy. For some of these, biopsy of systemic sites allows for diagnostic assessment at light microscopic, ultrastructural, and biochemical levels, again obviating the need for CNS biopsy. It is anticipated that, as precise biochemical and genetic definitions emerge for all of the metabolic diseases of the nervous system, CNS biopsy will become even rarer.

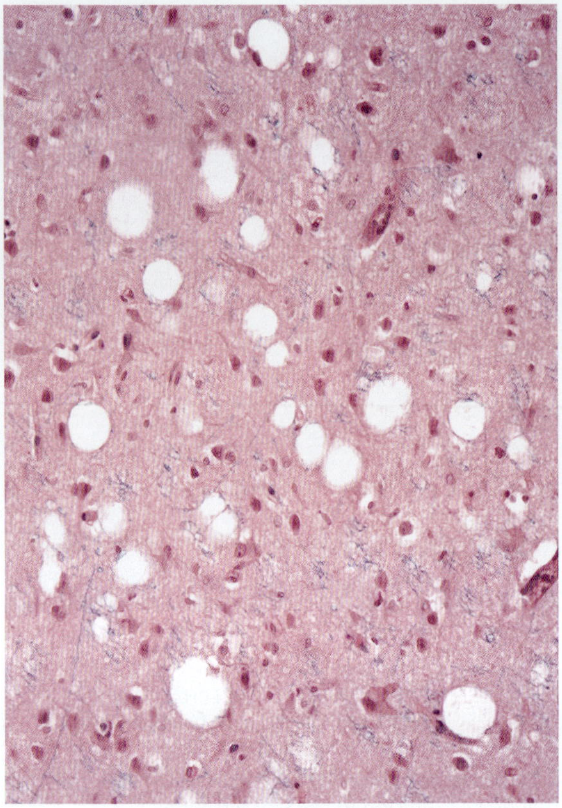

Figure 12-38

MITOCHONDRIAL DISEASE

Vacuolation may affect the gray matter (as in this section of cerebral cortex) or the white matter (Luxol fast blue-H&E stain).

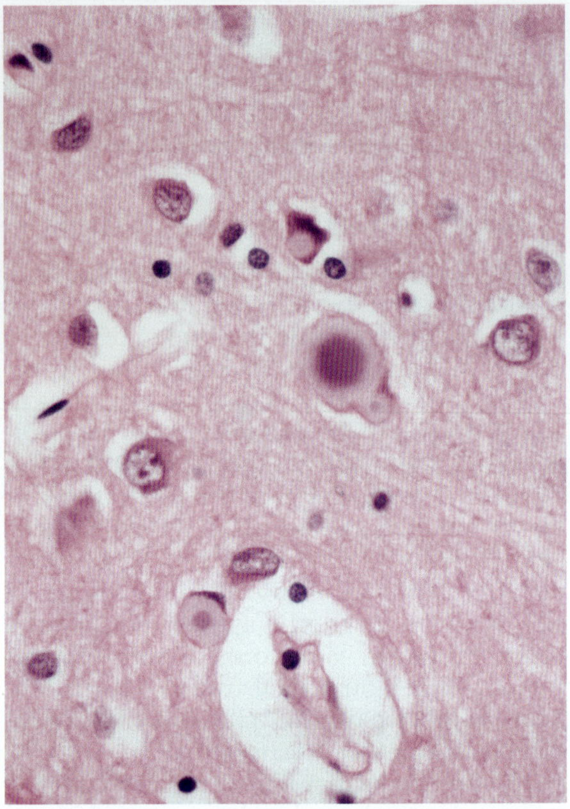

Figure 12-39

LAFORA BODY DISEASE

A laminated basophilic body is in a cortical neuron.

Lafora body disease is a rare autosomal recessive form of myoclonic epilepsy, characterized by so-called Lafora bodies in the CNS and a variety of systemic organs, including skin appendages, liver, and skeletal and cardiac muscle. Lafora bodies appear histologically identical to the corpora amylacea that are found commonly in astrocytic foot processes, often surrounding the ventricles of older persons. Lafora bodies and corpora amylacea are round, basophilic deposits, composed of polyglucosans, that range from a few to 30 µm in size (figs. 12-39, 12-40). Lafora bodies are PAS positive and diastase resistant; they are also Alcian blue positive and stain metachromatically with methyl violet stains on frozen tissue. They are found in neurons throughout the brain, with many found in the cerebellum. The disease has recently been found to arise from mutations in the *EPM2A* gene on 6q24, which encodes laforin, a protein tyrosine phosphatase (92) or from mutations in the *NHLRC1* gene on 6p22, which encodes for malin, a zinc finger protein with possible ubiquitin ligase function (93). A number of cases of Lafora body disease have been diagnosed by brain biopsy, with the characteristic bodies noted in the cerebrum or cerebellum (94–97).

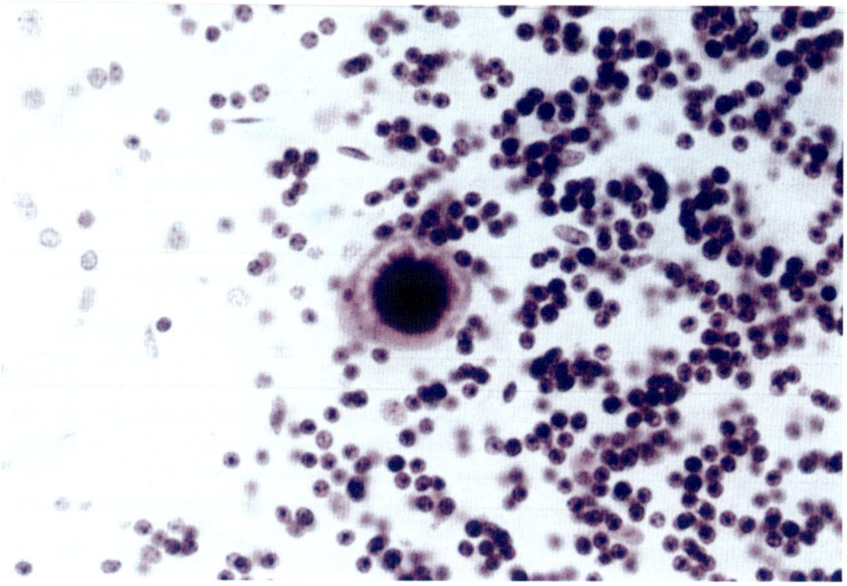

Figure 12-40

LAFORA BODY DISEASE

A Lafora body is in a Purkinje cell (Nissl stain).

REFERENCES

1. Love S, Louis DN, Ellison DW, eds. Greenfield's neuropathology, 8th ed. London: Hodder Arnold; 2008.
2. Ceuterick-de Groote C, Martin JJ. Extracerebral biopsy in lysosomal and peroxisomal disorders. Ultrastructural findings. Brain Pathol 1998;8:121-132.
3. Scriver CR, Beaudet AL, Valle D, et al. The metabolic and molecular bases of inherited disease, 8th ed. New York: McGraw-Hill; 2001.
4. Suzuki K, Suzuki K. Lysosomal diseases. In: Graham DI, Lantos PL, eds. Greenfield's neuropathology, Vol 1. London: Arnold; 2002:653-735.
5. Volk BW, Wallace BJ, Adachi M. Infantile Gaucher's disease: electron microscopic and histochemical studies of a cerebral biopsy. J Neuropathol Exp Neurol 1967;26:176-177.
6. Haltia M. The neuronal ceroid-lipofuscinoses. J Neuropathol Exp Neurol 2003;62:1-13.
7. Tyynela J, Suopanki J, Baumann M, Haltia M. Sphingolipid activator proteins (SAPs) in neuronal ceroid lipofuscinoses (NCL). Neuropediatrics 1997;28:49-52.
8. Lake BD, Hall NA. Immunolocalization studies of subunit c in late-infantile and juvenile Batten disease. J Inherit Metab Dis 1993;16:263-266.
9. Nijssen PC, Ceuterick C, van Diggelen OP, et al. Autosomal dominant adult neuronal ceroid lipofuscinosis: a novel form of NCL with granular osmiophilic deposits without palmitoyl protein thioesterase 1 deficiency. Brain Pathol 2003;13:574-581.
10. Augustine A, Fricchione G, Woznicki R, Broberg D, Holt J. Adult neuronal ceroid lipofuscinosis presenting with psychiatric symptoms: a case report. Int J Psychiatry Med 1993;23:315-322.
11. Hammersen S, Brock M, Cervos-Navarro J. Adult neuronal ceroid lipofuscinosis with clinical findings consistent with a butterfly glioma. Case report. J Neurosurg 1998;88:314-318.
12. Sinha S, Satishchandra P, Santosh V, Gayatri N, Shankar SK. Neuronal ceroid lipofuscinosis: a clinicopathological study. Seizure 2004;13:235-240.
13. Callagy C, O'Neill G, Murphy SF, Farrell MA. Adult neuronal ceroid lipofuscinosis (Kufs' disease) in two siblings of an Irish family. Clin Neuropathol 2000;19:109-118.
14. Carlen B, Englund E. Diagnostic value of electron microscopy in a case of juvenile neuronal ceroid lipofuscinosis. Ultrastruct Pathol 2001;25:285-288.
15. Goebel HH. Morphologic diagnosis in neuronal ceroid lipofuscinosis. Neuropediatrics 1997;28:67-69.
16. Batzdorf U, Sarlieve LL, Gold VA, Menkes JH. Tay-Sachs disease. Demonstration of the stored ganglioside in cultured cells from brain biopsy. Arch Neurol 1969;20:650-652.
17. de Baecque CM, Suzuki K, Rapin I, Johnson AB, Whethers DL. GM2-gangliosidosis, AB variant: clinico-pathological study of a case. Acta Neuropathol (Berl) 1975;33:207-226.

18. Pullarkat RK, Reha H, Beratis NG. Accumulation of ganglioside Gm2 in cerebrospinal fluid of a patient with the variant AB of infantile Gm2 gangliosidosis. Pediatrics 1981;68:106-108.
19. Suzuki K. Neuropathology of late onset gangliosidoses. A review. Dev Neurosci 1991;13:205-210.
20. Hulette CM, Earl NL, Anthony DC, Crain BJ. Adult onset Niemann-Pick disease type C presenting with dementia and absent organomegaly. Clin Neuropathol 1992;11:293-297.
21. Epstein MA, Zimmerman RA, Rorke LB, Sladky JT. Late-onset globoid cell leukodystrophy mimicking an infiltrating glioma. Pediatr Radiol 1991;21:131-132.
22. Stephenson DJ, Bezman L, Raymond GV. Acute presentation of childhood adrenoleukodystrophy. Neuropediatrics 2000;31:293-297.
23. Larner AJ. Adult-onset dementia with prominent frontal lobe dysfunction in X-linked adrenoleukodystrophy with R152C mutation in ABCD1 gene. J Neurol 2003;250:1253-1254.
24. Weller M, Liedtke W, Petersen D, Opitz H, Poremba M. Very-late-onset adrenoleukodystrophy: possible precipitation of demyelination by cerebral contusion. Neurology 1992;42:367-370.
25. Esiri MM, Hyman NM, Horton WL, Lindenbaum RH. Adrenoleukodystrophy: clinical, pathological and biochemical findings in two brothers with the onset of cerebral disease in adult life. Neuropathol Appl Neurobiol 1984;10:429-445.
26. Schaumburg HH, Powers JM, Raine CS, Suzuki K, Richardson EP Jr. Adrenoleukodystrophy. A clinical and pathological study of 17 cases. Arch Neurol 1975;32:577-591.
27. Kurihara M, Kumagai K, Yagishita S, et al. Adrenoleukomyeloneuropathy presenting as cerebellar ataxia in a young child: a probable variant of adrenoleukodystrophy. Brain Dev 1993;15:377-380.
28. Salmon E, Van der Linden M, Maerfens Noordhout A, et al. Early thalamic and cortical hypometabolism in adult-onset dementia due to metachromatic leukodystrophy. Acta Neurol Belg 1999;99:185-188.
29. Felice KJ, Gomez Lira M, Natowicz M, et al. Adult-onset MLD: a gene mutation with isolated polyneuropathy. Neurology 2000;55:1036-1039.
30. Bostantjopoulou S, Katsarou Z, Michelakaki H, Kazis A. Seizures as a presenting feature of late onset metachromatic leukodystrophy. Acta Neurol Scand 2000;102:192-195.
31. Henderson RD, MacMillan JC, Bradfield JM. Adult onset Krabbe disease may mimic motor neuron disease. J Clin Neurosci 2003;10:638-639.
32. Kolodny EH, Raghavan S, Krivit W. Late-onset Krabbe disease (globoid cell leukodystrophy): clinical and biochemical features of 15 cases. Dev Neurosci 1991;13:232-239.
33. Harzer K, Knoblich R, Rolfs A, Bauer P, Eggers J. Residual galactosylsphingosine (psychosine) beta-galactosidase activities and associated GALC mutations in late and very late onset Krabbe disease. Clin Chim Acta 2002;317:77-84.
34. De Gasperi R, Gama Sosa MA, Sartorato EL, et al. Molecular heterogeneity of late-onset forms of globoid-cell leukodystrophy. Am J Hum Genet 1996;59:1233-1242.
35. Farina L, Bizzi A, Finocchiaro G, et al. MR imaging and proton MR spectroscopy in adult Krabbe disease. AJNR Am J Neuroradiol 2000;21:1478-1482.
36. Brockmann K, Dechent P, Wilken B, Rusch O, Frahm J, Hanefeld F. Proton MRS profile of cerebral metabolic abnormalities in Krabbe disease. Neurology 2003;60:819-825.
37. Mimault C, Giraud G, Courtois V, et al. Proteolipoprotein gene analysis in 82 patients with sporadic Pelizaeus-Merzbacher disease: duplications, the major cause of the disease, originate more frequently in male germ cells, but point mutations do not. The Clinical European Network on Brain Dysmyelinating Disease. Am J Hum Genet 1999;65:360-369.
38. Woodward K, Kendall E, Vetrie D, Malcolm S. Pelizaeus-Merzbacher disease: identification of Xq22 proteolipid-protein duplications and characterization of breakpoints by interphase FISH. Am J Hum Genet 1998;63:207-217.
39. Woodward K, Palmer R, Rao K, Malcolm S. Prenatal diagnosis by FISH in a family with Pelizaeus-Merzbacher disease caused by duplication of PLP gene. Prenat Diagn 1999;19:266-268.
40. Begleiter ML, Harris DJ. Autosomal recessive form of connatal Pelizaeus-Merzbacher disease. Am J Med Genet 1989;33:311-313.
41. Cassidy SB, Sheehan NC, Farrell DF, Grunnet M, Holmes GL, Zimmerman AW. Connatal Pelizaeus-Merzbacher disease: an autosomal recessive form. Pediatr Neurol 1987;3:300-305.
42. Sasaki A, Miyanaga K, Ototsuji M, et al. Two autopsy cases with Pelizaeus-Merzbacher disease phenotype of adult onset, without mutation of proteolipid protein gene. Acta Neuropathol (Berl) 2000;99:7-13.
43. Saito Y, Ando T, Doyu M, Takahashi A, Hashizume Y. [An adult case of classical Pelizaeus-Merzbacher disease--magnetic resonance images and neuropathological findings]. Rinsho Shinkeigaku 1993;33:187-193. [Japanese]
44. Nance MA, Boyadjiev S, Pratt VM, Taylor S, Hodes ME, Dlouhy SR. Adult-onset neurodegenerative disorder due to proteolipid protein gene mutation in the mother of a man with Pelizaeus-Merzbacher disease. Neurology 1996;47:1333-1335.

45. Cailloux F, Gauthier-Barichard F, Mimault C, et al. Genotype-phenotype correlation in inherited brain myelination defects due to proteolipid protein gene mutations. Clinical European Network on Brain Dysmyelinating Disease. Eur J Hum Genet 2000;8:837-845.
46. Johnson AB. Alexander disease: a leukodystrophy caused by a mutation in GFAP. Neurochem Res 2004;29:961-964.
47. Gorospe JR, Naidu S, Johnson AB, et al. Molecular findings in symptomatic and pre-symptomatic Alexander disease patients. Neurology 2002;58:1494-1500.
48. Li R, Messing A, Goldman JE, Brenner M. GFAP mutations in Alexander disease. Int J Dev Neurosci 2002;20:259-268.
49. Probst EN, Hagel C, Weisz V, et al. Atypical focal MRI lesions in a case of juvenile Alexander's disease. Ann Neurol 2003;53:118-120.
50. Namekawa M, Takiyama Y, Aoki Y, et al. Identification of GFAP gene mutation in hereditary adult-onset Alexander's disease. Ann Neurol 2002;52:779-785.
51. Stumpf E, Masson H, Duquette A, et al. Adult Alexander disease with autosomal dominant transmission: a distinct entity caused by mutation in the glial fibrillary acid protein gene. Arch Neurol 2003;60:1307-1312.
52. Wilson SP, Al-Sarraj S, Bridges LR. Rosenthal fiber encephalopathy presenting with demyelination and Rosenthal fibers in a solvent abuser: adult Alexander's disease? Clin Neuropathol 1996;15:13-16.
53. Riggs JE, Schochet SS Jr, Nelson J. Asymptomatic adult Alexander's disease: entity or nosological misconception? Neurology 1988;38:152-154.
54. Martidis A, Yee RD, Azzarelli B, Biller J. Neuro-ophthalmic, radiographic, and pathologic manifestations of adult-onset Alexander disease. Arch Ophthalmol 1999;117:265-267.
55. Johnson AB. Alexander disease: a review and the gene. Int J Dev Neurosci 2002;20:391-394.
56. Sistermans EA, de Coo RF, van Beerendonk HM, Poll-The BT, Kleijer WJ, van Oost BA. Mutation detection in the aspartoacylase gene in 17 patients with Canavan disease: four new mutations in the non-Jewish population. Eur J Hum Genet 2000;8:557-560.
57. Wittsack HJ, Kugel H, Roth B, Heindel W. Quantitative measurements with localized 1H MR spectroscopy in children with Canavan's disease. J Magn Reson Imaging 1996;6:889-893.
58. Matalon R, Kaul R, Casanova J, et al. SSIEM Award. Aspartoacylase deficiency: the enzyme defect in Canavan disease. J Inherit Metab Dis 1989;12(Suppl 2):329-331.
59. Schiffmann R, Tedeschi G, Kinkel RP, et al. Leukodystrophy in patients with ovarian dysgenesis. Ann Neurol 1997;41:654-661.
60. Schiffmann R, Moller JR, Trapp BD, et al. Childhood ataxia with diffuse central nervous system hypomyelination. Ann Neurol 1994;35:331-340.
61. Schiffmann R, van der Knaap MS. The latest on leukodystrophies. Curr Opin Neurol 2004;17:187-192.
62. Fogli A, Wong K, Eymard-Pierre E, et al. Cree leukoencephalopathy and CACH/VWM disease are allelic at the EIF2B5 locus. Ann Neurol 2002;52:506-510.
63. van der Knaap MS, Barth PG, Gabreels FJ, et al. A new leukoencephalopathy with vanishing white matter. Neurology 1997;48:845-855.
64. Prass K, Bruck W, Schroder NW, et al. Adult-onset leukoencephalopathy with vanishing white matter presenting with dementia. Ann Neurol 2001;50:665-668.
65. Ohtake H, Shimohata T, Terajima K, et al. Adult-onset leukoencephalopathy with vanishing white matter with a missense mutation in EIF2B5. Neurology 2004;62:1601-1603.
66. Biancheri R, Rossi A, Di Rocco M, et al. Leukoencephalopathy with vanishing white matter: an adult onset case. Neurology 2003;61:1818-1819.
67. van der Knaap MS, Leegwater PA, van Berkel CG, et al. Arg113His mutation in eIF2Bepsilon as cause of leukoencephalopathy in adults. Neurology 2004;62:1598-1600.
68. Wong K, Armstrong RC, Gyure KA, et al. Foamy cells with oligodendroglial phenotype in childhood ataxia with diffuse central nervous system hypomyelination syndrome. Acta Neuropathol (Berl) 2000;100:635-646.
69. Seiser A, Jellinger K, Brainin M. Pigmentary type of orthochromatic leukodystrophy with early onset and protracted course. Neuropediatrics 1990;21:48-52.
70. Constantinidis J, Wisniewski TM. The dominant form of the pigmentary orthochromatic leukodystrophy. Acta Neuropathol (Berl) 1991;82:483-487.
71. Calandriello L, Matteucci C, Bertini E, et al. Biopsy diagnosis of a case of adult onset orthochromatic leukodystrophy. Clinical and brain biopsy findings. Ital J Neurol Sci 1992;13:787-792.
72. Shannon P, Wherrett JR, Nag S. A rare form of adult onset leukodystrophy: orthochromatic leukodystrophy with pigmented glia. Can J Neurol Sci 1997;24:146-150.
73. Dousset V, Tison F, Vital A, Henry P. [Fulminant orthochromatic leukodystrophy in an adult]. Rev Neurol (Paris) 1998;154:415-418. [French]

74. Marotti JD, Tobias S, Fratkin JD, Powers JM, Rhodes CH. Adult onset leukodystrophy with neuroaxonal spheroids and pigmented glia: report of a family, historical perspective, and review of the literature. Acta Neuropathol (Berl) 2004;107:481-488.
75. van der Knaap MS, Naidu S, Kleinschmidt-Demasters BK, Kamphorst W, Weinstein HC. Autosomal dominant diffuse leukoencephalopathy with neuroaxonal spheroids. Neurology 2000;54:463-468.
76. Olivier M, Lenard HG, Aksu F, Gartner J. A new leukoencephalopathy with bilateral anterior temporal lobe cysts. Neuropediatrics 1998;29:225-228.
77. Harbord MG, Harden A, Harding B, Brett EM, Baraitser M. Megalencephaly with dysmyelination, spasticity, ataxia, seizures and distinctive neurophysiological findings in two siblings. Neuropediatrics 1990;21:164-168.
78. van der Knaap MS, Barth PG, Vrensen GF, Valk J. Histopathology of an infantile-onset spongiform leukoencephalopathy with a discrepantly mild clinical course. Acta Neuropathol (Berl) 1996;92:206-212.
79. Ben-Zeev B, Gross V, Kushnir T, et al. Vacuolating megalencephalic leukoencephalopathy in 12 Israeli patients. J Child Neurol 2001;16:93-99.
80. Leegwater PA, Yuan BQ, van der Steen J, et al. Mutations of MLC1 (KIAA0027), encoding a putative membrane protein, cause megalencephalic leukoencephalopathy with subcortical cysts. Am J Hum Genet 2001;68:831-838.
81. Leegwater PA, Boor PK, Yuan BQ, et al. Identification of novel mutations in MLC1 responsible for megalencephalic leukoencephalopathy with subcortical cysts. Hum Genet 2002;110:279-283.
82. Mejaski-Bosnjak V, Besenski N, Brockmann K, Pouwels PJ, Frahm J, Hanefeld FA. Cystic leukoencephalopathy in a megalencephalic child: clinical and magnetic resonance imaging/magnetic resonance spectroscopy findings. Pediatr Neurol 1997;16:347-350.
83. Mejaski-Bosnjak V, Besenski N. Megalencephalic leukoencephalopathy: a further case of a new neurodegenerative white matter disease. Dev Med Child Neurol 1997;39:561-563.
84. Simon DK, Rodriguez ML, Frosch MP, Quackenbush EJ, Feske SK, Natowicz MR. A unique familial leukodystrophy with adult onset dementia and abnormal glycolipid storage: a new lysosomal disease? J Neurol Neurosurg Psychiatry 1998;65:251-254.
85. van der Knaap MS, Naidu S, Pouwels PJ, et al. New syndrome characterized by hypomyelination with atrophy of the basal ganglia and cerebellum. AJNR Am J Neuroradiol 2002;23:1466-1474.
86. van der Knaap MS, van der Voorn P, Barkhof F, et al. A new leukoencephalopathy with brainstem and spinal cord involvement and high lactate. Ann Neurol 2003;53:252-258.
87. Kaye EM. Update on genetic disorders affecting white matter. Pediatr Neurol 2001;24:11-24.
88. Johns DR, Stein AG, Wityk R. MELAS syndrome masquerading as herpes simplex encephalitis. Neurology 1993;43:2471-2473.
89. Gilchrist JM, Sikirica M, Stopa E, Shanske S. Adult-onset MELAS. Evidence for involvement of neurons as well as cerebral vasculature in strokelike episodes. Stroke 1996;27:1420-1423.
90. Kang PB, Hunter JV, Kaye EM. Lactic acid elevation in extramitochondrial childhood neurodegenerative diseases. J Child Neurol 2001;16:657-660.
91. Goto Y, Nonaka I, Horai S. A mutation in the tRNA(Leu)(UUR) gene associated with the MELAS subgroup of mitochondrial encephalomyopathies. Nature 1990;348:651-653.
92. Minassian BA, Lee JR, Herbrick JA, et al. Mutations in a gene encoding a novel protein tyrosine phosphatase cause progressive myoclonus epilepsy. Nat Genet 1998;20:171-174.
93. Chan EM, Young EJ, Ianzano L, et al. Mutations in NHLRC1 cause progressive myoclonus epilepsy. Nat Genet 2003;35:125-127.
94. Drury I, Blaivas M, Abou-Khalil BW, Beydoun A. Biopsy results in a kindred with Lafora disease. Arch Neurol 1993;50:102-105.
95. Elliott EJ, Talbot IC, Pye IF, Hodges S, Swift PG, Tanner MS. Lafora disease: a progressive myoclonus epilepsy. J Paediatr Child Health 1992;28:455-458.
96. Busard HL, Renier WO, Gabreels FJ, et al. Lafora disease: a quantitative morphological and biochemical study of the cerebral cortex. Clin Neuropathol 1987;6:1-6.
97. Yerby MS, Shaw CM, Watson JM. Progressive dementia and epilepsy in a young adult: unusual intraneuronal inclusions. Neurology 1986;36:68-71.

13 SEIZURE DISORDERS AND MALFORMATIONS

Neuropathologists are frequently called upon to evaluate specimens from patients with a history of seizures or congenital malformations. These specimens are obtained through resections to treat intractable epilepsy or from diagnostic biopsies, since a wide range of both neoplastic and non-neoplastic diseases are associated with seizures. While some congenital malformations are associated with seizures, specimens in these cases are more frequently obtained from surgical repairs. This chapter addresses the major conditions encountered in surgical neuropathology practice that are associated with seizures (hippocampal sclerosis, malformations, hamartomas, neurocutaneous syndromes, autoimmune disease) and congenital malformations (neural tube and related defects).

While there is a diversity of histopathologic findings associated with seizures, a few common themes emerge in the evaluation of these specimens. Reviewing the clinical information is an essential step in the diagnostic evaluation of such specimens; the histopathologic findings alone may be insufficiently sensitive or specific to establish the correct diagnosis. It is also imperative to review the neuroimaging studies for the location and appearance of the affected brain regions. In many cases, this provides correlative gross pathology for the neuropathologist. Some conditions, including heterotopias and hamartomas, may not be readily recognizable solely on microscopic review. Finally, it is important to keep in mind the limitations imposed by sampling and anatomy. Disorders such as Rasmussen syndrome may show wide temporal and spatial variation in histopathologic appearance. Other processes, including cortical dysplasia, tuberous sclerosis, and hemimegalencephaly, may have overlapping histopathologic characteristics. The descriptive histopathology of these lesions is a strong starting point, but adequate sampling, a complete clinical history, and pertinent neuroimaging studies are often essential in establishing the correct diagnosis.

HIPPOCAMPAL SCLEROSIS

Definition. *Hippocampal sclerosis* is cell loss and gliosis in the hippocampus associated with temporal lobe epilepsy (TLE), and sometimes extratemporal epilepsy. Many terms have been applied to the selective loss of neurons in the hippocampus in association with seizures. This variable terminology includes *incisural sclerosis, mesial temporal sclerosis, Ammon's horn sclerosis,* and *end folium sclerosis*. While it is indisputable that hippocampal sclerosis is associated with TLE, it remains an ongoing debate whether hippocampal sclerosis is the cause or the consequence of chronic seizures in these patients. Regardless of the dispute, resection of these lesions is associated with significant clinical improvement in patients with TLE (1).

Clinical Features. The frequency of hippocampal sclerosis varies in patients with TLE, but is reported in up to 65 percent (2). Other causes of TLE include focal lesions in the mesial temporal lobe structures such as tumors, vascular malformations, and hamartomas (3). TLE is one of the most common and well-characterized epilepsy syndromes. It is also strikingly refractory to medical therapy, and surgical resection is typically required for seizure control (4). This type of epilepsy is often accompanied by a history of febrile seizures or traumatic injury in childhood (although febrile seizures, which are quite common, usually do not result in TLE) and is sometimes associated with subsequent spontaneous afebrile seizures in later childhood (2). The seizures, while initially responsive to medical therapy, progress to become intractable, usually by early adulthood. The seizures are usually complex partial seizures and are preceded by an aura, most often epigastric, but also autonomic or emotional. Characteristically, there is a postictal phase with amnesia and, if involving the language-dominant hemisphere, dysphasia. Seizures may be accompanied by depression and other behavioral disturbances (4). A family history of seizures is often encountered, but TLE does not appear to have a significant genetic component (1,4). There is a genetic predisposition to febrile seizures, however, which is one of the important causes of hippocampal injury leading to TLE (5).

Radiologic Findings. The structural changes associated with hippocampal sclerosis are readily appreciated by magnetic resonance imaging (MRI). In fact, neuroimaging techniques are often the primary diagnostic tools for this disorder. Axial T1- and T2-weighted images are often used to identify hippocampal anatomy. Images from either of these sequences can be used to recognize the presence of hippocampal atrophy. A common finding on T1-weighted images is the loss of internal structures of the hippocampus on the affected side in patients with TLE. Gradient echo T1-weighted images can identify the gray-white matter interface and are useful for identifying areas of cortical dysplasia. Fluid-attenuated inversion recovery (FLAIR) sequences are also useful for identifying both epileptogenic cortical foci and pathologic changes in the hippocampus. The key combination of imaging features is atrophy of the hippocampus and an increased T2-weighted signal in mesial temporal structures. The latter may reflect the severity of neuronal loss and gliosis, but is not specific. The radiologic changes described above are typically unilateral, but may be bilateral in up to 15 percent of cases (4,6).

Gross Findings. *Gross Anatomy of the Hippocampus.* Standard surgical approaches for hippocampal resection typically yield two specimens: 1) a portion of anterolateral temporal cortex, often 4 to 5 cm, and 2) the hippocampus. Depending on the surgeon, the hippocampus is received in fragments or as an en bloc resection, which is better as it allows orientation for optimal sectioning. In intact specimens, the orientation of the hippocampus is the essential step in producing sections that show the characteristic changes of hippocampal sclerosis. Fragmented or poorly oriented sections are still interpretable, but finer details concerning the involvement of specific hippocampal regions may be lost.

In situ, the rostral extent of the hippocampus begins at the level of the mamillary body and anterior commissure. The hippocampus extends to the caudal end of the corpus callosum (fig. 13-1). Given this course, it is not surprising that the resected hippocampus is typically somewhat curved. The key to handling the gross specimen is to recognize the distinctive surface anatomy of this structure. The rostral end of the hippocampus is the widest and has slightly bulbous undulations, described as a cat's paw appearance, or hippocampal digitations. The hippocampus tapers toward the caudal end. A second anatomic hallmark that can be used to establish the proper orientation of the specimen is the dorsal, or ventricular, surface of the hippocampus. The hippocampus has a smooth white surface due to the myelinated fibers (the alveus) that run along the ventricular surface. These are collected into a large band of fibers to form the fimbria of the hippocampus. The fimbria extends along the dorsal aspect of the hippocampus until it exits, just below the corpus callosum, as the fornix.

When intact specimens are received, use should be made of these surface features to properly orient the hippocampus so that it can be serially sectioned perpendicular to its long axis. Only if this is done will the neuropathologist receive frontal sections of the hippocampus that show the characteristic hippocampal cortex forming an inwardly rolled up band, Ammon's horn (fig. 13-1, inset).

Gross Pathology of the Hippocampus and Medial Temporal Lobe. The ability to recognize gross pathologic changes in these specimens is related to both the severity of the disease and the intactness of the specimen. In intact hippocampal resection specimens from severely affected patients, variable degrees of shrinkage and flattening of the hippocampal outline may be appreciated. The tissue may be firm to touch and show effacement of normal surface anatomy landmarks with gray-brown discoloration, changes consistent with gliosis.

Because of the frequency of dual pathology (see below) in patients with TLE, the gross sections of the temporal lobe resection must be carefully examined. The most common finding in these sections is normal cortex and subcortical white matter. Focal processes, including glioneuronal tumors and vascular malformations, can also be identified. Because of the frequency with which cortical dysplasia is encountered in these sections, properly oriented full-thickness (extending from the pial surface to the subcortical white matter) sections are especially important.

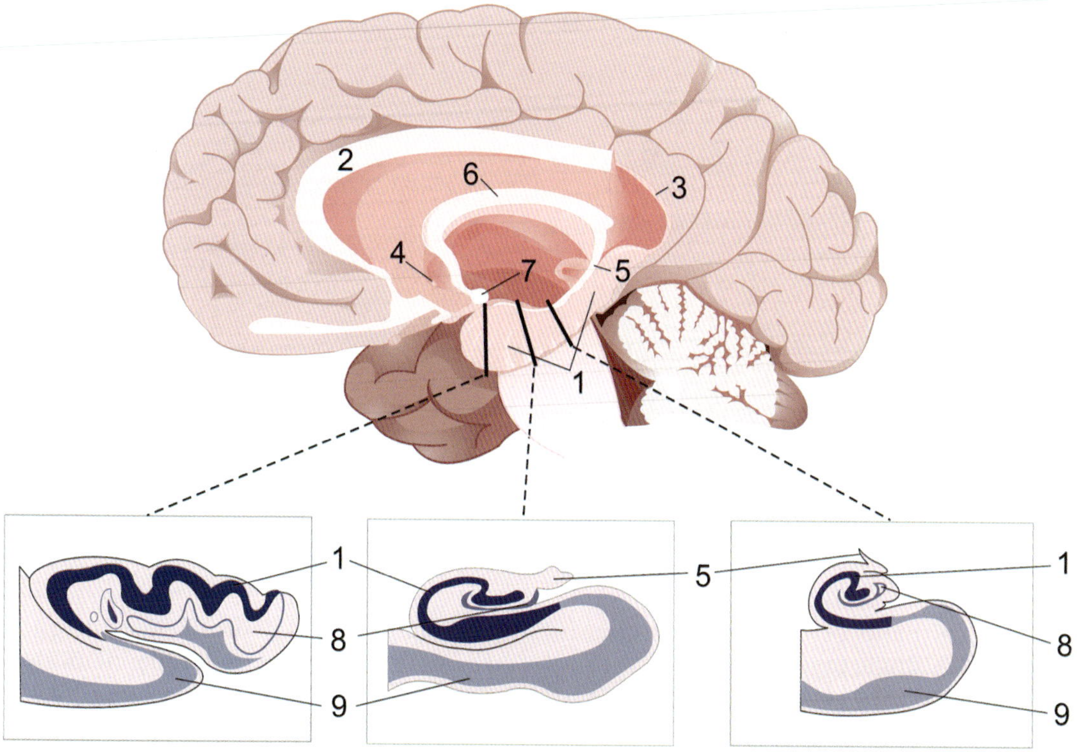

Figure 13-1

HIPPOCAMPUS: GROSS ANATOMY

Hippocampus in situ following removal of overlying left cerebral hemisphere. Inset shows varying profiles of Ammon's horn and dentate nucleus when the hippocampus is sectioned at different levels. Structures: 1 = hippocampus; 2 = corpus callosum; 3 = indusium griseum; 4 = anterior commissure; 5 = fimbria of the hippocampus; 6 = fornix; 7 = mamillary body; 8 = dentate gyrus; 9 = parahippocampal gyrus. (Illustration by Dr. Amy Noffsinger.)

Intraoperative Findings. When hippocampal sclerosis is the cause of the seizures of TLE, intraoperative consultation is rarely needed. From time to time, however, a focal lesion is the cause of the seizures. These most often are low-grade tumors, usually glioneuronal, such as ganglioglioma and dysembryoplastic neuroepithelial tumor. Other focal lesions that may be encountered are vascular malformations and hamartomas. Such lesions are generally readily distinguishable from the changes associated with hippocampal sclerosis, described below.

Microscopic Findings. *Microscopic Anatomy of the Hippocampus*. The diagnosis of hippocampal sclerosis requires familiarity with the microscopic anatomy of this structure (fig. 13-2). While the exact appearance of sections of the hippocampus varies depending on where along the hippocampus the section is taken, most of the structures can be identified if care is taken to orient and section en bloc specimens properly. When the specimen is fragmented or not properly oriented or sectioned, identification of the microscopic anatomy can be challenging.

Since the hippocampus is part of the archicortex, its cortical band does not have the same six-layered structure seen in other supratentorial regions, including the temporal lobe neocortex, which may also be part of the resection specimen. Instead, the structures of the hippocampus are three-layered, with a superficial molecular layer, a deep polymorphic layer, and an intermediate layer containing the pyramidal and granule cells that are the most distinctive histologic features of the hippocampus. Immediately adjacent to the hippocampal cortex is the subiculum which forms a transitional zone between the three-layered hippocampus and the six-layered entorhinal cortex.

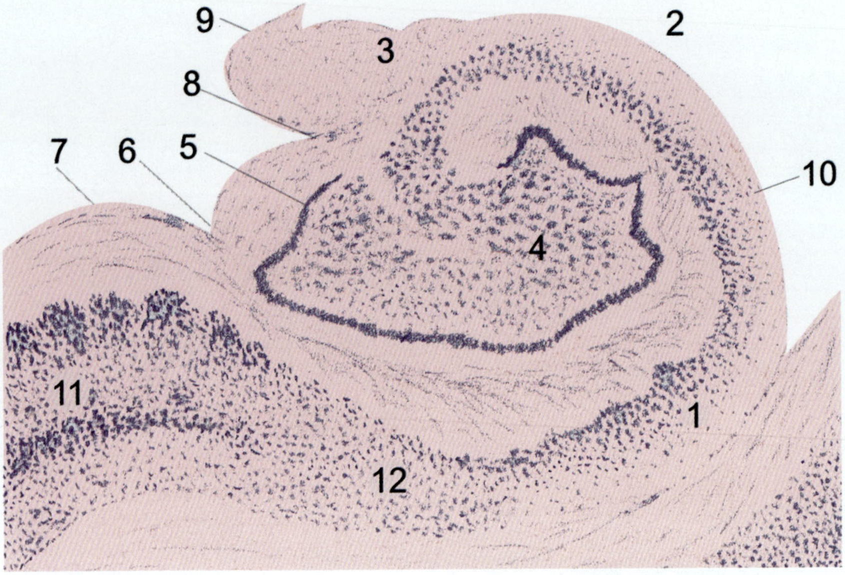

Figure 13-2

HIPPOCAMPUS: MICROSCOPIC ANATOMY

Ammon's horn, frontal section through the hippocampus. Structures: 1 = CA1; 2 = CA2; 3 = CA3; 4 = CA4; 5 = dentate gyrus (fascia dentata); 6 = parahippocampal sulcus; 7 = parahippocampal gyrus; 8 = fimbriodentate sulcus; 9 = fimbria of the hippocampus; 10 = alveus of the hippocampus; 11 = entorhinal cortex; 12 = subiculum. (Illustration by Dr. Amy Noffsinger.)

The cortical band of the hippocampus is composed of a single layer of pyramidal cells that are divided into sectors or fields on the basis of size and cell density: CA1 contains small pyramidal cells, CA2 features a narrow densely packed collection of large pyramidal cells, CA3 is characterized by a broad loose band of pyramidal cells, and the endplate, or CA4 field, is a loosely structured zone that contains both large and small pyramidal cells. The orientation and morphology of the neurons in this region can sometimes be diverse. The CA4 field is enclosed by a densely packed collection of small granular neurons, the dentate gyrus. Within the limitations of sampling and specimen orientation, it is often possible to identify the CA1 region approximately by considering the dentate gyrus as a broad arrow pointing to it.

Overlying these structures is the alveus. This is the major efferent pathway leaving the hippocampus, imparting to the dorsal or ventricular surface of the hippocampus its shiny white appearance. The alveus forms a distinctive landmark of microscopic anatomy: a superficially situated white matter tract with an overlying ependymal lining. In addition to microscopic orientation, the recognition of this structure, or parts of it, in a biopsy specimen obtained for other reasons, may be helpful in establishing a hippocampal location.

Pathologic Changes in the Hippocampus. Hippocampal sclerosis is defined by the presence of strikingly focal neuronal loss and gliosis (fig. 13-3). Typically, the pyramidal neurons of CA1 (Sommer sector) are most severely affected, with this field showing extensive neuronal loss. Neuronal loss is also typically seen in CA3 and CA4 (hilus). The pyramidal cells of CA2, by contrast, are often relatively preserved (2). In some patients with less extensive pathology, changes are confined to the CA3 and CA4 regions, a pattern of injury which has been described as *end folium sclerosis* (7). In cases with at least moderately severe pathology, gliosis with greater than 50 percent neuronal loss may be seen (7).

Classic descriptions of hippocampal sclerosis have focused on the pathology of the pyramidal neurons and emphasized the relative preservation of the granular neurons of the dentate. However, the functional relationship between the granular neurons and pyramidal cells of the CA3 and CA4 regions makes it unlikely that this area is completely spared in hippocampal sclerosis. Indeed, published series that have carefully examined this region have demonstrated that almost 50 percent of cases have dentate abnormalities that range from granular cell dispersion (bilaminar arrangement of the neurons) to granular cell loss with gliosis (2). Associated with neuronal loss is reactive astrocytosis. Typically these changes are readily appreciable by routine hematoxylin and eosin (H&E) staining. They can be dramatically highlighted by the use of neurofilament protein or NeuN staining for

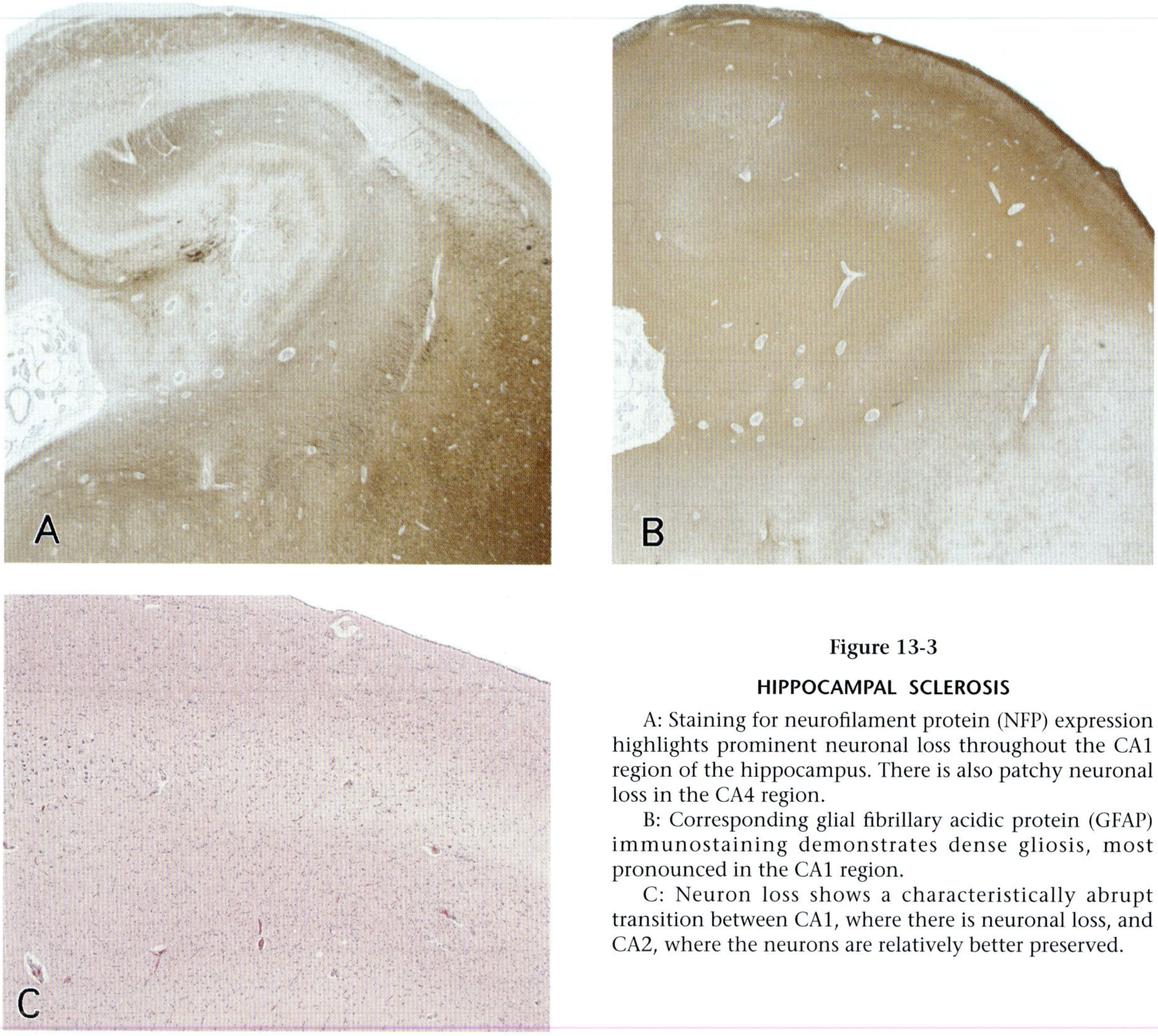

Figure 13-3

HIPPOCAMPAL SCLEROSIS

A: Staining for neurofilament protein (NFP) expression highlights prominent neuronal loss throughout the CA1 region of the hippocampus. There is also patchy neuronal loss in the CA4 region.

B: Corresponding glial fibrillary acidic protein (GFAP) immunostaining demonstrates dense gliosis, most pronounced in the CA1 region.

C: Neuron loss shows a characteristically abrupt transition between CA1, where there is neuronal loss, and CA2, where the neurons are relatively better preserved.

neurons and glial fibrillary acidic protein (GFAP) for reactive astrocytes. Neurofilament protein and NeuN immunostaining may also be useful in highlighting pyramidal neurons in specimens that have been extensively fragmented.

Pathologic Changes in the Temporal Lobe. In a subset of patients with hippocampal sclerosis, TLE is associated with a second pathologic process or lesion (dual pathology). The frequency of this is variable but in large series ranges from just over 6 to 15 percent of cases. The focal lesions associated with this dual pathology are often, but not exclusively, found in the accompanying temporal lobe resection specimens. The most common pathologic processes are cortical dysplasia and other lesions that are typically associated with neurodevelopmental insults (porencephalic cysts and reactive gliosis), but low-grade tumors, vascular malformations, and hamartomas are also identified (8).

Differential Diagnosis. The correct diagnosis of hippocampal sclerosis is significantly aided by awareness of the radiographic findings and clinical presentation. A wide range of neoplastic and non-neoplastic lesions are associated with TLE. Only an infiltrating glioma that has extended to involve the hippocampus, however, is likely to leave the overall structures and anatomy relatively intact. This is not a common issue, particularly when the clinical and radiographic findings are known. Careful attention to features not seen in hippocampal sclerosis, such as increased cellularity, formation of Scherer secondary structures, and cytologic atypia of individual cells, should be sufficient to clarify this diagnosis.

Treatment and Prognosis. Despite ongoing debate about the exact nature of hippocampal sclerosis in TLE, the data clearly demonstrate that TLE is the epileptic syndrome most commonly and effectively treated by surgical resection, with 80 to 90 percent of patients becoming seizure free after surgery (4).

MALFORMATIVE LESIONS

Developmental brain abnormalities are an important cause of seizures. There are four broad types of events that underlie the myriad specific pathways and processes of cerebral cortical development: cell proliferation, apoptosis, neuronal migration, and cortical organization (9). In the broadest terms, central nervous system (CNS) development begins with the emergence of neuroepithelial progenitor cells from the periventricular zone. The migration of these cells outward along radial glia and other processes populates the cortical plate in a characteristic inside-out fashion to produce the six-cell layer neocortex (10). Migration of neurons into the cortex begins around 7 weeks, peaks at 11 to 15 weeks, and is largely completed by approximately 24 weeks of gestation (11). Disruptions of the various steps involved in this complex process produce symptomatic malformations.

Malformations of cortical development can be broadly classified by the putative or known disruption of one of these fundamental processes. The malformations most commonly encountered in surgical neuropathology are cortical dysplasia, cerebral heterotopia, and hemimegalencephaly. One or more of the developmental processes outlined above have been implicated in each of these malformations. In cortical dysplasia, this includes abnormal neuroglial progenitor proliferation, apoptosis, and cortical organization. In cerebral heterotopia, disruption of normal neuronal migration has been strongly implicated. Hemimegalencephaly may involve both abnormal neuronal and glial proliferation and abnormal apoptosis (9).

The major clinical manifestations of these malformations include epilepsy, mental retardation, and developmental delay. The exact process by which these lesions cause epilepsy in most cases is unknown. Studies involving a range of malformations have identified some basic changes that are common to many of these lesions: an increased number of excitatory pyramidal neurons and a decreased number or functionality of inhibitory interneurons. These observations suggest that an imbalance between excitation and inhibition within and around areas of malformed brain tissue may be an important cause of the epilepsy associated with these malformations (12).

Most of these malformative and hamartomatous lesions are relatively infrequent in surgical neuropathology practice and are more commonly encountered in large epilepsy centers. As these lesions are most commonly resected for the treatment of intractable epilepsy, intraoperative evaluation is rarely needed. The features of some of these lesions, however, particularly cortical dysplasia, may be associated with low-grade neuroglial neoplasms and may be appreciated on frozen sections from such specimens. Each of the entities within this section requires careful gross examination, description, and blocking, since well-oriented specimens are essential for accurate diagnosis of these often subtle malformative processes.

Cortical Dysplasia

Definition. *Cortical dysplasia* is a common finding in surgical resection specimens for intractable epilepsy. Cortical dysplasia is a subtle malformation of the cortex that is typically characterized by a disruption of the neocortical architecture and organization (dyslamination), abnormal clusters of cells, ectopically placed neurons in the molecular layer or subcortical white matter, and the presence of abnormal cells (giant cells, ballooned cells, dysmorphic neurons). Cortical dysplasia may be focal, multifocal, or diffuse.

Clinical Features. The reported incidence of cortical dysplasia varies widely but is as high as 60 percent in patients with intractable childhood epilepsy with verified pathologic findings (14–17). The exact incidence of cortical dysplasia is difficult to determine due to a longstanding lack of consensus on the exact histopathologic features that comprise the entity and the nomenclature that should be used to describe the pathologic changes observed in these malformations. In addition, it has not always been possible to recognized cortical dysplasia on routine preoperative imaging studies.

Seizures associated with cortical dysplasia often begin in the first decade of life, but may also present as infantile seizures or later, even in adulthood (17). There is no reported sex predilection. A wide range of seizure types are associated with cortical dysplasia. The clinical phenotype is not predicted by the specific histopathologic features of the cortical dysplasia, although this may change with improvement in the classification of cortical dysplasias (17,18). The location of the dysplastic lesion in the brain, however, may correlate with the seizure type and symptoms. Subdural electroencephalogram (EEG) monitoring may provide detailed localization of areas of seizure activity associated with focal cortical dysplasia. Less common are more severe clinical conditions such as mental retardation and hemiparesis (19).

Radiologic Findings. Improvements in MRI have made the detection of subtle cortical abnormalities feasible, and increasing numbers of cases of cortical dysplasia are detectable by this technique. Blurring of the gray-white junction, thickening of the cortical ribbon, and T2-weighted signal changes in gray matter are abnormalities found in association with cortical dysplasia (19). T2 signal change and reduced white matter volume are also common (19,20). Frontal and temporal lobe involvement is most common, but any lobe can be affected (13).

Gross Findings. The ability to detect gross pathologic changes in cortical dysplasia is strongly influenced by the extent of the surgical resection, the completeness of the specimens available for review, and the care taken by the neuropathologist to orient the specimen. Particular attention should be paid to preparing sections that show the cortex and subcortical white matter in a well-oriented, full-thickness plane. Because of variations in gyral surface anatomy and fragmentation of specimens, orientation of the specimen for processing should by done by the pathologist. In centers where patients are preoperatively studied with subdural EEG monitoring, gross photographs may allow for the later correlation of microscopic findings to EEG data.

Large en bloc resections need to be examined to ascertain increased firmness of the tissue, corresponding to gliosis, or subtle abnormalities of the gyral pattern (e.g., wider than normal gyri). Cross sections of specimens may, in a few cases, reveal an abnormally thickened cortical ribbon or an indistinct interface between the cortex gray matter and subcortical white matter. In many cases, however, gross abnormalities are inapparent in focal cortical dysplasia.

Intraoperative Findings. There is little use for routine intraoperative evaluation of cortical dysplasia. Histologic features common to both cortical dysplasia and hemimegalencephaly (see below) are encountered with some frequency in surgical resection specimens of low-grade neoplasms, particularly gangliogliomas and dysembryoblastic neuroepithelial tumors (DNETs). These tumors are often accompanied by dysplastic changes in the adjacent cerebral tissue. The significance of these findings is uncertain. The nature of the relationship between dysplastic changes and neoplasia in these cases is unclear, and occasionally challenging diagnostic issues arise as a result (see Differential Diagnosis).

Microscopic Findings. The histopathologic features that comprise cortical dysplasia have not been widely agreed upon. There is general agreement that routine histopathologic and immunohistochemical studies can define several basic types of findings that fall under the general heading of cortical dysplasia. There is an emerging consensus that there are basic hallmarks of cortical dysplasia which should be described with standardized and reproducible terminology.

Abnormalities of the molecular layer are frequently observed. These include heterotopic or excessive neurons, with or without accompanying gliosis (13,21,22). The significance of this finding is uncertain, but published studies have suggested a relationship with both epilepsy and behavior or cognitive difficulties (18). A similar finding, reported as part of cortical dysplasia in many published series, is the presence of increased numbers of white matter neurons. Neurons are normally found in the white matter of all four lobes and are most numerous in temporal lobe white matter. However, it is abnormal to see more than 4 neurons/20X field in temporal lobe white matter, or more than 1 neuron/20X field in nontemporal lobe white matter (23,24). The presence of more than 10 neurons/high-power field in temporal lobe white matter has been reported to correlate with a worse postoperative outcome (25).

In Taylor's original report of the pathology of 10 patients with intractable epilepsy, particular note was taken of three histopathologic features that are widely accepted as evidence of cortical dysplasia: disorganized cortical architecture, neuronal cytomegaly, and ballooned cells (26). In various degrees and combinations, subsequent reports of cortical dysplasia have consistently identified these features, as well as cytoarchitectural abnormalities in cortical neurons, which may or may not be enlarged. In any case, one or more of these features are usually evident and, in combination, allow the diagnosis of cortical dysplasia to be made. The lack of an established consensus in the nomenclature of cortical dysplasia has somewhat obscured the significance of the individual findings within and between cases, however.

The routine use of H&E and Nissl stains helps in the recognition of several of the characteristic features of cortical dysplasia (fig. 13-4). Beginning at the molecular layer, hypercellularity may be appreciated. With careful examination it is readily evident that in addition to gliosis, many cases of cortical dysplasia show increased numbers of neurons in layer 1 of the cortex (13). This finding may be less prominent in cortical dysplasia with ballooned cells, and more evident in other types of cortical dysplasia (21). It is unclear whether these neurons, believed to be residual Cajal-Retzius cells, play any role in the development of seizures or are simply markers of other events and processes more central to the development of cortical dysplasia (21).

Examination of the cortex at low power frequently reveals dyslamination, disruption of the normal laminar architecture of the six-layered neocortex (22), which may be due to abnormal clustering of cells within the cortical layers. These clusters may contain neurons and glia, and are often haphazardly arranged. Hypocellular areas may be appreciated around these clusters (13). In other cases, the borders between laminae are effaced by the haphazard distribution of neurons throughout the neocortex, which is often due to either large pyramidal cells present in layers 2 and 4, or to diffusely distributed dysmorphic neurons and cells with immature neuronal features (13,22). Even with routine stains it is often apparent that these cells are misshapen and abnormally oriented. The cells described as immature neurons are often round to oval, with a large nucleus and thin rim of cytoplasm (18).

In a subset of cortical dysplasia cases, ballooned cells are identified. These striking cells may be found at all levels of the section and are often randomly distributed. Ballooned cells are large (80 to 100 μm) and reminiscent of gemistocytic astrocytes. They are also virtually identical to the dysmorphic cells seen in tuberous sclerosis. They may be single or multinucleated, but frequently the nuclei are eccentrically positioned and contain nucleoli. The abundant cytoplasm is eosinophilic and glassy (18,27,28). Finally, careful examination frequently demonstrates the presence of increased numbers of neurons scattered within the subcortical white matter.

While not necessary for the recognition of focal cortical dysplasia, the use of immunohistochemical or silver stains aids substantially in the recognition of several of the changes characteristic of this disorder. The abnormal cellular morphology hinted at by routine stains is related to marked cytoskeletal disarray, with loss of the normal shape, size, and orientation of neuronal processes (18,27). These changes are highlighted by both silver impregnation and immunohistochemical staining to demonstrate abnormal accumulation of neurofilament proteins (NFP) (22,29). The abnormal accumulation of microtubule-associated binding proteins (MAP) is also characteristic of dysplastic neurons and can be highlighted by staining with the MAP1B and MAP2 (29). In normal controls and unaffected regions in resection specimens, NFP staining at low power highlights the orderly parallel arrays of apical dendritic processes that point toward the pial surface. The loss of this staining (fig. 13-5) indicates laminar disruption. NeuN, which highlights the nuclei of cortical neurons, can also be effective for revealing disruption in the laminar architecture. In most cases, accumulation of NFPs highlights both the large pyramidal type neurons misplaced in various laminae, as well as dysmorphic neurons. The latter show a bewildering diversity of morphology but are generally characterized by increased size (evident with the abundant perikaryal accumulation of NFPs highlighted by this staining), and

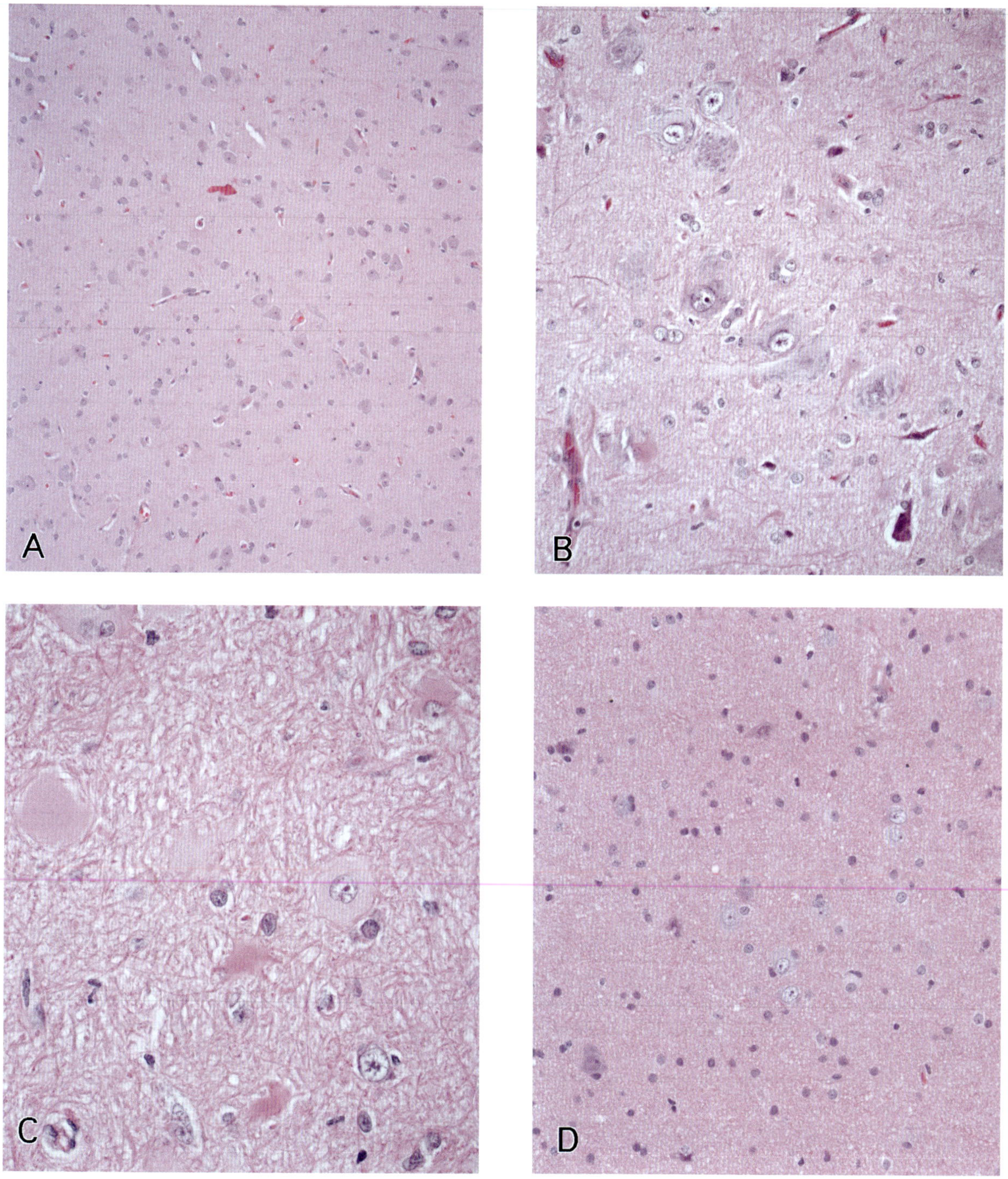

Figure 13-4

FOCAL CORTICAL DYSPLASIA

A: Loss of normal laminar architecture due to clusters of haphazardly arranged neurons.

B: Neurons in cortical dysplasia may be dysmorphic, with abundant, irregularly distributed cytoplasm and loss of normal orientation. There is often accompanying reactive gliosis.

C: Ballooned cells are seen in some cases of cortical dysplasia. These cells may be multinucleated and have abundant eosinophilic glassy cytoplasm.

D: In many cases, an increased number of neurons is appreciated in the subcortical white matter.

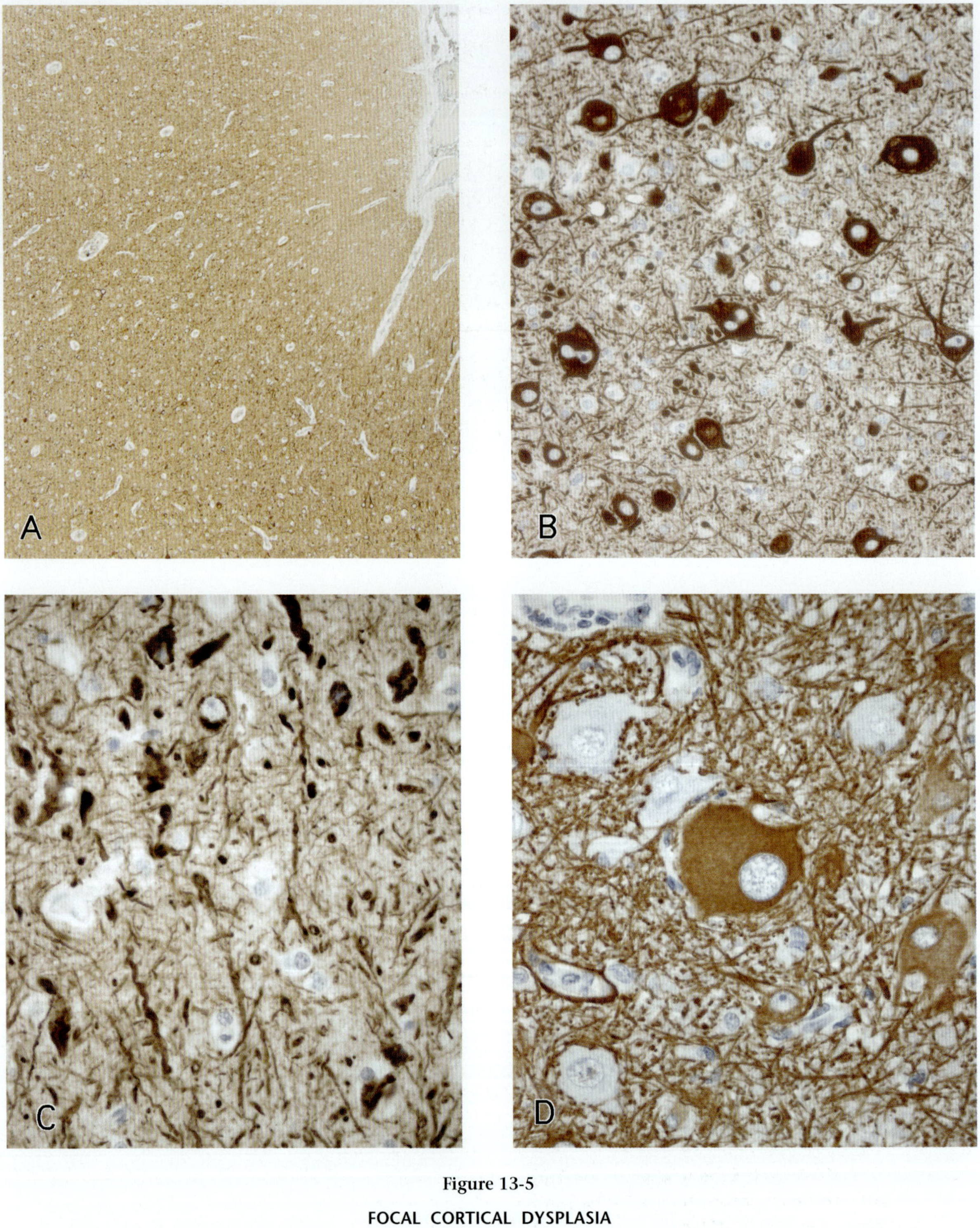

Figure 13-5

FOCAL CORTICAL DYSPLASIA

A: Immunohistochemical staining for NFP expression highlights the laminar disruption characteristic of cortical dysplasia. Haphazardly arranged and maloriented neurons fill the cortex.

B: Staining for NFP also highlights large abnormal neurons and many of the ballooned cells.

C: The intervening neuropil is filled with numerous maloriented and misshapen dystrophic neuritic processes, which can be seen in both longitudinal and cross-sectional profiles.

D: Some ballooned cells express GFAP.

the presence of numerous maloriented and misshapen dendritic processes. The latter can be seen both in longitudinal and cross-sectional profile and frequently are associated with a coarsening of the background neuropil. Recognition of these processes and neuropil changes may aid in the detection of subtle cortical dysplasia. When present, a subset of ballooned cells may express neuronal (NFP, synaptophysin) or glial (GFAP) differentiation markers. These cells frequently express vimentin, and coexpression of these markers has been reported (30).

Classification Systems. Recognizing the frequency of the various pathologic changes described above, and the inability to effectively study clinicopathologic correlation in the absence of standardized nomenclature, many classifications for cortical dysplasia have been proposed. A histologic-based grading system from Palmini et al. (18) is used in many centers. This system recognizes three broad categories of cases. Malformations caused by abnormalities of cortical development (MCD) are cases in which the histologic changes are limited to ectopically placed neurons. MCD is further subdivided into those cases in which pathology is limited to ectopically placed neurons in the molecular layer (mild MCD I) or outside the molecular layer (mild MCD II).

In the Palmini scheme, cortical dysplasias are termed focal cortical dysplasias (FCD) and are separated into those cases characterized primarily by dysplastic cortex without dysmorphic large neurons or ballooned cells (type I) and those cases with these features (type II). Each of the categories can be further subdivided. FCD type I is limited to isolated architectural abnormalities (IA) or is associated with giant or immature, but not dysmorphic, neurons (type IB). FCD type II encompasses the pathologic features of the "Taylor type focal cortical dysplasia" and includes dysmorphic large neurons (type IIA) and/or ballooned cells (type IIB). Based on these criteria, there is some evidence of regional variation in the type of cortical dysplasia encountered in resection specimens. FCD type I appears to be more common in the temporal lobes and is associated with hypoplasia of the temporal pole and a poorly defined increased subcortical white matter signal; FCD type II appears more often outside the temporal lobe, predominantly in the frontal lobe or adjacent frontocentral or perirolandic cortices, and may be associated with more specific and well-localized EEG findings (18).

Differential Diagnosis. The major entities in the differential diagnosis of cortical dysplasia are intracortical low-grade tumors that are frequently associated with TLE and in which dysplastic changes in the adjacent brain tissue may be encountered, and tuberous sclerosis (28). Gangliogliomas are typically low-grade (World Health Organization [WHO] grade I) tumors composed of neuronal elements, most often neurons with ganglion-like features, admixed with a variably prominent glial component, generally with features of low-grade astrocytoma. In classic examples, the associated findings include microcalcifications, granular bodies, and perivascular lymphocytic cuffing (2). While the ganglion cells of gangliogliomas may show similar cytoarchitectural abnormalities to those encountered in cortical dysplasia, the presence of a neoplastic glial component often leaves the diagnosis of ganglioglioma in little doubt. When the glial component is relatively inapparent (or perhaps not resected), however, distinguishing these entities can be difficult, especially because frank cortical dysplasia may coexist with ganglioglioma (31). Review of the MRI studies may clarify the diagnosis as classic gangliogliomas are associated with a cyst and mural nodule.

By contrast, DNETs are multilobulated intracortical tumors with microcysts formed from oligodendroglial-like cells that rest in a mucinous background. Neurons appear to float within mucinous pools in these microcystic areas and the oligodendroglial-like cells may align along the axonal processes of these cells (32). The neuronal elements of DNET do not show any cytoarchitectural abnormalities. Adjacent to the intracortical microcystic areas, however, extensive areas of cortical dysplasia are frequently identified (32). Because the imaging findings significantly overlap with those of cortical dysplasia, particularly if the cystic component of these lesions is not well developed, it is possible to overlook the low-grade neoplastic component of these lesions.

In some cases of cortical dysplasia, particularly those with a prominent ballooned cell component, differentiation from tuberous sclerosis is difficult. The clinical features that are characteristic of tuberous sclerosis are reviewed later in this chapter. Awareness of the medical history, clinical findings, and imaging results help resolve the diagnosis. In some cases, however, children lacking any obvious clinical features of tuberous sclerosis undergo surgery for intractable epilepsy and the resulting resection specimen shows prominent ballooned cells. In these cases, it may be impossible to determine with certainty on histologic grounds alone whether a lesion represents an isolated cortical tuber or cortical dysplasia. While more frequent and uniform expression of vimentin is seen in the ballooned cells of tuberous sclerosis, this and other routine immunohistochemical markers are unreliable for resolving the diagnosis. Staining for hamartin and tuberin has been demonstrated in both the dysplastic neurons and ballooned cells of cortical dysplasia (27). There is evidence that immunohistochemical staining for phosphorylated-p70S6K in the PI3kinase-Akt/PKB-mTOR-p70S6K-S6 pathway may help to distinguish tubers, in which this molecule accumulates in its phosphorylated state, from cortical dysplasia, in which phosphorylation of this molecule is far less frequently observed (33). Further studies may confirm the utility of this approach in resolving this difficult differential diagnosis.

Treatment and Prognosis. Surgery for the refractory seizures caused by cortical dysplasia is an effective treatment that frequently results in improved seizure control and, in many instances, complete absence of seizures. In individual cases, however, firm conclusions about prognosis and clinical outcomes are difficult to draw because of the lack of widely accepted histopathologic grading criteria. This has resulted in a poor correlation between pathology and outcome data. With the application of the grading criteria outlined above, such correlations may improve.

Patients with cortical dysplasias classified as MCD or FCD I may have epilepsy or mild cognitive impairment. Some series have reported better postsurgical seizure control among patients with these types of pathology (34). By contrast, those patients with cortical dysplasias classified as FCD II have more extensive and severe pathology which often, although not always, is associated with more severe seizures and related clinical findings. While the pathologic changes are most severe in cortical dysplasias classified as FCD IIB, there may be slightly better postoperative seizure control among these patients, which may reflect the fact that the pathologic changes in cases with ballooned cells are more likely focal than diffuse (19). The overall rate of seizure freedom (with varying postoperative follow-up) is up to 75 percent in patients with cortical dysplasia (17,35).

Cerebral Heterotopia

Definition. *Cerebral heterotopias* are malformations characterized by the presence of collections of neurons and glia in various abnormal locations. These sometimes striking malformations include *leptomeningeal heterotopia, subcortical heterotopia*, and *subependymal (periventricular) heterotopia*. *Subcortical band heterotopia*, also referred to as *double cortex*, has similar features to these cerebral heterotopias, but has recently been classified as part of the spectrum of lissencephalies, more extensive malformations of cortical development. While many of the cerebral heterotopias are associated with seizures, they are not as commonly encountered as focal cortical dysplasia in surgical neuropathology practice.

Clinical and Radiologic Findings. While there have been many pathologic descriptions of the various cerebral heterotopias, greater awareness and systematic classification of these lesions have been facilitated by the widespread availability of MRI (36). Most are readily detectable with T1-weighted images; T2 imaging may define additional related white matter changes (36). While described as extremely rare, MRI has revealed that these lesions are common malformations that may be encountered in patients with seizures, neurodevelopmental abnormalities, or as unexpected incidental findings (36).

Based on the combination of clinical features, imaging results, and genetic studies, classification of these lesions has been proposed around known and presumed pathogenetic processes. Many of these lesions represent failure of the normal developmental process of neuronal migration, either at the level of initiation, impaired motility, or appropriate stopping (37). In addition, there is evidence that some of these lesions, particularly leptomeningeal and, occasionally, periventricular heterotopias are also produced by epigenetic insults including trauma, hemorrhage, or hypoxic ischemia (38,39).

Leptomeningeal heterotopia, also referred to as *marginal glioneuronal heterotopia*, is one of the most commonly encountered malformations of the brain and has been reported in up to 31 percent of infant autopsies (40). It is commonly associated with other malformations and may also be a manifestation of destructive lesions during development in the mid-fetal period (38). It has also been suggested that these lesions represent neuroblast overmigration (36). Leptomeningeal heterotopia is rarely detectable by imaging studies. Since leptomeningeal heterotopia is most commonly encountered in conjunction with other malformations and lesions, the clinical significance of an isolated lesion is unknown (39).

Subependymal heterotopia, also referred to as *periventricular nodular heterotopia*, is the most commonly identified cerebral heterotopia in clinical neurology and by neuroimaging. The lesion can be further classified as unilateral, bilateral, or diffuse. The unilateral, sparsely scattered heterotopia is typically sporadic (9), whereas the bilateral and diffuse forms are typically X-linked, with a consequent female predominance. In particular, many are associated with mutations in *FLN1 (FLNA)* on Xq28, disrupting neuroblast migration and leading to the development of subependymal heterotopia (37). Mutations in other non-X-linked genes have also been identified in cases of subependymal heterotopia (37). These lesions are formed early in development, and have been detected as early as 21 weeks, but do not often present with seizures until the second decade (36,41).

Subcortical heterotopia is less common than subependymal heterotopia. Manifestations range from apparently normal patients to individuals with hemiplegia and mild mental retardation. Epilepsy is seen in virtually all patients and develops during the first or second decades of life. The severity of the symptoms shows some correlation to the degree (thin versus thick) and extent (unilateral versus bilateral) of the subcortical heterotopia, as well as the associated abnormalities of the overlying cortex. The most common of these associated abnormalities is agenesis or thinning of the corpus callosum, present in up to 70 percent of cases. Other commonly associated abnormalities include thinning of the overlying cortex with small gyri and shallow sulci, as well as a reduction in white matter volume. This heterotopia is generally sporadic.

Subcortical band heterotopia is one of the most striking cerebral malformations encountered in patients with seizures, but is less frequent than the cerebral heterotopia described above. Patients with subcortical band heterotopia have a highly variable symptomatology. They frequently have seizures beginning in childhood and a variable degree of cognitive disability. As with the subcortical heterotopia, there is some correlation between the severity of the symptoms and the thickness of the heterotopic bands. The strong female predominance and familial X-linked inheritance are due to the strong association (over 75 percent of familial cases) with mutations in *DCX* (Xq22.3-q23). Mutations of the *LIS1* gene (17p13.3) have also been identified in subcortical band heterotopia. Both of these genes encode proteins that regulate microtubules and are critical for normal neuroblast migration (37). These mutations correspond to different distributions of subcortical band heterotopia, which can be appreciated by MRI or direct gross examination of the brain at autopsy: subcortical bands that show a predominately parietal and occipital distribution are more commonly associated with *LIS1*mutations, while *DCX* mutations tend to show the most severe pathology in a frontal distribution. The rare males with subcortical band heterotopia have milder mutations of the same genes that presumably allow for some residual function of these proteins (42). Deletions of *LIS1* have been shown to cause, based on the extent of the deletion of the surrounding genomic regions, either lissencephaly with an associated unique set of facial features (Miller-Dieker syndrome) or isolated lissencephaly (43). Mutations in *DCX* are associated with isolated lissencephaly in males, while heterozygous females most commonly exhibit subcortical band heterotopia (37). It has been proposed that, although the features of subcortical band heterotopia are similar to those of cerebral heterotopia, these cases should more appropriately be classified within the spectrum of lissencephaly rather than cerebral heterotopia (9).

Figure 13-6

CEREBRAL HETEROTOPIA

A: Heterotopic gray matter occasionally is arranged in subcortical bands that follow the contour of the overlying cortical tissue.

B,C: More commonly, heterotopic neurons are multinodular subependymal collections along the ventricular surface (B), or isolated nodules within the subcortical white matter (C). (A,B: courtesy of Dr. Lucy Rorke-Adams, Philadelphia, PA; C: courtesy of Dr. Jeffrey Golden, Philadelphia, PA.)

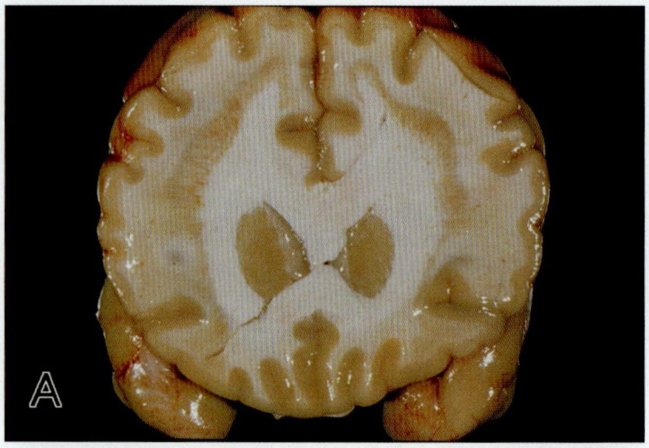

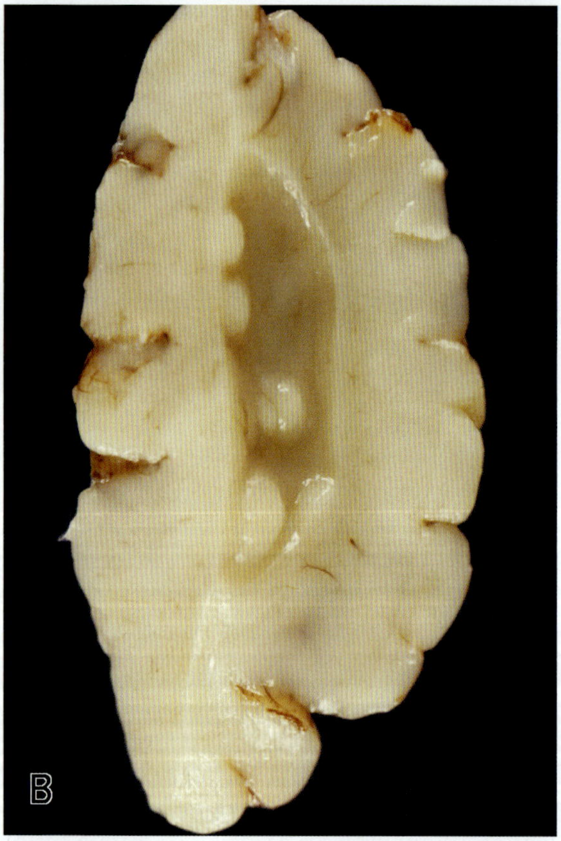

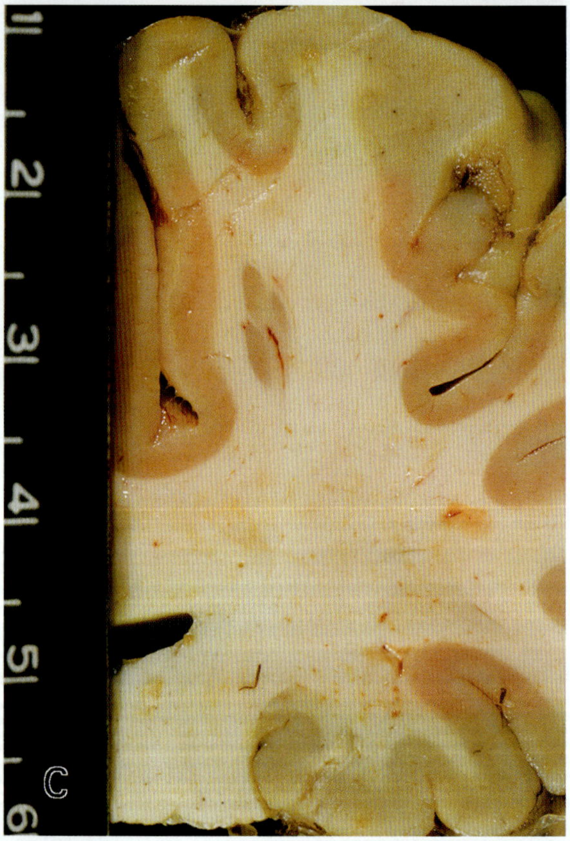

Gross Findings. Leptomeningeal heterotopia is not generally detectable by direct gross examination. The other cerebral heterotopias are generally well defined by imaging studies so that direct gross examination is rarely the first time that their presence is appreciated. Even in well-oriented specimens, an apparent cerebral heterotopia can be "created" by a tangential cut that leaves a portion of a normal gyrus isolated by the surrounding subcortical white matter. While sometimes confusing, these pseudoheterotopias can be recognized by their superficial location and close association with the overlying cortex. Close examination of the gyral pattern in adjacent sections can help distinguish a true heterotopia from a deep sulcus.

Cerebral heterotopias are most commonly located in a periventricular distribution, at the corners of the ventricles or closely hugging the ependymal surface (fig. 13-6). Depending on the size and number, these can be small, almost granular lesions beneath the ependymal surface,

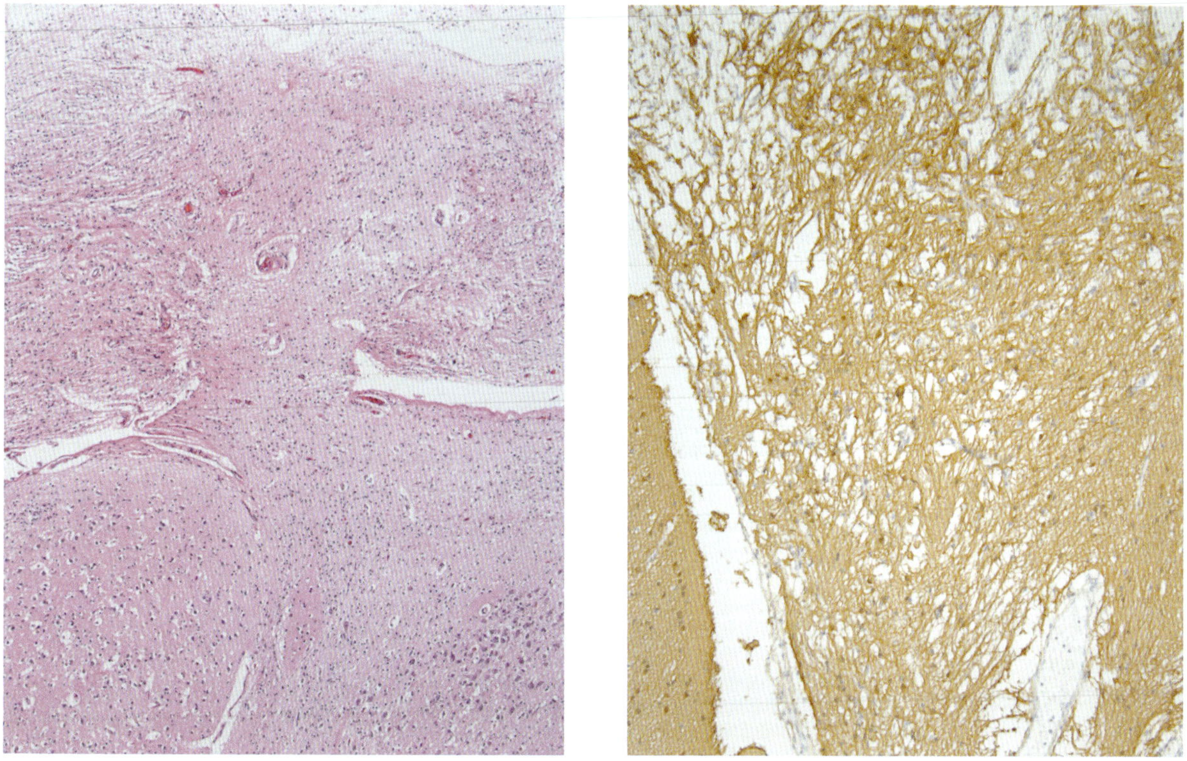

Figure 13-7

LEPTOMENINGEAL HETEROTOPIA

Left: The lesions often are associated with small bridges that connect the pial surface to the abnormal collection of neurons and glia within the overlying leptomeninges.

Right: Strong GFAP expression is characteristic in the heterotopic tissue.

or large nodules that indent and distort the ventricular surface or extend to a variable degree into the subcortical white matter. They may also be identified within the subcortical white matter, where they may be single or multiple, unilateral or bilateral nodules. In all locations, they have the same gross appearance as cortex and tend to form clusters of rounded irregular nodules that may be separated from each other by myelinated fibers (44). The most striking gross pattern is that seen in subcortical band heterotopia, which often form smoothly marginated bands of gray matter that follow the contour of the underlying ventricle and overlying cortex, giving the appearance of a second band of cortical tissue buried deep within the subcortical white matter. In most cases, these lesions are readily appreciated by MRI. Careful correlation with imaging studies aids in interpreting the more limited and fragmented specimens likely to be received at the surgical pathology lab.

Depending on the exact type of cerebral heterotopia, the overlying cortex can also show pathologic changes that are grossly appreciable. These vary from normal to agyric cortex in subcortical band heterotopia to focal areas of gyral thinning with small gyri and shallow sulci in subcortical heterotopia (36).

Intraoperative Findings. There is little use for routine intraoperative evaluation of cerebral heterotopia.

Microscopic Findings. Leptomeningeal heterotopia is recognizable as collections of neurons and glia that appear to extend as small excrescences from the pial surface upward to the overlying leptomeninges (fig. 13-7). The glial tissue typically predominates, and it is not absolutely necessary to identify a neuronal component when making this diagnosis. Careful examination often reveals small bridges connecting the heterotopic tissue to the underlying marginal zone. These bridges may be associated with the

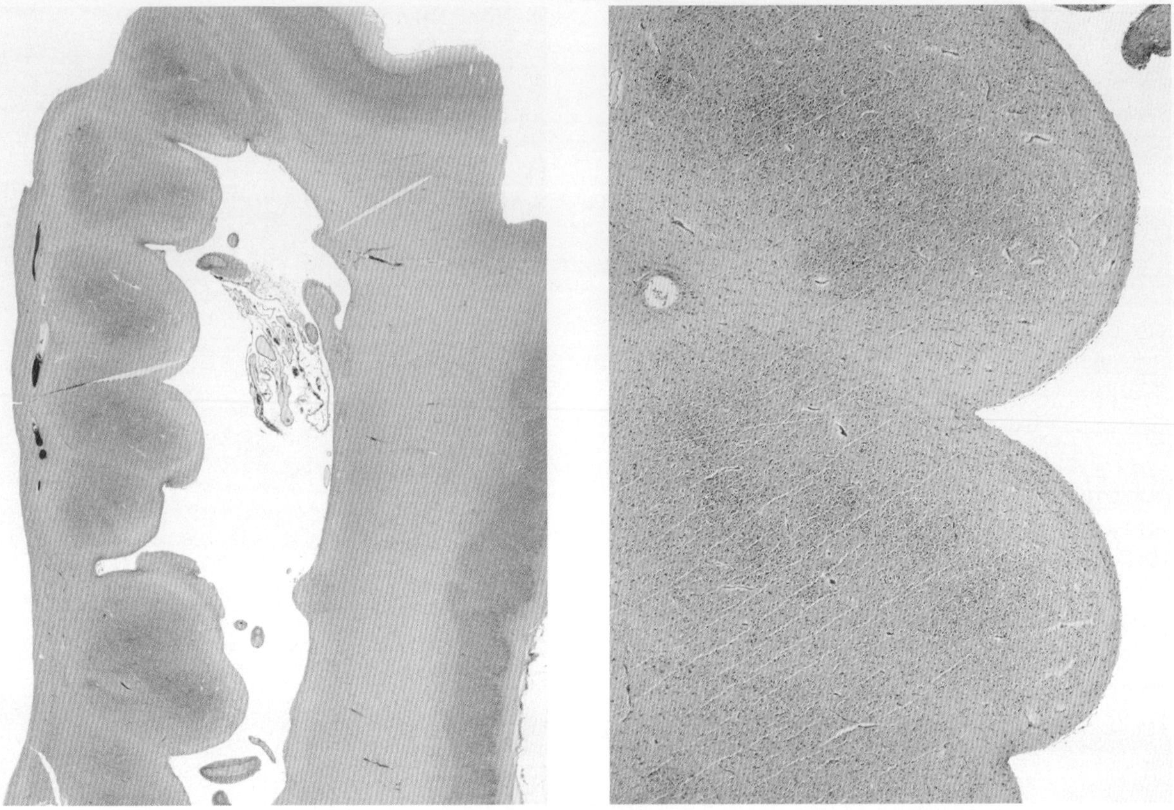

Figure 13-8

CEREBRAL HETEROTOPIA

Left: Nodular collections of subependymal gray matter create an irregular ventricular contour.

Right: The nodules consist of disorganized collections of neurons and glial. (Courtesy of Dr. Lucy Rorke-Adams, Philadelphia, PA.)

small vessels; immunohistochemical staining with GFAP may highlight the accompanying glial tissue that protrudes from the underlying marginal zone along the vessels (38).

Regardless of location (subependymal, subcortical), the remaining cerebral heterotopias show essentially similar features (fig. 13-8). The lesions are well circumscribed from the adjacent tissue, usually white matter. The heterotopias may be individual nodules or collections of nodules that coalesce to form irregular masses, or they may be symmetric with a grossly laminar configuration, depending on the specific type of cerebral heterotopia. In all cases, however, the heterotopias are composed of pyramidal and nonpyramidal neurons that are admixed with glial cells and embedded in a variably well-formed neuropil. Generally, well-formed laminar architecture is not present.

Immunohistochemical staining with markers of neuronal differentiation, including neurofilaments, NeuN, and synaptophysin, generally highlights the neurons within these lesions. In some cases, otherwise normal-appearing neurons fail to stain with these markers. Astrocytes within these lesions express GFAP. Myelin staining may highlight abnormalities in the white matter surrounding these lesions, as well as the presence of small bundles of myelinated fibers within these lesions. In some fetal cases, staining for vimentin has highlighted disorganized radial glial processes around the lesions (41).

Differential Diagnosis. While imaging studies generally resolve the specific diagnostic issues in most cases, tangential and poorly oriented sections may occasionally produce pseudoheterotopias in otherwise normal sections. It is important to recognize that cerebral heterotopias are not often situated at the junction of the subcortical white matter and cortex, whereas artefactual heterotopias are usually produced in this region. In addition, while a pseudoheterotopia may appear somewhat disorganized due to the plane of section, careful examination generally reveals some evidence of underlying laminar architecture, which is uncommon in a true heterotopia.

Treatment and Prognosis. The outcomes associated with resection of these lesions in patients with seizures are mixed (36). Within the heterotopic tissue there is some indirect evidence to suggest the presence of functional neuronal circuitry, with both excitatory pyramidal neurons and inhibitory gamma-aminobutyric acid (GABA)ergic interneurons (45). Some studies have suggested that there is abnormal development of both neuronal populations in heterotopia (12,45). There is evidence of at least limited connectivity between neurons within heterotopic nodules and beyond these lesions (12,45). The relationship between heterotopia and adjacent abnormal and apparently normal overlying cortex remains to be fully elucidated. It also remains unclear what precise role the cerebral heterotopias play in seizures and whether the seizures are related to other brain regions in patients with cerebral heterotopia (36).

Hemimegalencephaly

Definition. Cerebral asymmetry is the hallmark of *hemimegalencephaly* (HME). This rare cerebral malformation is associated with severe epilepsy and characterized by diffuse hypertrophy of one cerebral hemisphere. HME may occur sporadically or in association with neurocutaneous syndromes, including epidermal nevus syndrome, hypomelanosis of Ito, Proteus syndrome, and Klippel-Trenaunay-Weber syndrome. Less frequently, HME has been reported in association with neurofibromatosis type 1 and tuberous sclerosis (46). The affected hemisphere frequently shows changes that are similar to those described in the cortical dysplasias, but are more extensive. The grossly unaffected hemisphere may be normal or may show cortical dysplasia (47).

Clinical Features. HME is often associated with severe early onset, occasionally infantile, seizures. Cranial asymmetry or macrocephaly may be apparent on clinical examination. Additional clinical findings include developmental delay, mental retardation, and hemiparesis (48). There is no clear evidence of sex predilection in this disorder. Given the strong association with neurocutaneous syndromes, patients in whom HME is suspected should be carefully examined for the characteristic clinical features of these disorders. A distinctive and much less common variant is so-called *total HME* in which there is accompanying enlargement of the ipsilateral brain stem and cerebellum (49). While HME is a rare disorder, the relative severity of the seizures and the importance of early surgical intervention make this condition over-represented in pediatric surgical neuropathology practice.

Radiologic Findings. Imaging studies are required to confirm the diagnosis of HME. MRI is the modality of choice for demonstrating both the gross structural asymmetry of the hemispheres as well as other accompanying cortical malformations (50). Enlargement of one or more lobes of one hemisphere is generally accompanied by ventricular asymmetry and midline shift. Abnormalities of the cortical ribbon may be focal or diffuse but typically take the form of irregular thickening. Associated with this may be other, more severe, abnormalities in the gyral pattern including lissencephaly, pachygyria, and polymicrogyria. T2 and FLAIR studies highlight white matter abnormalities such as altered myelination patterns and a poorly demarcated gray-white matter interface. Neuronal heterotopia may also be detected in the subcortical white matter.

Gross Findings. Most specimens are from hemispherectomies or multilobar cerebral cortical resections. Intact gross specimens should be carefully oriented so that they can be sectioned perpendicular to the cortical surface. Careful inspection shows the characteristic features of HME: an irregularly thickened cortical ribbon with a poorly defined to absent cortex-white matter junction (fig. 13-9). Consistent with the frequent finding of pachygyria in these cases, gyri are often reduced in number and those that are present may be shallow and poorly formed.

Intraoperative Findings. There is little use for routine intraoperative evaluation of HME. An awareness of the features of HME is important, however, when asked to evaluate frozen

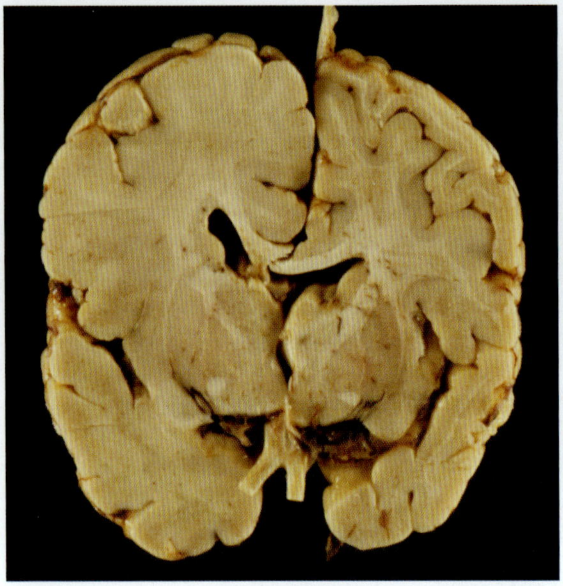

Figure 13-9

HEMIMEGALENCEPHALY

The grossly enlarged hemisphere is associated with an irregularly thickened cortical ribbon and ill-defined gray-white matter junction. Sulci are shallow or poorly formed. Compare with corresponding structures from the opposite hemisphere. (Courtesy of Dr. Lucy Rorke-Adams, Philadelphia, PA.)

sections for suspected gliomatosis cerebri. At least superficially, these conditions may have overlapping clinical and radiographic features, and recognition of the dysplastic features of HME is occasionally useful in resolving this differential diagnosis.

Microscopic Findings. There is substantial overlap in the histopathology of HME and cortical dysplasia. Both cortical and subcortical abnormalities, however, are present in HME (51). HME is characterized by focal or diffuse disruption of the normal laminar architecture (fig. 13-10). This ranges from simple disorganization of the cerebral cortex to areas with cortical architecture similar to that described in polymicrogyria. Corresponding to the infrequent and shallow sulci observed in gross sections, excessive folding and fusion across the superficial lamina is seen microscopically. The blurring of the gray-white junction seen grossly reflects the presence of heterotopic gray matter in the subcortical white matter. Some reports have also emphasized the presence of leptomeningeal glioneuronal heterotopia in HME (52).

Four distinct cell types are observed in HME: astrocytes, neurons, giant neurons, and ballooned cells. Apparently normally formed neurons may comprise the bulk of the disorganized cortex. Scattered among these cells and extending into the subcortical white matter, both singly and as heterotopia, are pleomorphic giant neurons (5 to10 times the size of normal neurons) with characteristic peripheralization of Nissl substance. These cells may also show cytoplasmic vacuolation (53). These giant neurons are frequently maloriented and have both cytoskeletal and dendritic abnormalities, with abnormal neurofilament accumulations, fibrillary disarray, and a paucity of axosomatic synaptic connections noted on ultrastructural examination (52). Coarse cytoplasmic neurofibrils may accumulate in these cells, which can by highlighted by silver impregnation or by expression of various neurofilament epitopes (52). They also express MAP2, MAP1B, nestin, and ubiquitin (29,54).

Ballooned cells can be distributed anywhere throughout the abnormal cortex and subcortical white matter. They are indistinguishable at the light microscopic level from similar-appearing cells within the cortical tubers of tuberous sclerosis and focal cortical dysplasia (54). Like the giant neurons, these cells are large, and have abundant eosinophilic cytoplasm and an eccentrically positioned nucleus; multinucleation is uncommon. The nuclei often have a vesicular chromatin pattern with a prominent nucleolus. Despite their histologic similarity to the cells seen in tuberous sclerosis, some ultrastructural differences have been reported: ballooned cells of tuberous sclerosis have abundant lysosomes, microfilaments, and microtubules, while these are much less abundant in the ballooned cells of HME (54). The ballooned cells in HME generally fail to express markers that are seen in similar-appearing cells in tuberous sclerosis lesions; in particular, vimentin, a primitive intermediate filament in the CNS that is expressed in tuberous sclerosis, is reportedly not expressed in HME (54).

Extensive gliosis with large atypical astrocytes is a variable feature of HME. In some cases, there may be minimal astrocytic proliferation and in other cases, prominent cells in both the gray and white matter are reminiscent of gemistocytic astrocytes. These cells may express both GFAP and vimentin (54). In the white matter,

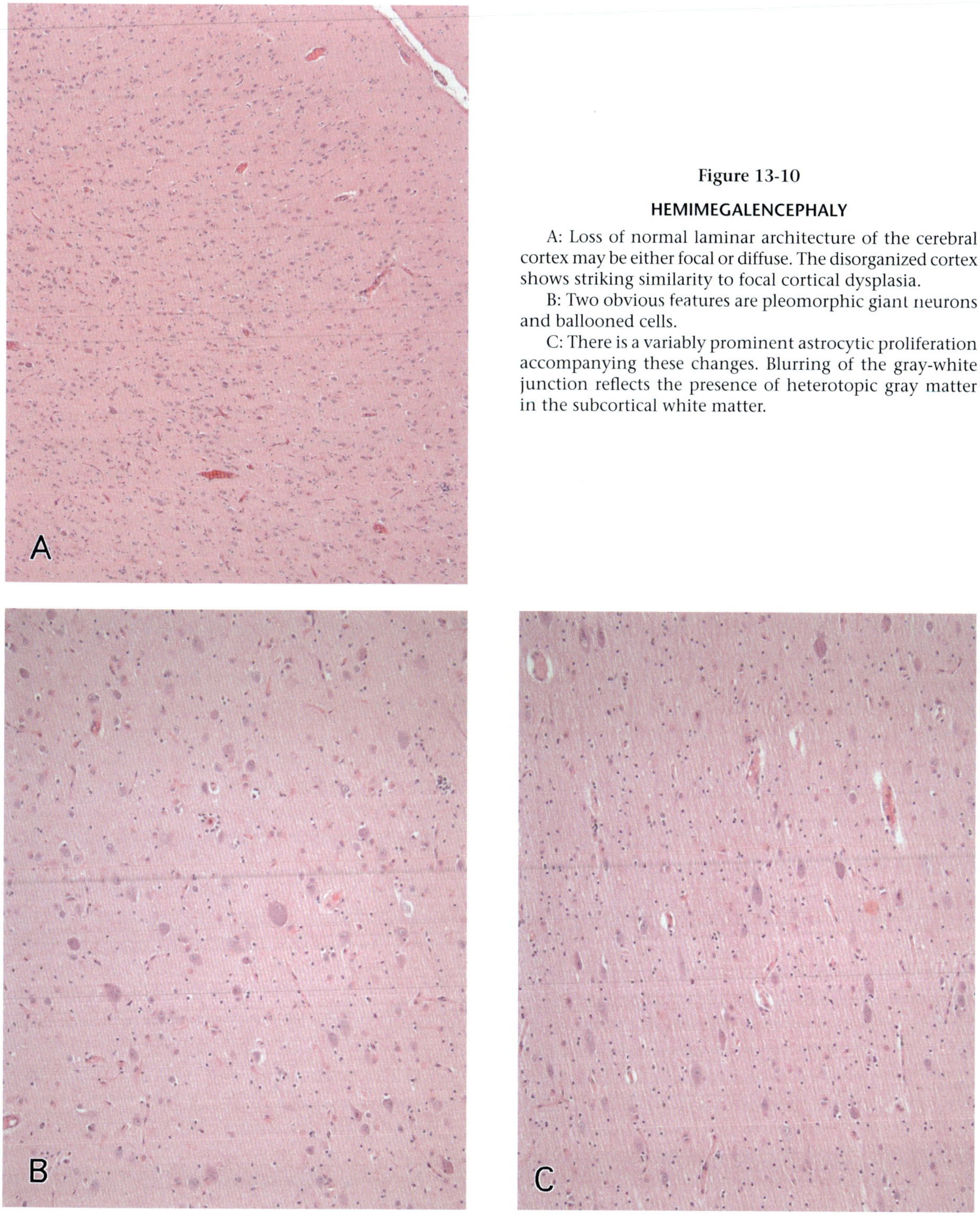

Figure 13-10

HEMIMEGALENCEPHALY

A: Loss of normal laminar architecture of the cerebral cortex may be either focal or diffuse. The disorganized cortex shows striking similarity to focal cortical dysplasia.

B: Two obvious features are pleomorphic giant neurons and ballooned cells.

C: There is a variably prominent astrocytic proliferation accompanying these changes. Blurring of the gray-white junction reflects the presence of heterotopic gray matter in the subcortical white matter.

in addition to heterotopia, HME may be associated with hypomyelination, gliosis, dystrophic calcification and, occasionally, Rosenthal fiber deposition (53).

Differential Diagnosis. The entities in the pathologic differential diagnosis of HME include extensive cortical dysplasia, pachygyria and polymicrogyria, and tuberous sclerosis.

Distinction from cortical dysplasia on histologic grounds alone is not possible and HME may represent the extreme end of the spectrum of changes seen in cortical dysplasia (27). The clinical presentation, including the age of the patient, and the imaging findings should resolve these difficulties. While the laminar disruption in HME may be associated with focal areas of pachygyria and polymicrogyria, the presence of giant neurons and ballooned cells is not typical for those malformations.

The ultrastructural and immunophenotypic differences between the ballooned cells of HME and those of tuberous sclerosis are described above. While HME has rarely been reported in association with tuberous sclerosis, and may occur in conjunction with various phakomatosis, the various lesions associated with tuberous sclerosis (see below) are not typically seen in conjunction with HME (55). Infarction, ischemia, and conditions such as Sturge-Weber disease may cause a relative atrophy of one hemisphere, leaving the normal unaffected hemisphere to appear to be hypertrophic. Finally, as mentioned above (see Intraoperative Findings), HME may have overlapping clinical and radiographic features with gliomatosis cerebri, but these can be readily distinguished histologically.

Treatment and Prognosis. Surgical intervention, hemispherectomy as a general rule, is required for seizure control in patients with HME. This may be accomplished by large brain excision or, increasingly, by smaller resections with hemispheric disconnection (46). Early surgical intervention in this disease is important for three reasons. First, untreated HME is associated with significant morbidity and mortality. Second, surgery provides the best opportunity for many patients to achieve seizure freedom or experience significant reductions in seizure frequency. Third, because of the greater capacity for neuroplasticity in the younger brain, the chances for successful rehabilitation are better. Reported rates of postoperative seizure freedom range from 30 to 50 percent; in those patients who continue to have seizures, meaningful improvement in both seizure frequency and quality of life are reported (46,48). Surgical intervention is also reported to improve cognitive and behavioral development (48).

MENINGIOANGIOMATOSIS

Definition. *Meningioangiomatosis* (MEAN) is a plaque-like growth of small blood vessels and perivascular spindle cells, usually involving the cerebral cortex. The exact nature of this lesion is unclear, but it has many features to suggest a hamartomatous origin. Some cases are associated with overlying meningiomas (56).

Clinical Features. Initially described as an incidental autopsy finding in patients with neurofibromatosis type 2 (NF2), MEAN has subsequently been recognized as an infrequent cause of refractory epilepsy in both children and adults. MEAN most often presents sporadically, but in approximately 25 percent of cases is associated with NF2. These forms differ in both their clinical manifestations and histopathologic findings. The median age of diagnosis for MEAN is 17 years (for sporadic cases) and 25 years (for those associated with NF2), with the difference perhaps reflecting the preponderance of autopsy reports of this entity in earlier series (56,57). MEAN associated with NF2 is virtually always asymptomatic and frequently multifocal. Sporadic MEAN, by contrast, is associated with seizures or vaguely defined neurologic symptoms. Both forms show a striking male predominance as well as an unexplained predisposition for the right cerebral hemisphere, where it is most common in the frontal and parietal lobes (56).

MEAN tissue in patients with NF2 is associated with mutations in the *NF2* gene. Genetic analysis of the *NF2* gene in sporadic MEAN has demonstrated no evidence of mutation in almost all cases; a single case of sporadic MEAN in which loss of heterozygosity for microsatellite makers of *NF2* has been described (58,59). Since symptomatic cases as a general rule are sporadic, MEAN in patients with neurologic symptoms and without clinical or pathologic evidence of NF2 is not considered a forme fruste of NF2 (56).

Radiologic Findings. MEAN appears as a variably calcified mass lesion on computerized tomography (CT) scans (60). With MRI, the lesions are hypointense to isointense on T1-weighted sequences. T2-weighted sequences highlight the gyriform appearance of MEAN and usually demonstrate a heterogeneous mass with areas of increased signal intensity. Dense calcifications in these lesions produce

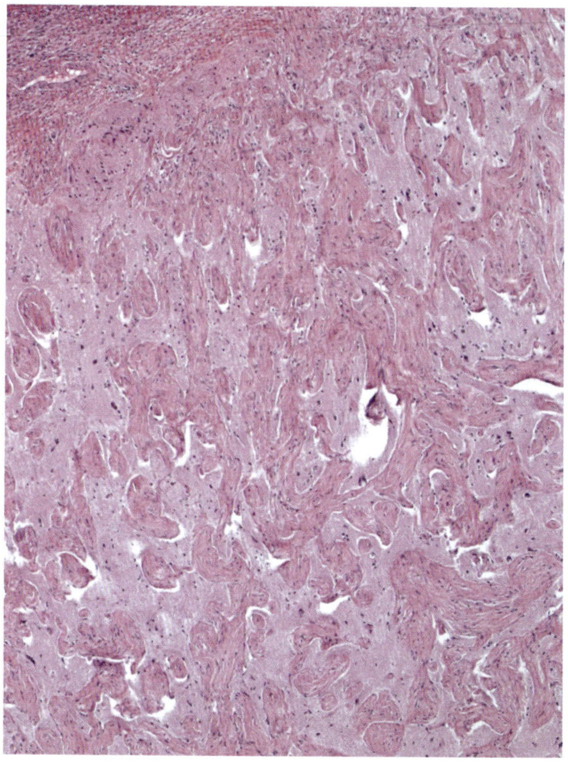

Figure 13-11

MENINGIOANGIOMATOSIS

Left: These superficially situated lesions ramify downward through the superficial cortex and, in some cases, extend into the subcortical white matter.

Below: The lesions are composed of abnormal, variably hyalinized blood vessels surrounded by a perivascular proliferation of spindle cells. This process divides the cortical tissue into islands, which may have prominent gliosis and microcalcification or psammoma body formation.

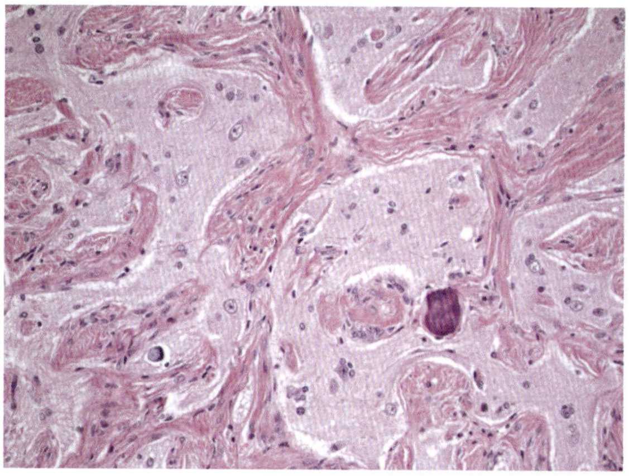

areas of low signal intensity on both T1- and T2-weighted sequences. MEAN may be contrast enhancing. While most often cortically based, it has also been reported in the third ventricle, cerebral peduncle, corpus callosum, and medulla (57).

Gross Findings. MEAN is suspected intraoperatively by a surgeon who encounters a firm, gritty, superficial mass or expanded gyrus, with or without leptomeningeal involvement (60). En bloc resections show a plaque-like superficial and intracortical lesion that follows and expands the cortical ribbon (56). Pale discoloration and a gritty texture due to microcalcifications are other distinctive gross features. These specimens are often firm, even rubbery, and difficult to cut.

Intraoperative Findings. A complicating factor at the time of intraoperative consultation is the tendency for MEAN to present in association with other pathologic processes, most commonly meningiomas (56,60). This is particularly true in children and young adults. The exact nature of the relationship between these processes is discussed below. In such instances, it is important to review the imaging studies and obtain the surgeon's intraoperative impression of the relationship between the MEAN and the meningioma or other apparent secondary processes.

Microscopic Findings. MEAN has a striking histopathologic appearance that, once seen, is readily recognized (fig. 13-11). All MEAN lesions represent variable combinations of two basic elements, vascular proliferation and spindle cells. MEAN is characterized by an abnormal proliferation of small blood vessels that ramify from the superficial cortex through the deeper layers and, in some cases, into the underlying subcortical white matter. These blood vessels show variable degrees of hyalinization and calcification. Accompanying these vessels is a perivascular proliferation of spindle cells. These cells exhibit some histologic features reminiscent of meningothelial cells and often form nests and whorls, with occasional psammoma bodies (56,61). Nuclear pseudoinclusions, however, are not a major feature of MEAN (57).

The intervening cortex becomes entrapped between these abnormal blood vessels and proliferative perivascular spindle cells, forming islands of neuropil with irregular geographic boundaries.

Within entrapped cortex are reactive gliosis and microcalcification. Degenerative changes are sometimes found within entrapped neurons, including the presence of neurofibrillary tangles, threads, granulovacuolar degeneration, and Pick-like inclusion bodies (56).

The histopathologic features of sporadic MEAN and NF2-associated MEAN are similar, although NF2-associated cases may demonstrate extensive hyalinization of the vessels, as well as abundant hyalinized scar tissue replacing much of the cortex. In addition, careful review of the adjacent and remote cortex frequently discloses the presence of the glial microhamartomas (see below), which are pathognomonic for NF2 (56).

Histochemical staining demonstrates abundant reticulin deposition, and may be used to highlight neurodegenerative neuronal pathology (59). Despite the widely held belief that these lesions arise from meningothelial cells, only 25 percent express epithelial membrane antigen (EMA) and often such expression is weak or focal. Cytokeratins are inconsistently expressed and MIB1 or Ki-67 labeling is usually less than 1 percent (56,57,61). Despite strong presumptive histologic evidence, immunohistochemical staining and ultrastructural studies have so far failed to definitively establish a meningothelial origin for the perivascular spindle cells (57).

Differential Diagnosis. MEAN may occur in association with a number of other lesions including arteriovenous malformations, encephalocele, encephalomalacia, cortical dysplasia, and oligodendroglioma. The most common process, by far, seen in association with MEAN is meningioma. While MEAN is not a common lesion, it is often associated with meningiomas in children and young adults. Meningiomas associated with MEAN have similar patterns of gene deletion (*NF2/4.1B*), protein loss (merlin/protein 4.1B), and progesterone receptor expression in both the meningioma and MEAN components (56). These results suggest that in cases where a meningioma is present along with apparent MEAN, the latter is actually a histologic mimic of MEAN caused by the spread of the meningioma along the Virchow-Robin spaces (56). It is important to note the excellent prognosis associated with these cases and caution against misinterpreting the MEAN pattern as a form of brain invasion (62).

Other entities in the differential diagnosis include desmoplastic infantile astrocytoma and ganglioglioma. These are tumors have a peak incidence in children under 24 months. These superficial low-grade neoplasms typically have different radiographic findings than MEAN, being most often associated with an enhancing cyst mural nodule configuration. While the desmoplastic changes and ganglion cell component may mimic MEAN, the vascular proliferation that is so prominent in MEAN is not seen in these tumors.

MEAN may also be confused with Sturge-Weber syndrome. The features of Sturge-Weber disease are addressed below, but one helpful feature in distinguishing these two entities on morphologic grounds is that Sturge-Weber disease is typically associated with cortical atrophy, which is not a feature of MEAN.

Treatment and Prognosis. Complete excision is usually curative and associated with complete resolution of symptoms (61). One large retrospective series reported that seizure control is not always achieved, however, with less than half (43 percent) of patients becoming seizure free postoperatively, and many patients requiring continued antiepileptic medications (57). This is consistent with EEG data in one series that suggest that the focus of epileptogenic activity may not be restricted to the MEAN lesion, and may be in the perilesional cortex, or even in remote sites (57).

OTHER HAMARTOMAS

In addition to MEAN, there are three other types of CNS hamartomas that can be encountered in routine surgical neuropathology practice. Some of these lesions result in seizure activity and all most likely arise as a result of maldevelopmental processes similar to those that generate the lesions discussed in this chapter. For this reason, they are included briefly at this point.

Neurofibromatosis 2-Related Hamartomas. In patients with NF2, small focal collections of dysplastic-appearing neuroglial cells may be seen in the cortex. These cells have enlarged, occasionally multilobed nuclei with vesicular chromatin and variable amounts of amphophilic cytoplasm (56,63). These are assumed to be clinically incidental findings, and have not been associated with seizures or with mental retardation.

Sporadic Cortical Hamartomas. Hamartomatous lesions have been reported as a sporadic finding in patients with epilepsy. In these cases, the lesions typically are composed of well-circumscribed collections of disorganized glial, predominantly astrocytic, cells. Occasionally, a neuronal component is present. Reactive parenchymal changes, including eosinophilic granular bodies and microcalcifications, may also be present. A frequent association with cortical dysplasia, particularly the architectural disorganization of the surrounding cortex, has been noted. The major differential diagnostic issue is to distinguish these lesions from low-grade neoplasms. While this may be challenging, the lack of cytologic atypia and absence of evidence of active proliferation or necrosis are reassuring features characteristic of these lesions (64).

Hypothalamic Hamartomas. Hypothalamic hamartomas are uncommon congenital nonneoplastic collections of hypothalamic tissue that may be associated with precocious puberty (65). Hypothalamic hamartomas are most often an isolated finding, but may also be part of syndromic conditions including Pallister-Hall, oral-facial-digital, and Bardet-Biedel syndromes (66). Typically located in the region of the floor of the third ventricle, these lesions may be sessile (generally intrahypothalamic) or pedunculated (frequently parahypothalamic) (65,67,68). Hypothalamic hamartomas are often associated with gelastic seizures, characterized by ictal laughter. The localization of these seizures has been controversial but there is evidence that these arise within the hamartomatous tissue. The sessile lesions are more likely to be associated with neurologic symptoms at presentation; precocious puberty is a common symptom regardless of the type of lesion (68). Untreated, this may progress to other seizure types, with accompanying cognitive decline and psychiatric deterioration (69).

The seizures are typically refractory and treatment requires resection (68). Resections of these lesions contain a mixed population of large neurons, glia, and intervening neuropil. The appearance is that of somewhat disorganized hypothalamic tissue containing neurons, glia, and intervening myelinated and unmyelinated fibers (fig. 13-12). These lesions may be difficult to recognize in the absence of a clinical history and radiographic findings.

TUBEROUS SCLEROSIS

Definition. *Tuberous sclerosis complex* (TSC) is an autosomal dominant hereditary hamartoma syndrome characterized in the CNS by tubers, subependymal nodules, and subependymal giant cell tumors. The prevalence of TSC is about 1 to 6/10,000 (70,71). TSC shows variable penetrance, and approximately two thirds to three fourths of cases arise via spontaneous mutation (71,72).

General Comments. TSC results from a mutation in one of two genes: *TSC1* (9q34, hamartin) and *TSC2* (16p13.3, tuberin) (73). Multiple mutations have been identified in each of these genes (72). The phenotypic features of TSC are not clearly separable based on the specific gene mutations; however, mutations of *TSC1* are more often associated with familial TSC, while *TSC2* mutations are much more common in patients with sporadic TSC, and may be associated with more severe neurologic symptoms (71,72).

The hamartin-tuberin complex regulates mTOR activity through multiple signal transduction pathways (73). Mutations in *TSC1* and *TSC2* result in lost or reduced function of this complex, with abnormal activation of mTOR signaling in affected tissues (73). This has been confirmed by the detection of abnormal accumulations of phosphorylated proteins downstream of mTOR in both tubers and subependymal giant cell tumors (74). This dysfunction affects the regulation of several signaling pathways (PI3K, WNT, RAS). The net effect of reduced or lost function of this protein complex appears to be increased constitutive signaling along these pathways that promote cell growth, cell proliferation, and nuclear transcription, among other things (72).

Clinical Features. The clinical features of TSC are highly variable in affected individuals, even within the same family. Of the many systemic manifestations of TSC, the following are either among the more common or more important for the surgical neuropathologist to be aware of when considering the diagnosis. Cutaneous lesions occur in more than 95 percent of patients, usually as hypomelanic macules (90 percent), facial angiofibromas (also known as adenoma sebaceum; 50 percent), periungual or subungual fibromas, and fibrous hamartomas (also known as shagreen patches). Cardiac rhabdomyomas

Figure 13-12

HYPOTHALAMIC HAMARTOMA

A: Typically, these lesions project from the floor of the third ventricle and appear as rounded, smooth-contoured masses that are sometimes pedunculated.

B: Hamartomas often have a multinodular appearance when examined at low magnification. Note the typical position of this lesion (lower left) situated below the third ventricle, and adjacent to the mamillary body and optic radiations (lower right).

C: Hamartomas contain a disorganized collection of large neurons, glial cells, and neuropil.

D: Gliosis is common (GFAP immunohistochemistry).

E: Immunostaining for NFP highlights the abnormal arrangement of large neurons.

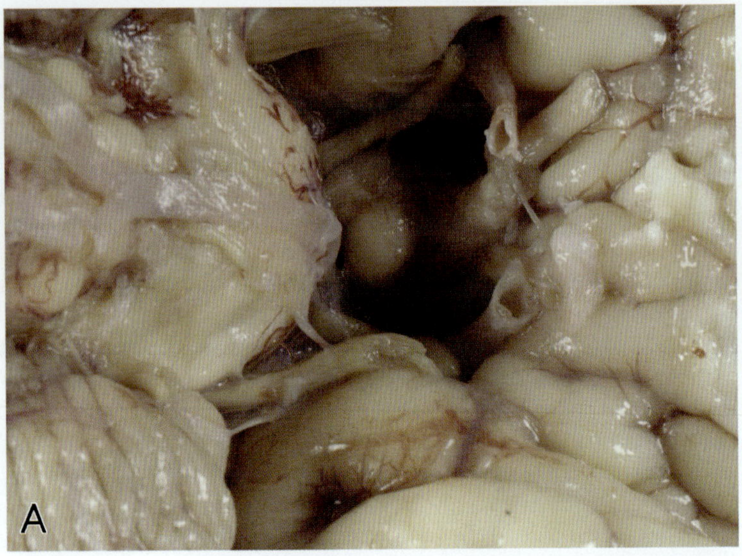

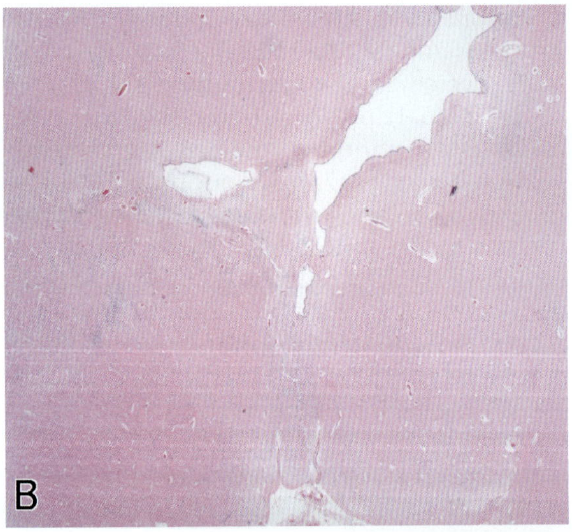

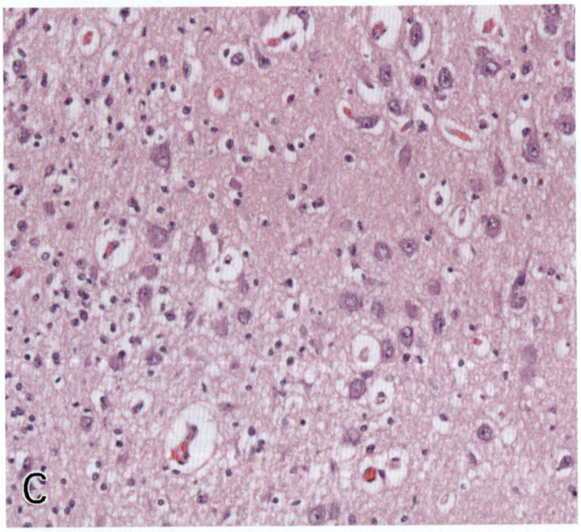

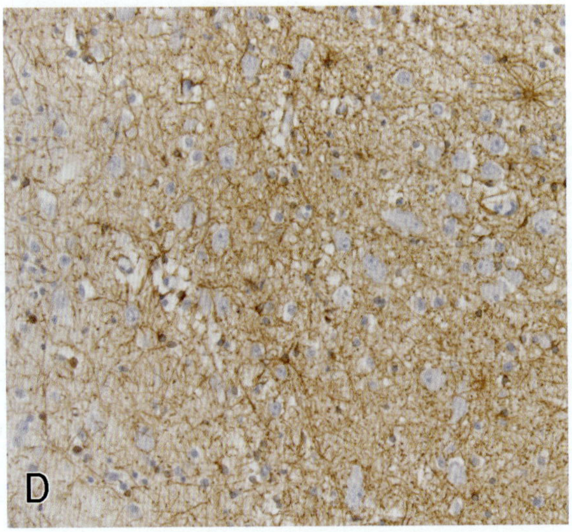

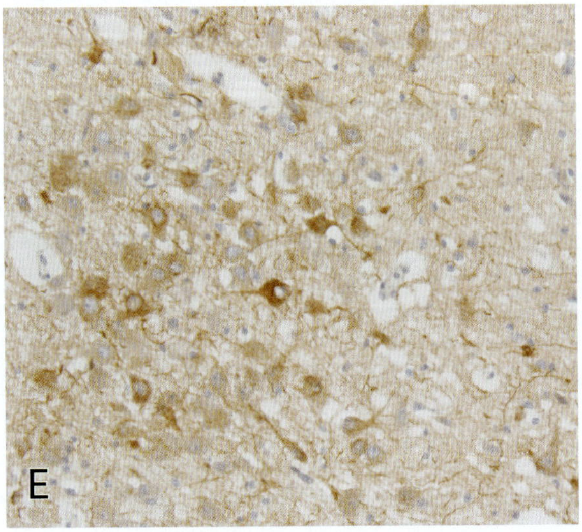

(50 percent) are frequently asymptomatic, but may be associated with significant cardiac dysfunction and sudden death. Renal manifestations include angiomyolipomas (75 to 80 percent), which are more frequent in women, and cysts (10 to 20 percent). Pulmonary disease, in the form of lymphangiomyomatosis, although infrequent, is more common in women and may be severe (70,72).

Currently, clinical criteria are used to establish the diagnosis of TSC. These criteria divide the manifestations of TSC into major (this includes but is not limited to cortical tubers, subependymal nodules, subependymal giant cell astrocytomas, and pathologic lesions in other organ systems) and minor (bone cysts, gingival fibromas, multiple renal cysts, nonrenal hamartomas) features. A diagnosis is classified as definite with either 2 major features or 1 major and 2 minor features; probable with 1 major and 1 minor feature; and possible with either 1 major or 2 or more minor features. No single lesion is pathognomonic for TSC (75). Genetic testing for TSC is available, but has limited diagnostic utility due to a high (about 30 percent) false negative rate (75).

The neurologic manifestations of TSC can be considered in three broad categories: seizures, including infantile spasms; mental retardation; and hydrocephalus. The latter is most commonly encountered as a complication of subependymal giant cell tumors and is associated with the symptoms typical of obstructive hydrocephalus. The frequency and severity of both seizures and mental retardation vary widely in published reports but range up to 90 percent for seizures and 50 percent for mental retardation (70). Seizure onset usually occurs within the first year of life, and shows the highest incidence between 4 and 5 months (76). The likelihood of developing both seizures and mental retardation is correlated with the number of cortical tubers (70).

Radiologic Findings. MRI is effective for demonstrating the characteristic CNS lesions of TSC. Until approximately 12 months of age, tubers are characterized by a high T1-weighted signal; after that, they are more readily appreciated with T2-weighted sequences; FLAIR sequences are particularly sensitive for detecting the tubers (70). After myelination has occurred, T2-weighted sequences may also highlight the hypomyelination of the subcortical white matter underlying the tubers. These lesions are often wedge shaped, with a broad cortical surface showing increased signal that may narrow toward the subcortical white matter. The abnormal signal often trails down to the edge of the ventricle.

Neuroimaging highlights subependymal nodules in up to 80 percent of TSC patients (70,72). These nodules are located along the wall of the lateral ventricles, most commonly around the caudate nucleus and along the groove between the caudate nucleus and thalamus. They are similar in signal intensity to gray matter, but may appear hypointense on T2-weighted images due to calcification; they are frequently enhancing (70). Subependymal giant cell tumors develop in up to 15 percent of patients, typically around the foramen of Monro. Radiologically, these lesions are distinguished from subependymal nodules by size (greater than 15 mm) and an association with ventricular obstruction (70).

Gross Findings. Tubers are circumscribed areas of the gyral surface that are firm to palpation (sclerosis), whitish, and slightly raised above the cortical surface (tuberous). Tubers, particularly in fresh specimens, are often readily appreciated by palpation. They may be single, but are often multiple, and range in size from a few millimeters to lesions that span several gyri. They can expand and distort the normal gyral surface architecture (fig. 13 13). As with other disorders described in this chapter, well-oriented sections are essential to evaluate the pathologic findings. These sections confirm the expansion and distortion of the gyral architecture in the region of the tuber, and typically show blurring of the gray-white junction.

While subependymal nodules may be present in the vast majority of TSCs, it is unlikely that they are encountered in routine surgical neuropathology practice unless they enlarge substantially and become obstructive lesions, which are generally considered to be subependymal giant cell tumors. When encountered in gross specimens, subendymal nodules are typically distributed along the walls of the lateral and third ventricle, where they form whitish rounded excrescences of varying sizes that protrude out into the ventricle in a fashion

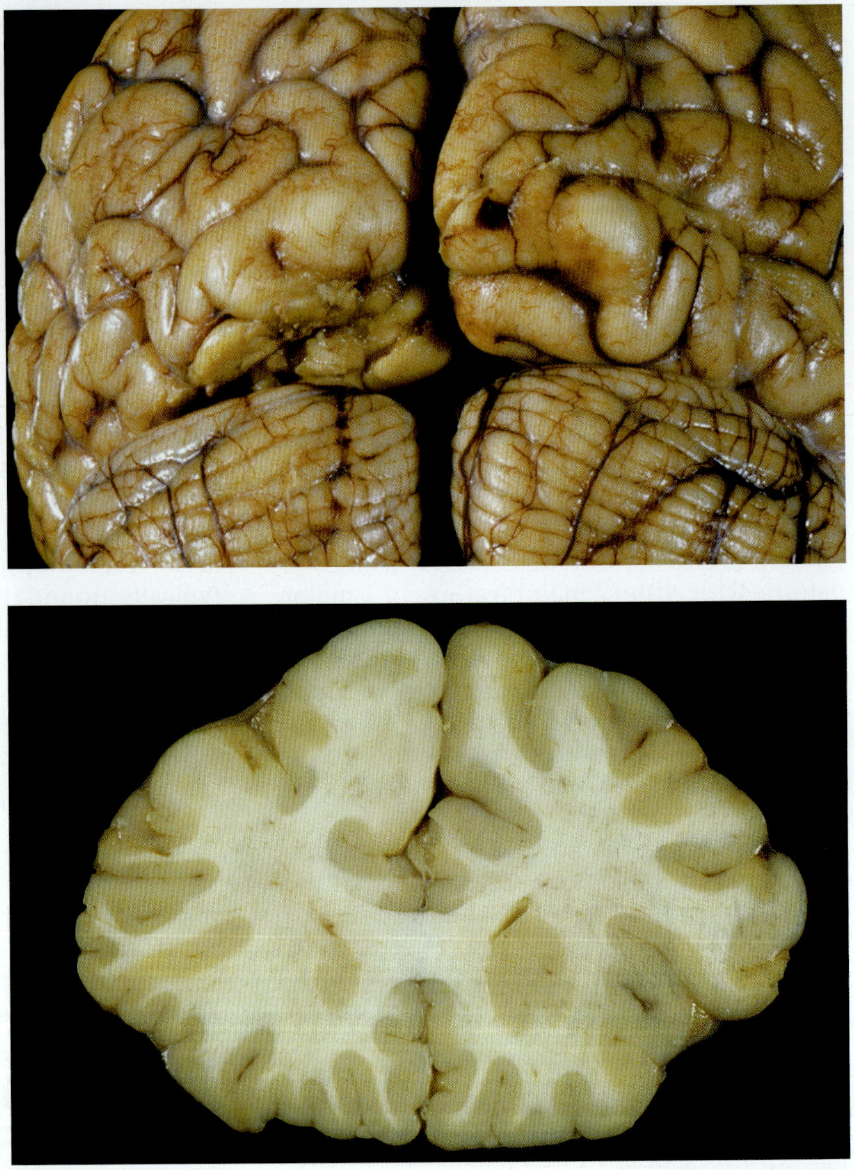

Figure 13-13

TUBEROUS SCLEROSIS

Top: Tubers are circumscribed areas that expand and distort the normal gyral surface architecture, as seen here at the occipital poles.

Bottom: On cut section, tubers are characterized by expansion of the gyri, loss of well-defined cortical ribbon, and blurring of the gray-white junction. (Courtesy of Dr. Jeffrey Golden, Philadelphia, PA.)

described as candle gutterings. They are frequently calcified. As previously noted, they have a particular predilection for the caudothalamic groove, and are often seen in proximity to the foramen of Monro (77).

Intraoperative Findings. Frozen sections from tubers are rarely requested to guide intraoperative decisions. Subependymal nodules and subependymal giant cell tumors, however, are more frequently encountered in surgical neuropathology. Awareness of the neuroimaging results and clinical history aids in the proper diagnosis on frozen section. In the absence of this information, the major challenge on frozen section is to avoid making the diagnosis of a malignant glioma on the basis of the large atypical and gemistocytic-appearing cells.

Microscopic Findings. *Tubers.* Tubers are characterized by the disruption of the normal laminar architecture of the neocortex or the trilayer architecture of the cerebellum. The disruption is caused by the effacement of the normal architecture by large cells with features that are histologically reminiscent of both neurons and glia (TS cells) and randomly distributed dysmorphic neurons (fig. 13-14). Like neurons, the striking TS cells often have large nuclei with prominent nucleoli; multinucleation is common

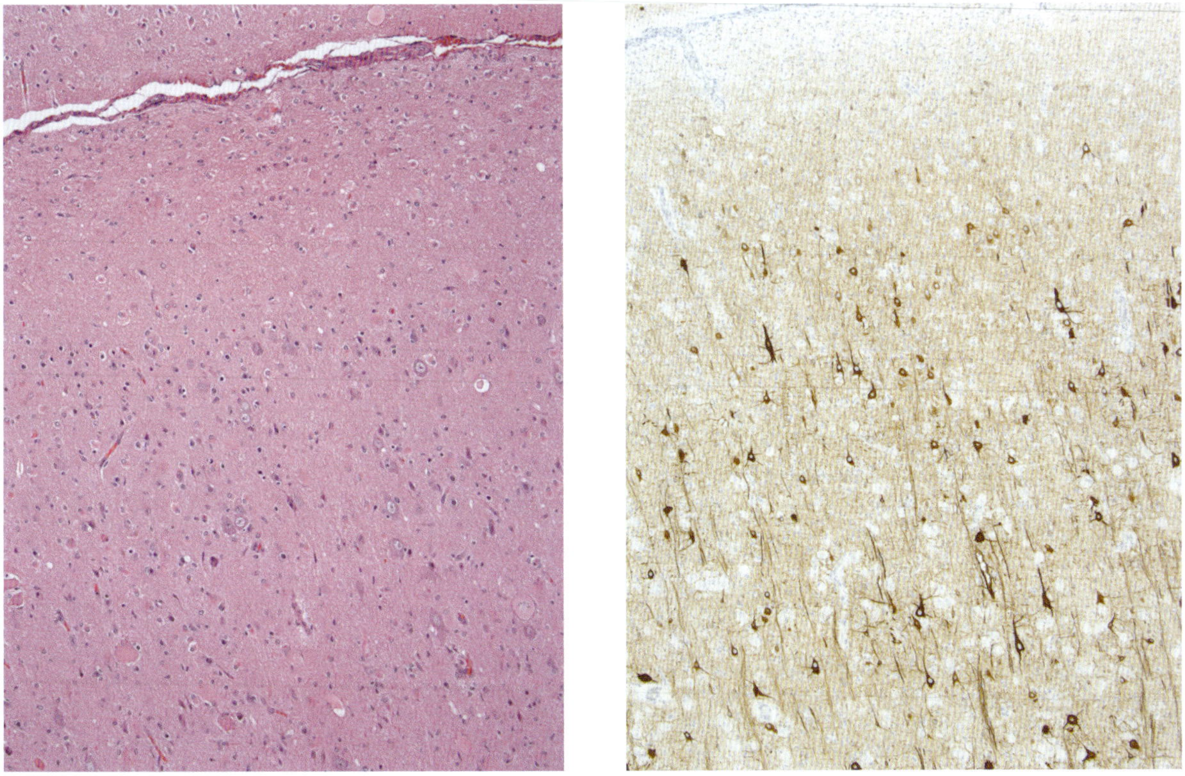

Figure 13-14

TUBEROUS SCLEROSIS

Left: Disruption of the normal laminar architecture by large cells and dysmorphic neurons is characteristic of tubers. Right: Immunohistochemical staining for NFP highlights the dysmorphic neurons and laminar disruption.

(fig. 13-15). Similar to astrocytes, TS cells have abundant pale, glassy eosinophilic cytoplasm. These cells are widely distributed throughout the cortex, at any layer, and characteristically stream into the subcortical white matter toward the underlying ventricle.

Dysmorphic neurons with many of the same features described in cortical dysplasia are also a component of the tuber. These cells are recognized by their enlarged size, bizarre shape and orientation relative to their position in the cortex, and abnormal randomly oriented processes. These changes are accompanied by striking gliosis both in the cortex and subcortical white matter (77).

Myelin staining demonstrates hypomyelinated cores where the tuber extends into the subcortical and periventricular white matter. These cores are filled with a mixture of heterotopic neurons, large astrocytes, and abnormal giant cells (77). Tubers in the cerebellum generally have a similar histologic appearance to those in the cerebrum (77).

Immunohistochemical staining can help elucidate the extent of involvement of the cortex and highlight the disruption of the underlying cortical architecture. Not surprisingly, TS cells that have neuroglial features show a variable immunohistochemical phenotype (fig. 13-16). Many of these cells express vimentin, which may represent an early, uncommitted state of phenotypic differentiation. Consistent with this is the variable expression of GFAP and NFP, as well as other neuronal markers including synaptophysin, MAP2, and class III beta-tubulin by a smaller subset of these abnormal cells (78,79). NFP expression also demonstrates the presence of dysmorphic neurons within these lesions. These cells are characterized by bizarre cytoarchitectural forms with malformed, misshapen and randomly oriented processes quite reminiscent of those observed in the abnormal

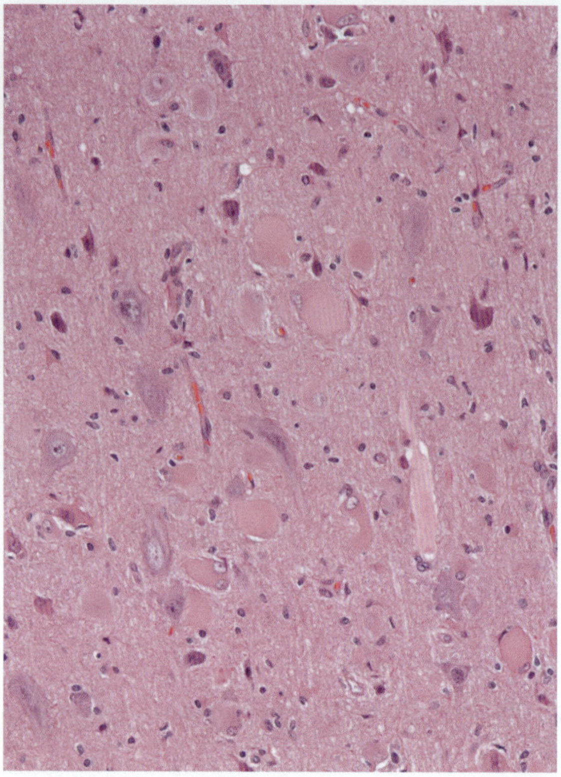

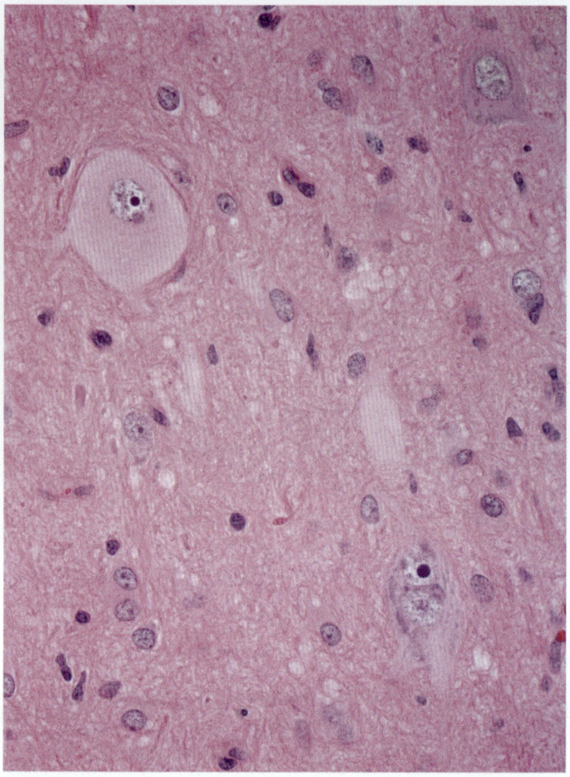

Figure 13-15

TUBEROUS SCLEROSIS

Left: Tubers are composed of a mixture of dysmorphic neurons and large cells, with features suggestive of both neuronal and glial differentiation (tuberous sclerosis [TS] cells); not infrequently the latter are multinucleated.

Right: These cells typically have large nuclei with prominent nucleoli, as well as abundant eosinophilic cytoplasm.

neurons of cortical dysplasia. GFAP expression also highlights the presence of numerous fibrillary reactive astrocytes throughout the affected cortex and subcortical white matter.

Immunohistochemical staining for hamartin and tuberin is positive and frequently colocalizes within the tubers. Detection of this expression with antibodies for these proteins does not generally contribute to the diagnosis of TSC (79); however, the accumulation of the phosphorylated forms of proteins downstream of mTOR, i.e., phospho-S6, and p70S6K, may be a sensitive and relatively specific marker of the abnormal neuroglial cells of TSC (33).

Subependymal Nodules and Subependymal Giant Cell Tumors. Subependymal nodules are distinguished from subependymal giant cell tumors primarily on the basis of size. Subependymal nodules are composed of the same cells with the prominent, eccentrically positioned nuclei, often large nucleoli, and abundant eosinophilic cytoplasm that are found in cortical tubers. These features are even more striking when these cells are present in a subependymal nodule where they are all compressed together within a fibrillary and vascular background (77,79). Subependymal nodules are slow-growing lesions that are frequently calcified. They may extend to a limited degree into the nuclei of the underlying gray matter, but tend to grow outward into the ventricles (77). As they enlarge and cause obstructive symptoms they frequently come to surgical attention. These larger lesions are described as subependymal giant cell tumors or astrocytomas (fig. 13-17).

Subependymal giant cell tumors often have a prominent second component that has generally similar nuclear features, but a more spindle and elongated morphology. The cells may even form areas with vascular pseudorosettes. Cells with

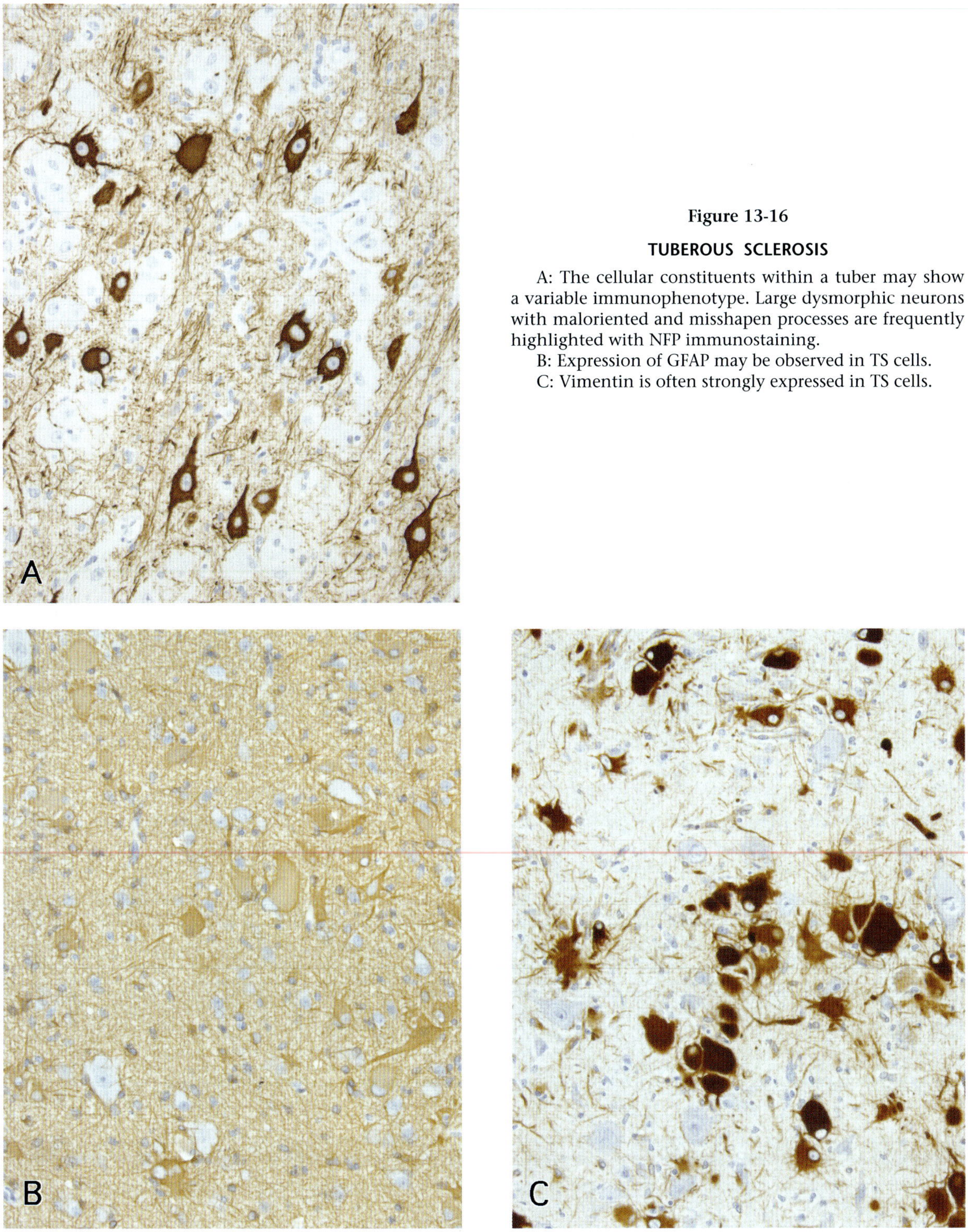

Figure 13-16

TUBEROUS SCLEROSIS

A: The cellular constituents within a tuber may show a variable immunophenotype. Large dysmorphic neurons with maloriented and misshapen processes are frequently highlighted with NFP immunostaining.

B: Expression of GFAP may be observed in TS cells.

C: Vimentin is often strongly expressed in TS cells.

ganglionic and more vaguely neuronal features are frequently encountered within these lesions. Multinucleated cells and calcification are common. Cells with features of gemistocytic astrocytes are seen in both subependymal nodules and subependymal giant cell tumors.

Occasional mitoses and areas of necrosis do not represent evidence of malignant degeneration or a propensity for more aggressive biological behavior in these lesions (79).

Immunohistochemical staining confirms that the nomenclature of subependymal giant cell "astrocytoma" is one of historical convenience rather than biological relevance. These lesions clearly include multiple cell types, including those with histologic evidence of both neuronal and glial differentiation. While variable GFAP expression is observed in the cells with gemistocytic and indeterminate features, the spindle cell component of these lesions frequently expresses GFAP (79). A subset of cells within these lesions frequently shows evidence of neuronal differentiation by expression of synaptophysin and neurofilament protein (79). MIB1 labeling is minimal, typically around 1 percent, confirming the slow-growing nature of the lesion (80).

Differential Diagnosis. The major entity in the differential diagnosis of tubers in TSC is cortical dysplasia. There are several overlapping features in the histopathology of these two disorders which have been noted above. The diagnosis is challenging when cortical dysplasia with ballooned cells is considered, given the essentially similar histologic features of ballooned cells and the large cells with indeterminate neuroglial features common in TSC. Awareness of the imaging studies and clinical features of any particular case generally resolves these challenges. Reliance upon the histopathologic features alone to distinguish a tuber from cortical dysplasia may be difficult. Some clues support the diagnosis of a tuber over cortical dysplasia. First, there are often differences in the distribution of the large abnormal cells in TSC and the ballooned cells of cortical dysplasia. In general, ballooned cells are typically present in the deeper layers of the cortex and superficial subcortical white matter. By contrast, the large abnormal cells characteristic of TSC are widely distributed throughout the cortex and extend into the deeper subcortical white matter. These cells frequently extend to the ventricle, an unusual event in cortical dysplasia. Second, while both TSC and cortical dysplasia are characterized by dysregulation of the insulin signaling pathway, there appear to be different causes in each disorder. TSC and cortical dysplasia accumulate phospho-S6, a molecule downstream of mTOR in the insulin signaling pathway. In TSC this is due to the constitutive activation of p70S6K, detectable by immunohistochemical staining for cytoplasmic accumulation of phospho-p70S6K. In cortical dysplasia, such activation of p70S6K is not observed and the ballooned cells are negative by immunohistochemical staining for phospho-p70S6K (33).

The subependymal nodules and giant cell tumors of TSC raise two other possible differential diagnoses. These lesions are readily recognized when their location and clinical setting is appreciated, but may be mistaken for a malignant glioma, particularly a gemistocytic astrocytoma, by pathologists who are unfamiliar with them. Malignant gliomas are typically seen in adults, rather than children, and are more commonly parenchymal with white matter infiltration, rather than well-circumscribed lesions with intraventricular extension (81). Pathologic features that distinguish malignant gliomas include: nuclear atypia and vascular proliferation, frequent mitosis, and necrosis, which are not seen in subependymal nodules and giant cell tumors of TSC. The distinctive biphenotypic immunohistochemical profile of these tumors should eliminate any remaining doubt about the true diagnosis.

By location, nodular heterotopia could be entertained in the differential diagnosis of subependymal nodules of TSC. Nodular heterotopia is rarely calcified and histologically resembles disorganized gray matter rather than hamartomatous elements.

Treatment and Prognosis. The major treatable manifestations of TSC are seizures and, when it occurs, obstructive hydrocephalus due to subependymal giant cell tumors. Those patients with the earliest onset of seizures are more likely to have intractable epilepsy (76). Surgery for intractable epilepsy associated with TSC is effective in patients with well-defined foci of seizure activity associated with a tuber (70,76,82). Not surprisingly, however, most of the epilepsy associated with TSC is complex and multicentric. The effectiveness of surgical intervention in these patients is less clear and long-term data on clinical improvement in seizure control are not yet available (82).

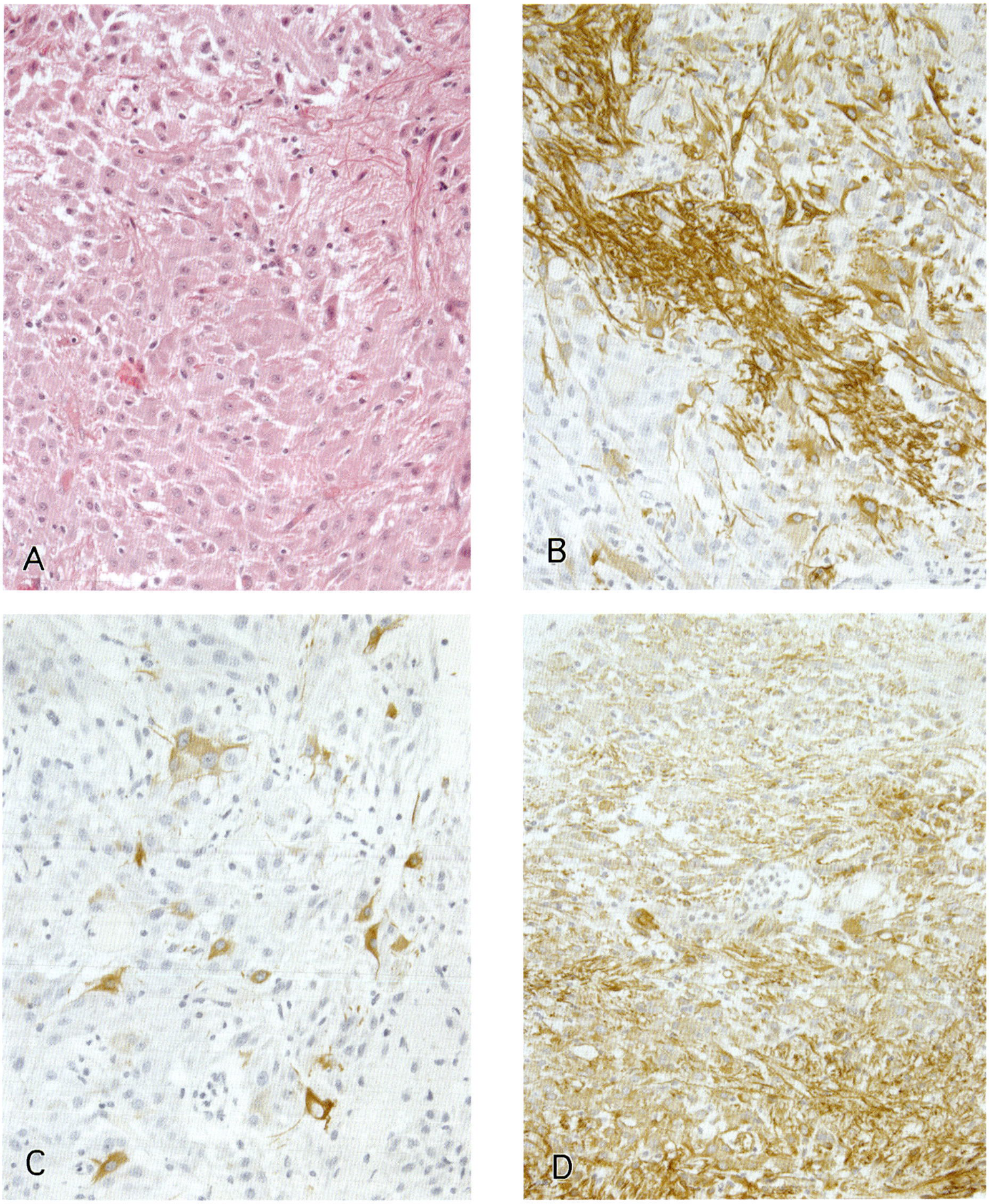

Figure 13-17

SUBEPENDYMAL GIANT CELL TUMOR

A: Large cells with abundant eosinophilic cytoplasm and eccentrically positioned nuclei are characteristically admixed with spindled and elongated cells.

B: Expression of GFAP is seen in a subset of larger cells, as well as in the spindled component of these lesions.

C,D: Some cells express NFP (C) and vimentin (D).

STURGE-WEBER SYNDROME

Definition. *Sturge-Weber syndrome* (SWS) is a rare sporadic neurocutaneous syndrome of leptomeningeal angiomatosis and ipsilateral facial cutaneous vascular malformation, typically distributed along the ophthalmic division of the trigeminal nerve. SWS is often associated with a variety of other neurologic manifestations (83).

General Comments. SWS is an uncommon, sporadically occurring congenital disorder, classified as a phakomatosis (84). The estimated frequency is 1/50,000 live births (83). Unlike other phakomatoses, SWS is not associated with an increased risk of malignancy (84). The fundamental disorder in this syndrome appears to be an abnormality in the postcapillary circulation, specifically, abnormal venous drainage, most likely representing a developmental failure of embryonic vessels, resulting in impaired blood flow to the brain. While the exact pathogenesis of SWS is not understood, the underlying events are hypothesized to occur early in development (first trimester), at a time when the structures affected in SWS (ipsilateral occipital lobe, eye, upper face) are all relatively close together (84,85).

Clinical Features. Typical of SWS is the presence at birth of a facial cutaneous vascular malformation (nevus flammeus or "portwine stain"), generally involving the upper half of the face and following the distribution of the ophthalmic division of the trigeminal nerve (84). This lesion consists of dilated veins or telangiectasias that are filled with deoxygenated blood, imparting the characteristic dark color (86). This finding is neither sensitive nor specific; it is estimated that the overall risk of SWS is only 8 percent in individuals with a facial nevus (83). Ocular manifestations of SWS include choroidal, scleral, or episcleral telangiectasia (86). Glaucoma is the most frequent complication of ocular involvement and is seen in 30 to 70 percent of patients (83).

Because facial nevi are common, the intracranial lesions are considered by most authors to be the key diagnostic feature of SWS (83,86). SWS is characterized by regions of abnormal venous drainage from the cerebral hemispheres, most often involving the occipital and parietal lobes (83). This abnormal circulation is associated with chronic hypoperfusion and progressive cerebral atrophy with loss of white matter (86). An associated secondary change is focal calcification in the leptomeninges and cortex, which gives rise to the distinctive radiographic appearance described below.

The most common symptom in patients with SWS is seizure (84). Seizures affect up to 90 percent of patients and typically begin in childhood, often within the first 2 years of life. In unilateral SWS, seizures characteristically affect the side of the body contralateral to the facial lesion (84). In addition to seizures, patients with SWS develop a number of other variably severe neurologic complications including vascular headache (30 to 45 percent), developmental delay and mental retardation (50 to 75 percent), hemianopsia (40 to 45 percent) and hemiparesis (25 to 60 percent), and stroke-like episodes (83,86).

Radiologic Findings. The most common imaging feature of SWS is dense calcifications that follow the gyral contours (fig. 13-18) (84). These may form parallel calcified lines in the cortical gyri, giving rise to "tram-track" calcifications. They are detected on CT scan as well as on MRI, where they appear hypodense on T1-weighted images. Contrast-enhanced T1-weighted studies are useful for identifying the characteristic leptomeningeal angiomatosis which typically appears as extensive leptomeningeal enhancement. T1-weighted studies are also useful for documenting the presence and extent of cortical atrophy; T2-weighted studies may highlight the presence of white matter atrophy (83,86).

Gross Findings. Gross examination of resection specimens from affected SWS brain tissue reveals thickening of the leptomeninges. The dark discoloration and granular appearance are due to an extensive leptomeningeal vascular network covering the cortical surface (fig. 13-19) (87). Coronal sections show dusky congestion of the thickened leptomeninges and often demonstrate areas of narrowed cortical ribbon due to atrophy. These changes may extend into the subcortical white matter. The presence of gliosis and calcification may render the tissue firm and gritty (83).

Intraoperative Findings. Intraoperative evaluation of specimens resected from SWS patients is not required, but the changes described below are also readily appreciated on frozen section.

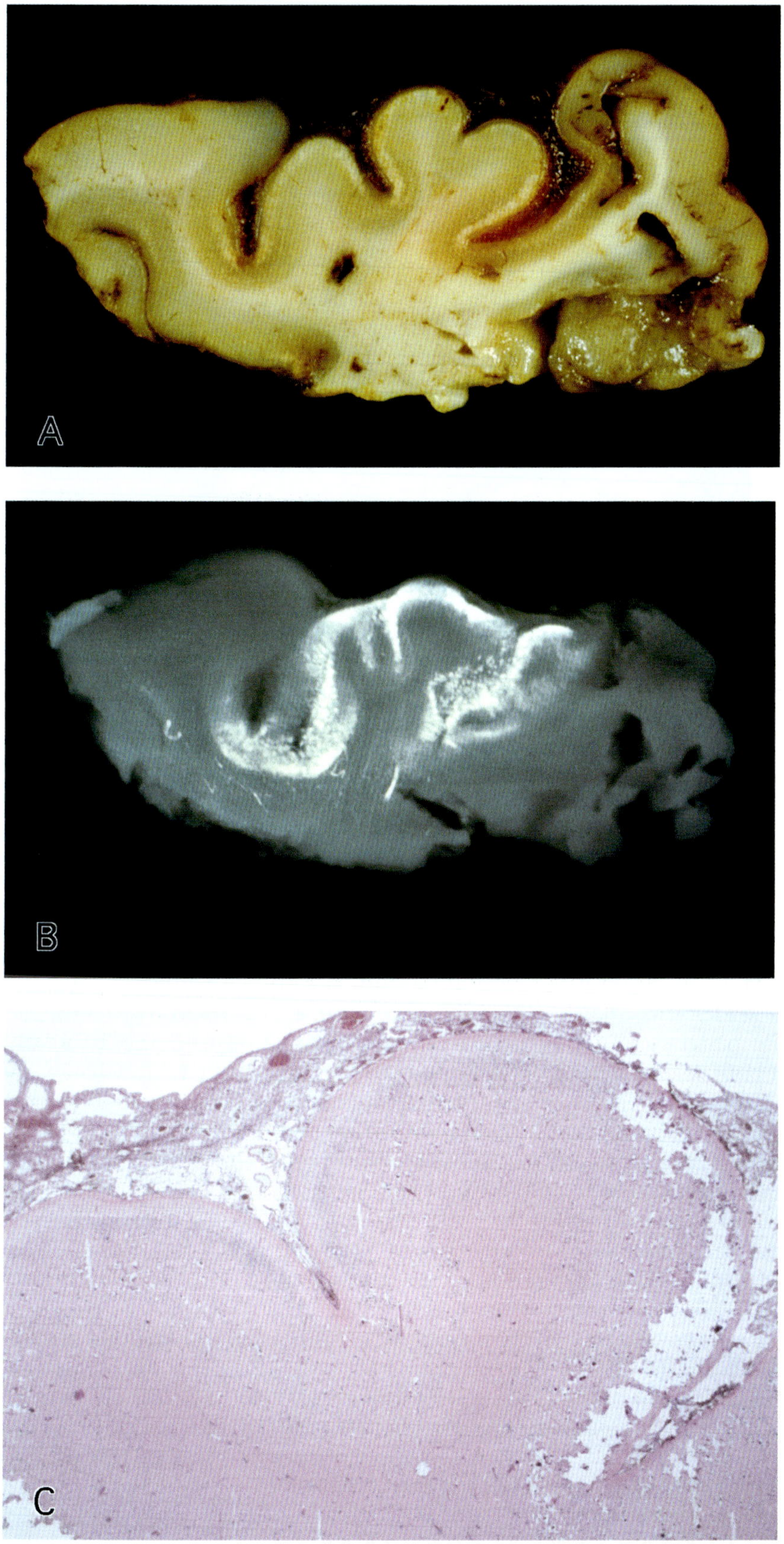

Figure 13-18

STURGE-WEBER SYNDROME

A: Dense calcification following the gyral contours is common in Sturge-Weber syndrome.

B: Calcification is readily appreciated on specimen X ray.

C: Histologic sections demonstrate a corresponding band of parenchymal calcification in the superficial layers of the cortex. (Courtesy of Dr. Jeffrey Golden, Philadelphia, PA.)

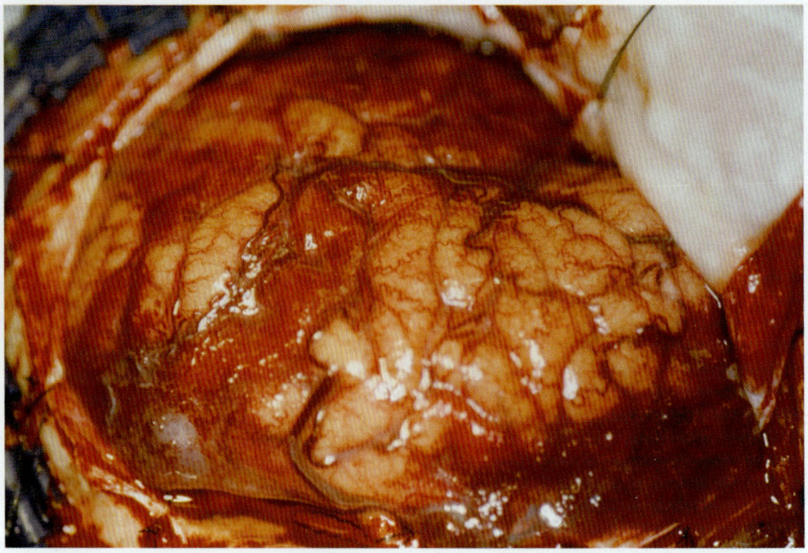

Figure 13-19

STURGE-WEBER SYNDROME

There is subarachnoid congestion over the cerebral hemispheres in regions with an extensive leptomeningeal vascular network. (Courtesy of Dr. Jeffrey Golden, Philadelphia, PA.)

Microscopic Findings. The most significant histopathologic change in SWS is the striking proliferation of leptomeningeal vessels (fig. 13-20). These dilated, thin-walled vessels have a single layer of endothelial cells and a thin layer of connective tissue, are variably calcified, and are associated with subpial gliosis (85,87,88). The vessels extend into the underlying cortex and subcortical white matter (89). The cortex itself is typically normally formed, but association with polymicrogyria has been noted (90). The cortex is atrophied, however, with diffuse neuronal dropout and gliosis, changes presumed to be due to chronic tissue anoxia associated with the abnormal vessels in SWS (83). Typically, there is calcification of the superficial layers of the cortex; this may extend into the subcortical white matter (87). This calcification takes the form of both perivascular encrustation and parenchymal deposits; these calcifications may also be laminated (87). With careful examination, most parenchymal deposits can be demonstrated to have a perivascular component (87,91).

Ultrastructural studies have identified calcium deposits within vessel walls as well as in perithelial cells and the perivascular space (87,91). Calcifications and other parenchymal changes all appear to increase with age (87). The etiology of the calcifications is unclear, but they are regarded by most authors as a secondary dystrophic change (91).

Differential Diagnosis. The characteristic clinical and histopathologic changes of SWS are not readily confused with the other phakomatoses. There are, however, rare reported cases in which features of SWS and other phakomatoses are combined, including SWS and neurofibromas, adenoma sebaceum, and von Hippel-Lindau disease (84). While vascular lesions may be part of the differential diagnosis, the presence of fairly uniform-appearing venous structures in the subarachnoid space, with accompanying superficial cortical calcification, is unique to SWS.

Treatment and Prognosis. The treatment of the seizures is one of the primary objectives in the clinical management of SWS. This is particularly important because prevention of seizures is believed to limit the effects of hypoperfusion and hypometabolism that underlie SWS (83). Children with SWS and intractable seizures are considered candidates for epilepsy surgery, most often hemispherectomy or subtotal hemispherectomy (89). Small series and case reports suggest that surgical resection is effective in not only controlling seizures, but also in stopping or even reversing developmental deterioration (83,92).

The overall prognosis of patients with SWS varies widely. Patients with the most widespread hemispheric or bihemispheric disease are believed to be at the greatest risk for neurologic complications. While there are many patients who are severely affected with mental retardation, seizures, and other serious neurologic sequelae, there are also patients with normal cognitive function and neurologic status (83).

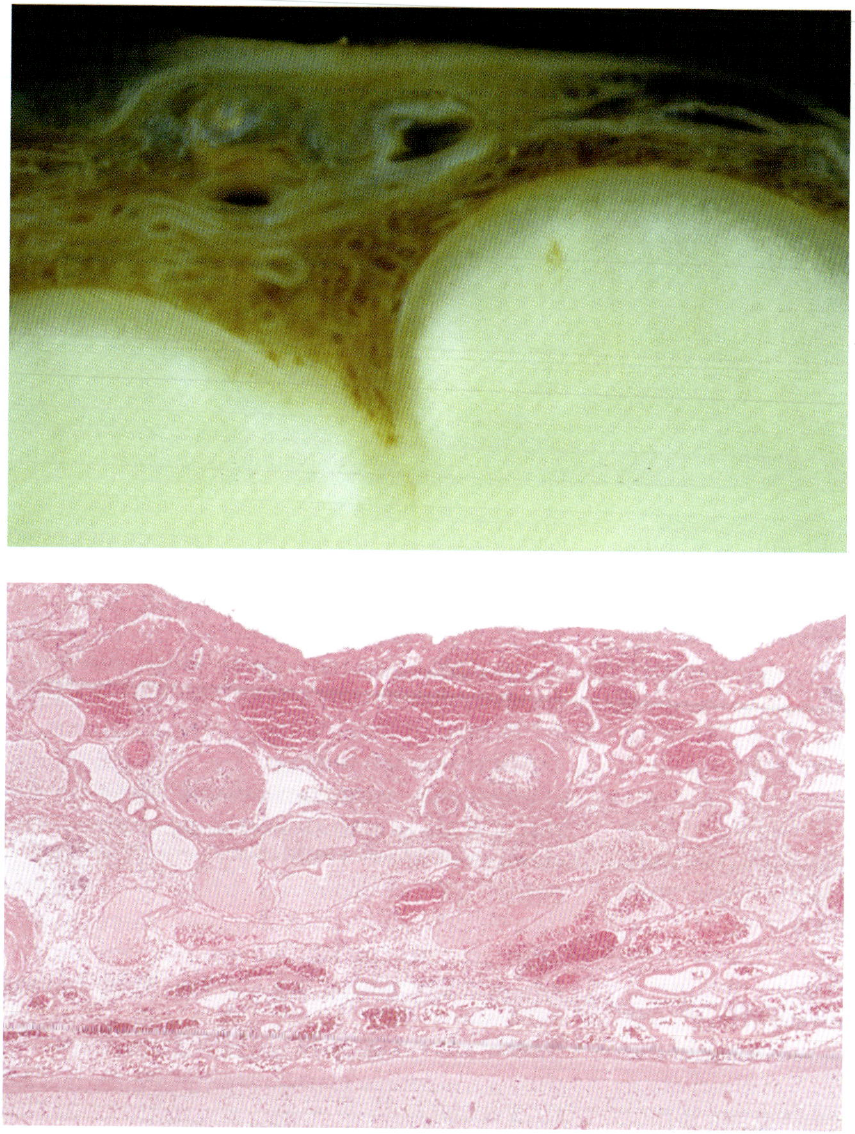

Figure 13-20

STURGE-WEBER SYNDROME

Top: The thickened leptomeninges are darkly discolored and have a granular appearance due to an extensive vascular network.

Bottom: There is a striking proliferation of dilated, thin-walled leptomeningeal vessels. The associated subpial gliosis is prominent. (Courtesy of Dr. Jeffrey Golden, Philadelphia, PA.)

RASMUSSEN SYNDROME

Definition. *Rasmussen syndrome* (RS) is an autoimmune disorder that produces progressive multifocal encephalopathy associated with unilateral cortical atrophy and progressive neurologic deterioration in children (93,94).

General Comments. RS is a rare condition that generally presents in childhood. It was initially described in a small series of patients who were felt to have focal seizures due to chronic localized encephalitis (96). Some of these patients had a nonspecific history of preceding infection or inflammation which suggested an infectious etiology (96).

Clinical Features. RS has a characteristic clinical presentation: acute onset of focal seizures in childhood. These seizures remain focal or multifocal and are always unilateral. Epilepsia partialis continua develops in half of the patients at some point in this progressive disorder. The intractable seizures are associated with progressive injury of the involved hemisphere.

The other symptoms associated with RS are hemiparesis, hemianopia, cognitive impairment, and dysphasia when the dominant hemisphere is involved (93). Progression of symptoms can be rapid, and most of the brain damage occurs in the first 8 to 12 months after

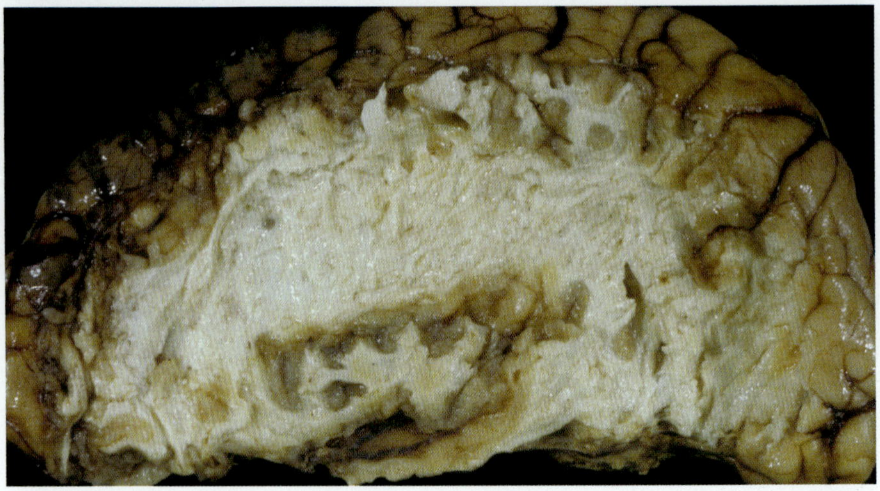

Figure 13-21

RASMUSSEN SYNDROME

In advanced disease, cortical resection specimens show evidence of atrophy and gliosis of the affected regions. (Courtesy of Dr. Jeffrey Golden, Philadelphia, PA.)

the onset of disease (95). Involvement of the motor cortex is inevitable and commonly occurs early in the course of the disease. Hemiparesis occurs within a year of onset in about 40 percent of patients, followed by cognitive and behavioral changes. These may progress over a variable period of months to up to 10 years (96). The clinical symptoms are accompanied by unilateral cortical atrophy.

Radiologic Findings. Neuroimaging studies are essential for excluding other disease processes that may also be associated with intractable epilepsy, such as tumor, cortical dysplasia, or vascular malformations. Both CT and MRI demonstrate the structural changes of cortical atrophy and hydrocephalus associated with the progression of RS. Even early in the course of the disease, the MRI may show focal cortical atrophy and ipsilateral ventricular dilatation. White matter hyperintensity on T2-weighted images is characteristic of affected regions (97).

Gross Findings. Since RS is a condition in which the age of onset and the duration of the disease both significantly influence the extent of pathology, the gross features discernable in cortical resection specimens vary widely. Advanced disease features cortical scarring and spongiosis (fig. 13-21). In such cases, cortical atrophy and gliosis may be readily apparent. In less severely involved brain regions, gross changes may be less or inconspicuous (98).

Intraoperative Findings. Because the pathologic changes may be quite focal and variable in severity, biopsies may or may not accurately represent the extent and severity of the underlying disease process. For this reason, it has been suggested that brain biopsy is not routinely indicated in making the diagnosis of RS (93,94). In any event, the changes described below should be readily appreciable on frozen section. Awareness of the clinical presentation and radiographic findings is essential in making the correct diagnosis.

Microscopic Findings. The histopathologic changes may vary considerably based on the extent and age of the lesion being sampled. The changes of RS are readily recognized by neuropathologists as those of a chronic encephalitic process: lymphocytic cuffing and parenchymal infiltrates, microglial nodules, neuronophagia, and reactive gliosis (fig. 13-22). Most lesions exist somewhere along a spectrum of active disease to end-stage changes (93). Recognizing this, a four-stage classification scheme is used to describe these lesions. Early in the course of the disease (stage 1), there are mild to moderate lymphocytic infiltration and perivascular cuffing, focal microglial nodules and activation, mild to focal gliosis, and minimal neuronal loss. The intermediate stage (stage 2) features more diffuse cortical inflammation and gliosis, marked lymphocytic infiltrates and perivascular cuffs, microglial activation, and more widely distributed nodules. Moderate to severe neuronal loss and marked reactive gliosis are present. Necrosis and cavitation are typically seen in at least one affected gyrus. Later, in stage 3, a mixture of active and remote disease is evident, with areas that show cortical degeneration and gliosis with severe neuronal loss. These features may be accompanied by patchy lymphocytic

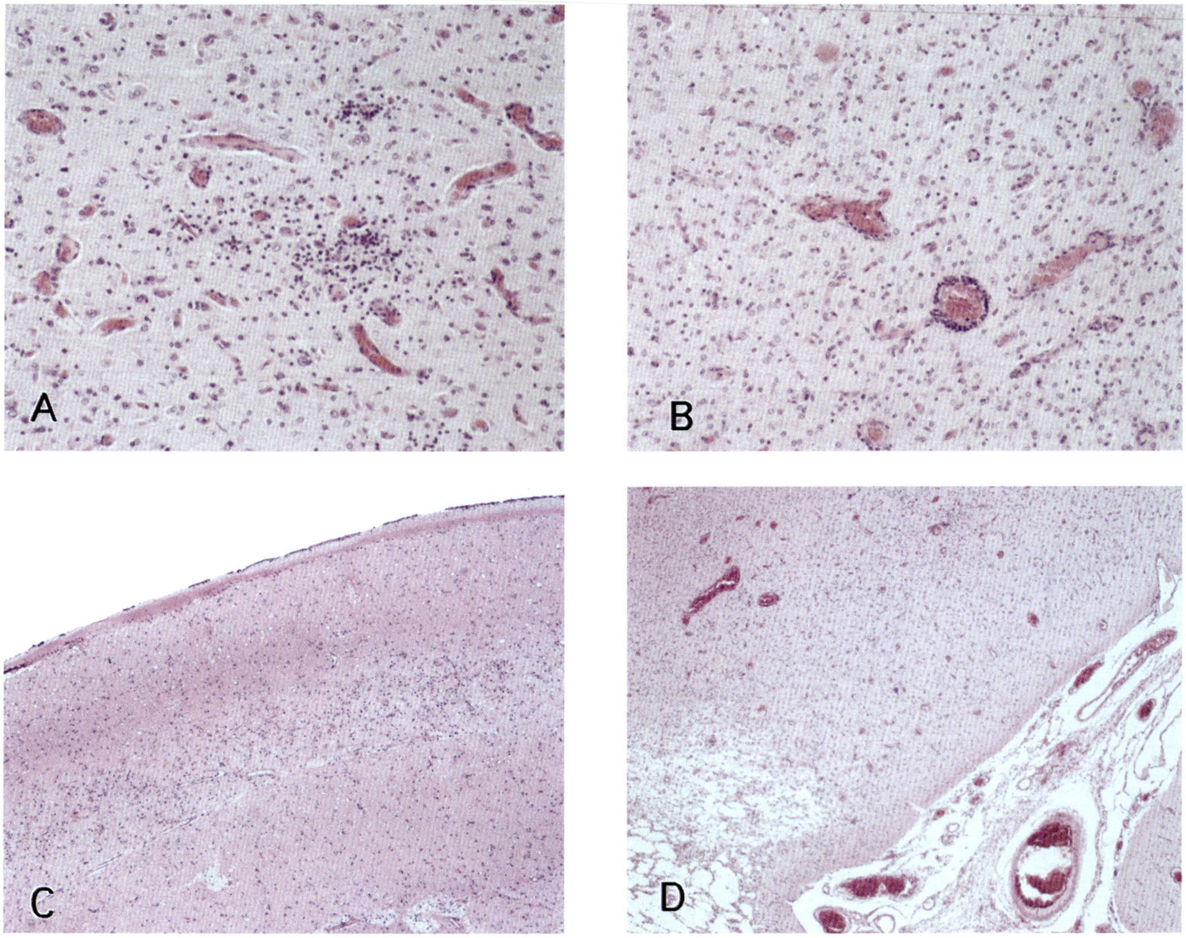

Figure 13-22

RASMUSSEN SYNDROME

A,B: Encephalitic changes, including lymphocytic perivascular cuffing, infiltrates, and microglial nodules, are characteristic of this chronic process.

C: Lesions may show various states of progression, with more diffuse cortical gliosis and neuronal drop-out appearing later in the course of the disease.

D: In end-stage lesions there is more extensive neuronal loss, gliosis, and cortical cavitation. (A,B,D: courtesy of Dr. Jeffrey Golden, Philadelphia, PA; C: courtesy of Dr. Lucy Rorke-Adams, Philadelphia, PA.)

infiltrates and variable degrees of microglial activation. Finally, in the end stage (stage 4), the changes are fairly nonspecific, consisting mainly of cortical cavitation, extensive gliosis and neuronal loss, and rare lymphocytic infiltrates with few to no microglial nodules (96). Careful examination typically reveals no evidence of viral cytopathic changes.

Immunohistochemical stains for viral antigens are generally negative. Staining with GFAP highlights the presence of reactive astrocytes. Immunostaining with markers for B lymphocytes and plasma cells confirm the paucity of these cells in RS. T cells (CD3 positive) predominate in the lymphocytic infiltrates; the majority of these cells are CD8 positive and express GrB-positive granules, consistent with a cytotoxic T-cell reaction directed against neurons. The majority of cells that express HAM56 or CD68 have morphologic features of microglia rather than macrophages (94). There are a small number of reported cases in which the typical clinical and pathologic findings of RS are combined with a second pathologic process, including vascular abnormalities, neoplasia, cortical dysplasia, and tuberous sclerosis (99,100).

Differential Diagnosis. Since the most striking features of RS are those characteristically associated with chronic encephalitis, the differential diagnosis includes a number of infectious conditions. These can often be eliminated on the basis of the strictly unilateral involvement and characteristic clinical features of RS. When considering the diagnosis of RS, however, care should be given to examining the tissues closely for evidence of viral cytopathic effect and antigens in order to rule-out acute viral meningoencephalitis. A number of less commonly encountered infectious agents, including measles (subacute sclerosing panencephalitis) and rubella, are also considered. These can be eliminated by bilateral involvement and recognition of the Cowdry A inclusions (subacute sclerosing panencephalitis) or a characteristic pattern of cortical sparing and necrotizing vasculitis in white matter and deep gray matter (rubella).

In resections from later stages of RS, cystic destruction, spongiosis, and gliosis may predominate. These features may overlap somewhat with those associated with prion disease. The presence of even scant inflammation in late RS and the lack of amyloid plaques are features that are helpful in distinguishing RS from prion disease (101).

Based on the clinical presentation, a number of other conditions are simulated that can be readily eliminated by examination of tissue sections. Unihemispheric epileptic syndromes are seen in association with cortical dysplasia, HME, tuberous sclerosis, and Sturge-Weber syndrome. The characteristic features of each of these are addressed elsewhere in this chapter. Epilepsia partialis continua may also be associated with metabolic disorders. Finally, mitochondrial disorders may be associated with progressive neurologic disease that occasionally is mistaken for RS (94).

Treatment and Prognosis. Since the original description of this disorder, numerous studies and accumulated clinical experience have proven that the only treatment for RS is hemispherectomy. Partial resections are ineffective because RS will develop in the residual tissue of the hemisphere. Hemispherectomy has proven safe and effective in treating RS. In one large center, up to 65 percent of patients were reported seizure free following hemispherectomy; patients in whom significant residual seizures were observed reportedly were those in whom hemispherectomy was incomplete. Importantly, in addition to offering the only effective means of seizure control, hemispherectomy does not appear to create additional neurologic problems for individuals with this progressive encephalopathy (93).

CHASLIN GLIOSIS, ALEXANDER DISEASE, AND TRAUMA

Three other pathologic lesions are widely associated with seizures and may be encountered, with varying frequency, in resection or biopsy specimens from patients with epilepsy. *Chaslin gliosis* is a descriptive term for the presence of subpial gliosis in patients with longstanding epilepsy. *Alexander disease* is a leukodystrophy associated with megalencephaly (described in chapter 12) that, in its infantile form, is often associated with seizures. *Traumatic brain injury* results from contusions and other lesions (described in chapter 11) and may be a cause of seizures.

In Chaslin gliosis, subpial gliosis expands the glia limitans (102). The changes are nonspecific and not restricted to particular brain regions (fig. 13-23). This change is believed to be the consequence rather than the cause of seizure activity (103). Chaslin gliosis is a fairly common finding in many resection specimens from patients with seizures. With the increasing frequency of intracortical EEG monitoring for several days or weeks preoperatively, care must be taken to recognize the potential contribution of iatrogenic factors to this histopathologic finding.

In the original description of Alexander disease, an infantile presentation with seizures, enlarging head size, and developmental delay were noted (104). Clinical descriptions of Alexander disease now include rarer juvenile and adult forms. Seizures are a prominent clinical finding in infantile cases (age under 2 years), along with megalencephaly, spasticity, and developmental delay (105). Seizures are rarely encountered in the juvenile and adult forms of the disease (106). Imaging studies demonstrate widespread white matter abnormalities, with the greatest involvement in the frontal lobes and typically associated with low T1- and high T2-weighted signals (107). The presence of subpial, perivascular, or subependymal Rosenthal fibers and astrocytic inclusions (see chapter 12), should suggest the possibility of this diagnosis in infants presenting with seizures and widespread white matter signal abnormalities.

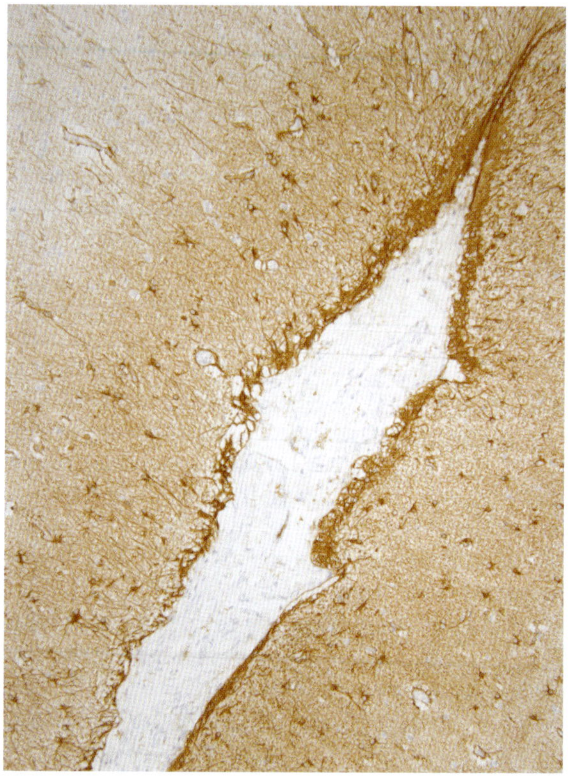

Figure 13-23

CHASLIN (SUBPIAL) GLIOSIS

Gliosis of the subpial space is a common change in many resection specimens from patients with seizures (GFAP stain).

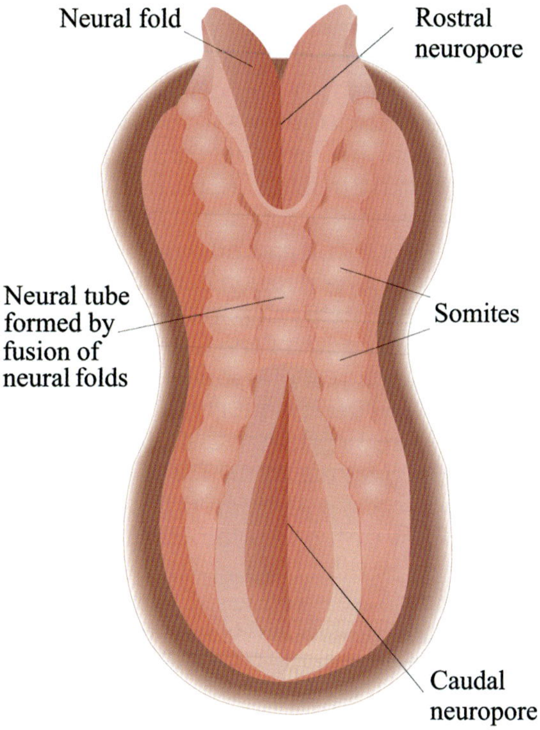

Figure 13-24

PRIMARY NEURULATION

Formation of the neural tube: neural folds have fused near the middle of the embryo to form the neural tube. Still open are the rostral and caudal neuropores, which correspond to the head and spinal regions, respectively. (Illustration by Dr. Amy Noffsinger.)

Traumatic brain injury is estimated to account for up to 20 percent of patients with symptomatic epilepsy. The onset of these seizures may be delayed following injury, but the vast majority of those affected develop seizures within 2 years of injury (108). The likelihood of developing post-traumatic seizures is significantly associated with the presence of multiple brain contusions, particularly when bilateral (108). The clinical course is difficult to predict, as some patients develop seizures that are limited in number and ultimately transient, while others require medical treatment. In a minority of cases, intractable epilepsy develops (109). Because of this, resections from patients with subacute and remote traumatic brain injury are seen by the pathologist. The histopathologic features of contusions, particular those with chronic changes, should be sought in these specimens. For a complete description of the histopathology of these lesions, see chapter 11.

NEURAL TUBE CLOSURE ABNORMALITIES

Defects in neural tube closure and closely related developmental processes are responsible for several lesions encountered in surgical neuropathology. Neural tube closure abnormalities are second only to congenital heart defects in frequency and affect 1/1,000 births in American Caucasians. These defects are associated with events early in development. The formation and closure of the neural tube occur between 18 and 26 days postconception. Neurulation, or the formation of the neural tube, occurs in both primary and secondary phases. Primary neurulation is the process by which the brain and the spinal cord are formed (fig. 13-24). During this process, the neural folds form, converge toward the midline and, at a single point, fuse to initiate formation of the neural tube. Fusion of the neural folds proceeds from this point both rostrally and caudally. The ends of the neural tube remain open. Designated the rostral and caudal neuropores, these areas roughly correspond to the head and spinal regions, respectively. Closure of the neuropores occurs at the end of this developmental process around day 26. Structures in the sacrococcygeal region derive from the tail bud, a separate stem cell population that arises distal to the closure of the caudal neuropore. Through the process of secondary neurulation, these cells proliferate and condense to form a solid structure, which then cavitates to produce a tube that gives rise to the tissue types found in the sacrococcygeal region (110).

Regardless of the location along the developing neural tube, two general patterns of malformation are encountered. In the first, there is a failure of the developing neural tube to close properly, with secondary disruption of the axial mesoderm. This results in abnormal neuroectodermal tissue protruding to a variable degree through a secondary defect in mesenchymal structures. Examples of this include encephalocele (rostral neural tube) and myelomeningocele (caudal neural tube). In the second pattern of malformation, the underlying embryonic defect is primarily in the development of the axial mesoderm. These lesions are associated with a closed neural tube. Only a portion of this structure, the membranes and cerebrospinal fluid (CSF), herniates through the defect to produce a meningocele. Meningoceles develop along both the rostral (cranial meningoceles) and caudal (spinal meningoceles) neural tube. Abnormalities in the developmental sequence of the tail bud give rise to a distinct but related group of lesions that often result in tethered cord syndrome.

Anterior Neural Tube Closure Abnormalities: Cephalocele, Encephalocele, and Nasal Glioma

Definition. *Cephalocele* is a general term used to describe a congenital defect of the skull with herniation of any intracranial structures (111). When both meninges and brain tissue herniate through a mesenchymal defect, the lesion is called an *encephalocele*. If the lesion consists of meninges and CSF, without neural tissue, it is referred to as a *cranial meningocele*.

Encephaloceles occur both anteriorly and posteriorly, and are further classified by their position. Anterior encephaloceles are generally sphenoidal or frontal-ethmoidal in location while posterior encephaloceles are most often occipital and can involve both supratentorial and infratentorial structures. Occipital encephaloceles that contain only cerebellar tissue are also classified as *Chiari III malformations*.

Encephaloceles in the nasal region, as well as so-called *nasal gliomas*, are believed to arise from aberrations of the normal developmental sequence that occurs around the end of the second month of gestation. During this period, there is a transiently present prenasal space through which a diverticulum of dura extends along the foramen cecum outward to the nose. In normal development, this dural projection regresses and the foramen cecum is filled in with fibrous tissue (fig. 13-25). Encephaloceles in the nasal region, as well as nasal gliomas, arise when cerebral tissue herniates into this dural projection. When there is regression of the proximal portion of the projection, the more distal elements may remain in the nasal cavity, separated from the intracranial space, forming a nasal glioma (fig. 13-25). In up 15 percent of these lesions some connection with intracranial structures persists (112).

Clinical Features. The incidence of encephaloceles is approximately 1/5,000 live births (113). These lesions are much less common than those along the posterior or spinal segment of the neuraxis. There are marked differences in the distribution of these lesions between the sexes. Posterior, particularly occipital, encephaloceles are far more common in females, whereas anterior encephaloceles are more common in males (113). There are also wide geographic variations in the distribution of these lesions. Posterior encephaloceles are more common among individuals of white European and North American extraction, while anterior encephaloceles predominate among Southeast Asians (114). In North America, 70 to 90 percent of encephaloceles are occipital (115).

Most encephaloceles are sporadic and not part of an associated syndrome. Encephaloceles may be encountered, however, in multiple syndromes with variably severe associated malformations, including Meckel-Gruber, Dandy-Walker, Walker-

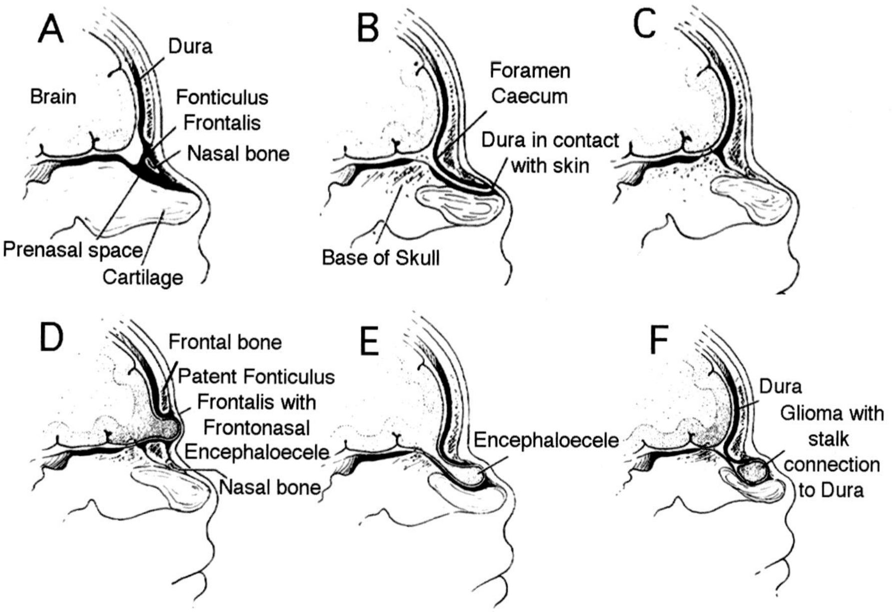

Figure 13-25

DEVELOPMENT OF BASE OF SKULL AND PRENASAL SPACE

A–C: Normal developmental sequence of the nasal region.

D–F: Formation of encephaloceles and nasal gliomas. (Modified from figs. 15 and 16 from Barkovich AJ, Vandermarck P, Edwards MS, Cogen PH. Congenital nasal masses: CT and MR imaging features in 16 cases. AJNR Am J Neuroradiol 1991; 12:113, 114.)

Warburg, Joubert, and Roberts syndromes, among others. Encephaloceles associated with these syndromes show distinct patterns of frontal (Roberts) or occipital (Meckel-Grubera, Walker-Warburg) distribution (116).

Anterior encephaloceles are often associated with a visible facial deformity such as hypertelorism, frontal mass, or labial fissure. Other symptomatic abnormalities include nasal or pharyngeal obstruction, optic nerve abnormalities, coloboma, and endocrinopathies. CSF leakage and recurrent meningitis (chemical and infectious) may be present. Anterior encephaloceles are frequently associated with agenesis of the corpus callosum (115). Occipital encephaloceles may be associated with Chiari II and Dandy-Walker malformations (114). Encephaloceles in either location are associated with seizures (117).

Radiologic Findings. Radiologic studies are used for both recognition and delineation of these lesions. Most cephaloceles are detected by prenatal ultrasound, which is sensitive for the bony cranial defects associated with these lesions, as well as other related CNS abnormalities. During the postnatal period, both skull films and CT scans are effective in defining the extent of these defects. CT scans also demonstrate the presence and amount of cerebral tissue and CSF contained within these lesions. MRI is the preferred modality for delineating the exact nature and relationship of the tissues within these lesions, as well as identifying connections with the intracranial compartment (113,115).

Gross Findings. During the surgical repair of these lesions, the encephalocele sac is generally resected. The lesion may be sessile or pedunculated and vary widely in size. Many specimens show at least partial coverage by normal skin; other areas of the surface are enclosed by a covering membrane of variable thickness (fig. 13-26). Posterior encephaloceles are often covered by normal scalp or, particularly when larger, by abnormal skin with an accompanying angioma. In addition to CSF, the sac may contain a variable amount of cerebral tissue; in occipital lesions this may include cerebrum and cerebellum (118). Care should be taken to sample these specimens adequately to maximize the chance of identifying any brain parenchyma that is present, since this has significant prognostic implications.

Intraoperative Findings. There is little use for routine intraoperative evaluation of these lesions. Rarely, frozen section of a nasal glioma may be submitted for evaluation. These lesions show the microscopic features described below.

Microscopic Findings. These lesions are characteristically covered by variably intact skin or membranous tissue. In the central area overlying the lesion, careful examination may reveal diminished to absent dermal appendages and an

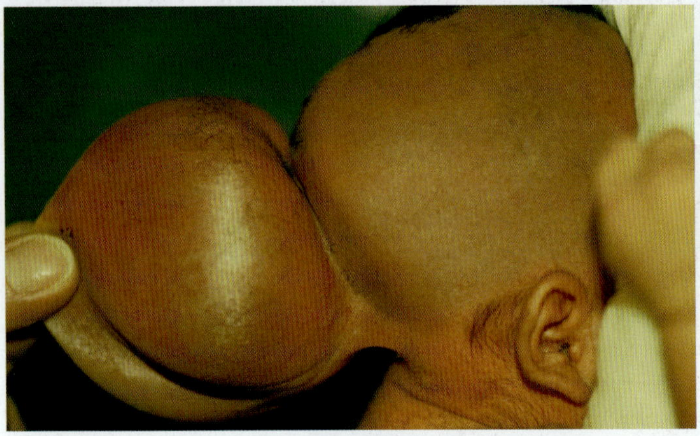

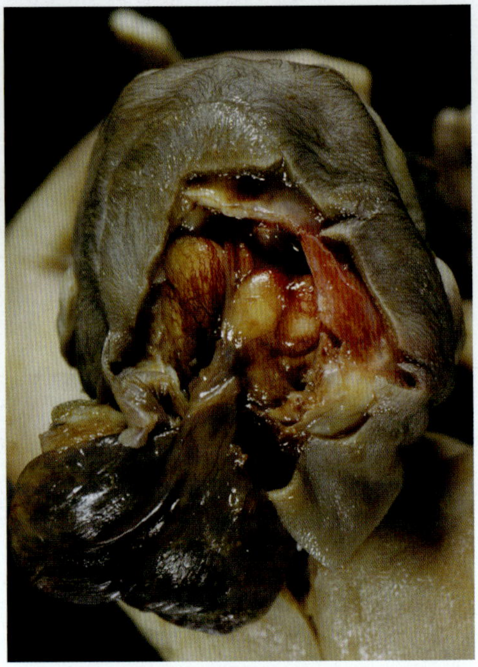

Figure 13-26

ENCEPHALOCELE

Above: These defects may be completely or partially covered by intact skin. (Courtesy of Dr. Lucy Rorke-Adams, Philadelphia, PA.)

Right: The lesions are frequently pedunculated and extend through a bony defect to communicate with the intracranial compartment. (Courtesy of Dr. Jeffrey Golden, Philadelphia, PA.)

abnormal accumulation of blood vessels in the underlying dermis (fig. 13-27). Cells with meningothelial features may be admixed within the fibrocollagenous tissue of the deep dermis or, in the case of a meningocele, line a cavitary space within the deep dermis. Immunohistochemical staining with vimentin and EMA aids in the detection and recognition of these cells.

In approximately one third of cases, the brain tissue within the lesion resembles normal cerebral cortex, often with a leptomeningeal covering. In the rest of the cases, the tissue within the lesion is dysplastic and arranged as an irregular mass of cerebral tissue (119). The latter often lacks a well-defined leptomeningeal covering and extends upward to the overlying connective tissue and epidermis. In lesions that are occipital and cervical, it is possible to identify brain stem and cerebellar tissue. Generally, cerebellar tissue is present both as fragments of necrotic cerebellum and larger intact pieces with normally developed cerebellar architecture and leptomeninges, including the typically rich vasculature of the subarachnoid space seen in the perinatal period (119). Neural tissue within these lesions is often quite gliotic and shows signs of degeneration.

Ependymal-lined spaces are present in up to a third of the lesions. Choroid plexus, often with reactive changes including fibrosis and hemosiderin accumulation, may be present. Immunohistochemical staining for GFAP, neurofilaments, and synaptophysin highlights the presence of neuroglial tissue within these lesions.

The histopathologic features of nasal gliomas are not significantly different from those seen in frontal encephalocele and range from well-differentiated glial tissue to dysplastic neuroglial tissue. There may be a prominent fibrovascular stroma in these lesions, as well as associated respiratory epithelium and glandular elements. A variable chronic inflammation may be present.

Differential Diagnosis. With a proper clinical history, a diagnosis can be made readily and without consideration of other entities. In the problematic situation of a pathologist encountering one of these specimens without adequate clinical information, the hypercellularity and disorganization of the neuroepithelial elements may raise the possibility of a low-grade glioneuronal tumor. Even in this situation, however, the usual finding of dermal, meningothelial, and choroid plexus components should enable the pathologist to avoid a misdiagnosis of neoplasia.

Treatment and Prognosis. The treatment of cephaloceles is surgical. The outcome is dependent on the nature and extent of the lesion, particularly the amount of brain tissue involved

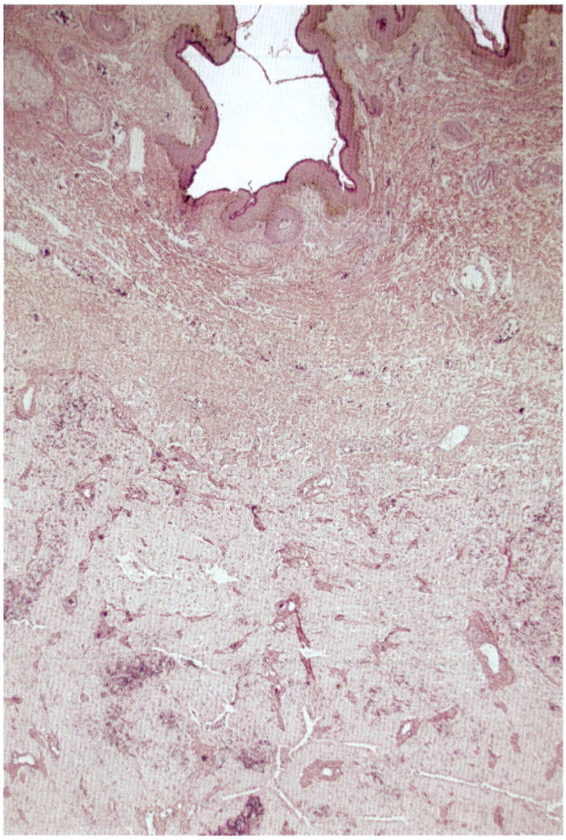

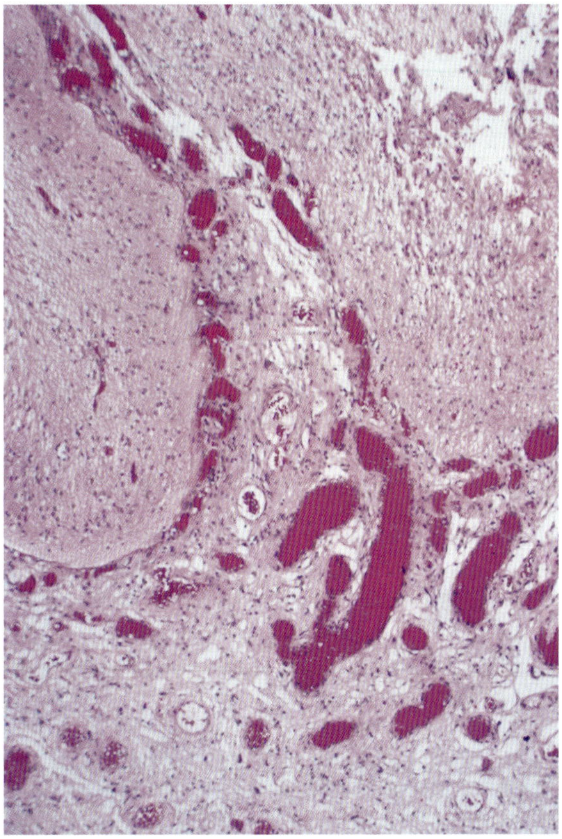

Figure 13-27

ENCEPHALOCELE

Left: Skin overlying these lesions typically shows absent or reduced dermal appendages and disruption of the normal dermal architecture. In this case, disorganized neuroglial tissue is also present within the deep dermis. (Courtesy of Dr. Jeffrey Golden, Philadelphia, PA.)

Right: Disorganized gliotic cerebellar folia and leptomeninges with prominent vasculature from a cervical encephalocele. (Courtesy of Dr. Lucy Rorke-Adams, Philadelphia, PA.)

in the defect, and the presence of associated CNS malformations. Patients whose lesions contain only a leptomeningeal sac without cerebral tissue (meningocele) have a better prognosis than those whose lesions contain cerebral tissue. Of lesions that contain cerebral tissue, anterior encephaloceles, particularly those that are frontal-ethmoidal, are often associated with both good surgical outcome and an excellent prognosis. Nasal gliomas also fall into this category. A major treatment issue for these lesions is the presence of any intracranial connection to the nasal glioma, since this creates a risk for CSF leak and other complications. This issue is typically resolved by imaging studies rather than histopathologic findings. It is incumbent upon the pathologist to discuss this with the operating physician, as nasal gliomas are often not suspected preoperatively. This overall favorable picture is in contrast to that for patients with the more commonly encountered posterior encephaloceles, which have a questionable prognosis, significant mortality, and, in many cases, severe morbidity and complications despite surgical correction (113,116).

Caudal Neural Tube Closure Abnormalities: Myelomeningocele and Spinal Meningocele

Definition. *Spinal dysraphism* includes both *spina bifida cystica* (*myelomeningocele* and *meningocele*), also known as *spina bifida aperta* or *open spina bifida*, and *spina bifida occulta* (*tethered cord* and *lipoma*), discussed separately below. Myelomeningocele is the most commonly encountered neural tube closure abnormality

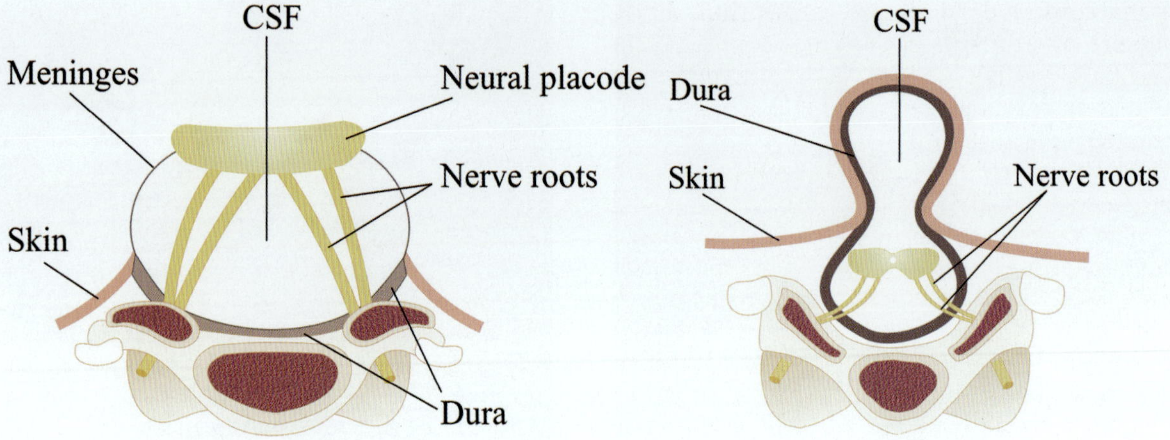

Figure 13-28

SPINA BIFIDA CYSTICA (MYELOMENINGOCELE AND MENINGOCELE)

Left: Schematic diagram illustrating key features of myelomeningocele.
Right: Schematic diagram illustrating key features of meningocele. (Illustration by Dr. Amy Noffsinger).

and the predominate form of spina bifida cystica (116). There is a spectrum of findings in these lesions and a variety of terms used to describe them. All are characterized by the failure of the superficial ectoderm to separate properly from the neural ectoderm and the persistence of the neural placode, a flat plate of unneurulated tissue, in place of the normal spinal cord at the level of the lesion (115). Most of these lesions are bulging, but when the neural placode opens directly onto and is flush with the skin surface, the lesion may be referred to as *myelocele* or *myeloschisis* (120).

These lesions show a slight female predominance and wide geographic and ethnic variance in frequency (0.3 to 2.92/1,000 live births) (122). Neural tube defects are believed to arise from the complex interaction of genetic and environmental factors. There are currently no well-established genetic loci for this disorder and most cases are sporadic; however, siblings and relatives of affected individuals are at a significantly increased risk (110). In addition, there are three well-established risk factors for myelomeningocele: 1) maternal pregestational diabetes; 2) inadequate maternal intake of folic acid; and 3) in utero exposure to antiepileptic drugs. It is estimated that adequate periconceptual folic acid supplementation alone could produce up to a 70 percent reduction in the risk of developing spina bifida and other neural tube defects (122).

Congenital spinal meningoceles are characterized by a vertebral defect with an associated cystic lesion containing herniated dura and arachnoid; the underlying spinal cord remains normally positioned (fig. 13-28) (118). These lesions are relatively rare, occurring 1/10,000 live births, and are without any gender predilection. They account for approximately 10 percent of all cases of spina bifida cystica, occur in the same distribution as myelomeningocele, and are rarely associated with other anomalies (121). Acquired meningoceles are a complication of spinal surgery, such as laminectomy, and are more common in adult populations (118).

Clinical Features. The clinical manifestations of myelomeningocele are diverse, owing both to the significant effect played by the location and extent of the lesion, as well as the specific associated abnormalities seen along with the myelomeningocele. Chiari II malformation is the most common associated abnormality, encountered in more than 95 percent of cases of myelomeningocele (123). A wide range of other CNS anomalies has been described, including hypoplasia or aplasia of cranial nerve nuclei, cerebellar dysplasia, thalamic fusion, agenesis of the corpus callosum, and complete or partial agenesis of the olfactory tract and bulb (124). Hydromyelia and syringomyelia are common in the spinal cord rostral to the lesion, as is diplomyelia and diastematomyelia (see below);

spinal cord caudal to the lesion may show diplomyelia or multiple ependymal canals (120). Most individuals with myelomeningocele are of normal intelligence but may have neurologic or cognitive difficulties due to complications from the myelomeningocele, as well as from any associated abnormalities (122).

The common clinical manifestations of myelomeningocele are divided into those that are a direct consequence of the spinal malformation and those due to Chiari II and related hindbrain malformations. An immediate clinical consequence of the spinal lesion is an increased susceptibility to CNS infection due to a poorly formed and frequently ulcerated skin or cystic covering at the site of the myelomeningocele (125). The other effects of the spinal lesion are variable, depending on the level and extent of the lesion. Most lesions are found in the lumbosacral spine (125). Lower extremity sensory and motor function can range from normal or near normal in low sacral lesions, to paraplegia for lesions above L3 (116). Sphincter disturbances are seen in all cases. Bladder outlet obstruction, chronic urinary tract infection, and pyelonephritis are major sources of morbidity and mortality in myelomeningocele patients (116). The clinical manifestations of Chiari II malformation and the associated hydrocephalus do not differ between patients with myelomeningocele and other patients.

Symptoms are encountered in up to a third of myelomeningocele patients and include apnea, cyanotic episodes, swallowing difficulties, impaired head control, upper extremity weakness, and coordination or balance difficulties. Brain stem dysfunction related to these abnormalities is a major cause of mortality in patients with myelomeningocele, particularly over the first two decades of life (121). Impaired cognition is linked directly to the degree and management of hydrocephalus as well as the incidence of CNS infection (116). By contrast, patients with meningocele are neurologically normal. Meningoceles are not typically associated with hydrocephalus. Because of the intact skin covering, the incidence of CNS infections in these patients is not increased.

Radiologic Findings. Most of these lesions are first detected by screening maternal serum alpha-fetoprotein and prenatal ultrasound; diagnosis is typically confirmed with amniocentesis combined with detailed ultrasound examination. This approach is effective for detecting both the spinal defect and the associated Chiari II malformation. Ultrasound studies are also used to assess spontaneous lower extremity movement. Prenatal MRI with T2-weighted sequences can provide detailed structural information that may be useful in predicting neurologic function (122).

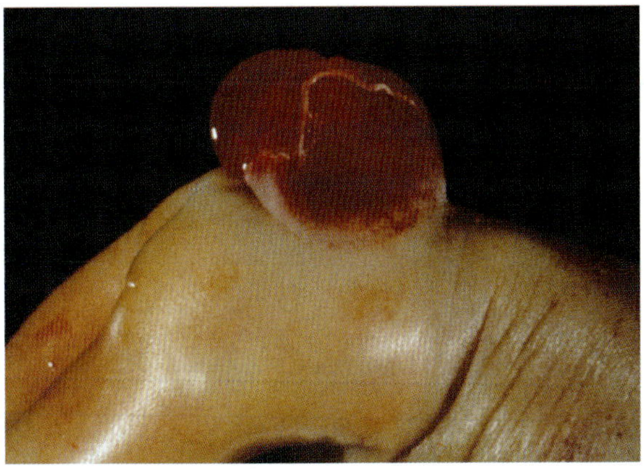

Figure 13-29

MYELOMENINGOCELE

This bulging sac-like structure is situated along the posterior midline. Along the lateral surface, there is a border between the cyst membrane (which is congested) and the skin. (Courtesy of Dr. Jeffrey Golden, Philadelphia, PA.)

Gross Findings. The intact myelomeningocele is a sac-like structure typically situated along the posterior midline (fig. 13-29). It is covered by a combination of variably intact skin and cyst membrane, which is often disrupted or absent due to breakdown. The neural placode may be evident as a flat mass positioned near the center of the cystic lesion. The cyst wall is formed by arachnoid, which is adherent to the neural placode, dura, and skin (fig. 13-28). In addition to meninges and CSF, the myelomeningocele sac typically contains nerve roots from the neural placode and cauda equina (121). The neural placode has been described as having the appearance of an open book in which the two leaves are comprised of the relatively intact anterior columns and the disrupted remnants of the dorsal spinal cord structures. Between these runs a midline neural groove and caudal central canal. The dorsal nerve roots exit the

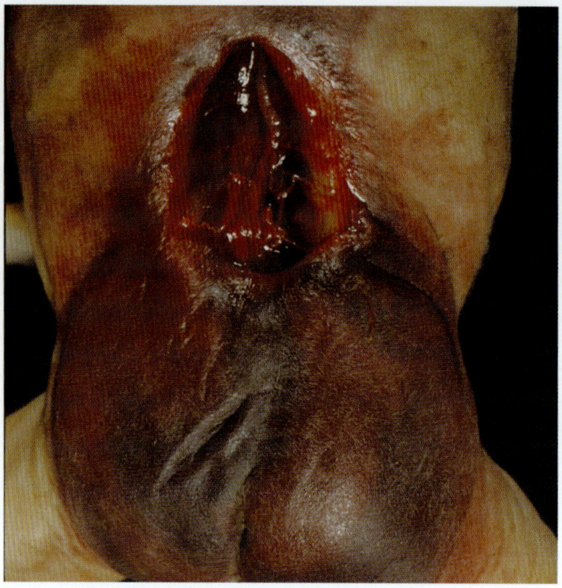

Figure 13-30

MYELOMENINGOCELE: NEURAL PLACODE

This abnormally formed remnant of spinal cord tissue is markedly congested, splayed open along the midline, and associated with multiple abnormally situated nerve roots. (Courtesy of Dr. Jeffrey Golden, Philadelphia, PA.)

neural placode laterally and the ventral roots medially (121). Myeloceles appear as flat open lesions with an area of disrupted skin covering in which sits the neural placode. In both myelomeningocele and myeloceles, this structure appears as a round, highly vascular mass, also referred to as the area medullovasculosa. This area may weep and discharge CSF and may be partially epithelialized (118). This is in contrast to meningoceles in which the spinal cord is normally formed and tissue herniating through the posterior defect is meninges covered with skin.

From the point of view of surgical pathology, neither the neural placode nor nerve roots are typically included in specimens since spinal tissue is most often left in situ by the surgeon. The pathology specimens generally consist of a roughly circular disc of soft tissue that is covered by skin and/or membrane. Ulceration of the surface is common, particularly in myelomeningocele. When present, the neural placode often appears as a highly vascular spongy tissue (fig. 13-30). The deep surfaces of these specimens generally contain some admixture of subcutaneous tissues and smooth membrane from the cystic sac (120).

Intraoperative Findings. There is little use for routine intraoperative evaluation of these specimens.

Microscopic Findings. Both meningocele and myelomeningocele are characterized by changes in the overlying skin. Skin from the center of these lesions often has a decreased number of dermal appendages and scar-like fibrosis; this contrasts with skin peripheral to the lesions which often has increased dermal appendages. The spinal meningocele itself is typically composed of bands of collagen fibers that are lined by meningothelial cells, with small interfiber spaces and clefts that are probably filled with CSF. Associated with this tissue are small bands of smooth muscle, and occasionally, abundant collections of small nerves, lymphatics, and blood vessels, the latter probably representing a vascular malformation or hamartoma (120).

The surface covering of myelomeningocele sac is composed of a variable combination of skin, cyst wall, and occasionally, neural elements from the neural placode (fig. 13-31). In grossly ulcerated areas, the surface may be covered by degenerating keratin debris and inflammatory cells. If the neural placode extends to the surface, there may be a combination of epidermis and a superficial plaque of abnormal neuroglial tissue, often with at least focal areas of ependymal differentiation. While some lesions extend to the surface, in most cases the abnormal tissue is more deeply situated beneath a fibrotic dermis. Here, abnormal collections of glial and neuroglial tissue can be seen in various configurations. Among the most common patterns is a deep plaque of glial tissue surrounded by connective tissue and situated in the subcutis; however, many different arrangements of this abnormal tissue have been described (120). Regardless of the histologic pattern, neurons are commonly encountered in these lesions.

While the neuronal and glial elements are often readily appreciated by routine histologic examination, the use of immunohistochemical stains for GFAP and neurofilaments or NeuN help better define the various tissue elements found in these lesions (fig. 13-32). In some cases, the extent, if not the presence, of these tissues may be underestimated without immunohistochemical staining. Abnormal bundles

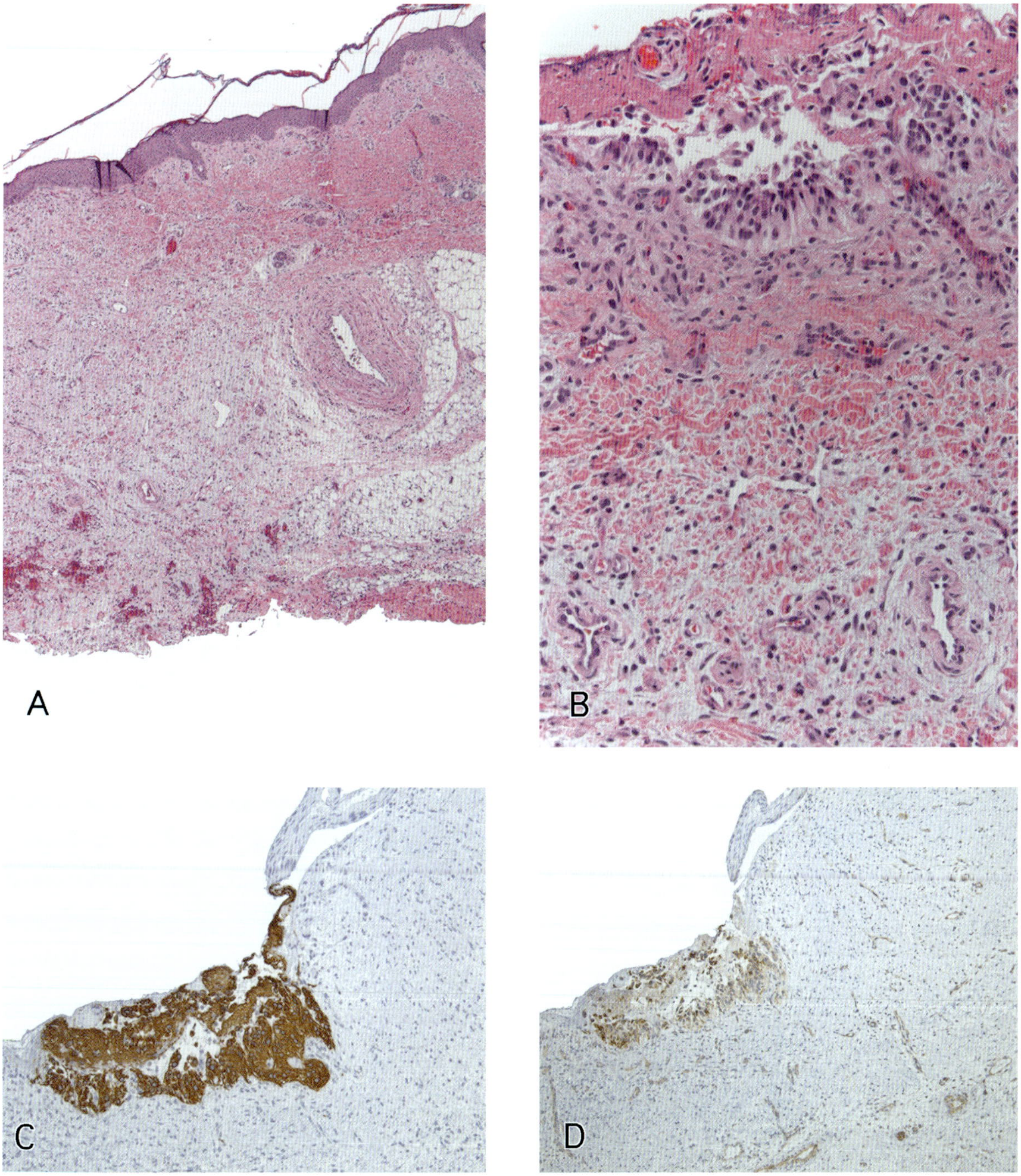

Figure 13-31

MYELOMENINGOCELE

A: Skin from the area around a myelomeningocele shows several characteristic changes including loss of normal dermal appendages, fibrosis and disruption of the normal dermal collagen, abnormal thick-walled blood vessels in the deep dermis and subcutaneous tissue, and abnormal collections of smooth muscle.

B: When present at the surface, the neural placode is often associated with ulceration and inflammation. The cells typically have features of glial (often ependymal) differentiation.

C,D: Immunohistochemical staining for GFAP (C) and NFP (D) confirms the neuroglial nature of these lesions.

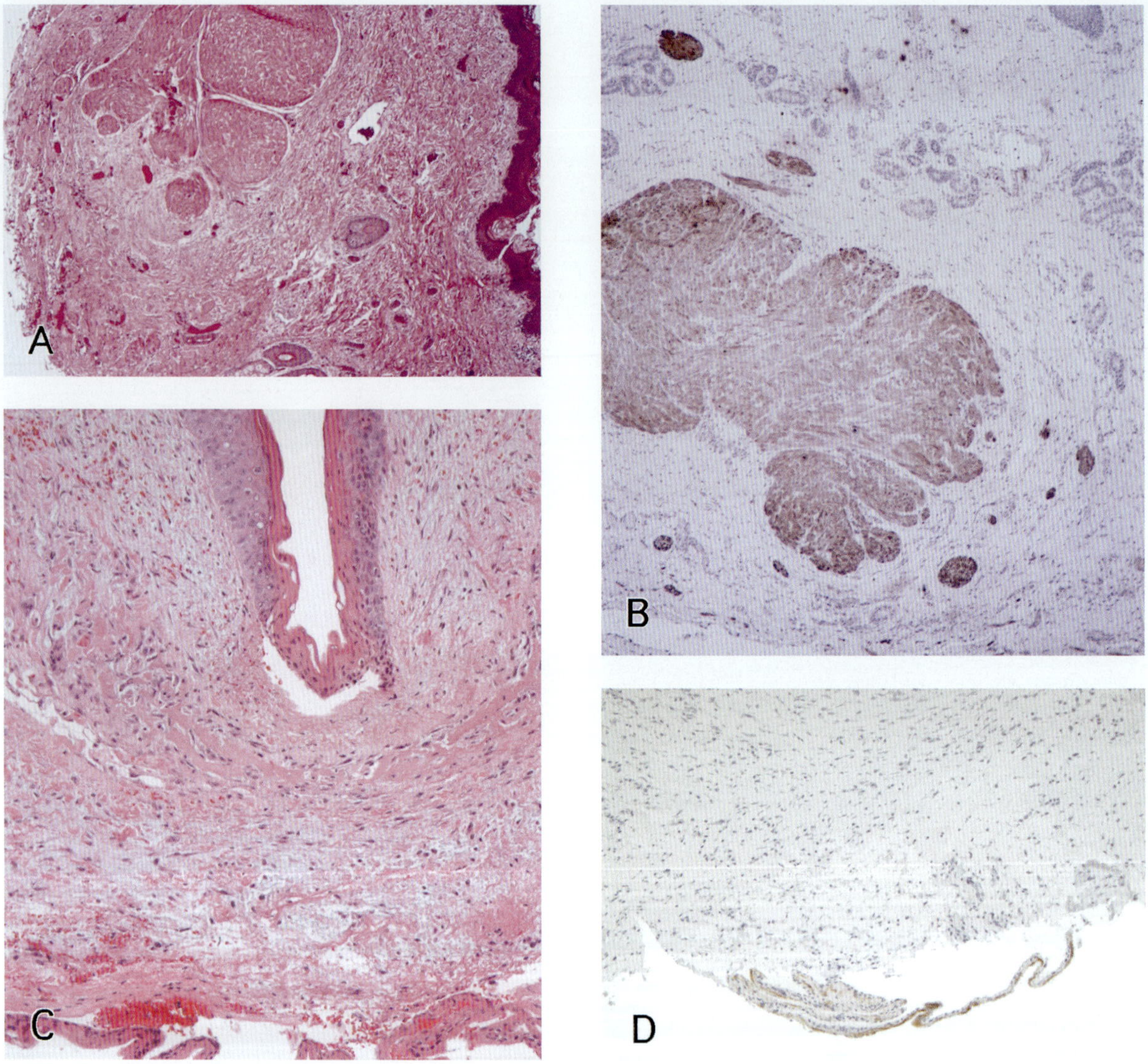

Figure 13-32

MYELOMENINGOCELE

A: The presence of large bundles of smooth muscle within the dermis is a clue to the presence of a myelomeningocele. (A-C: Courtesy of Dr. Lucy Rorke-Adams, Philadelphia, PA.)

B: These bundles are readily highlighted with immunostain for desmin.

C: Occasionally, fragments of leptomeninges are incorporated in these lesions, often adherent to or admixed within the deep dermis and subcutaneous tissue.

D: When present, leptomeningeal elements can be readily recognized with the assistance of epithelial membrane antigen (EMA) immunohistochemical staining.

of smooth muscle are readily demonstrated by staining for smooth muscle actin (SMA) or desmin expression. SMA also highlights the rich vasculature seen in many of these lesions. In addition to highlighting areas of ependymal differentiation, EMA demonstrates the presence of meningothelial cells.

Differential Diagnosis. Teratomas can occur in the sacrococcygeal region and are important to distinguish from myelomeningocele. As with myelomeningocele, teratomas are often present at birth and show a female predominance. They are most often postsacral in location and are slow growing. A cystic postsacral teratoma,

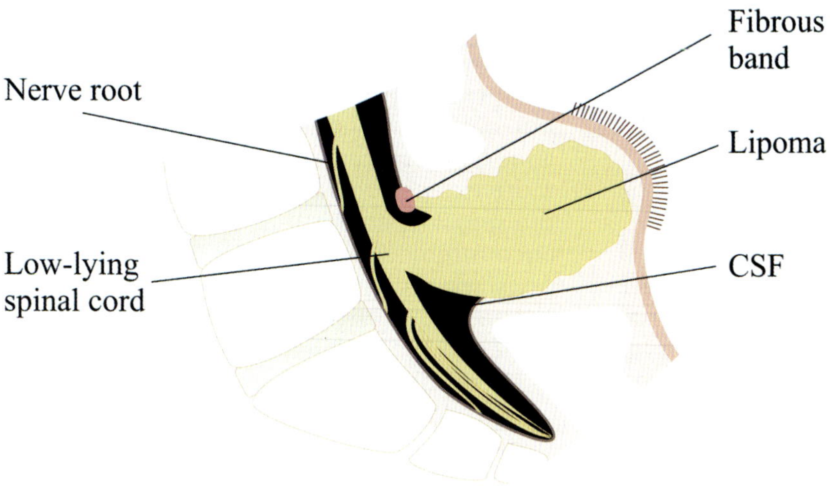

Figure 13-33

SPINA BIFIDA OCCULTA (LIPOMYELOMENINGOCELE)

Lipoma overlies the disrupted dorsal surface of a low-lying tethered spinal cord. Lipomas are frequently associated with a meningocele and protrude into the lumbosacral region where they merge with normal subcutaneous fat. (Illustration by Dr. Amy Noffsinger.)

particularly when associated with spinal anomalies, may be mistaken for myelomeningocele on clinical examination. The presence of cysts, glands, and ducts as well as mesenchymal tissue, particularly skeletal muscle, bone, and cartilage, would support the diagnosis of a teratoma (120).

Treatment and Prognosis. The goal of postnatal surgical repair of myelomeningocele is to preserve motor and sensory function of the spinal cord and to prevent CNS infection (121). Recently, techniques for in utero repair of these lesions have been developed. Initial studies have demonstrated that in utero repair is associated with significant improvement in the incidence of hydrocephalus and hindbrain abnormalities with a decreased requirement for shunting (122). The 1-year survival rate of patients with myelomeningocele is about 87 percent, decreasing to about 78 percent by 17 years (122). Complications due to the neurologic and other structural abnormalities discussed above are the major reason for both excess morbidity and mortality. By contrast, meningoceles do not require immediate repair and elective closure later in childhood is the rule. These lesions are not associated with the severe neurologic complications of myelomeningocele.

Spina Bifida Occulta: Tethered Cord Syndrome, Dermal Sinuses, and Spinal Lipomas

Definitions. *Spina bifida occulta* refers to spinal dysraphisms and associated abnormalities that occur without herniation of neural tissue or coverings. These lesions are most common in the lumbosacral region and are associated with less severe clinical manifestations than other spinal dysraphisms. The normal structures in the lumbosacral region develop from the tail bud, an initially solid collection of stem cells at the caudal end of the neural tube. The tail bud gives rise to all three germ cell layers through a process of secondary neurulation.

Many of the lesions within spina bifida occulta arise from abnormalities in this process. Examples of such lesions include *hydromyelia, diplomyelia* (duplication of the spinal cord), *diastematomyelia* (splitting of the spinal cord associated with a collagen or bone spur), *dermal sinuses* and their associated dermoid/epidermoid cysts, and some *spinal lipomas* (116,118,120). Other more commonly encountered lesions of spina bifida occulta, including intradural spinal lipomas and lipomyelomeningocele, probably arise from other embryologic mechanisms (fig. 13-33). *Lipomyelomeningocele* is a myelomeningocele with a superimposed lipoma and connective tissue capsule that rests beneath an intact skin covering (115). These are the most common form of spinal lipoma and account for up to half of the cases of spina bifida occulta (125). Intradural lipomas are relatively uncommon and typically involve the cervical and thoracic spine (125). These lesions are characterized by a posteriorly opened or unfused spinal cord with a lipoma situated within the incompletely fused segment (115).

These diverse lesions are often minimally symptomatic, but may share a common complication that brings them to surgery: abnormal fixation or tethering of the distal end of the spinal cord. This causes *tethered cord syndrome* with which one or more of these abnormalities are associated, with a low or dilated conus medullaris and thickening of the filum terminale, in combination with a characteristic clinical presentation as discussed below (125).

Clinical Features. These lesions are often initially asymptomatic, although the presence of cutaneous abnormalities in the lumbosacral region, including hypertrichosis, midline dimples, or soft fluctuant subcutaneous masses, may signal their presence to the astute clinician. Because tethering of the spinal cord causes stretching of the lumbosacral cord and nerve roots, lesions that result in tethering are associated with a characteristic clinical presentation. Disproportionate growth of the vertebral column relative to the spinal cord produces progressively increasing tension on these structures. The result is lower extremity motor and sensory deficits and impaired bowel and bladder control (120). Over time, many patients develop abnormal spinal curvature. Onset and severity of these symptoms is highly variable; progression is the rule and severe impairment can result in cases that are left untreated (125).

In addition to causing spinal cord tethering, dermal sinuses frequently extend into the dura and become intraspinal. Many dermal sinsuses are also associated with dermoid or epidermoid cysts that may be intraspinal or adjacent to the spine. Because they may provide a connection between the skin surface, associated cystic structures, and the spinal canal, dermal sinuses are associated with both chemical and infectious meningitis. Dermal sinus is an important entity in the differential diagnosis of occult meningitis (120,125).

Radiologic Findings. Imaging findings in cases of spina bifida occulta are variable, depending on the associated specific dysraphic malformation. Plain films or CT may demonstrate relatively subtle bone abnormalities of the spine. In patients with suspected tethered cored syndrome, T2-weighted MRI studies can demonstrate the presence of the spinal cord at lower than normal levels, as well as the presence of lipomas, which appear as high signal intensity lesions (115). Other structural defects and abnormalities of the spinal cord, such as hydromyelia, diplomyelia, and diastematomyelia, are readily identified by MRI.

Gross Findings. Since the goal of surgery in most cases is the release of the abnormal fixation of the distal end of the spinal cord from the abnormal structure to which it is attached, the more extensive abnormalities associated with the spinal dysraphism in these cases are rarely encountered in surgical pathology. In most cases, resection is limited to the filum terminale, connective tissue, and affixed tissues that are related to the tethered cord (fig. 13-33).

Often, these specimens consist of a portion of skin with attached subcutaneous and connective tissue. Careful inspection of the skin may demonstrate lesions such as a central dimple or, in the case of dermoid sinus, an ostium. Other abnormalities include skin tags, nevi, hypertrichosis, and hemangioma. Lipomas of the filum are very common in tethered cord syndrome. These may be difficult to distinguish grossly from mature subcutaneous adipose tissue. Heterotopic bone or cartilage may be encountered in the lipomas (120). Occasionally, atrophied nerve roots are admixed with the resection tissue. Filum terminale may be difficult to recognize or distinguish but in the gross state has the appearance of a thin strand of connective tissue (fig. 13-34).

Intraoperative Findings. There is little use for routine intraoperative evaluation of these lesions. Occasionally, frozen sections may be sought to rule out a teratoma in this location.

Microscopic Findings. Examination of the skin in resection specimens often demonstrates changes consistent with the gross findings described above, such as an increased number of dermal appendages in cases with hypertrichosis. In cases with a sinus tract, dermoid cyst, or epidermoid cyst, serial sections may be necessary to fully demonstrate the lesion. The sinuses may be continuous or discontinuous, extending from the intradural space into the subcutaneous tissue, or even to the epidermis (fig. 13-35). Intraspinal connections are common, accounting for the frequent association with tethered cords (120). Dermoid and epidermoid cysts have the characteristic histologic features described for these lesions in other locations. Both cysts and sinuses are often associated with secondary changes, including abundant keratinous debris,

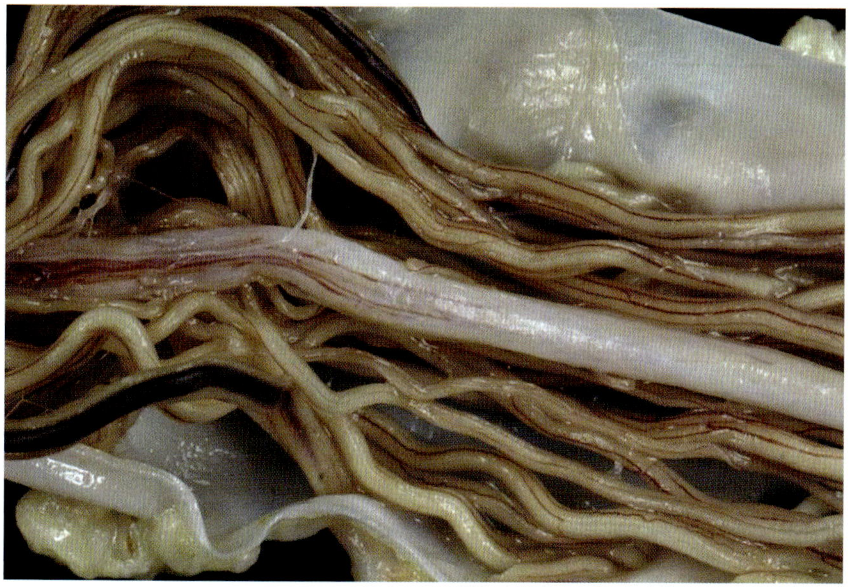

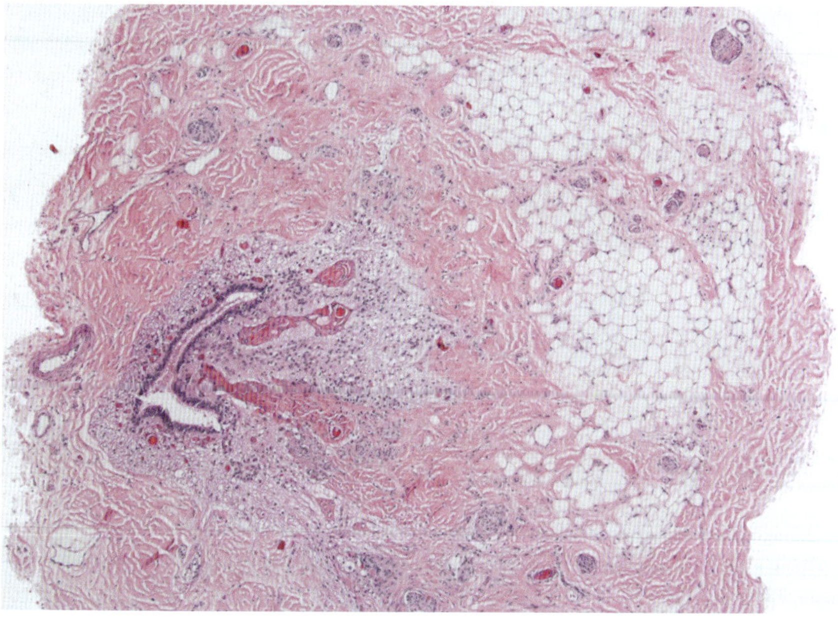

Figure 13-34

FILUM TERMINALE

Top: The filum terminale extends from the caudal tip of the spinal cord. The intradural portion of the filum is here situated among the nerve roots of the cauda equina.

Bottom: The filum terminale typically contains a mixture of dense collagenous tissue, small nerve roots, and adipose tissue. Ependymal canals, either continuous or interrupted, are frequently seen in sections of filum.

giant cell reaction, and inflammatory infiltrates. A distinctive feature of these lesions in the spinal cord is the occasional presence of the meningeal tissue that ensheathes these lesions as they extend into the subcutaneous tissue or dermis (120). In cases in which these lesions have become involuted, no cyst or obvious sinus may be detectable, but there may be clues to the original lesion in the form of an irregular fibrous mass, keratinaceous debris, or hair (120).

In instances in which the spinal cord is anchored by an attachment of the filum terminale, resection specimens may include a portion of this structure. The normal filum terminale extends from the caudal end of the spinal cord (conus medullaris), passes among the roots of the cauda equina, and normally penetrates the spinal dura. It exits at the sacral hiatus, where it terminates in the subcutaneous tissue posterior to the coccyx, sometimes demarcated by a post-anal pit (120). Cross sections of normal filum terminale consist primarily of a fascicle of dense collagenous connective tissue and blood vessels. Well-preserved specimens occasionally have a

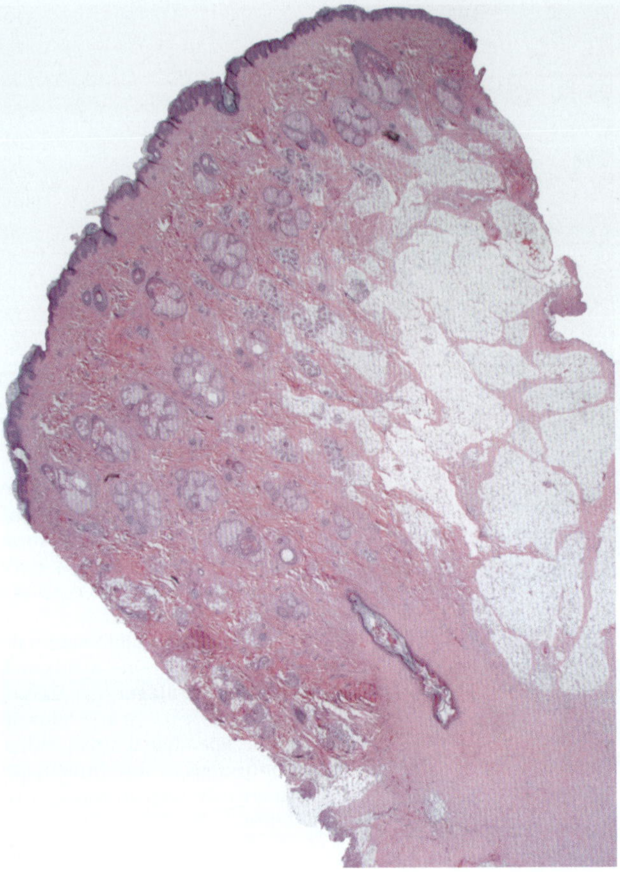

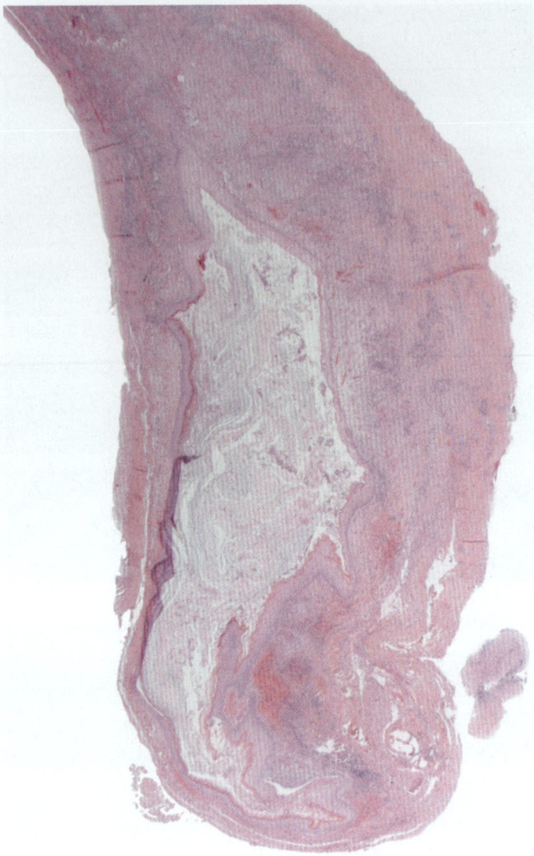

Figure 13-35

DERMAL SINUS TRACT

Top: Sinuses may be encountered in the epidermis or subcutaneous tissue, where they are characterized by a well-differentiated squamous epithelial lining.

Bottom: These lesions are associated with prominent secondary changes including abundant keratinous debris and inflammatory infiltrates.

dilated ependymal-lined space that is a remnant of the central canal, called the ventriculus terminalis (126). Specimens from a tethered cord resection may show all of these features. In many cases, however, these specimens consist simply of a fascicle of dense collagenous connective tissue (44).

Differential Diagnosis. Most resection specimens for tethered cord are fairly straightforward. There are, however, both normal structures and other developmental abnormalities that occur in this region which may lead to confusion. First, it is important to recognize that the subcutaneous terminus of the normal filum terminale consists chiefly of glioependymal rests and leptomeningeal tissue. The presence of these structures alone in subcutaneous tissue of the lumbosacral region should not be mistaken for spina bifida occulta (120). Rarely, these structures give rise to subcutaneous ependymomas in this location.

If the spinal cord is tethered to a lipoma, or if one of the other types of spinal lipoma is resected, the specimen will be composed predominantly of mature adipose tissue with wide fibrous septa and occasional excess nerves and Paccinian corpuscles. Heterotopic bone and cartilage may be encountered in these specimens. In resections where there is a lipomyelomeningocele, the specimen typically contains neuroglial and/or meningeal tissue in addition to the lipomatous elements (120).

Teratomas also occur in the sacrococcygeal region, most often as a postcoccygeal mass. Usually, teratomas are not associated with spina bifida. Vertebral abnormalities have been reported in up to 16 percent of cases, however, as well as a small number of associated meningoceles, myelomeningoceles and lipomyelomeningoceles (120). The most commonly encountered, and frequently predominate, element in sacrococcygeal teratomas is neuroglial tissue. Cysts, glands and ducts, adipose tissue, and striated muscle are also frequently present. The presence of nephrogeneic tissue or anything resembling Wilms tumor is unusual in a sacrococcygeal teratoma and should suggest an extrarenal nephroblastic proliferation. This entity is associated with both spinal dysraphism and extrarenal sacrococcygeal Wilms tumor (127). The differential diagnosis of teratoma and myelomeningocele is discussed in the preceding section. The distinction between lipomyelomeningocele and sacrococcygeal teratoma may be particularly challenging. Myelomeningoceles frequently contain muscles; therefore, a lesion that contains adipose tissue, smooth muscle, and neuroglial tissue, but no cysts, glands, or ducts, is most likely to be a lipomyelomeningocele.

Finally, enteric malformations, while more common in the thoracic spine, also occur in the sacrococcygeal region. There is a broad spectrum of hindgut malformations. In several types, hindgut sinuses or loops of rectum pass through lumbosacral defects and extend into the subcutaneous tissue. In the process, connections are formed with the spinal canal and/or sacral skin. As with dermal sinus tracts, these structures may lead to meningitis. Often, these lesions are associated with both spinal cord and vertebral abnormalities. Histologically, the specimens may contain any of the normal types of gastrointestinal mucosa, as well as occasionally ciliated or bronchial mucosa. In rare cases, pancreatic and adipose tissues are present. The presence of a well-defined muscularis mucosa, even focally, is an important clue to the true nature of these lesions. These lesions may occasionally be difficult to distinguish from a sacrococcygeal teratoma, although the prevalence of well-differentiated enteric structures and the absence of prominent neuroglial elements are clues. Additional clinical history and imaging studies often suggest the diagnosis (120).

Treatment and Prognosis. In contrast to the other spinal dysraphisms, patients with spina bifida occulta have less severe morbidity and mortality. While neurologic impairment due to spinal cord tethering may not be reversible, progression can be halted with surgical treatment. With the exception of dermoid cysts and sinuses, many of the other lesions discussed above may not be symptomatic beyond the tethered cord syndrome.

REFERENCES

1. Blumcke I, Beck H, Lie AA, Wiestler OD. Molecular neuropathology of human mesial temporal lobe epilepsy. Epilepsy Res 1999;36:205-223.
2. Blumcke I, Thom M, Wiestler OD. Ammon's horn sclerosis: a maldevelopmental disorder associated with temporal lobe epilepsy. Brain Pathol 2002;12:199-211.
3. Wolf HK, Wiestler OD. Surgical pathology of chronic epileptic seizures disorders. Brain Pathol 1993;3:371-380.
4. Engel J Jr. Mesial temporal lobe epilepsy: what have we learned? Neuroscientist 2001;7:340-352.
5. Cendes F. Febrile seizures and mesial temporal sclerosis. Curr Opin Neurol 2004;17:161-164.
6. Kido DK, Tien RD, Lee B, Bahn MM. Hippocampal pathology. Neuroimaging Clin N Am 1997;7:51-65.
7. Wyler AR, Dohan FC, Schweitzer JB, Berry AD. A grading system for mesial temporal pathology (hippocampal sclerosis) from anterior temporal lobectomy. J Epilepsy 1992;5:220-225.
8. Prayson RA, Reith JD, Najm IM. Mesial temporal sclerosis. A clinicopathologic study of 27 patients, including 5 with coexistent cortical dysplasia. Arch Pathol Lab Med 1996;120:532-536.
9. Barkovich AJ, Kuzniecky RI, Jackson GD, Guerrini R, Dobyns WB. Classification system for malformations of cortical development: update 2001. Neurology 2001;57:2168-2178.
10. Walsh C, Cepko CL. Widespread dispersion of neuronal clones across functional regions of the cerebral cortex. Science 1992;255:434-440.
11. Marin-Padilla M. Origin, formation, and prenatal maturation of the human cerebral cortex: an overview. J Craniofac Genet Dev Biol 1990;10:137-146.
12. Hannan AJ, Servotte S, Katsnelson A, et al. Characterization of nodular neuronal heterotopia in children. Brain 1999;122(Pt 2):219-238.
13. Prayson RA, Estes ML. Cortical dysplasia: a histopathologic study of 52 cases of partial lobectomy in patients with epilepsy. Hum Pathol 1995;26:493-500.
14. Duchowny M, Levin B, Jayakar P, et al. Temporal lobectomy in early childhood. Epilepsia 1992;33:298-303.
15. Paolicchi JM, Jayakar P, Dean P, et al. Predictors of outcome in pediatric epilepsy surgery. Neurology 2000;54:642-647.
16. Sisodiya SM. Surgery for malformations of cortical development causing epilepsy. Brain 2000;123(Pt 6):1075-1091.
17. Thom M. Epilepsy part I: cortical dysplasia. In: Golden JA, Harding BN, eds. Pathology & genetics. Developmental neuropathology. Basel: ISN Neuropath Press; 2004:61-66.
18. Palmini A, Najm I, Avanzini G, et al. Terminology and classification of the cortical dysplasias. Neurology 2004;62(Suppl 3):S2-8.
19. Lawson JA, Birchansky S, Pacheco E, et al. Distinct clinicopathologic subtypes of cortical dysplasia of Taylor. Neurology 2005;64:55-61.
20. Colombo N, Tassi L, Galli C, et al. Focal cortical dysplasias: MR imaging, histopathologic, and clinical correlations in surgically treated patients with epilepsy. AJNR Am J Neuroradiol 2003;24:724-733.
21. Garbelli R, Frassoni C, Ferrario A, Tassi L, Bramerio M, Spreafico R. Cajal-Retzius cell density as marker of type of focal cortical dysplasia. Neuroreport 2001;12:2767-2771.
22. Mischel PS, Nguyen LP, Vinters HV. Cerebral cortical dysplasia associated with pediatric epilepsy. Review of neuropathologic features and proposal for a grading system. J Neuropathol Exp Neurol 1995;54:137-153.
23. Emery JA, Roper SN, Rojiani AM. White matter neuronal heterotopia in temporal lobe epilepsy: a morphometric and immunohistochemical study. J Neuropathol Exp Neurol 1997;56:1276-1282.
24. Rojiani AM, Emery JA, Anderson KJ, Massey JK. Distribution of heterotopic neurons in normal hemispheric white matter: a morphometric analysis. J Neuropathol Exp Neurol 1996;55:178-183.
25. Kasper BS, Stefan H, Buchfelder M, Paulus W. Temporal lobe microdysgenesis in epilepsy versus control brains. J Neuropathol Exp Neurol 1999;58:22-28.
26. Taylor DC, Falconer MA, Bruton CJ, Corsellis JA. Focal dysplasia of the cerebral cortex in epilepsy. J Neurol Neurosurg Psychiatry 1971;34:369-387.
27. Vinters HV. Histopathology of brain tissue from patients with infantile spasms. Int Rev Neurobiol 2002;49:63-76.
28. Frater JL, Prayson RA, Morris IH, Bingaman WE. Surgical pathologic findings of extratemporal-based intractable epilepsy: a study of 133 consecutive resections. Arch Pathol Lab Med 2000;124:545-549.
29. Crino PB, Trojanowski JQ, Eberwine J. Internexin, MAP1B, and nestin in cortical dysplasia as markers of developmental maturity. Acta Neuropathol (Berl) 1997;93:619-627.
30. Englund C, Folkerth RD, Born D, Lacy JM, Hevner RF. Aberrant neuronal-glial differentiation in Taylor-type focal cortical dysplasia (type IIA/B). Acta Neuropathol (Berl) 2005;109:519-553.
31. Prayson RA, Khajavi K, Comair YG. Cortical architectural abnormalities and MIB1 immunoreactivity in gangliogliomas: a study of 60 patients with intracranial tumors. J Neuropathol Exp Neurol 1995;54:513-520.

32. Daumas-Duport C. Dysembryoplastic neuroepithelial tumours. Brain Pathol 1993;3:283-295.
33. Miyata H, Chiang AC, Vinters HV. Insulin signaling pathways in cortical dysplasia and TSC-tubers: tissue microarray analysis. Ann Neurol 2004;56:510-519.
34. Fauser S, Schulze-Bonhage A, Honegger J, et al. Focal cortical dysplasias: surgical outcome in 67 patients in relation to histological subtypes and dual pathology. Brain 2004;127(Pt 11):2406-2418.
35. Prayson RA, Frater JL. Cortical dysplasia in extratemporal lobe intractable epilepsy: a study of 52 cases. Ann Diagn Pathol 2003;7:139-146.
36. Barkovich AJ, Kuziecky RI. Gray matter heterotopia. Neurology 2000;55:1603-1608.
37. Mochida GH, Walsh CA. Genetic basis of developmental malformations of the cerebral cortex. Arch Neurol 2004;61:637-640.
38. Iida K, Hirano S, Takashima S, Miyahara S. Developmental study of leptomeningeal glioneuronal heterotopia. Pediatr Neurol 1994;10:295-298.
39. Monuki ES, Ligon KL. Cerebral hetetotopia. In: Golden JA, Harding BN, eds. Pathology & genetics. Developmental neuropathology. Basel: ISN Neuropath Press; 2004:52-60.
40. Hirano S, Houdou S, Hasegawa M, Kamei A, Takashima S. Clinicopathologic studies on leptomeningeal glioneuronal heterotopia in congenital anomalies. Pediatr Neurol 1992;8:441-444.
41. Santi MR, Golden JA. Periventricular heterotopia may result from radial glial fiber disruption. J Neuropathol Exp Neurol 2001;60:856-862.
42. Pilz DT, Kuc J, Matsumoto N, et al. Subcortical band heterotopia in rare affected males can be caused by missense mutations in DCX (XLIS) or LIS1. Hum Mol Genet 1999;8:1757-1760.
43. Cardoso C, Leventer RJ, Ward HL, et al. Refinement of a 400-kb critical region allows genotypic differentiation between isolated lissencephaly, Miller-Dieker syndrome, and other phenotypes secondary to deletions of 17p13.3. Am J Hum Genet 2003;72:918-930.
44. Friede RL. Developmental neuropathology, 2nd ed. New York: Springer-Verlag; 1989.
45. Tassi L, Colombo N, Cossu M, et al. Electroclinical, MRI and neuropathological study of 10 patients with nodular heterotopia, with surgical outcomes. Brain 2005;128(Pt 2):321-337.
46. Gupta A, Carreno M, Wyllie E, Bingaman WE. Hemispheric malformations of cortical development. Neurology 2004;62(Suppl 3):S20-26.
47. Jahan R, Mischel PS, Curran JG, Peacock WJ, Shields DW, Vinters HV. Bilateral neuropathologic changes in a child with hemimegalencephaly. Pediatr Neurol 1997;17:344-349.
48. Devlin AM, Cross JH, Harkness W, et al. Clinical outcomes of hemispherectomy for epilepsy in childhood and adolescence. Brain 2003;126(Pt 3):556-566.
49. Flores-Sarnat L. Hemimegalencephaly: part 1. Genetic, clinical, and imaging aspects. J Child Neurol 2002;17:373-384.
50. Broumandi DD, Hayward UM, Benzian JM, Gonzalez I, Nelson MD. Best cases from the AFIP: hemimegalencephaly. Radiographics 2004;24:843-848.
51. Crino PB, Miyata H, Vinters HV. Neurodevelopmental disorders as a cause of seizures: neuropathologic, genetic, and mechanistic considerations. Brain Pathol 2002;12:212-233.
52. De Rosa MJ, Secor DL, Barsom M, Fisher RS, Vinters HV. Neuropathologic findings in surgically treated hemimegalencephaly: immunohistochemical, morphometric, and ultrastructural study. Acta Neuropathol (Berl) 1992;84:250-260.
53. Thom M. Epilepsy part I: hemimegalencephaly. In: Golden JA, Harding BA, eds. Pathology & genetics. Developmental neuropathology. Basel: ISN Neuropath Press; 2004:67-72.
54. Arai Y, Edwards V, Becker LE. A comparison of cell phenotypes in hemimegalencephaly and tuberous sclerosis. Acta Neuropathol (Berl) 1999;98:407-413.
55. Griffiths PD, Gardner SA, Smith M, Rittey C, Powell T. Hemimegalencephaly and focal megalencephaly in tuberous sclerosis complex. AJNR Am J Neuroradiol 1998;19:1935-1938.
56. Perry A, Kurtkaya-Yapicier O, Scheithauer BW, et al. Insights into meningioangiomatosis with and without meningioma: a clinicopathologic and genetic series of 24 cases with review of the literature. Brain Pathol 2005;15:55-65.
57. Wiebe S, Munoz DG, Smith S, Lee DH. Meningioangiomatosis. A comprehensive analysis of clinical and laboratory features. Brain 1999;122(Pt 4):709-726.
58. Stemmer-Rachamimov AO, Horgan MA, Taratuto AL, et al. Meningioangiomatosis is associated with neurofibromatosis 2 but not with somatic alterations of the NF2 gene. J Neuropathol Exp Neurol 1997;56:485-489.
59. Takeshima Y, Amatya VJ, Nakayori F, Nakano T, Sugiyama K, Inai K. Meningioangiomatosis occurring in a young male without neurofibromatosis: with special reference to its histogenesis and loss of heterozygosity in the NF2 gene region. Am J Surg Pathol 2002;26:125-129.
60. Tien RD, Osumi A, Oakes JW, Madden JF, Burger PC. Meningioangiomatosis: CT and MR findings. J Comput Assist Tomogr 1992;16:361-365.
61. Prayson RA. Meningioangiomatosis. A clinicopathologic study including MIB1 immunoreactivity. Arch Pathol Lab Med 1995;119:1061-1064.
62. Giangaspero F, Guiducci A, Lenz FA, Mastronardi L, Burger PC. Meningioma with meningioangiomatosis: a condition mimicking invasive meningiomas in children and young adults: report of two cases and review of the literature. Am J Surg Pathol 1999;23:872-875.

63. Wiestler OD, von Siebenthal K, Schmitt HP, Feiden W, Kleihues P. Distribution and immunoreactivity of cerebral micro-hamartomas in bilateral acoustic neurofibromatosis (neurofibromatosis 2). Acta Neuropathol (Berl) 1989;79:137-143.
64. Volk EE, Prayson RA. Hamartomas in the setting of chronic epilepsy: a clinicopathologic study of 13 cases. Hum Pathol 1997;28:227-232.
65. Nguyen D, Singh S, Zaatreh M, et al. Hypothalamic hamartomas: seven cases and review of the literature. Epilepsy Behav 2003;4:246-258.
66. Biesecker LG. Heritable syndromes with hypothalamic hamartoma and seizures: using rare syndromes to understand more common disorders. Epileptic Disord 2003;5:235-238.
67. Jung H, Parent AS, Ojeda SR. Hypothalamic hamartoma: a paradigm/model for studying the onset of puberty. Endocr Dev 2005;8:81-93.
68. Kerrigan JF, Ng YT, Chung S, Rekate HL. The hypothalamic hamartoma: a model of subcortical epileptogenesis and encephalopathy. Semin Pediatr Neurol 2005;12:119-131.
69. Striano S, Striano P, Sarappa C, Boccella P. The clinical spectrum and natural history of gelastic epilepsy-hypothalamic hamartoma syndrome. Seizure 2005;14:232-239.
70. Kandt RS. Tuberous sclerosis complex and neurofibromatosis type 1: the two most common neurocutaneous diseases. Neurol Clin 2003;21:983-1004.
71. Roach ES, Sparagana SP. Diagnosis of tuberous sclerosis complex. J Child Neurol 2004;19:643-649.
72. Au KS, Williams AT, Gambello MJ, Northrup H. Molecular genetic basis of tuberous sclerosis complex: from bench to bedside. J Child Neurol 2004;19:699-709.
73. Inoki K, Corradetti MN, Guan KL. Dysregulation of the TSC-mTOR pathway in human disease. Nat Genet 2005;37:19-24.
74. Crino PB. Molecular pathogenesis of tuber formation in tuberous sclerosis complex. J Child Neurol 2004;19:716-725.
75. Hyman MH, Whittemore VH. National Institutes of Health consensus conference: tuberous sclerosis complex. Arch Neurol 2000;57:662-665.
76. Romanelli P, Verdecchia M, Rodas R, Seri S, Curatolo P. Epilepsy surgery for tuberous sclerosis. Pediatr Neurol 2004;31:239-247.
77. Richardson EP Jr. Pathology of tuberous sclerosis. Neuropathologic aspects. Ann N Y Acad Sci 1991;615:128-139.
78. Hirose T, Scheithauer BW, Lopes MB, et al. Tuber and subependymal giant cell astrocytoma associated with tuberous sclerosis: an immunohistochemical, ultrastructural, and immunoelectron and microscopic study. Acta Neuropathol (Berl) 1995;90:387-399.
79. Vinters HV, Miyata H. Tuberous sclerosis. In: Golden JA, Harding BH, eds. Pathology & Genetics. Developmental neuropathology. Basel: ISN Neuropath Press; 2004:79-88.
80. Gyure KA, Prayson RA. Subependymal giant cell astrocytoma: a clinicopathologic study with HMB45 and MIB-1 immunohistochemical analysis. Mod Pathol 1997;10:313-317.
81. Ironside JW, Moss TH, Louis DN, Lowe JS, Weller RO. Diagnostic pathology of nervous system tumours. Philadelphia: Churchill Livingstone; 2002.
82. Weiner HL, Ferraris N, LaJoie J, Miles D, Devinsky O. Epilepsy surgery for children with tuberous sclerosis complex. J Child Neurol 2004;19:687-689.
83. Thomas-Sohl KA, Vaslow DF, Maria BL. Sturge-Weber syndrome: a review. Pediatr Neurol 2004;30:303-310.
84. Griffiths PD. Sturge-Weber syndrome revisited: the role of neuroradiology. Neuropediatrics 1996;27:284-294.
85. Comi AM. Pathophysiology of Sturge-Weber syndrome. J Child Neurol 2003;18:509-516.
86. Smirniotopoulos JG. Neuroimaging of phakomatoses: Sturge-Weber syndrome, tuberous sclerosis, von Hippel-Lindau syndrome. Neuroimaging Clin N Am 2004;14:171-183, vii.
87. Norman MG, Schoene WC. The ultrastructure of Sturge-Weber disease. Acta Neuropathol (Berl) 1977;37:199-205.
88. Prayson RA. Clinicopathological findings in patients who have undergone epilepsy surgery in the first year of life. Pathol Int 2000;50:620-625.
89. Hoffman HJ, Hendrick EB, Dennis M, Armstrong D. Hemispherectomy for Sturge-Weber syndrome. Childs Brain 1979;5:233-248.
90. Simonati A, Colamaria V, Bricolo A, Bernardina BD, Rizzuto N. Microgyria associated with Sturge-Weber angiomatosis. Childs Nerv Syst 1994;10:392-395.
91. Di Trapani G, Di Rocco C, Abbamondi AL, Caldarelli M, Pocchiari M. Light microscopy and ultrastructural studies of Sturge-Weber disease. Childs Brain 1982;9:23-36.
92. Ito M, Sato K, Ohnuki A, Uto A. Sturge-Weber disease: operative indications and surgical results. Brain Dev 1990;12:473-477.
93. Freeman JM. Rasmussen's syndrome: progressive autoimmune multi-focal encephalopathy. Pediatr Neurol 2005;32:295-299.
94. Bien CG, Granata T, Antozzi C, et al. Pathogenesis, diagnosis and treatment of Rasmussen encephalitis: a European consensus statement. Brain 2005;128(Pt 3):454-471.
95. Bien CG, Urbach H, Deckert M, et al. Diagnosis and staging of Rasmussen's encephalitis by serial MRI and histopathology. Neurology 2002;58:250-257.
96. Hart Y. Rasmussen's encephalitis. Epileptic Disord 2004;6:133-144.
97. Granata T, Gobbi G, Spreafico R, et al. Rasmussen's encephalitis: early characteristics allow diagnosis. Neurology 2003;60:422-425.

98. Rasmussen T. Further observations on the syndrome of chronic encephalitis and epilepsy. Appl Neurophysiol 1978;41:1-12.
99. Hart YM, Andermann F, Robitaille Y, Laxer KD, Rasmussen T, Davis R. Double pathology in Rasmussen's syndrome: a window on the etiology? Neurology 1998;50:731-735.
100. Palmer CA, Geyer JD, Keating JM, et al. Rasmussen's encephalitis with concomitant cortical dysplasia: the role of GluR3. Epilepsia 1999;40:242-247.
101. Cross H. Epilepsy part II: Rasmussen syndrome, hippocampal sclerosis, granule cell dysplasia. In: Golden JA, Harding BH, eds. Pathology and genetics. Developmental neuropathology. Basel: ISN Neuropath Press; 2004:73-78.
102. Hardiman O, Burke T, Phillips J, et al. Microdysgenesis in resected temporal neocortex: incidence and clinical significance in focal epilepsy. Neurology 1988;38:1041-1047.
103. Honavar M, Meldrum BS. Epilepsy. In: Graham DI, Lantos PL, eds. Greenfield's neuropathology, Vol I, 7th ed. New York: Arnold; 2002:899-941.
104. Alexander WS. Progressive fibrinoid degeneration of fibrillary astrocytes associated with mental retardation in a hydrocephalic infant. Brain 1949;72:373-381.
105. Johnson AB. Alexander disease: a review and the gene. Int J Dev Neurosci 2002;20:391-394.
106. Li R, Johnson AB, Salomons G, et al. Glial fibrillary acidic protein mutations in infantile, juvenile, and adult forms of Alexander disease. Ann Neurol 2005;57:310-326.
107. van der Knaap MS, Naidu S, Breiter SN, et al. Alexander disease: diagnosis with MR imaging. AJNR Am J Neuroradiol 2001;22:541-552.
108. Englander J, Bushnik T, Duong TT, et al. Analyzing risk factors for late posttraumatic seizures: a prospective, multicenter investigation. Arch Phys Med Rehabil 2003;84:365-373.
109. Caveness WF. Epilepsy, a product of trauma in our time. Epilepsia 1976;17:207-215.
110. Detrait ER, George TM, Etchevers HC, Gilbert JR, Vekemans M, Speer MC. Human neural tube defects: developmental biology, epidemiology, and genetics. Neurotoxicol Teratol 2005;27:515-524.
111. Martinez-Lage JF, Poza M, Sola J, et al. The child with a cephalocele: etiology, neuroimaging, and outcome. Childs Nerv Syst 1996;12:540-550.
112. Barkovich AJ, Vandermarck P, Edwards MS, Cogen PH. Congenital nasal masses: CT and MR imaging features in 16 cases. AJNR Am J Neuroradiol 1991;12:105-116.
113. Humphreys RP. Encephalocele and dermal sinuses. In: Cheek WR, ed. Pediatric neurosurgery: surgery of the developing nervous system. Philadelphia: W. B. Saunders; 1994:96-103.
114. Naidich TP, Altman NR, Braffman BH, McLone DG, Zimmerman RA. Cephaloceles and related malformations. AJNR Am J Neuroradiol 1992;13:655-690.
115. Osborn AG. Diagnostic neuroradiology. Philadelphia: Mosby; 1994.
116. Aicardi J. Diseases of the nervous system in childhood. New York: Cambridge Univeristy Press; 1992.
117. Folkerth RD. Congenital malformations, perinatal diseases, and phacomatoses. In: Prayson RA, ed. Neuropathology. Philadelphia: Elsevier Churchill Livingstone; 2005:95-180.
118. Copp AJ, Harding BH. Neural tube defects. In: Golden JA, Harding BH, eds. Pathology and genetics. Developmental neuropathology. Basel: ISN Neuropath Press; 2004:2-13.
119. Emery JL, Kalhan SC. The pathology of exencephalus. Dev Med Child Neurol Suppl 1970;22(Suppl 22):51+.
120. Bale PM. Sacrococcygeal developmental abnormalities and tumors in children. Perspect Pediatr Pathol 1984;8:9-56.
121. Reigel DH, Rotenstein D. Spina bifida. In: Cheek WR, ed. Pediatric neurosurgery: surgery of the developing nervous system, 3rd ed. Philadelphia: W. B. Saunders; 1994:51-76.
122. Mitchell LE, Adzick NS, Melchionne J, Pasquariello PS, Sutton LN, Whitehead AS. Spina bifida. Lancet 2004;364:1885-1895.
123. Golden JA. Chiari malformations. In: Golden JA, Harding BH, eds. Pathology and genetics. Developmental neuropathology. Basel: ISN Neuropath Press; 2004:90-94.
124. Gilbert JN, Jones KL, Rorke LB, Chernoff GF, James HE. Central nervous system anomalies associated with meningomyelocele, hydrocephalus, and the Arnold-Chiari malformation: reappraisal of theories regarding the pathogenesis of posterior neural tube closure defects. Neurosurgery 1986;18:559-564.
125. Reigel DH, McLone DG. Tethered spinal cord. In: Cheek WR, ed. Pediatric neurosurgery: surgery of the developing nervous system, 3rd ed. Philadelphia: WB Saunders; 1994:77-95.
126. Fuller GN, Burger PC. Central nervous system. In: Sternberg SS, ed. Histology for pathologists, 2nd ed. Philadelphia: Lippincott-Raven; 1997:243-284.
127. Abrahams JM, Pawel BR, Duhaime AC, Sutton LN, Schut L. Extrarenal nephroblastic proliferation in spinal dysraphism. A report of 4 cases. Pediatr Neurosurg 1999;31:40-44.

14 REACTION TO NEOPLASMS AND ANTINEOPLASTIC THERAPIES

The brain and meninges may react markedly to adjacent or infiltrating neoplasms and to antineoplastic therapies. These reactive changes figure prominently in the differential diagnosis in two settings. If a mass lesion is biopsied under the suspicion of neoplasia, the prominent reactive changes may distract the pathologist from recognizing the underlying neoplasm, resulting in an erroneous diagnosis of a non-neoplastic condition. Also, for neoplasms that have been treated, prior steroid therapy may lyse lymphoma cells and complicate the diagnosis and prior radiation therapy may confuse the diagnosis of recurrent malignant glioma. Knowledge of the reactive patterns that are found adjacent to intracranial tumors and in response to certain therapies should force the pathologist to weigh clinical, radiologic, and histopathologic data before diagnosing a lesion.

REACTION TO GLIOMAS

The brain and meninges react in stereotypical ways to glial brain tumors, but the degree of response varies from tumor to tumor. The diffuse gliomas present the most diagnostic challenges in terms of distinguishing gliotic response from tumor, since these tumors are so infiltrative and low-grade astrocytomas and gliosis may have histologically similar features. The circumscribed gliomas (e.g., pilocytic astrocytoma) present less of a diagnostic problem since their sharp margins allow easy distinction of tumor from reactive brain; however, biopsies that only sample the non-neoplastic edge of a circumscribed glioma may be diagnostically misleading. The involved brain itself may provide a clue to distinguishing a diffuse from a circumscribed glioma. This is most readily demonstrated with neurofilament immunohistochemistry (fig. 14-1). Diffuse gliomas display many entrapped axons, whereas circumscribed gliomas generally exclude axons from the tumor mass.

Diffuse Gliomas

The common diffusely infiltrating astrocytic, oligodendroglial, and oligoastrocytic gliomas often elicit a reactive astrocytic response, which is microscopically most apparent toward the

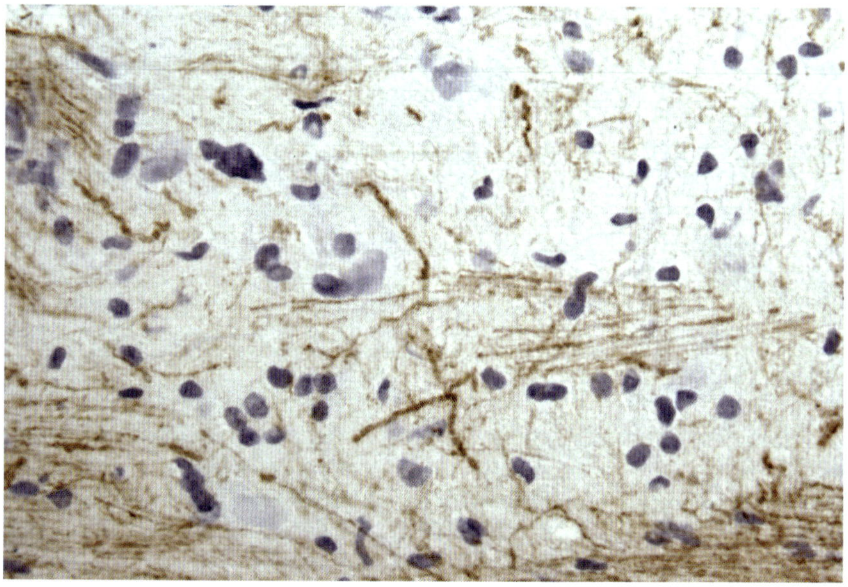

Figure 14-1

REACTION TO DIFFUSE GLIOMA

Axons are entrapped in an infiltrating glioma (neurofilament immunohistochemistry).

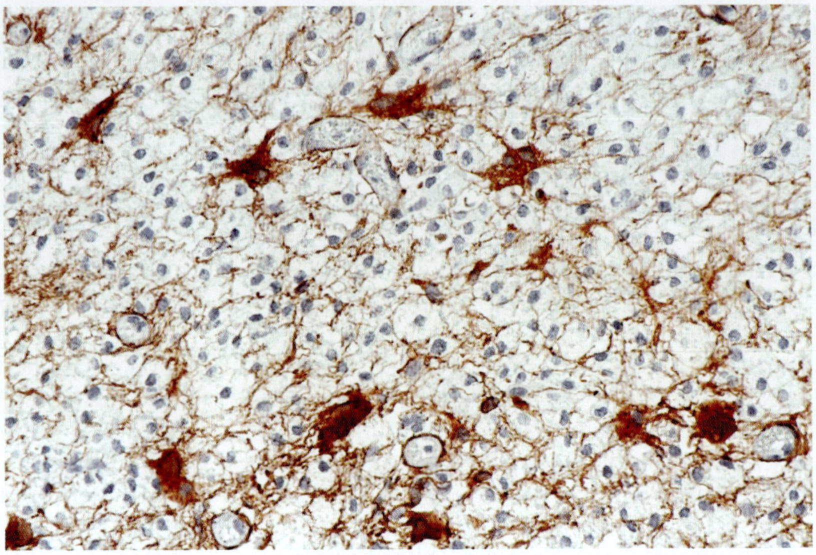

Figure 14-2

REACTION TO DIFFUSE GLIOMA

Reactive astrocytes are seen (glial fibrillary acidic protein [GFAP] immunohistochemistry).

invasive edges (fig. 14-2). Reactive changes, however, may also occur within the bulk of the tumor; these are most often inflammatory in nature and tend to be more prominent in treated gliomas.

Reactive astrocytes dominate as the response of the normal brain to diffuse glioma invasion. These reactive cells are classic in their appearance (see chapter 2), with oval euchromatic nuclei having prominent nucleoli as well as copious eosinophilic cytoplasm tapering into multiple long processes. Glial fibrillary acid protein (GFAP) immunohistochemistry highlights the typical reactive astrocytic shapes, since these cells are strongly GFAP positive (fig. 14-2). Often, the strength of the reaction with GFAP contrasts with that of neoplastic glial cells, which rarely stain as strongly.

When reactive astrocytes are seen in the center of cellular malignant gliomas, they are most often ignored by the pathologist, who is rightly focusing on the nature of the neoplastic component. At the invasive edges, however, reactive cells may constitute a significant percentage of the total cellular population. As a result, they catch the eye and suggest a diagnosis of reaction versus neoplasm. This situation can be particularly tricky in a small stereotactic biopsy that samples only the edge of a tumor. Attention to the cytologic features of the neoplastic cells and knowledge that reactive cells can occur at the edges of malignant gliomas allow the correct diagnosis.

Invasion into the surrounding brain by diffuse gliomas produces "secondary structures" of Scherer (1,2). These include perineuronal satellitosis, perivascular satellitosis, and subpial spread, architectural features that are diagnostically useful. Because these structures are intrinsic to the manner in which the neoplastic cells interface with the native brain parenchyma, they are not covered here and the reader is referred to standard textbooks on brain tumor pathology (3,4). The central nervous system (CNS) may react to the presence of tumor by eliciting desmoplastic responses, however; such responses have been termed "tertiary structures" by Scherer (1). Desmoplasia is particularly pronounced when gliomas involve the subarachnoid space, presumably as a result of a reaction by leptomeningeal cells, including fibroblasts. Standard trichrome and reticulin stains are adequate for highlighting such changes. Generally, such phenomena are not of substantial clinicopathologic significance, but the pathologist must be cautious not to misinterpret leptomeningeal desmoplasia with the more fulminant fibroblast-like alterations of gliosarcoma.

Well-Demarcated Gliomas

The well-demarcated gliomas that are commonly encountered by the pathologist include pilocytic astrocytomas and ependymomas, with ganglion cell tumors, pleomorphic xanthoastrocytomas, chordoid gliomas, and subependymal giant cell astrocytomas being less common. Most

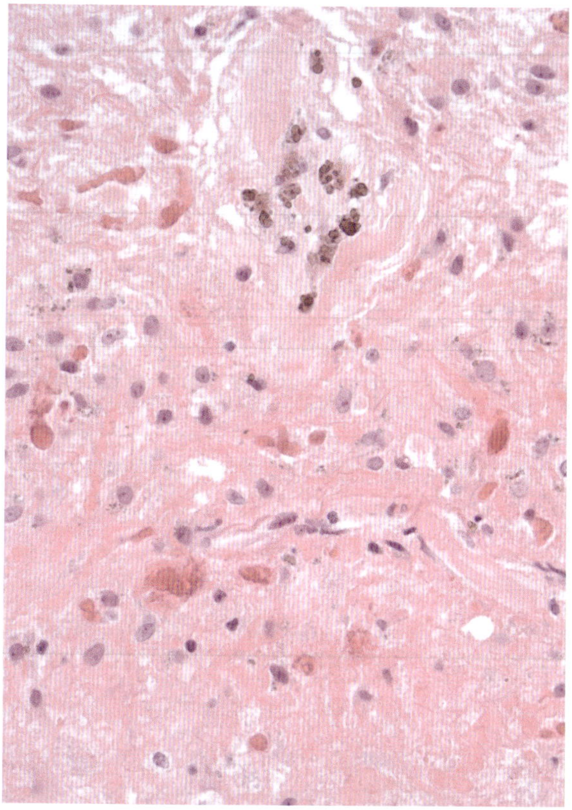

Figure 14-3

REACTION TO CIRCUMSCRIBED GLIOMA

Chronic gliosis, Rosenthal fibers, and hemosiderin deposits are adjacent to an ependymoma.

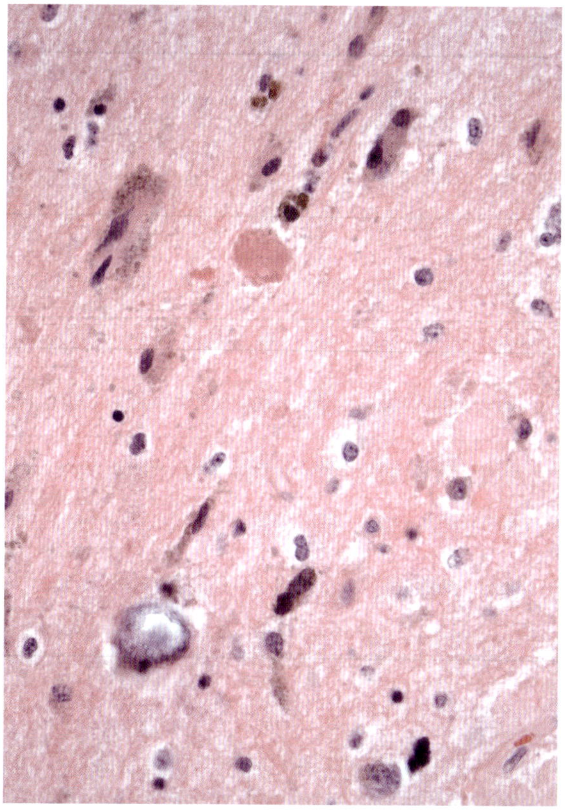

Figure 14-4

REACTION TO CIRCUMSCRIBED GLIOMA

Chronic gliosis, eosinophilic granular bodies, and hemosiderin are adjacent to an oligodendroglioma with a "pushing" border.

of these tumors have "pushing" margins that compress rather than invade the adjacent brain. All of these tumor types, however, can have moderately infiltrative margins. In our practice, we draw attention to the presence of infiltrating margins in the setting of glioma types that are expected to have circumscribed growth patterns since this may alert the clinician to provide closer follow-up to detect recurrence. In many cases, the neurosurgeon has already been alerted to this possibility if the tumor is less easily separable from the surrounding brain.

The response of the adjacent brain to circumscribed gliomas is similar to that of other tumor types with pushing margins (see Reaction to Other Neoplasms, below), but tends to be less marked (figs. 14-3, 14-4). Reactive astrocytes are present. Given the indolent nature of many of these tumors, the gliosis is often chronic, with elongated astrocytes without prominent eosinophilic cytoplasm. Rosenthal fibers and eosinophilic granular bodies may be present (figs. 14-3, 14-4), but these are typically far fewer than found at the margins of other neoplasms, such as hemangioblastomas or craniopharyngiomas (figs. 14-5, 14-6). Inflammation may be prominent, both within the tumors (as in gangliogliomas) and in the adjacent brain (chordoid gliomas of the third ventricle). Inflammation is most often perivascular collections of small lymphocytes with bland nuclei, but plasma cells are present as well.

Optic Nerve Glioma

Optic nerve gliomas usually involve the subarachnoid space surrounding the optic nerve, but do not transgress the dural sheath. Typically, involvement of the subarachnoid space expands the intradural contents, but does not elicit a specific response aside from some desmoplasia.

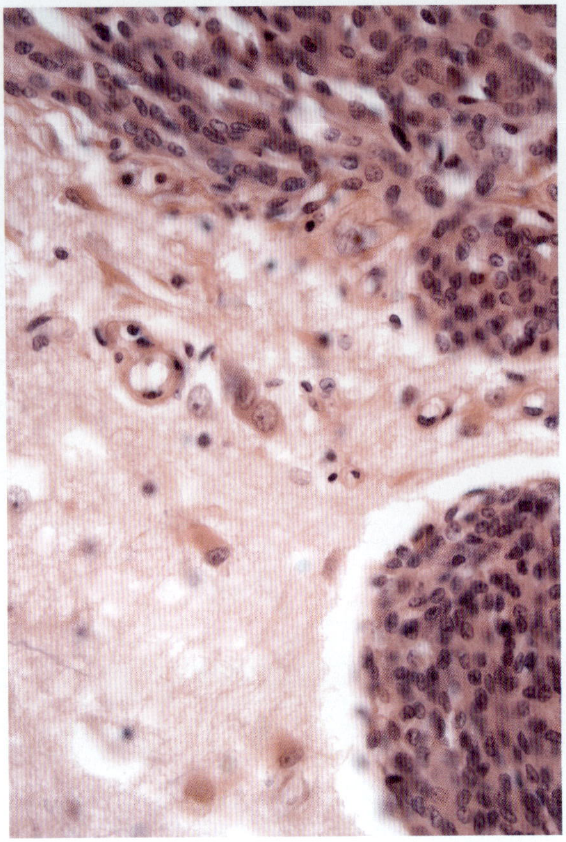

Figure 14-5

REACTION TO MENINGIOMA

Reactive astrocytosis in the cerebral cortex.

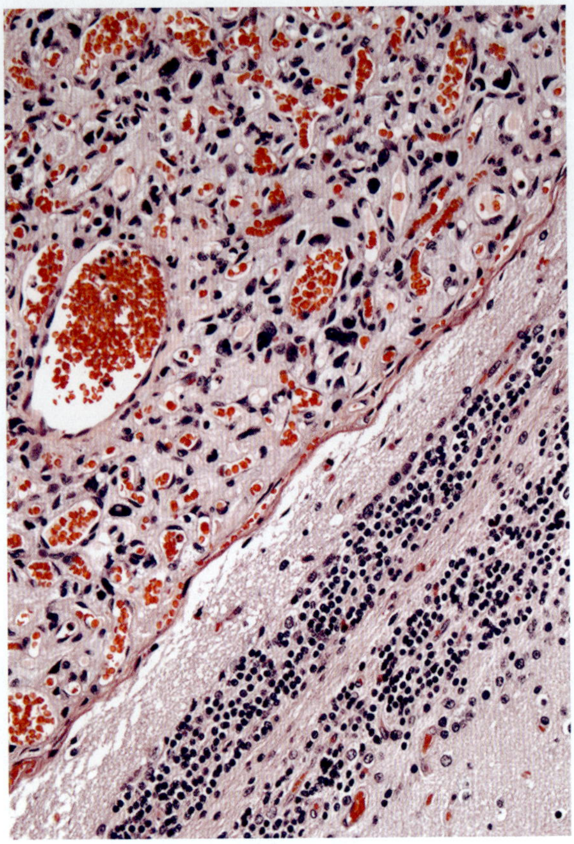

Figure 14-6

REACTION TO HEMANGIOBLASTOMA

The adjacent cerebellum is atrophied.

Occasionally, there may be prominent arachnoidal hyperplasia in response to an optic nerve glioma. The arachnoid proliferates in response to adjacent neoplastic or inflammatory processes, with the minute arachnoidal nests forming small nodules that are histologically indistinguishable from meningothelial meningiomas. Biopsies of such nodules that miss the adjacent, inciting process may yield a false diagnosis of meningioma. The finding of areas resembling meningothelial meningioma from the optic nerve region in a patient thought to have an optic nerve glioma on neuroimaging should prompt a consultation between the neurosurgeon, neuroradiologist, and neuropathologist to determine whether such a lesion is more likely to be arachnoidal hyperplasia overlying a glioma or a true optic nerve meningioma. The clinical features of the case may also help, since optic nerve gliomas are typically tumors of children or young adults while optic nerve meningiomas more often affect middle-aged and elderly patients. A further distinction must be made in patients with neurofibromatosis; patients with neurofibromatosis 1 (NF1) often develop optic nerve gliomas, while patients with NF2 develop multiple meningiomas, including those of the optic nerve. As a result, the diagnosis of optic nerve meningothelial meningioma should be carefully reconsidered in a young patient or a patient with NF1, since it may reflect misinterpretation of arachnoidal hyperplasia.

REACTION TO LYMPHOMA AND STEROID THERAPY

Primary CNS lymphomas (PCNSL) are moderately common in large neuropathology practices. With occasional exceptions, these are large B-cell tumors, characterized by prominent nucleoli, considerable nuclear irregularity, and

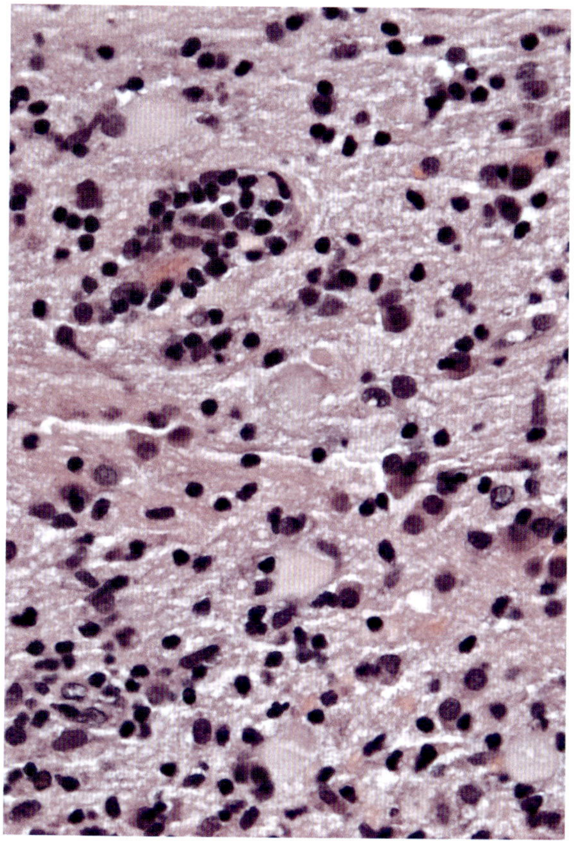

Figure 14-7

STEROID THERAPY OF PRIMARY CENTRAL NERVOUS SYSTEM LYMPHOMA (PCNSL)

A chronic inflammatory infiltrate is present.

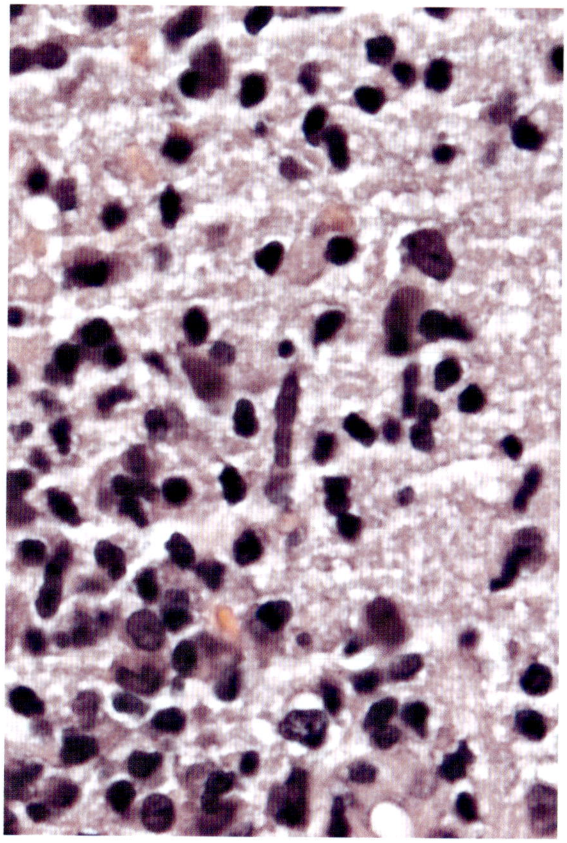

Figure 14-8

STEROID THERAPY OF PCNSL

Lymphocytes and microglia are present.

hyperchromasia. Both within the tumors and at the edges of the lesions, PCNSL is attended by numerous reactive cells, primarily reactive astrocytes, small benign T lymphocytes, and scattered macrophages. Within the tumor, in light of the large neoplastic cells, the reactive cells generally fail to catch much of the pathologist's attention. At the edges and in the setting of prior steroid therapy (see below), however, reactive cells can constitute the majority or the entirety of the cell population, necessitating careful searches at the histologic, immunohistochemical, and molecular levels for rare PCNSL cells. Reactive cells can be highlighted immunohistochemically with T-cell markers, CD68 for macrophages and GFAP for astrocytes; they contrast with the large, irregular neoplastic cells that stain for B-cell markers.

PCNSL, particularly in immunocompetent patients, may be remarkably steroid sensitive. Within a day, there may be a dramatic response of PCNSL to steroids, as demonstrated with neuroimaging. Indeed, it has been suggested that a marked response to steroids in a lesion initially suspected (based on the anatomic distribution and imaging characteristics) to be PCNSL is strong evidence for a diagnosis of PCNSL. Given that many patients with intracranial mass lesions are treated with steroids to control mass effect, some patients may be biopsied after steroids have been administered. In that setting, it is not unusual for the pathologist to have difficulty finding neoplastic B cells. The specimen may consist entirely of reactive cells (figs. 14-7–14-9). Demyelination may be present (fig. 14-10). Given the clinical question of PCNSL, it is necessary for the pathologist to entertain the possibility of tumor, but usually the specimens are not diagnostic. It is also imperative, given the

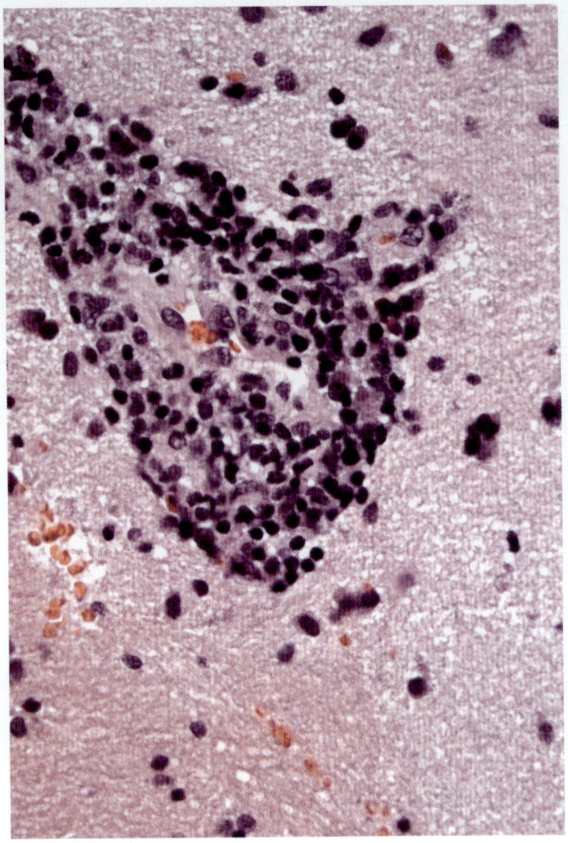

Figure 14-9

STEROID THERAPY OF PCNSL

Lymphocytes cluster around blood vessels.

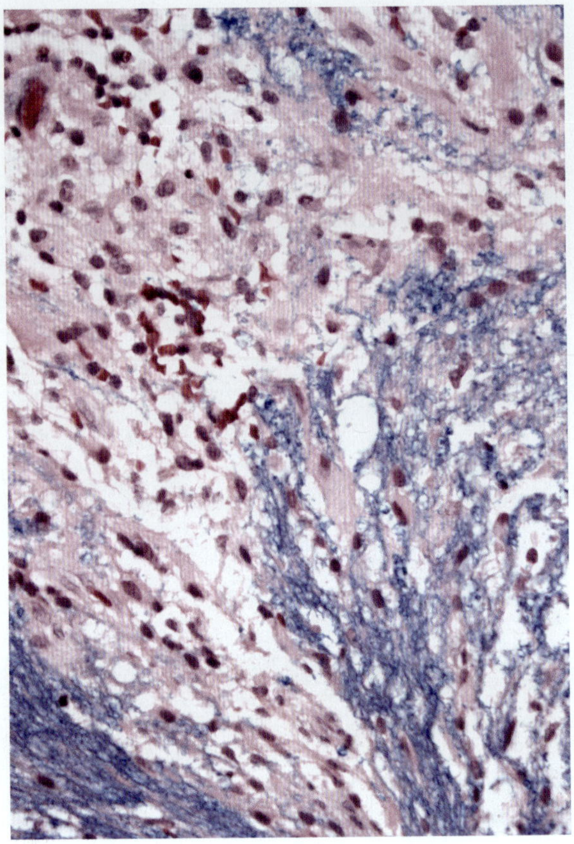

Figure 14-10

STEROID THERAPY OF PCNSL

Frank demyelination may occur (Luxol fast blue-hematoxylin and eosin [H&E] stain).

primarily "inflammatory" nature of these biopsies, to exclude infectious or other inflammatory etiologies (fig. 14-10). If such a nondiagnostic biopsy is encountered, the typical course of action is to withdraw steroids once mass effect has been controlled, and to follow the patient carefully with neuroimaging. If PCNSL was present prior to steroid therapy, it will recur and possibly be amenable to biopsy at that time.

As mentioned, some patients ultimately diagnosed with PCNSL have transient symptomatic contrast-enhancing lesions with nondiagnostic histopathologic features that antedate their diagnoses of PCNSL (fig. 14-11). We refer to these antecedent processes as "sentinel lesions" (5). We initially reported (5) four immunocompetent middle-aged patients with contrast-enhancing intraparenchymal brain lesions that, on biopsy, consisted of demyelination with axonal sparing in two patients (fig. 14-10), nonspecific inflammation in one, and normal brain in the last. All four patients recovered within 2 to 4 weeks after the initial biopsy and imaging studies revealed resolution of the lesions. After 7 to 11 months, however, each patient developed symptomatic lesions in a different region of the brain, which were biopsy-proven B-cell PCNSLs (fig. 14-12). We have subsequently seen a few similar cases in our consultation practice. Such sentinel lesions of PCNSL should be considered in patients with contrast-enhancing focal parenchymal lesions that show nonspecific or demyelinating histopathologic changes. Close clinical and radiographic follow-up is essential in such cases.

REACTION ADJACENT TO MENINGIOMAS

The reaction of the adjacent brain to meningiomas can be divided into the reaction to

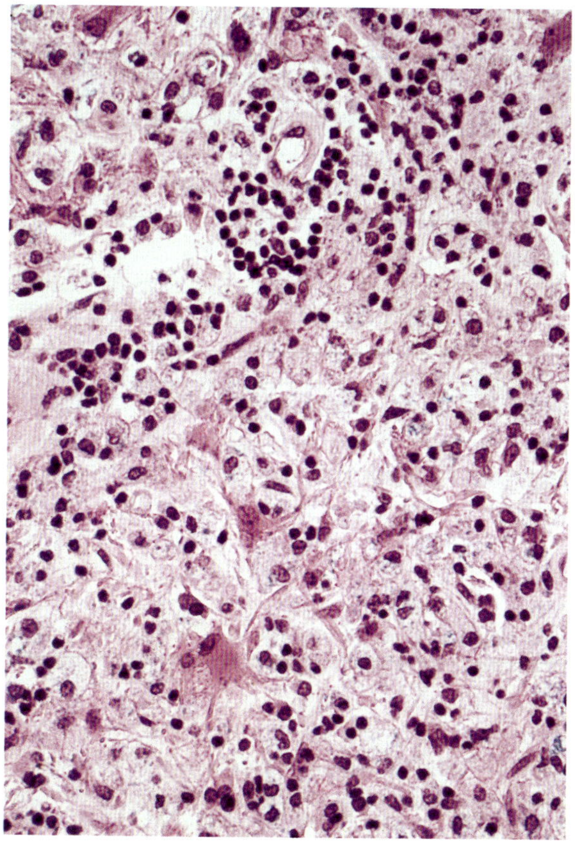

Figure 14-11

STEROID THERAPY OF PCNSL

"Sentinel lesions" show reactive changes, including gliosis and a chronic inflammatory infiltrate.

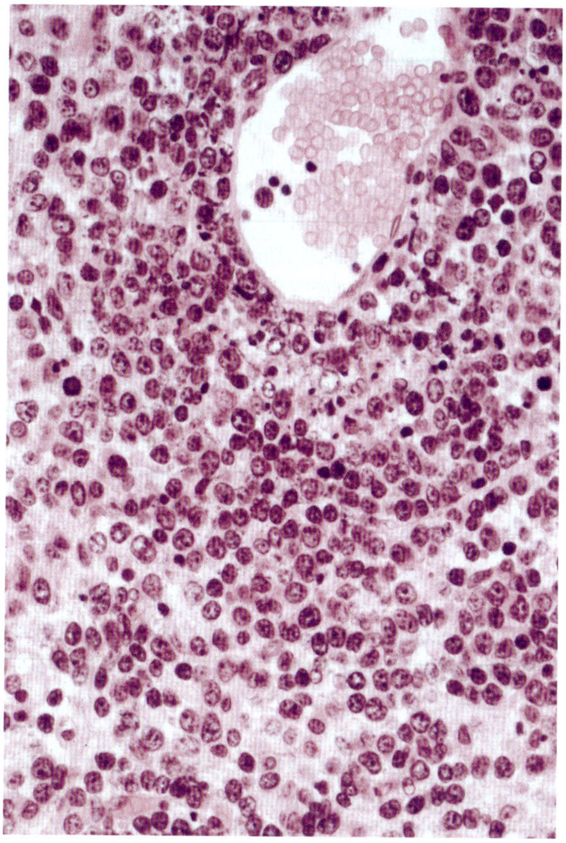

Figure 14-12

RECURRENT PCNSL

PCNSL recurred after biopsy of an inflammatory sentinel lesion.

adjacent meningioma and the reaction to invading meningioma. The meninges themselves often show little, if any, reaction to an adjacent meningioma. The dura mater is often sampled or removed during meningioma surgery. In most cases, the dura mater is not involved by meningioma, with the tumor plastered just below the dura. Some meningiomas invade the dura, usually as moderate-sized lobules of tumor rather than as single cells. In these situations, the dura mater looks unperturbed by the tumor.

The leptomeninges are not often sampled during meningioma surgery, but may contain a "tail" of loose, granulation-like tissue at the edge of the tumor. This is more often encountered by the pathologist at autopsy examination of incidental meningiomas. The meninges may demonstrate evidence of past hemorrhage or prior surgery, with hemosiderin debris and reaction to foreign material, respectively.

The brain reacts to invading meningioma with reactive gliosis, which may be marked (fig. 14-5). The most prominent astrocytic response occurs in the setting of frank brain invasion, rather than simple involvement of Virchow-Robin spaces. Indeed, the finding of prominent reactive gliosis in a fragment of brain removed with a meningioma should prompt a detailed search for brain invasion elsewhere.

REACTION TO OTHER NEOPLASMS

The response of the CNS to slowly growing, well-demarcated lesions such as craniopharyngiomas, hemangioblastomas, and syringomyelia is somewhat stereotypical and is similar to the response to well-demarcated gliomas (fig. 14-6). Given the relatively common nature of some of the slowly growing, well-demarcated tumors, these reactive changes are often seen in surgical neuropathology practice. The often deep-seated location of these lesions may make neurosurgical access more difficult and may result in small biopsies that sample the reactive edges of such lesions rather than the lesions themselves. As a result, knowledge of these reactive changes is critical in surgical neuropathology.

Because these are slowly growing tumors, the gliotic response is chronic. In addition, because most of these lesions are deep seated, the gliotic response features numerous Rosenthal fibers (see fig. 14-3). As a result, the reactive brain tissue surrounding craniopharyngiomas, hemangioblastomas, and syringomyelic cavities often demonstrates many Rosenthal fibers in a densely and coarsely fibrillary background. The differential diagnosis includes pilocytic astrocytoma, but the reactive changes actually feature more Rosenthal fibers than in typical pilocytic astrocytoma. Indeed, it has been remarked that the finding of numerous Rosenthal fibers from a deep-seated lesion should initially suggest a diagnosis other than pilocytic astrocytoma. Because the cellularity of pilocytic astrocytoma may not be high and because the cellularity of reactive changes can be moderately high, the degree of cellularity may not be helpful in establishing the correct diagnosis. Similarly, the chronic reactive gliosis surrounding craniopharyngiomas, hemangioblastomas, and syringomyelic cavities may be "piloid" in nature. Thus, in the setting of a deep-seated lesion, the presence of numerous Rosenthal fibers should raise a "red flag." In this situation, discussion with the neurosurgeon about the exact anatomic origin of the specimen as well as correlation with neuroimaging findings can be crucial.

We have noted arachnoidal hyperplasia (see chapter 2, fig. 2-37) adjacent to sellar region neoplasms. Small biopsies that miss the adjacent tumor may be misinterpreted as meningothelial meningiomas. The possible diagnosis of meningothelial meningioma in a setting in which the clinical and radiologic features suggest a craniopharyngioma should raise the suspicion of arachnoidal hyperplasia and should prompt a request for additional diagnostic tissue. We have also observed arachnoidal hyperplasia in association with inflammatory meningeal masses such as Rosai-Dorfman disease.

REACTION TO ANTINEOPLASTIC THERAPIES

Cerebral Radiation Damage

Definition. *Cerebral radiation damage*, also referred to as *radiation effects, radiation necrosis*, or *radionecrosis*, is a necrotizing process of the brain or spinal cord that arises after therapeutic radiation.

After high doses of radiation, such as those used to treat astrocytomas or tumors adjacent to the brain, symptomatic radiation damage may follow. Late delayed radiation necrosis typically occurs at least 6 months after treatment, but radiation effects may be found on imaging earlier than 6 months. Because radiation is used in the treatment of many brain tumors, and in essentially all patients with common malignant gliomas, radiation effects are often encountered in neuro-oncology practices. The most common setting in which the surgical pathologist confronts the possibility of radiation necrosis is in patients with prior radiation therapy for malignant glioma, with the differential diagnosis involving recurrent glioma, radiation damage, or both.

Clinical and Radiologic Findings. Radiation damage occurs after therapeutic high-dose radiation of cerebral or other cranial neoplasms (6). In this setting, radiation damage presents either as a symptomatic mass lesion or as radiologic progression on routine follow-up neuroimaging. In both settings, the differential diagnosis is radiation damage versus neoplasm. If radiation has been given for primary glioma, the diagnostic considerations are radiation damage versus recurrent glioma; if radiation has been given for another intracranial mass, the diagnostic considerations are radiation damage versus radiation-induced malignant glioma. The former situation is more common. Unfortunately, radiation damage may clinically and radiologically resemble a recurrent high-grade tumor and, although modern neuroimaging techniques such as single photon emission tomography and magnetic resonance spectroscopy are proving useful in making the distinction between radiation necrosis and recurrent tumor (7), a biopsy is still necessary for a definite diagnosis.

Gross Findings. Macroscopic examination of radiated brain typically demonstrates yellowing of the intact white matter, which reflects the chronic gliotic response. If frank radiation

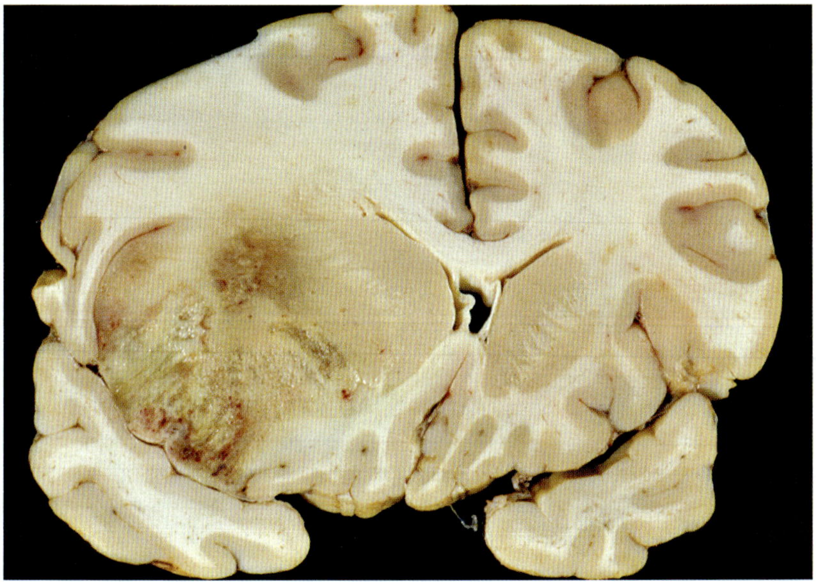

Figure 14-13

RADIATION DAMAGE

Postmortem radiation-damaged high-grade glioma. The white matter in the left hemisphere is yellow and granular.

necrosis has occurred, the parenchyma has a soft, tan, granular appearance, sometimes with regions of bright yellow (fig. 14-13). Foci of hemorrhage may punctuate the necrotic material. Mass effect may be present, although this is not appreciated in surgical biopsy or resection material. Macroscopic distinction from recurrent primary glioma may not be possible.

Intraoperative Findings. The distinction between radiation necrosis and recurrent or radiation-induced malignant glioma may need to be made in the frozen section laboratory. In particular, the decision between recurrent malignant glioma and radiation damage may affect the degree of resection attempted and may affect the patient's intraoperative therapy, for example, the application of chemotherapy wafers. The neurosurgeon may also want to make sure that diagnostic tissue has been acquired to make this distinction postoperatively, in order to decide on further therapy. In general, as discussed below (see Differential Diagnosis), the key distinction is between highly cellular, mitotically active, recurrent glioma and radiation damage. While one cannot exclude the presence of recurrent glioma in nonfrozen material, intraoperative consultation can document the presence of active malignant glioma when viable, highly cellular neoplasm is present; in such situations, the tumor cells are often small and anaplastic, and mitotic activity is usually easily detected.

Microscopic Findings. Radiation injury to the CNS is characterized histologically by preferential involvement of white matter structures (fig. 14-14) by coagulative necrosis and alterations of blood vessels and glia (figs. 14-15–14-23). The vasculature is thickened and hyalinized (figs. 14-15, 14-18, 14-19). Endothelial cells may appear activated, with enlarged nuclei and prominent nucleoli (fig. 14-19). In many cases, frank fibrinoid necrosis of vessels is present, and fibrin deposition is commonly seen surrounding damaged vessels. This is often accompanied by thrombosis. Occasionally, the response to vascular damage results in small malformative foci that resemble capillary telangiectasias. Astrocytes are reactive, but may be large, with copious eosinophilic cytoplasm and large, hyperchromatic, irregular nuclei (figs. 14-16, 14-17). As the process progresses, necrosis ensues. This is often coagulative in appearance, with numerous cellular "ghosts" as well as necrotic blood vessels (figs. 14-20, 14-21). Characteristically, but not invariably, there are fine calcifications within the necrotic regions (fig. 14-22). Inflammation is scant. When hemorrhage has occurred, there may also be clusters of macrophages with hemosiderin debris or areas with cholesterol clefts. There may be demyelination surrounding the necrotic foci, but this is usually obscured by the destructive changes.

Immunohistochemical Findings. Immunohistochemistry is not of diagnostic use for

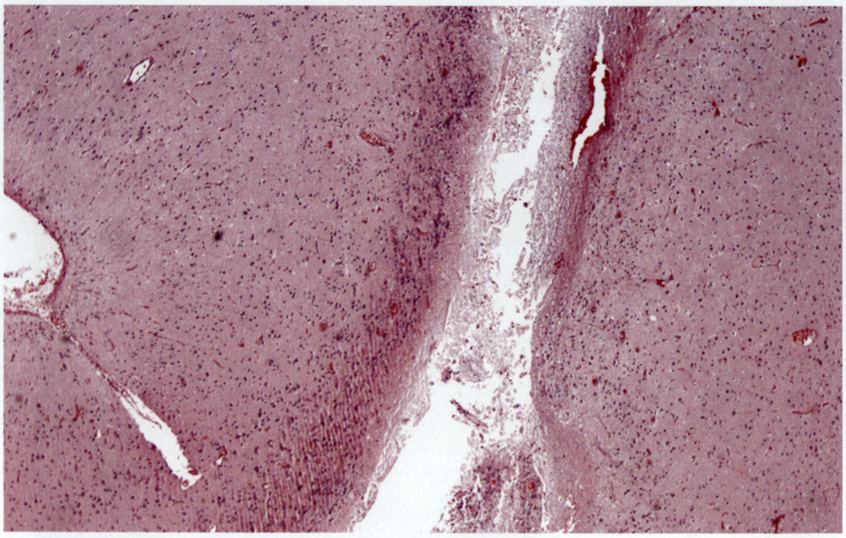

Figure 14-14

RADIATION DAMAGE

Preferential cavitation of white matter is noted between two sections of cerebral cortex.

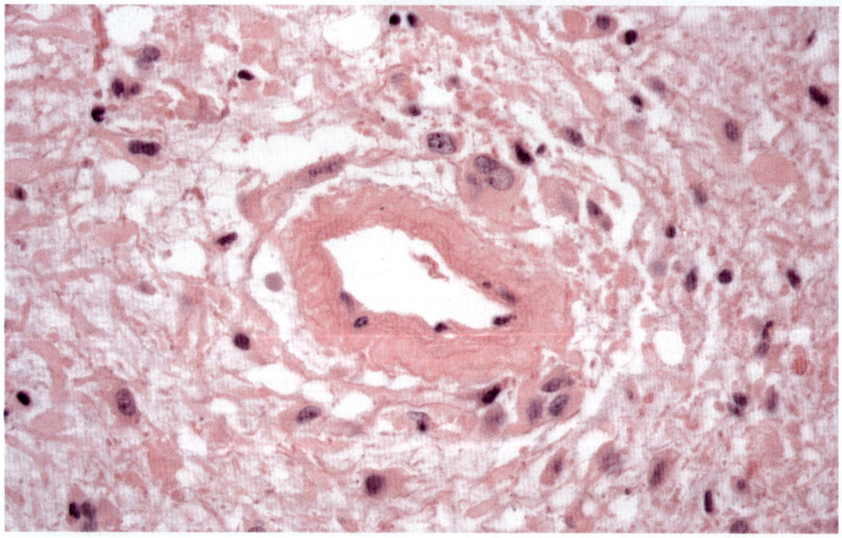

Figure 14-15

RADIATION DAMAGE

Atypical gliosis surrounds a hyalinized small vessel.

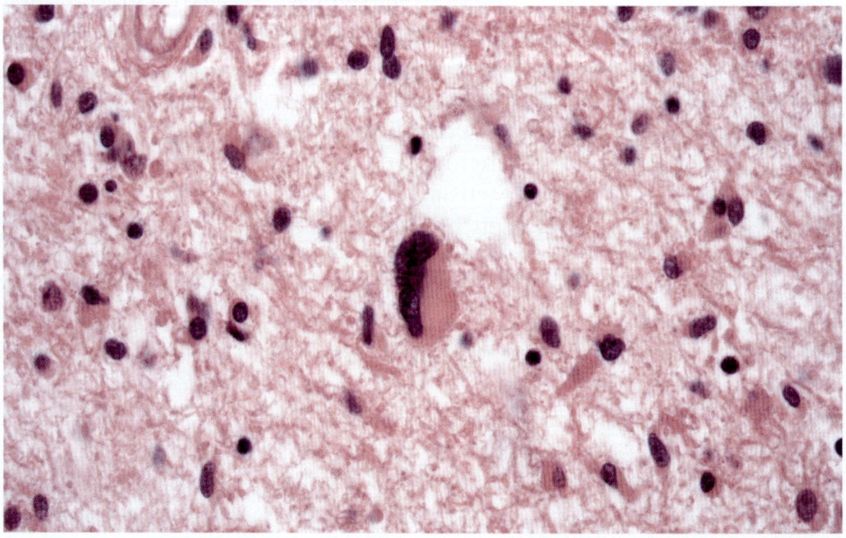

Figure 14-16

RADIATION DAMAGE

Astrocytes may be cytologically bizarre.

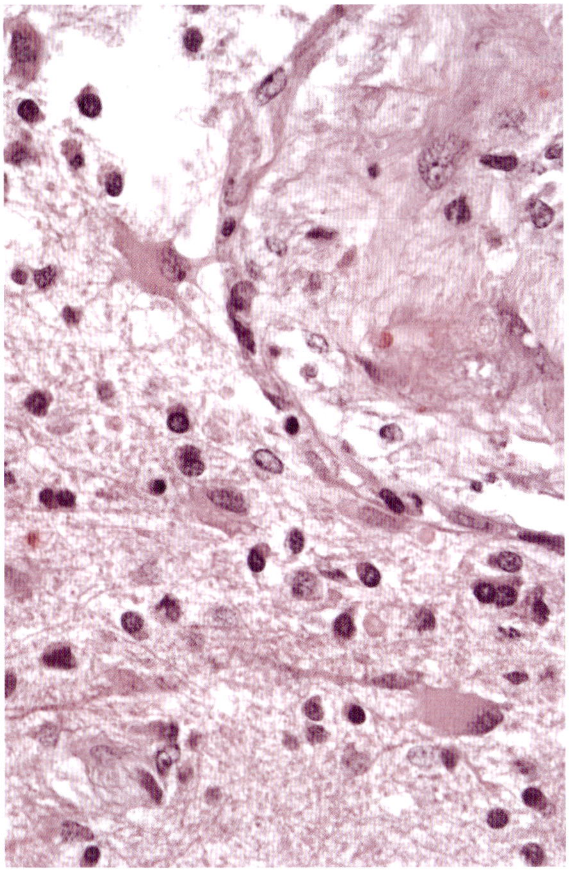

Figure 14-17

RADIATION DAMAGE

Atypical and reactive astrocytes surround a damaged medium-sized vessel.

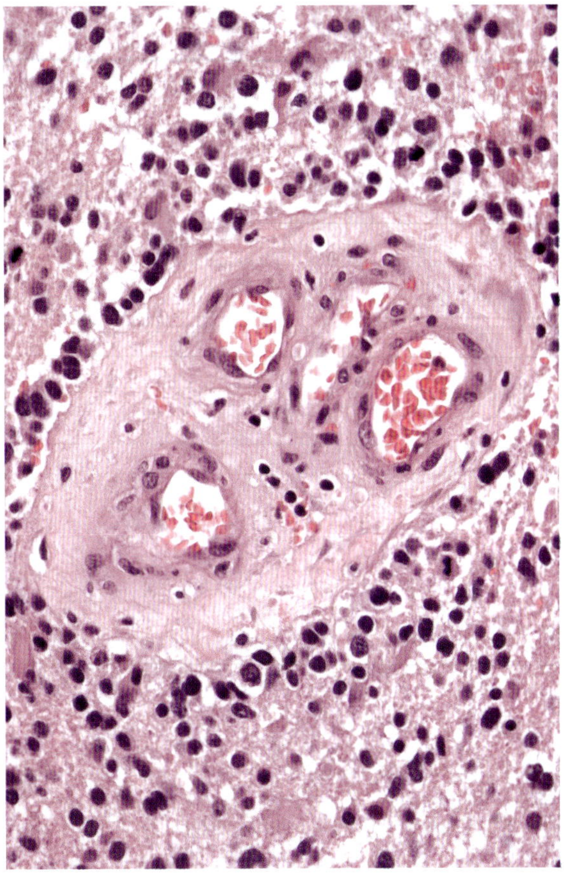

Figure 14-18

RADIATION DAMAGE

Marked vascular hyalinization in a radiated glioma.

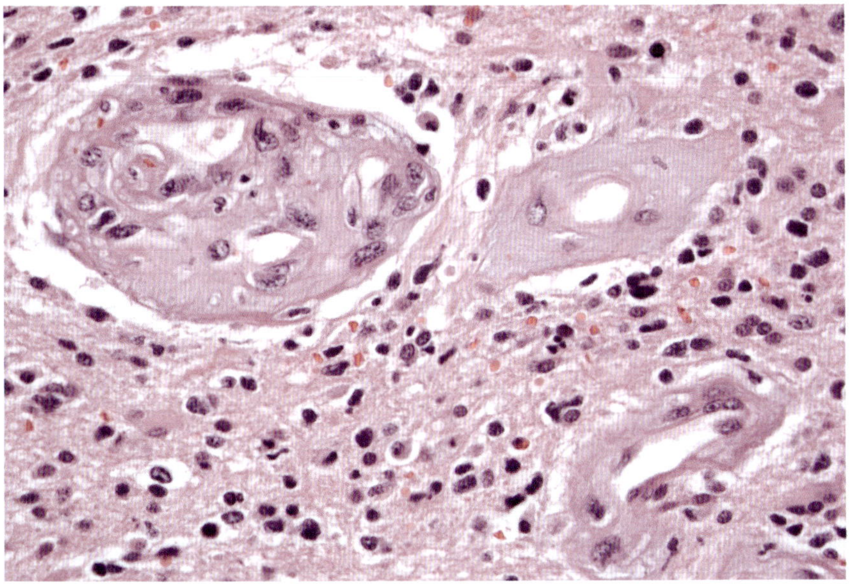

Figure 14-19

RADIATION DAMAGE

Vascular hyalinization with activated endothelial cells.

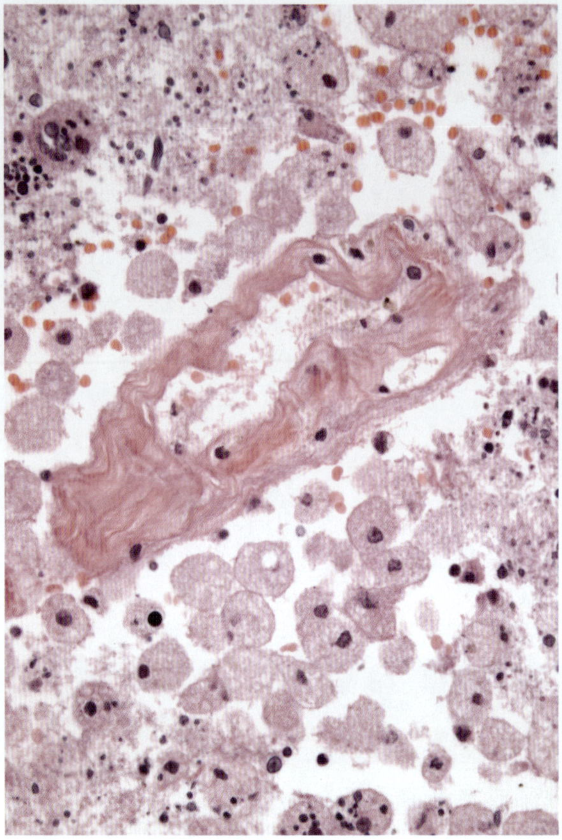

Figure 14-20

RADIATION DAMAGE

Necrosis with "ghost" vessel and numerous macrophages.

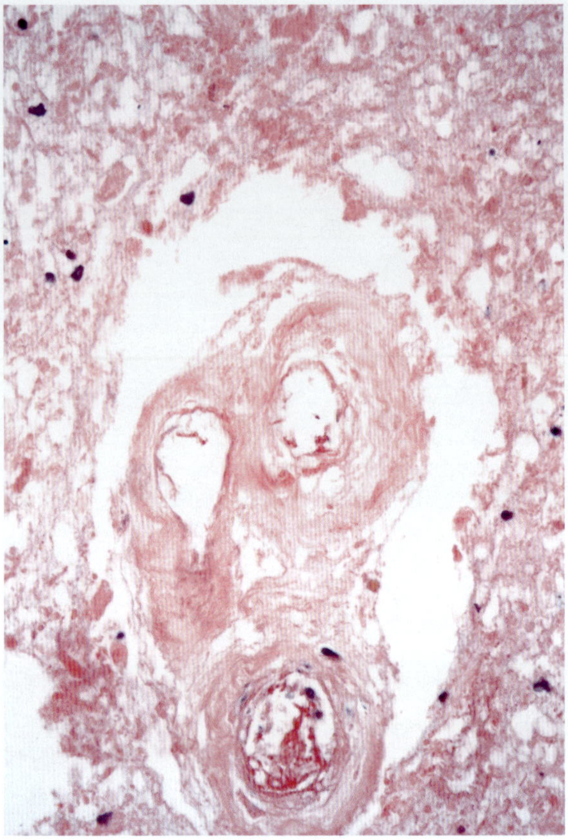

Figure 14-21

RADIATION DAMAGE

Necrosis with a typical ghost vessel.

Figure 14-22

RADIATION DAMAGE

Necrosis with punctate areas of mineralization.

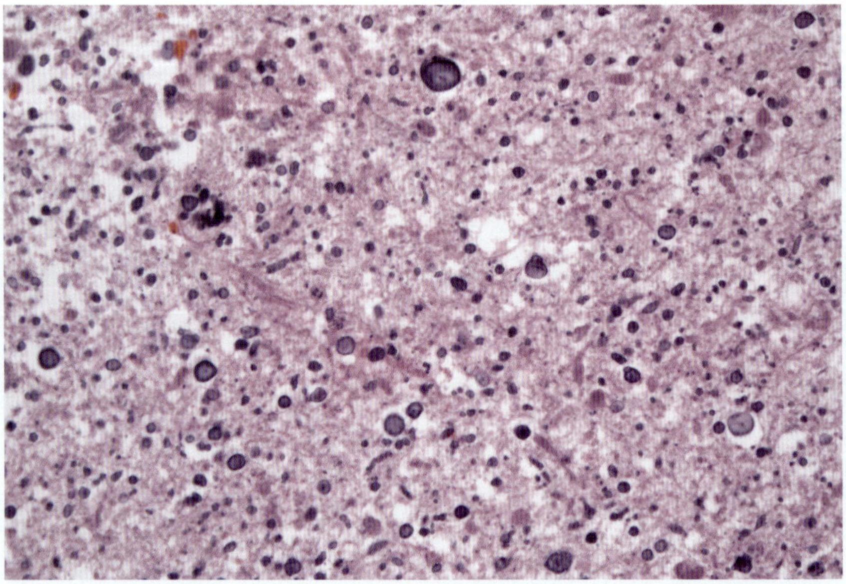

the diagnosis of radiation damage. Macrophage populations can be highlighted with CD68 stains, and reactive astrocytes with GFAP. MIB-1 is not of particular use, since reactive astrocytes may be proliferating.

Differential Diagnosis. With a history of radiation (which should be available to the pathologist), the differential diagnosis is narrowed to three conditions: recurrent tumor, residual tumor, and radiation necrosis. Recurrent tumor is defined as tumor that has arisen since therapy was last given. This diagnosis is the most straightforward histologically, featuring typical astrocytoma or glioblastoma, often with aggregates of small, anaplastic cells. Fortunately for the pathologist, the most important histologic decision is whether recurrent tumor is present. Residual tumor, on the other hand, is defined as tumor that was present at the time of radiation and is still present. It is thought that residual tumor cells are either not viable or not as viable as recurrent tumor. Residual tumor cells are enlarged, often with bizarre nuclei and eosinophilic cytoplasm, appearing cytologically similar to radiated tumor cells in other areas of the body. These are scattered throughout the biopsy, but are not densely aggregated. Often these cells accompany radiation necrosis, and it may be impossible to distinguish radiated residual tumor cells from bizarre radiated reactive astrocytes (fig. 14-23).

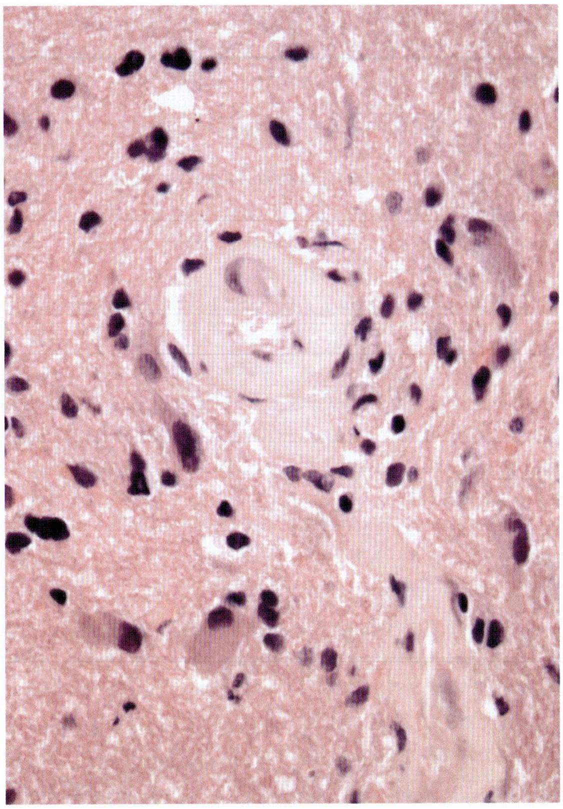

Figure 14-23

RADIATION DAMAGE

Atypical astrocytes of residual glioma are seen.

Treatment and Prognosis. Radiation necrosis is treated by surgical resection if the patient is symptomatic, or is simply followed neuroradiologically if the patient is asymptomatic. The prognosis of radiation necrosis is generally more favorable than that of recurrent malignant glioma or radiation-induced malignant glioma. Some cases of radiation necrosis may be progressive, however, with extension throughout the cerebral white matter, sometimes extending beyond the area exposed to radiation. In such cases, radiation necrosis itself may follow an aggressive course, leading to the death of the patient regardless of the state of the underlying neoplastic process.

Other Forms of Radiation and Radiation Damage. A number of novel approaches to radiation therapy have been developed and implemented. These include stereotactic radiosurgical approaches, proton beam therapy, and neutron boron capture therapy. Each of these may result in mass lesions for which the differential diagnosis includes recurrent tumor versus complications of therapy. The neuropathologic changes are similar to those observed in standard radiation damage, although they may be more extensive and more marked (8; DN Louis, unpublished observations).

Other Effects of Radiation on Nervous System-Related Structures. Radiation therapy may affect a number of structures related to the CNS and result in neurologic dysfunction. These include cranial and peripheral nerves adjacent to the CNS. Peripheral nerves may display epineurial fibrosis as well as vascular changes, degeneration of axons, and myelin loss. Large cerebral, cervical, and spinal arteries may be directly affected, with fibrosis and vascular wall damage that result in cerebrovascular complications. Surgical biopsy of radiated nerves and vessels, however, is uncommon and these entities are therefore only rarely encountered by the surgical pathologist.

Reaction to Chemotherapy

Although many medications used in the treatment of cancer produce neurologic side effects, histologically detectable reactions to chemotherapy are only rarely encountered in the examination of CNS tissues. (The particular effect of steroids on primary CNS lymphomas is discussed above.) In our experience, such effects only come to biopsy in the setting of widespread, diffuse changes of uncertain etiology that predominantly affect the white matter.

A few chemotherapeutic agents have been implicated in particular (9). Intraarterial administration of BCNU has resulted in necrotizing lesions histologically similar to disseminated necrotizing leukoencephalopathy (see below) (10). 5-fluorouracil/levamisole (11–17) and cisplatin have produced similar lesions as well (18), but these do not usually feature the conspicuous mineralization and axonal dilatation found in disseminated necrotizing leukoencephalopathy (see below). Demyelination with macrophage infiltration may also be a prominent component (19). Finally, the advent of direct release chemotherapy delivery systems, such as the wafers currently in clinical use, has resulted in biopsies to determine whether expanding lesions that occur with this treatment represent tumor recurrence or complications of therapy.

Disseminated Necrotizing Leukoencephalopathy

Definition. *Disseminated necrotizing leukoencephalopathy* (DNL) is a rare, focally necrotizing condition of the white matter that usually arises after combined chemotherapy and radiation therapy.

General Comments. DNL is a rare condition initially recognized in the late 1960s and early 1970s as a complication of combined cerebral radiation and chemotherapy for children with leukemia (20,21). Rare cases have also been reported following therapy for other neoplasms, including lymphomas and some visceral malignancies, and in adults (22,23). Similar toxic encephalopathies have been noted after intrathecal chemotherapy and whole-brain radiation for the treatment of leptomeningeal carcinomatosis (24), and after intraarterial BCNU and cerebral radiation for glioma therapy (10). The entity was particularly noted after prophylactic radiation therapy over 20 Gy that was given prior to or during chemotherapy, and particularly after intrathecal chemotherapeutic regimens that included methotrexate. Nonetheless, the condition has been noted with other chemotherapies, other routes of administration, and without additional radiation therapy. The entity follows a rapidly progressive course, with death typically following within 3 months.

Given the recognition of the dangers of the above combinations and timing of combined radiation and chemotherapy, DNL is now only exceptionally encountered. Furthermore, it is unusual for such patients to come to biopsy, with most cases diagnosed at postmortem examination. Nonetheless, because the condition most likely represents a common pathologic endpoint, it is possible that the surgical pathologist will encounter DNL in the future in the setting of other, new therapeutic regimens.

Clinical and Radiologic Findings. Patients most often present with neurologic decline, including mental status changes, lethargy, seizures, and eventually coma, with death occurring within a few months. Given the current rarity of the lesion, modern neuroimaging characteristics are not well described, and many imaging findings in such patients relate to other disease complications (25). Computerized tomography (CT) scans demonstrate low densities throughout the white matter (26). A unique pattern of white matter contrast enhancement on T1-weighted magnetic resonance images (MRI) has been described in two patients after high-dose methotrexate therapy for acute lymphoblastic leukemia; the enhancement in these two cases was more prominent near the base of the brain than at the vertex (27).

Gross Findings. The cerebral white matter is affected by multiple small, sometimes confluent areas of necrosis, some with petechial hemorrhage. Some cases show a predilection for the pons and rare cases have affected the spinal cord (22).

Intraoperative Findings. The unique histologic features, particularly the prominent axonal spheroids and mineralization, should prompt consideration of this entity on frozen section

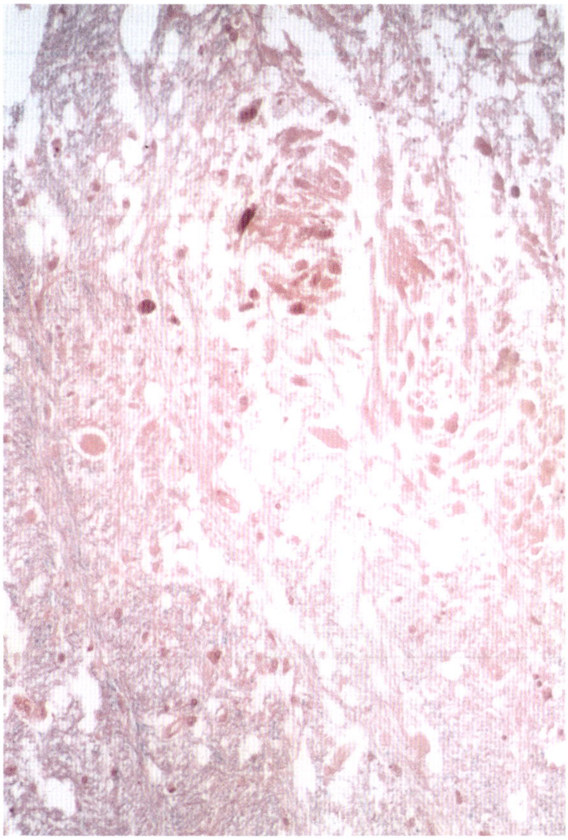

Figure 14-24

DISSEMINATED NECROTIZING LEUKOENCEPHALOPATHY

The neuropil is disrupted and numerous axonal spheroids are present (Luxol fast blue-H&E stain).

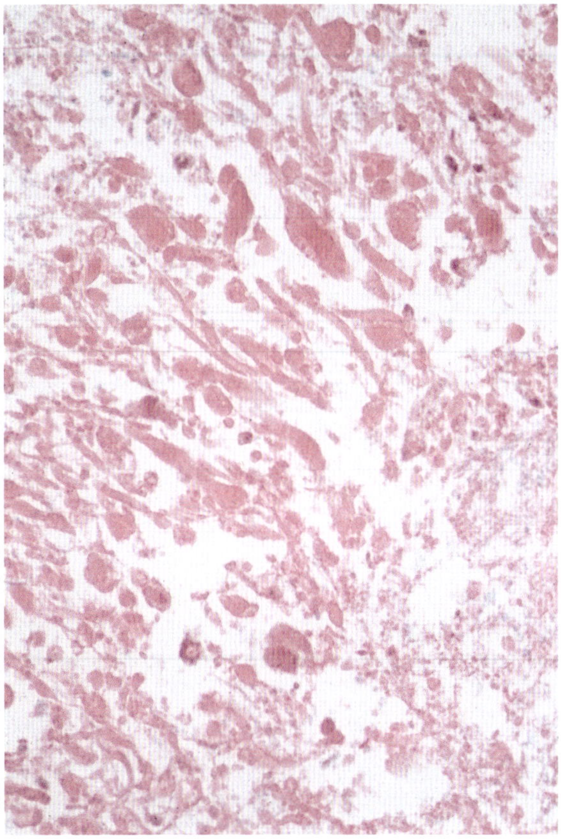

Figure 14-25

DISSEMINATED NECROTIZING LEUKOENCEPHALOPATHY

There are many axonal spheroids and loss of myelin (Luxol fast blue-H&E stain).

diagnosis in the appropriate clinical setting. Given the current rarity of this condition, it is unlikely that such lesions will be encountered for intraoperative diagnosis; nonetheless, recognition of the distinct histopathologic features of DNL is important if similar findings are encountered in the setting of novel therapeutic modalities and agents.

Microscopic Findings. The histologic features of DNL are unique. Multiple foci of bland, coagulative necrosis are associated with little tissue loss, but with marked myelin loss and with striking surrounding axonal damage (figs. 14-24–14-26). The axonal damage is characterized by numerous axonal spheroids, many of which exhibit dense mineralization. The axonal swellings are often found in a vacuolated neuropil, but without accompanying inflammatory cells and with only rare lipid-laden macrophages. These histologically distinct foci may coalesce, forming geographically irregular zones. Although vascular changes resembling those of radionecrosis may be present, these are typically not prominent and the necrotic zones do not appear vasculocentric. Myelin stains highlight the loss of myelin in and surrounding the necrotic foci, and silver impregnations demonstrate the axonal nature of the surrounding spheroids (fig. 14-26). Stains for calcium demonstrate the mineral deposition, but this is usually apparent with standard hematoxylin and eosin (H&E) stains.

Immunohistochemical Findings. Immunohistochemistry is not necessary for the diagnosis of DNL and most reports antedate the era of immunohistochemical investigation. Neurofilament immunohistochemistry can highlight the axonal swellings.

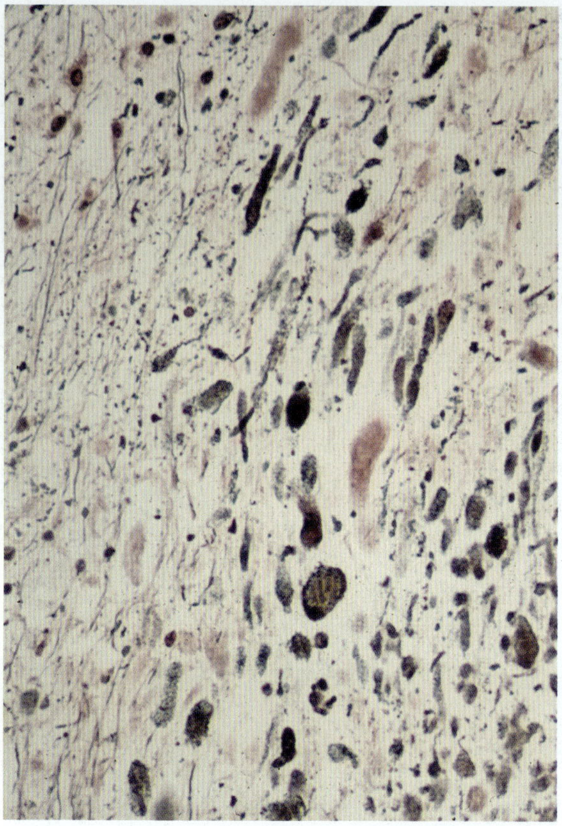

Figure 14-26

DISSEMINATED NECROTIZING LEUKOENCEPHALOPATHY

Axonal spheroids are highlighted on Bodian silver impregnation.

Ultrastructural Findings. Ultrastructural alterations are primarily related to the axonal spheroids. These swellings resembling those seen in other diseases that destroy axons: markedly expanded axons filled with a disorganized mass of intraaxonal organelles, including intermediate filaments, mitochondria, and a variety of autophagic vacuoles, vesicles, and dense bodies. Spiculated dense bodies, representative of mineralization, may also be present.

Differential Diagnosis. The differential diagnosis is narrow, given the unique histologic features of DNL. Consideration must be given to the more standard consequences of radiation damage to the brain, but the clinical and neuroimaging features help distinguish DNL from standard radiation damage. Changes similar to DNL have been found after intraarterial administration of BCNU. Since such changes most likely represent a common endpoint, it is likely that similar findings could arise as a result of a variety of therapeutic agents and modalities and routes of administration.

Treatment and Prognosis. The prognosis of patients with DNL is poor: most patients die a few months after the onset of neurologic problems. However, this may represent reporting bias, and it is possible that less extensive histologic effects of DNL occur. For example, the clinical impairment and imaging abnormalities seen in some survivors of childhood leukemia treated with similar regimens may represent subclinical forms of DNL (28–31).

Reaction to Gene Therapy

The use of viruses to deliver therapeutic genes to malignant gliomas has resulted in resection specimens seen by pathologists during clinical trials. The primary clinical question is whether the specimen represents recurrent tumor or the effects of therapy. Gene therapeutic approaches have not produced specific histologic findings that enable the pathologist to implicate gene therapy in a causative manner (32,33). In particular, encephalitic changes related to herpes vectors have not been noted (33). However, some reports of neuropathologic examination of patients treated with adenoviral vectors have found moderate amounts of chronic inflammation in the tumor beds after therapy, an unusual finding in the setting of standard radiation or chemotherapy (34; EA Chiocca and DN Louis, unpublished observations). The inflammatory infiltrates tend to be vasculocentric and composed of lymphocytes and plasma cells. Evidence of viral infection is not apparent.

REFERENCES

1. Scherer HJ. Structural development in gliomas. Am J Cancer 1938;34:333-351.
2. Scherer HJ. The forms of growth in gliomas and their practical significance. Brain 1940;63(Pt 1):1-35.
3. Burger PC, Scheithauer BW, Vogel FS. Surgical pathology of the nervous system and its coverings, 4th ed. New York: Churchill Livingstone; 2002.
4. Ironside JW, Moss TH, Louis DN, Lowe JS, Weller RO. Diagnostic pathology of nervous system tumours. London: Churchill Livingstone; 2002.
5. Alderson L, Fetell MR, Sisti M, Hochberg F, Cohen M, Louis DN. Sentinel lesions of primary CNS lymphoma. J Neurol Neurosurg Psych 1996;60:102-105.
6. Gutin PH, Liebel SA, Sheline GE. Radiation injury to the nervous system. New York: Raven Press; 1991.
7. Rabinov JD, Lee PL, Barker FG, et al. In vivo 3-T MR spectroscopy in the distinction of recurrent glioma versus radiation effects: initial experience. Radiology 2002;225:871-879.
8. Aziz T, Peress NS, Diaz A, Capala J, Chanana A. Postmortem neuropathological features secondary to boron neutron capture therapy for glioblastoma multiforme. J Neuropathol Exp Neurol 2000;59:62-73.
9. Cossaart N, SantaCruz KS, Preston D, Johnson P, Skikne BS. Fatal chemotherapy-induced encephalopathy following high-dose therapy for metastatic breast cancer: a case report and review of the literature. Bone Marrow Transplant 2003;31:57-60.
10. Rosenblum MK, Delattre JY, Walker RW, Shapiro WR. Fatal necrotizing encephalopathy complicating treatment of malignant gliomas with intra-arterial BCNU and irradiation: a pathological study. J Neurooncol 1989;7:269-281.
11. Budka H. Pathology of encephalopathies induced by treatment or prophylaxis of neoplastic lesions of the nervous system. In: Hildebrand J, Gangji D, eds. Treatment of neoplastic lesions of the nervous system. Oxford: Pergamon Press; 1982:45-50.
12. Recht LD, Primavera JM. Case records of the Massachusetts General Hospital. Weekly clinicopathological exercises. Case 24-1999. Neurologic disorder in a 65-year-old man after treatment of colon cancer. N Engl J Med 1999;341:512-519.
13. Kimmel DW, Wijdicks EF, Rodriguez M. Multifocal inflammatory leukoencephalopathy associated with levamisole therapy. Neurology 1995;45:374-376.
14. Figueredo AT, Fawcet SE, Molloy DW, Dobranowski J, Paulseth JE. Disabling encephalopathy during 5-fluorouracil and levamisole adjuvant therapy for resected colorectal cancer: a report of two cases. Cancer Invest 1995;13:608-611.
15. Fassas AB, Gattani AM, Morgello S. Cerebral demyelination with 5-fluorouracil and levamisole. Cancer Invest 1994;12:379-383.
16. Critchley P, Abbott R, Madden FJ. Multifocal inflammatory leukoencephalopathy developing in a patient receiving 5-fluorouracil and levamisole. Clin Oncol (R Coll Radiol) 1994;6:406.
17. Hook CC, Kimmel DW, Kvols LK, et al. Multifocal inflammatory leukoencephalopathy with 5-fluorouracil and levamisole. Ann Neurol 1992;31:262-267.
18. Bruck W, Heise E, Friede RL. Leukoencephalopathy after cisplatin therapy. Clin Neuropathol 1989;8:263-265.
19. Moore-Maxwell CA, Datto MB, Hulette CM. Chemotherapy-induced toxic encephalopathy causes a wide range of symptoms: a series of four autopsies. Mod Pathol 2004;17:241-247.
20. Rubinstein LJ, Herman MM, Long TF, Wilbur JR. Disseminated necrotizing leukoencephalopathy: a complication of treated central nervous system leukemia and lymphoma. Cancer 1975;35:291-305.
21. Rubinstein JL, Herman MM, Long TF, Wilbur JR. Leukoencephalopathy following combined therapy of central nervous system leukemia and lymphoma. Acta Neuropathol Suppl (Berl) 1975;(Suppl 6):251-255.
22. Russell DS, Rubinstein LJ. Pathology of tumours of the nervous system, 5th ed. London: E. Arnold; 1989.
23. Henson RA, Urich H. Cancer and the nervous system: the neurological manifestations of systemic malignant disease. Oxford: Blackwell Scientific; 1982.
24. Grossman SA, Krabak MJ. Leptomeningeal carcinomatosis. Cancer Treat Rev 1999;25:103-119.
25. Chen CY, Zimmerman RA, Faro S, Bilaniuk LT, Chou TY, Molloy PT. Childhood leukemia: central nervous system abnormalities during and after treatment. AJNR Am J Neuroradiol 1996;17:295-310.
26. Sakamaki H, Onozawa Y, Yano Y, et al. Disseminated necrotizing leukoencephalopathy following irradiation and methotrexate therapy for central nervous system infiltration of leukemia and lymphoma. Radiat Med 1993;11:146-153.

27. Laxmi SN, Takahashi S, Matsumoto K, et al. Treatment-related disseminated necrotizing leukoencephalopathy with characteristic contrast enhancement of the white matter. Radiat Med 1996;14:303-307.
28. Meadows AT, Evans AE. Effects of chemotherapy on the central nervous system. A study of parenteral methotrexate in long-term survivors of leukemia and lymphoma in childhood. Cancer 1976;37:1079-1085.
29. Peylan-Ramu N, Poplack DG, Pizzo PA, Adornato BT, Di Chiro G. Abnormal CT scans of the brain in asymptomatic children with acute lymphocytic leukemia after prophylactic treatment of the central nervous system with radiation and intrathecal chemotherapy. N Engl J Med 1978;298:815-818.
30. Wilson DA, Nitschke R, Bowman ME, Chaffin MJ, Sexauer CL, Prince JR. Transient white matter changes on MR images in children undergoing chemotherapy for acute lymphocytic leukemia: correlation with neuropsychologic deficiencies. Radiology 1991;180:205-209.
31. Laitt RD, Chambers EJ, Goddard PR, Wakeley CJ, Duncan AW, Foreman NK. Magnetic resonance imaging and magnetic resonance angiography in long term survivors of acute lymphoblastic leukemia treated with cranial irradiation. Cancer 1995;76:1846-1852.
32. Harsh GR, Deisboeck TS, Louis DN, et al. Thymidine kinase activation of ganciclovir in recurrent malignant gliomas: a gene-marking and neuropathological study. J Neurosurg 2000;92:804-811.
33. Markert JM, Medlock MD, Rabkin SD, et al. Conditionally replicating herpes simplex virus mutant, G207 for the treatment of malignant glioma: results of a phase I trial. Gene Ther 2000;7:867-874.
34. Trask TW, Trask RP, Aguilar-Cordova E, et al. Phase I study of adenoviral delivery of the HSV-tk gene and ganciclovir administration in patients with current malignant brain tumors. Mol Ther 2000;1:195-203.

Index*

*In a series of numbers, those in boldface indicate the main discussion of the entity.

C

D

E

F

G

H

I

J

K

L

M

N

O

P

R

S

V

W

Z